PENGUIN REFERENCE BOOKS

THE PENGUIN
MEDICAL ENCYCLOPEDIA

Peter Wingate was born in 1920 and spent part of his schooling in Switzerland and part at Malvern College. At Trinity College, Cambridge, he read medicine, qualifying as a doctor at St Bartholomew's Hospital. He then did three years' general practice, followed by eleven years' government service in Zambia and Malawi. Unlike general practice in this country, a colonial medical officer's duties ranged from school inspections to major surgery, and from psychiatry to the control of epidemics. For the first few years he was mainly occupied with surgery, but later more with public health education, which was in even more urgent need than a hospital service; and it was in this connection that he worked with the broadcasting corporation and the government's publications bureau.

After leaving Africa he spent four years as a medical adviser to a large drug company in Basle, and then joined the editorial staff of the *Lancet* for a time. He has also worked with the BBC on the television programme for doctors, *Medicine Today*. His publications include *Doctor Kalulu* (1956), a booklet on elementary hygiene for African schools; and a novel, *Rain Doctor* (1957). Research for the historical sections of this encyclopedia gave him the idea for his novel *The Heretics* (1975), in which the medical life of the sixteenth century plays an important part.

The Penguin
Medical Encyclopedia

PETER WINGATE

SECOND EDITION

PENGUIN BOOKS

Penguin Books Ltd, Harmondsworth, Middlesex, England
Viking Penguin Inc., 40 West 23rd Street, New York, New York 10010, U.S.A.
Penguin Books Australia Ltd, Ringwood, Victoria, Australia
Penguin Books Canada Limited, 2801 John Street, Markham, Ontario, Canada L3R 1B4
Penguin Books (N.Z.) Ltd, 182–190 Wairau Road, Auckland 10, New Zealand

—

First printed 1972
Reprinted 1974, 1975
Second edition 1976
Reprinted 1977, 1978 (twice), 1979, 1980, 1982, 1983, 1984, 1985, 1987

—

—

Made and printed in Great Britain by
Hazell Watson & Viney Limited,
Member of the BPCC Group,
Aylesbury, Bucks
Set in Monotype Times

INTRODUCTION

THE practice of medicine has changed almost beyond recognition in the thirty-odd years since my apprenticeship began.

Firstly, in the age-old struggle to promote medicine from a craft to a science there has been more progress in the past thirty years than in the previous two thousand. This progress is not as sudden as it seems. What is happening is that earlier discoveries about the natural history of health and disease are now being applied in the actual diagnosis and treatment of illness.

Secondly, the medical profession is learning to communicate with the general public. Many of the newer methods of treating and preventing illness depend on the patient's understanding and co-operation. Hippocrates, 24 centuries ago, said that a doctor must teach his patients to care for their own health, but until recently most doctors seem to have thought it was bad for patients to know too much.

Thirdly, the objectives of medical practice are being reappraised. I recently helped to produce a film on the diagnosis and treatment of angina pectoris. Three patients took part. One had recovered from a coronary thrombosis and was back at work. Another had only mild angina, although the X-rays showed that his coronary arteries were badly impaired. He had learnt to avoid anginal attacks, and was enjoying an active life. The third was a chronic invalid. The least exertion distressed him, and he spent much of his time awaiting sudden death. Some years before, he had been warned to take care of himself because of an abnormality in his electrocardiogram. That was all. His heart and arteries were in mint condition. The question is, which of the three was ill?

In the nineteenth century, which in medicine lasted until about 1935, the answers would have been clear. The first patient was lucky to be alive at all, the second had an incurable disease, and the third had nothing wrong with him. All this is largely true as far as it goes, but we now know that it does not go nearly far enough. Probably all three have incurable diseases. The first two have damaged arteries, and the third an intractable neurosis. But the first patient is working and doing what he can to avoid further attacks. If he had known sooner what he knows now he might have taken more exercise and less food in the past, and he might have avoided even one heart attack. Statistics show that the second patient is a relatively good risk. He has always been active and cheerful, and he has never smoked or put on weight. He fully understands his problem, and behaves almost as though he welcomed the challenge. One day, he will probably die of a heart attack, but in the meantime it is absurd to call him a sick man. It is the third patient, with the perfectly normal body, who really needs help. Health is not a matter of mere survival, but of being able to enjoy life. Many of our commonest diseases are in the old sense incurable, but if medicine can help the patient to lead a normal and happy life, then in my view he is as good as cured.

This book is concerned mainly with the scientific background to current medical opinion, and how it has evolved. In selecting the material I have put scientific interest before practical use. Books cannot teach much about the diagnosis and treatment of individual cases, but they should be able to explain the principles involved. Many statements are qualified with 'perhaps', 'probably', or 'it seems'. There are still not many certainties in medicine, and much of the book expresses no more than my opinion at the time of writing.

In compiling the book, I have plundered various text-books and journals, and for the historical data I have referred to original sources where I could. For this I have to thank the Librarians of the Wellcome Institute of the History of Medicine. The quotations from Hippocrates are from the translation by Francis Adams (London, 1843), except the Hippocratic Oath, prepared under the guidance of Miss Mary Hoskins.

Among the many people who have helped, I am especially grateful to Mrs Judith Wardman and Mr Richard Wingate for their patient and constructive criticism, and to Dr George Sacks, F.R.C.S., for suggesting that I should write the book in the first place and for his continuing encouragement.

Note to the Second Edition

I wish to thank the many people who have suggested improvements, in particular Mr F. D. Allen for advice about drugs and other matters, and Dr Penelope Leach, who helped to revise the whole book.

LIST OF ABBREVIATIONS

adj.	adjective	kg.	kilogram(s)
anat.	anatomy	Lat.	Latin
C.	centigrade	lb.	pound(s)
c.	*circa*, about	mm.	millimetre(s)
c.c.	cubic centimetre(s)	mV	millivolt(s)
cm.	centimetre(s)	n.	noun
cu.	cubic	oz.	ounce(s)
d.	died	path.	pathology
F.	Fahrenheit	pl.	plural
fl.	*floruit*, flourished	sq.	square
ft	foot, feet	surg.	surgery
g.	gramme(s)	WHO	World Health Organization
Gk	Greek	⬦	see
h.p.	horsepower	⬦⬦	see also
in., ins.	inch, inches		

A

abdomen (belly). The enclosed space belo the ◊ *thorax* (chest) and above the ◊ *pelvis.* Its roof, separating it from the thorax, is a dome-shaped muscle, the ◊ *diaphragm.* It has no floor; the cavity extends into the pelvis. Because the diaphragm is a dome the upper part of the abdomen is enclosed by the ribs. Behind, the abdomen is protected by the backbone with massive blocks of muscle on either side, as seen in a sirloin.

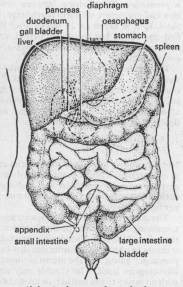

Abdominal organs from the front.

The front and sides of the abdominal wall are thin sheets of muscle covered with fat and skin, a flexible arrangement that facilitates breathing, eating, pregnancy etc. The weakest points are the groin, where the abdominal muscles meet those of the front of the thigh, and the openings in the diaphragm for the gullet and other structures (◊ *hernia*).

Immediately in front of the backbone are two huge blood vessels, both lying vertically: the *aorta*, and to its right the *vena cava.*

Each forms an inverted Y at the entrance to the pelvis to provide vessels for the legs. The two *kidneys* lie on the muscles to either side of the backbone; from each a thin pipe (*ureter*) runs down to the urinary *bladder* in the pelvis. A broad strip of soft glandular tissue, the *pancreas*, stretches from kidney to kidney across the front of the aorta and vena cava. Two smaller glands, the *adrenals*, perch on the kidneys, one to each side. All these structures are behind rather than within the cavity of the abdomen.

The abdomen proper is lined with a fine slippery membrane, the ◊ *peritoneum.* The abdominal organs grow into the cavity from behind, pushing a layer of peritoneum before them. Thus each organ acquires a smooth coat and can slide around without significant friction. This is as well, since the diaphragm pushes the organs down with every breath.

Much of the cavity is occupied by the digestive tract, a long tortuous tube entering through a hole in the diaphragm as the lower end of the *oesophagus* (gullet) and passing down into the pelvis as the large *intestine.* The *stomach* is the expanded part of the tube starting just below the diaphragm to the left of the midline, occupying much of the space protected by the lower left ribs, and narrowing to be continued as the intestine.

The *liver* fills the space below the right side of the diaphragm, down to the margin of the rib-cage, extending a little to the left of the midline. On the left, the *spleen* is tucked under the ribs beside the stomach.

A curtain of fatty tissue, the *omentum*, hangs from the stomach in front of the intestine.

1. ABDOMINAL SURGERY

The peritoneum is very susceptible to bacterial infection, and the consequent ◊ *peritonitis* is a most dangerous condition. Any wound – accidental or surgical – that enters the cavity of the abdomen is therefore dangerous unless care is taken to exclude bacteria, in fact so dangerous that abdominal surgery was impractical until Lister (1865) showed how to operate without infection. It is true that surgeons had been able to repair a hernia and remove a stone from the urinary bladder since antiquity, but these operations can be done without disturbing the peritoneum. Caesarean section is also an ancient operation, but until modern times it was done mainly to save the child when the mother's condition was already hopeless.

A second obstacle to abdominal surgery was the technical difficulty of working inside the cavity while the surrounding muscles were tense; this was overcome by the discovery of anaesthetics. (The more obvious advantage of anaesthesia is perhaps less important with the abdomen than with other parts of the body, because unless the peritoneum is stretched the abdominal organs do not give rise to pain.)

Within ten years of Lister's discovery abdominal operations were commonplace, and by the end of the 19th century abdominal surgery was very much as it is today. Many surgeons, including Lister himself, took part in this very rapid development, but the outstanding pioneer was Theodor Billroth (1829–94) of Vienna, who practically invented the whole of the surgery of the stomach and intestine.

The abdomen can be opened by various routes. If the surgeon knows in advance exactly what needs to be done he can cut through the abdominal wall over the organ to be treated and leave a small scar. But in many cases a complete diagnosis is impossible without actually seeing the affected organs. For instance, removing the appendix may be a ten-minute job with luck, or it may be a difficult and tedious operation if the appendix has become stuck to other organs; in either case the patient's symptoms may be the same. Even when the immediate diagnosis is certain the surgeon may wish to look at organs that are causing no symptoms at present but may show signs of impending trouble; thus he may save the patient a second operation later on. Hence operation scars are often larger than might seem necessary.

Provided that there is no infection, or that infection is overcome, abdominal injuries and operations heal remarkably well. Here, the most important factor is the ability of injured peritoneum to stick together. When intestine is cut and then stitched layer by layer, the peritoneal coat forms a watertight seal within a few minutes; the inner layers can heal in their own time without risk of leakage. Sometimes the rapid healing of peritoneum is a nuisance: areas that should be separate may join, and such *ad-hesions* occasionally cause symptoms and have to be divided surgically.

The abdominal wall is usually as good as new after an operation. It was once the rule to keep the patient lying in bed for two or three weeks with a tight binder to protect the wound. This was more likely to promote pneumonia than healing. Serious weakness of an operation scar is quite unusual, and the cause is more likely to be infection in the wound than getting up too soon after the operation.

abortion. Ending of pregnancy before the child has a reasonable chance of survival; delivery after this time but before full term is *premature*. The division between abortion and premature stillbirth is arbitrary; in the UK it is taken as 28 weeks after the first day of the last menstrual period, and in some other countries as 180 days after conception.

The distinction between *abortion* (up to 16 weeks) and *miscarriage* (16–28 weeks) is obsolete. Both are technically abortion, but social convention commonly calls accidental or spontaneous cases miscarriages and deliberately induced ones abortions.

1. Accidental Abortion (Miscarriage)

Nobody knows how many pregnancies end in miscarriage, if only because an early miscarriage can be mistaken for a delayed period. Estimates vary between 10 and 20 per cent of all pregnancies.

The commonest reason for miscarriage is something wrong with the development of the baby; if the baby dies during pregnancy it ceases to produce the hormones that keep pregnancy going, and the uterus automatically empties itself. The trouble may start with an injury to the mother, or an acute illness that also harms the baby; or general ill health or a structural defect can make it difficult for a woman to maintain pregnancy.

Known cases occur most often in the 3rd and 4th months of pregnancy.

The first symptom is bleeding, sometimes with pain. At any stage of pregnancy these symptoms need immediate attention, firstly because bleeding occasionally becomes severe, secondly because there may be a chance of continuing the pregnancy, and thirdly because the symptoms may have some other cause. At this stage abortion is said to be *threatened*. With rest and sedation all may still be well. Hormones (e.g. progesterone) are often given but their value is uncertain.

If the bleeding continues an abortion sooner or later becomes *inevitable*. The foetus (embryo) is too small to live independently and is no longer being kept alive by the mother's circulation. The only course is to get it over with as little further bleeding as possible. In most cases the pregnancy ends with little more trouble than an ordinary period, but if the embryo is not entirely detached bleeding can become serious and the abortion has to be completed surgically. The other possible danger is infection (of the same kind as ◊ *puerperal* fever). This is now rare except after unskilled interference.

Habitual abortion (defined as three or more consecutive miscarriages) may be due to remediable disorders of the uterus or of the endocrine glands (e.g. thyroid), or to chronic ill health of any kind. But in many cases no cause can be found. Treatment then has to be empirical. Hormones are often given and may help, but complete rest, especially during the hazardous 3rd and 4th months, seems to give the best chance of a live baby.

2. DELIBERATE ABORTION

Many drugs and poisons have a reputation for procuring abortion. They are either ineffective or dangerous. Drugs that stimulate the uterus during a natural confinement have little or no effect at any other stage of pregnancy. The few substances that may end a pregnancy do so by poisoning the embryo, and at the same time they poison the mother.

Mechanical insults such as falling downstairs are unlikely to disturb pregnancy unless they are severe enough to cause serious injury. Popular belief in such methods is nurtured by the large number of abortions that would have happened in any case and by their apparent success with women who were not pregnant at all.

Given the conditions of an operating theatre, with sterile instruments, trained assistance, and the means of dealing with complications, abortion is safe and easy in the early months of pregnancy. In nearly all countries there are laws against indiscriminate abortion, and laws tend to be vague about what is permissible because each case has to bej udged on its merits. Two independent medical opinions are generally required to justify the operation. ◊ *ethics*.

During the first three months of preg- nancy the simplest method of carrying out an abortion is to dilate the cervix, where the uterus opens into the upper end of the vagina, by inserting a series of curved metal rods, each slightly thicker than the last. The contents of the uterus are then removed with forceps. Instead of forceps a suction device can be used, with less risk of damaging the lining of the uterus. After the first three months of pregnancy the foetus will be too large for this method to be practicable. Abortion may then be carried out by injecting saline solution into the cavity of the uterus (not altogether reliable) or by performing an abdominal operation like a *Caesarean section*. A newer and safer method is to inject a ◊ *prostaglandin* through the cervix between the lining of the uterus and the enveloping membranes of the foetus.

abrasion. A graze; an injury caused by rubbing or scraping. ◊ *wound*.

abreaction ◊ *psychoanalysis*.

abscess. A collection of pus, a result of infection by bacteria. It represents an advanced stage of ◊ *inflammation*, which is itself a defensive reaction to infection. The formation of an abscess means that the defence has been partly successful. When the defence is more successful, bacteria are destroyed quickly and the inflammation proceeds straight to healing; when the defence completely fails, the infection spreads widely. An abscess represents an intermediate stage: it is surrounded by actively growing tissue like that of a healing wound, but the walls cannot grow together because of the pus in the centre, where bacteria are free to multiply and damage the surrounding tissue; the damage keeps pace with the attempt at repair.

An established abscess cannot heal until the pus has been released either by finding its own way to the surface and bursting through or by surgical operation.

The balance between infection and healing is not static. If tissue is destroyed faster than it can be replaced the abscess grows. Or with chronic (prolonged) infection such as tuberculosis healing may outpace damage, and a mass of unwanted new tissue is formed – a *granuloma*.

Abscesses cause symptoms locally by pressure on neighbouring structures. Other symptoms such as fever are due to poisons formed by bacteria and by damaged tissue.

In some places, notoriously between the liver and the diaphragm (*subphrenic abscess*), an abscess has room to expand without any local disturbance. An exact diagnosis is then difficult. The fever and the increase of white cells in the blood suggest that pus is being formed somewhere, but there is nothing to show precisely where. In other places the local effects of pressure are all-important. For instance, the skull cannot expand, and the great danger of an abscess there is injury to the brain by pressure. More familiar examples of abscesses confined by rigid walls, with no room for expansion, are small collections of pus in a tooth socket or inside the ear-drum, both excruciatingly painful.

In essence the treatment of all abscesses is the same: to release the pus, and to provide free drainage so that the opening does not heal before the walls have had time to grow together. If the second step is omitted, the abscess re-forms.

Antibiotic drugs have greatly improved the treatment of abscesses. If they are given in the early stages the infection may be overcome without any need for surgery, and in the later stages they at least prevent the infection from spreading.

The time-honoured ◊ *poultice* is useful only with abscesses very near the surface (◊ *boil*).

abstinence syndrome. Acute physical illness in a drug addict caused by sudden withdrawal of the drug. According to one definition, the abstinence syndrome distinguishes habit from true addiction; thus the habitual smoker may be very miserable without tobacco but is not physically ill, whereas a heroin addict is obviously and perhaps dangerously sick for a while when the drug is stopped (◊ *addiction*).

accidents. On an average day in England and Wales, accidents in the home and on the roads each claim about 20 lives, and accidents at work another three. For every death on the road, 50 people are injured. For every fatal industrial accident, 200 are injured at work. Nobody knows how many people are injured by accidents in the home.

More young men die in accidents than from all other causes together, and among them the motor cycle is the commonest single cause of death. Apart from road accidents, accidental death is commonest among the very young and the old. In babies, suffocation is the main cause; in old people, falls.

In a year, about 30,000 males die from strokes, and the same number from heart diseases other than coronary thrombosis. Only 10,000 die of accidents. But the average age of death is 73 with strokes and 75 with the heart diseases; it is 46 with accidents. Thus accidents account for more *lost years* than either of the other two causes. The prevention of accidents has become a major problem in public health.

The very word accident is dangerous, because it implies an event governed by chance and therefore inescapable. Yet in retrospect it is clear that few accidents could not have been prevented.

1. DANGEROUS SITUATIONS

Much research has gone into such matters as building safer homes and vehicles, removing hazards from old people's homes and nurseries, and safeguards in industry. Government departments and private organizations have published numerous reports on accident prevention. These are mainly concerned with reducing the number of situations where accidents become likely – with making the environment safer. In some cases, predisposing causes are actually outlawed: drunken driving, unprotected machinery, and inflammable nightdresses for children are illegal. But the precipitating cause of most accidents is human error, which neither advice nor legislation eliminates.

2. ACCIDENT-PRONENESS

If accidents really happen by chance, some people are remarkably unlucky, for with all classes of accident a few people suffer far more than their fair share. They are not necessarily clumsy or stupid; they are accident-prone. Against the concept of accident-proneness it has been argued that the number of serious accidents is not large enough for the statistics to mean anything – but if accidents are really not very common it is all the more remarkable that so many of them should involve so few people. Again, it has been said that people are not really accident-prone, but the after-effects of injury make them more liable to further accidents – but that is a possible explanation of accident-proneness, not an argument against it.

Personality is the primary factor. Hesitancy and aggression are easily recognized as dangers on the road and elsewhere, and either could be made worse by the memory of previous accidents. Aggression is closely linked to the male sexual drive, as are all forms of showing-off. Daring is a part of courtship, and the young Londoner's motor cycle is as much a symbol of virility as the young Zulu's spear. Young men who take unnecessary risks are not always trying to impress girls; they are as likely to be convincing themselves. At the opposite extreme is an urge to self-destruction. American police reports suggest that some road accidents are poorly disguised suicides. A subtler and commoner danger is a frame of mind where a person does not openly wish to kill himself but does not greatly care about surviving. Guilt with a desire for punishment and expiation is an important factor here.

These are all attitudes of normal people. In everyone there are dangerous forces that need expression, and society's problem is to find safe outlets for them. Sport, then, may be more than the pursuit of physical fitness.

Even slight and apparently harmless mental disorder adds greatly to the risk of accidents. The effects of alcohol are well known, but many other drugs can also impair judgement. Fatigue and minor illness can be dangerous, and the risk increases when external influences on the mind are combined. A couple of aspirins and a small whisky at the start of a cold can make a man as accident-prone as serious drinking at another time. Women are quite notoriously vulnerable just before a monthly period ($\diamond$ premenstrual tension), and in some industries accidents have been reduced by moving them to safer jobs at these times.

Psychopaths (roughly speaking, people with underdeveloped consciences) are a small but important group in this context. American records show two distinct classes of road accident. Firstly, most accidents seem due to misjudgement, a moment's inattention, or bad luck; and the people involved are a cross-section of the public (except that some are more prone than others). Secondly, a few accidents are due to breach of rules (e.g. disregard of signals, selfish overtaking); and a large number of these road-hogs are people who defy the law in other ways.

This account has dealt mainly with road accidents because there is most information

about them, but the principles of cause and prevention are the same with all classes of accident. The personal factor has been emphasized because of its medical overtones, but accidents pose equally important problems for employers, engineers, lawyers and many others.

accommodation. Focusing the eye. At rest a normal eye is focused at infinity, i.e. for distant vision. For near vision the *ciliary muscle* round the lens contracts, and the lens becomes rounder and optically more powerful. (A camera is focused by moving the lens; the eye, by adjusting the strength of the lens.) The lens begins to lose its flexibility quite early in life, and accommodation declines ($\diamond$ *vision*).

accoucheur. Obstetrician; specialist in midwifery.

acetabulum. Hemispherical socket in the bone at either side of the pelvis to fit the rounded upper end of the femur (thigh bone). This ball-and-socket arrangement gives the hip-joint great stability with a useful range of movement.

acetarsone. An organic compound of arsenic; it was originally intended to be given by mouth in the treatment of amoebic dysentery, but proved too poisonous to be used in this way. Pessaries of acetarsone can, however, be safely used for treating *trichomonas* infection.

acetyl choline. An ammonium derivative found in animals and plants. It is one of the chemical transmitters released at the ends of nerve fibres to set off an impulse in an adjacent nerve cell. Acetyl choline is also released by motor nerves to stimulate muscle fibres. (All nerve fibres outside the brain act by releasing acetyl choline, except sympathetic nerves, which release adrenaline and related compounds; there may well be other chemical transmitters in the brain.)

In 1914 (Sir) Henry Dale described some of the effects of acetyl choline, which he had extracted from ergot, on living organs. Many of them resembled the effects of stimulating the *vagus nerve*. In 1921 Otto Loewi slowed the beat of a frog's heart by stimulating its vagus nerve, and found that fluid passing through this heart picked up a substance that slowed a second frog's heart. The substance was later shown to be dentical with Dale's acetyl choline. Dale and Loewi shared the Nobel Prize for Medicine in 1936.

Acetyl choline sets off electrical impulses in nerve and muscle cells by making them permeable to electrically active atoms of sodium. The effect is very short-lived, because acetyl choline is rapidly destroyed by an enzyme, cholinesterase. The drug *eserine* interferes with this enzyme and so prolongs the effect of acetyl choline. On the other hand, *atropine* (belladonna) prevents the access of acetyl choline to various organs (e.g. heart; digestive system), and *curare* paralyses muscles in the same way.

acetylsalicylic acid. Aspirin; discovered in 1899 in Germany; one of the first synthetic drugs and still among the most popular (◊ *analgesic*).

Achilles tendon. Large tendon behind the ankle, formed from the soleus and gastrocnemius muscles in the calf and attached to the heelbone (calcaneum). It is subject to great stresses, and despite its strength it is occasionally torn and has to be repaired surgically.

achlorhydria. Lack of hydrochloric acid in the stomach. The digestive juice secreted by a normal stomach is strongly acidic (0·4 per cent hydrochloric acid) for the digestion of protein. The ability to form acid is lost with chronic diseases of the stomach, including pernicious ◊ *anaemia* (B.2). Various symptoms of indigestion are ascribed to achlorhydria; but some healthy people form no acid yet suffer no symptoms.

acholuric jaundice. ◊ *Jaundice* without bile in the urine. ◊◊ *anaemia* (A.2).

achondroplasia (Gk = 'non-growth of cartilage'). A hereditary disorder of the skeleton, transmitted as a *dominant* character (◊ *genetics* (2)). Bones formed in the embryo from simple connective tissue – those of the trunk and most of the skull – grow normally. But the bones of the limbs and the floor of the skull are first formed in cartilage, later converted to bone, and their growth is defective. This causes a characteristic type of dwarfism, with a protruding forehead (because the vault of the skull grows ahead of the face), a well developed trunk, and very short but strong limbs. Apart from their unusual bodily proportions these people are perfectly normal.

acidosis. Alteration of the acid/alkali balance of the blood and tissue fluid towards acidity. Even with severe acidosis these fluids do not become strictly acidic, but they become less alkaline than they should be. In health the slight alkalinity is held constant by the balance of dissolved carbon dioxide (acid) and sodium bicarbonate (alkali). The balance is regulated partly by the kidneys, from which acid or alkaline urine is secreted to correct any excess in either direction, and partly by the lungs, from which excessive carbon dioxide is eliminated by deeper breathing. Heavy breathing after exertion is a reflex response to the formation of acid in working muscle. The kind of acid does not matter; removing carbon dioxide (carbonic acid) by the lungs compensates for an excess of lactic acid in muscle, or an excess of any other acid.

Acidosis follows:

1. failure to eliminate carbon dioxide because of disorders of the lungs or muscles of breathing;

2. failure of the kidneys;

3. severe diarrhoea with loss of sodium bicarbonate through the intestine, leaving a relative excess of acid;

4. abnormal formation of acid through incomplete combustion of fat, with diabetes or malnutrition;

5. poisoning with acids, most commonly aspirin.

The condition popularly known as 'acidity', which is indigestion with regurgitation of acid from the stomach, has nothing to do with acidosis; nor has the excessive formation of acid in the stomach associated with duodenal ulcers. If anything, the formation of acid in the stomach tends to deplete the blood of acid; with severe vomiting this acid is lost and leads to the opposite state, *alkalosis*. Contrary to a common belief, children are not very prone to acidosis.

The alkalinity of the blood is easily measured in a hospital laboratory. The level can be adjusted with exact doses of sodium bicarbonate; but essentially the treatment of acidosis is the treatment of its cause. True acidosis is a dangerous condition in its own right, and treatment is a matter of some urgency.

acne (acne vulgaris). A disorder of the skin so common that it might be regarded as a normal state in adolescence. Basically, it is an excessive or perhaps abnormal activity of the sebaceous (grease) glands. The glands are most numerous in the skin of the face and back. At puberty they undergo rapid growth and may form so much grease that it blocks their openings. A characteristic sign of acne is a plug of partially dried greasy material in the opening of a sebaceous gland – a *comedo* or blackhead. In more severe cases, sebum trapped in some of the glands leaks between layers of the skin and forms rubbery lumps. These sheltered collections of inert matter are liable to incubate bacteria – sebum has antiseptic properties but certain fairly innocuous species of bacteria seem to thrive on it. They include *Staphylococcus albus* (found on most people's skin) and *Bacillus acnes*, once thought to be the cause of acne, but probably an innocent by-stander. These bacteria may produce small superficial abscesses (pimples). Occasionally the infection extends to the deeper layers of the skin and leaves scars.

Acne nearly always disappears when puberty and growth are over and the various endocrine glands have settled into their adult pattern; but this balance may be disturbed by hormone treatment of other disorders so that acne reappears in adult life. In some women menstruation has a similar effect.

In the more serious cases a hereditary factor appears to make the sebaceous glands over-sensitive to the influence of hormones.

Emotional stresses may aggravate acne, but more important is the emotional stress that acne *causes* to young people, and not only girls: adolescents of either sex can be acutely sensitive about their appearance. Their misery is often made worse by old wives' (or young boys') tales about the causes of acne.

Acne regularly improves in the summer, and sunlight is among the best forms of treatment. Artificial ultraviolet light is sometimes useful, and X-rays have also been recommended, but these are not suitable in every case. Blackheads can be removed with a special instrument; this needs some skill. Indiscriminate squeezing and pressing does more harm than good, increasing the risk of scars.

Various non-greasy pastes and lotions, some containing sulphur, are used. Most do at least some good, but none can be relied on in every case. Some promising new preparations are undergoing trials.

Diet was over-emphasized in the past, but in some cases of acne particular foods have an adverse effect. Chocolate seems to be the worst offender.

acquired. (Disorders) not present at birth, as opposed to *congenital*.

acriflavine. A yellow dye, strongly antiseptic but relatively harmless to human tissues.

acro-. Prefix = 'extremities'; hands and feet.

acromegaly. The term refers to the enlargement of the hands and feet which is one symptom of the disease. Acromegaly is a disorder of growth in adult life, i.e. of the process by which worn out tissues are constantly replaced. It is due to an excess of growth hormone from the pituitary gland. (A similar excess in childhood causes the child to grow into a ⟡ *giant*.) The bones cannot be made to grow longer when once growth has ceased, but growth hormone causes thickening of the skull, face, hands, and feet, and enlargement of various internal organs. There may be an excess of other pituitary hormones with complications such as diabetes and impotence. Acromegaly is treated by X-rays or surgery to the pituitary gland.

acromion. The point of the shoulder; an extension of the shoulder-blade over the top of the joint, giving anchorage to the deltoid muscle. ⟡ *scapula*.

ACTH. Adrenocorticotropic (-trophic) hormone; corticotrophin. Hormone formed in the anterior lobe of the ⟡ *pituitary body*, acting on the cortex of the ⟡ *adrenal* glands to promote the secretion of ⟡ *corticosteroids*. ACTH is sometimes used medicinally so that the patient, instead of being given corticosteroids directly, is stimulated to produce his own. Synthetic ACTH is less apt to cause allergic reactions than natural ACTH prepared from animal pituitary extracts. A solution of the hormone can be so prepared that it is only slowly assimilated from the site of injection. In this way a single dose can be made to last for several days.

actinomycosis. An uncommon disease due to infection with *Actinomyces*, a microbe intermediate between bacteria and fungi. The infection usually enters by the mucous membrane of the mouth (according to an ill-founded tradition, from sucking straws) and causes a chronic discharging abscess in the region of the jaw, or more rarely in some other part of the body. The infection responds slowly to penicillin. 'Lumpy jaw' is a similar and commoner disease of cattle.

acupuncture. Treatment of diseases by inserting needles through the skin at determined points, often remote from the actual disorder but said to affect it. ◊ Chinese medicine.

acute. (Disease) of rapid onset and generally of short duration, as opposed to ◊ chronic. Neither term describes the severity of a disease: the common cold and smallpox are both acute infections, and athlete's foot and leprosy are both chronic.

acute abdomen. Hospital jargon for any abdominal disorder needing urgent operation. It is a convenient diagnosis because the symptoms may not show precisely what is wrong. Hours could be wasted in trying to distinguish between a ruptured appendix and a perforated duodenal ulcer, but since in either case the abdomen has to be opened, the exact diagnosis can well wait until the surgeon actually sees the affected organ.

acute rheumatism = ◊ rheumatic fever.

addiction. According to a definition framed some years ago by the World Health Organization, true addiction to drugs (as opposed to mere habit) has four characteristics: (1) uncontrollable craving for the drug; (2) increasing tolerance to it; (3) physical dependence on it; (4) harmful effects on the subject and on society.
Craving is more than flabby self-indulgence; it is an urge that drives otherwise honest people to adopt any means, including crime, to get their supplies.
Tolerance means that larger and larger doses are needed for the same effect. An addict may stand doses large enough to kill several ordinary people. This means that new chemical processes are evolved in the body, or old ones adapted, for dealing with the drug.
Dependence is another sign of chemical adaptation. The drug becomes an integral part of some modified chemical process in the nervous system. The chemical balance is then disturbed when the drug is stopped,

with unpleasant and even dangerous withdrawal symptoms. This kind of physical illness is called abstinence syndrome. With opium narcotics (morphia, heroin) the symptoms of abstinence include restlessness and sweating, followed in severe cases by diarrhoea, fever, and rapid loss of weight. Barbiturates and some other hypnotics (sleeping pills) can lead to a different kind of abstinence syndrome with epileptic convulsions. The symptoms abate as soon as the drug is given again. More important, they are only mild if the drug is broken off gradually and not suddenly, or if it can be replaced by a less potent drug of the same type which can be stopped with less risk. An abstinence syndrome seldom lasts more than a week or ten days, but a few deaths have been recorded. The symptoms of abstinence strongly suggest poisoning of some kind. Poisoning by default is by no means impossible. The nervous system is regulated by highly poisonous substances such as adrenaline and acetyl choline which are automatically destroyed before they reach dangerous concentrations – unless the chemical balance is disturbed. If the balance is adapted to the presence of a drug, then absence of the drug could lead to a poisonous excess of normal substances.
Harmful effects are mainly on the addict's personality, though his physical health usually suffers to some extent. Since the drug becomes the centre of his life he may become virtually unemployable, and if he cannot afford food as well as the drug he will settle for the drug. Some drugs cause grave mental disorder; others do not. Since many addicts are unstable before they take to drugs it is difficult to say whether antisocial behaviour (apart from crimes committed to get the drugs) is due to addiction or to pre-existing tendencies.
Only a few drugs satisfy all four conditions. They include the narcotics derived from opium, of which morphia is the most important. Heroin (diacetyl morphine) is a synthetic compound of morphia, unhappily introduced to provide the medicinal effects of morphia without the danger of addiction; it is indeed the most effective pain-killing drug but also the most dangerous. With these drugs, addiction appears to be a property of the drug itself: anyone receiving them regularly will become an addict.
Most other drugs that are abused are not addictive in the strict sense of the word,

and some are not even really habit-forming but can be taken and given up at will. With some, dependence seems to arise from the character of the taker rather than from any inherent property of the drug itself. (This argument is confused by the fact that some drugs (e.g. alcohol) may weaken the power of making decisions.) As a rule these other drugs do not show all four characteristics; the desired dose may not increase, and there is no physical dependence in the sense of an abstinence syndrome. This is important because it means that the drug can be stopped without endangering the subject's health. But a few people develop true addiction to barbiturates, with an even more dangerous abstinence syndrome than that of opium.

Alcohol is not in the strictest (opium) sense a drug of addiction. Millions of regular drinkers do not increase the amount and can stop when they please. Dipsomania is quite unlike drug addiction, because between bouts of drinking, dipsomaniacs often abstain completely. The steady drinking of the chronic alcoholic is a disorder of personality. Although the drinker may lack the will to stop he is not physically ill when his supply is cut off. (*Delirium tremens* is not, as was once supposed, due to abstinence.)

Tobacco is also not a true drug of addiction. The heaviest smoker does not take to burglary if he runs out after closing time; most smokers consume the same amount year after year; there is no physical abstinence syndrome. But a confirmed smoker feels very wretched without tobacco; and the doctors who still smoke despite what they must know of the danger are silent witnesses to the grip of the habit. This is *psychic dependence* at its worst. As far as the habitué is concerned there is little to choose between physical and psychic dependence – between addiction and habituation.

Cocaine, hemp (*cannabis*), *amphetamine*, and *LSD* all lead to psychic dependence in susceptible subjects, but not to an abstinence syndrome. They cause various degrees of mental derangement, which may be lasting.

The distinction between 'true' addiction and habit is not always clear, and many people now feel that it is not worth making. 'Psychic' dependence could well be of the same nature as physical dependence, with the difference that the mechanism is more difficult to study. The chemistry of the brain is little understood, but the evidence at least shows that many mental disturbances are *associated with* and perhaps due to interference with certain chemicals: acetyl choline, adrenaline, serotonin and the like (◊ e.g., *depression*). Amphetamine and mescaline (a hallucinogen like *LSD*) are closely related to adrenaline. Cocaine mimics some effects of adrenaline. Bufotenin (another hallucinogen) resembles serotonin. Nicotine and LSD both disturb the transmission of impulses between nerve cells. Morphia, alcohol, and barbiturates all depress the activity of nerve cells. It is reasonable to suppose that all these drugs of 'addiction' or 'habit' act by altering the balance of chemical processes in the brain, some without greatly disturbing function and others with more serious consequences.

There are many obstacles to treatment. True addiction is in itself difficult to cure, and any drug habit is virtually incurable unless the patient is determined to give it up. Some addicts ask for treatment either in the hope of free supplies of the drug during the early stages, or because they think they will get more pleasure when they resume the habit after treatment.

Some form of behaviour therapy offers the best chance, but relapses are common, sometimes because an underlying personality disorder is harder to treat than the addiction itself.

The sudden spread of drug-taking from about 1960 took the medical profession unawares. In Britain and many other countries, doctors with little or no experience of the condition were consulted and sometimes pestered by young patients seeking a legitimate source of drugs and claiming to be 'registered addicts'. It was true that the Home Office kept a list of known addicts to certain drugs, but this form of registration in no way entitled anyone to have the drugs prescribed by a doctor. A few doctors were convicted of quite reckless prescribing, but many more prescribed in good faith, either because a regular if decreasing supply was needed in the early stages of treatment (as it sometimes is, but under the closest supervision) or in order to keep the addict out of the hands of criminals. In 1973 the restrictions were tightened so that addicts should be treated only by doctors with special training and experience.

Addison, Thomas (1793–1860). Physician at Guy's Hospital, one of the brilliant team led by Cooper. He described numerous diseases in terms of abnormalities of affected organs and not merely, as had been the custom, of symptoms. His is among the earliest recognizable accounts of appendicitis. He made a valuable study of the actions of poisons.

Addison is chiefly remembered for his descriptions of pernicious or Addisonian anaemia (◊ *anaemia* B.2), and of failure of the adrenal glands (Addison's disease).

Addison's disease. Deficiency of the adrenal glands. In 1855, when Addison's paper was published, the function of the adrenal glands (suprarenal capsules) was quite unknown. For years he had been studying 'a very remarkable form of general anaemia, occurring without any discoverable cause whatever' (pernicious anaemia), and 'whilst seeking in vain to throw some additional light upon this form of anaemia . . . stumbled upon [several cases of] anaemia, general languor and debility, remarkable feebleness of the heart's action, irritability of the stomach, and peculiar change of colour in the skin, occurring in connection with a diseased condition of the "supra-renal capsules"'. No more need be said about the symptoms of Addison's disease.

The ◊ *adrenal* is in two parts: the *medulla*, secreting adrenaline, and the *cortex*, secreting several hormones. Failure of the medulla does not matter because there are other sources of adrenaline. The symptoms are due to failure of the cortical hormones, which govern the rate at which sugar is made available, the amount of salt lost in the urine and other processes. The weakness is due both to deficiency of sugar in the blood and to disturbed balance of sodium and potassium through loss of salt. But loss of salt leads to loss of water, which in turn reduces the volume of blood; the circulation is then defective, while the heart itself is weakened like all the other muscles. Vomiting and diarrhoea, of which the cause is not clear, add to the dehydration. Anaemia, a shortage of red blood cells, may be due simply to reduced demand for oxygen and for the blood cells that carry oxygen. The pigmentation may be uniform (one of Addison's cases 'might have been mistaken for a mulatto'), but usually it is patchy. It is due to over-activity of the pituitary in an attempt to stimulate the adrenals.

Only about four people in a million develop Addison's disease today, and in three of them no cause can be found; their adrenals simply stop working. ◊ *Autoimmunity* has been suggested but not proved. The few remaining cases are mostly due to tuberculosis of the adrenal glands. Tuberculosis other than that of the lungs is now a rare disease, of which this is an unusual form. But a century ago all forms of tuberculosis were extremely common, and one can assume that most of Addison's cases were tuberculous.

The disease is effectively treated by replacing the missing hormones. Like a diabetic, the patient can lead a normal life if he has his daily injections. The only difficulty is that the demand is greatly increased in times of ◊ *stress*. If the patient has an injury or infection, his dose of hormones needs to be adjusted at once.

aden(o)-. Prefix = gland; glandular. *Adenitis* = inflammation, *adenoma* = tumour of a gland.

adenoid. Tissue resembling a lymph gland (lymph node) at the back of the nose, above and behind the soft palate (◊ *pharynx*).

adenovirus. A common virus, first discovered in adenoids removed surgically, a cause of sore throat and other symptoms much like those of the common cold.

ADH. Anti-diuretic hormone. ◊ *kidneys* (2).

adhesion. Sticking together of membranes as a result of inflammation.

Inflammation is both a defensive reaction to infection and the process by which healing takes place. The fluid in an inflamed region is derived from blood, and like blood can form a clot; connective tissue then grows into the clot. By this means moving surfaces such as those of joints, lungs or abdominal organs may become bound by *adhesions* if they have been inflamed.

adipose tissue. Connective tissue containing deposits of fat, forming a thick layer under the skin and serving as both insulator and fuel store (◊ *fat*).

adiposity. Excess of adipose tissue; fatness (◊ *obesity*).

adnexa. Appendages, especially those of the uterus (Fallopian tubes and ovaries).

adrenal. The adrenal glands (suprarenal bodies; suprarenal capsules) are a pair of small organs (each about ¼ oz.) at the back of the abdomen, against the upper ends of the two kidneys. An adrenal gland consists of two distinct organs: the *medulla* surrounded by the *cortex*. Their association is an accident of anatomy.

1. ADRENAL MEDULLA

The adrenal medulla is a unit of the ◊ *sympathetic* nervous system. Sympathetic nerves act by releasing minute amounts of *adrenaline* and *noradrenaline*. The effects include diversion of blood from skin and digestive organs to muscles, increased action of the heart, increased blood pressure, release of glucose (as ready fuel) from the liver into the blood-stream, and slowing of digestion. As a rule, the amount of adrenaline released at any one site is too small to affect other organs.

But when the adrenal medulla is stimulated by its sympathetic nerves, it pours a relatively large amount of adrenaline into the blood-stream. This circulates and produces 'sympathetic' effects throughout the body. In sum, these effects prepare the organs for physical effort. The muscles are supplied at the expense of functions such as digestion that can wait until the emergency is past. Although not strictly essential to life, the adrenal medulla has evolved as a useful mechanism in the struggle for survival.

Over- and under-activity of the adrenal medulla seem to play some part in emotional disorders; whether as cause or effect is not clear (◊, e.g., *anxiety*).

A rare tumour of the medulla (*phaeochromocytoma*) produces large quantities of noradrenaline, causing sudden attacks of very high blood pressure. The condition is cured by removing the tumour.

2. ADRENAL CORTEX

The adrenal cortex is an endocrine gland unconnected with the nervous system. It forms numerous hormones. Chemically these are closely related compounds – they are all ◊ *steroids* – but their biological properties are of three very different kinds: (1) *cortisol* (hydrocortisone) and similar hormones promote the synthesis and storage of glucose, suppress inflammation and the effects of allergy, and regulate the distribution of fat in the body; (2) *aldosterone* prevents excessive loss of salt and water through the

kidneys, and maintains the balance between sodium and potassium on which the activity of muscle depends; (3) *sex hormones*, male and female, are not important here because the testes and ovaries provide identical hormones. The adrenal sex hormones may represent an intermediate stage in the synthesis of cortisol.

Cortisol and aldosterone are essential to life. Hormones of this type (◊ *corticosteroids*) have a direct or indirect influence on many chemical processes in the body. The sum of their effects is to maintain the chemical *status quo* in a changing environment. Living tissue does not tolerate much change in its immediate surroundings, and the action of these hormones is important in preventing body chemistry from being disturbed by external influences or 'stresses'. In this context 'stresses' has a very wide meaning; it includes illness, injury, mental strain, and severe exertion. Without the adrenal cortex such stresses are lethal.

Some effects of cortisol seem paradoxical. Inflammation is a defensive reaction to infection and also the means of repairing injury, yet cortisol suppresses it. But inflammation becomes harmful if it runs riot, and cortisol keeps it within proper bounds. While other mechanisms deal with local problems, the adrenal cortex is concerned with the organism as a whole. Healthy functioning of the body is a balance between these (and many other) opposing forces.

The activity of the adrenal cortex is governed mainly by a hormone, ACTH, from the pituitary gland. By one of the many feed-back mechanisms of the body, secretion of ACTH is stimulated by a shortage of corticosteroids in the blood and suppressed by a surfeit. Stress evokes cortisol by stimulating the pituitary to secrete ACTH. (Aldosterone is regulated not by ACTH but by variations in the volume and salt content of body fluids.)

Corticosteroids and ACTH are widely used in medical treatment: ◊ *corticosteroids*.

3. DISORDERS

Deficiency of the adrenal cortex leads to ◊ *Addison's disease*, a fatal disorder if untreated, but remediable with regular doses of corticosteroids.

Three types of *over-activity* are described, due to excess of cortisol, aldosterone, or adrenal sex hormones; in practice these often overlap.

Excess of cortisol (*Cushing's syndrome*) may arise from overgrowth of the adrenal cortex, abnormal secretion of ACTH from a pituitary tumour, or prolonged medication with corticosteroids. The symptoms vary greatly. Since fat and carbohydrate are formed and stored at the expense of protein, there is loss of muscle and increase of fat. The fat has a characteristic distribution over the trunk but not the limbs; the neck is heavy and the face rounded. Bones and skin are both weakened. The disturbance of sugar chemistry sometimes goes as far as frank diabetes.

Excess of aldosterone alone (*Conn's syndrome*) causes retention of sodium and water with loss of potassium: the volume and pressure of the blood increase, and lack of potassium disturbs the working of muscle including heart muscle. This rare condition is due to a small tumour, which can be removed. More often the symptoms of Cushing's and Conn's syndromes are mixed.

Adrenogenital syndrome is another rare condition. The synthesis of corticosteroids is held up at the intermediate stage of sex hormones, which are secreted in great excess, and cause precocious sexual development with a tendency in either sex to develop male characters. Since there is a deficiency of cortisol, the adrenals are under constant stimulation by ACTH, and they can only respond by forming more and more sex hormones in an attempt to form cortisol. The disorder is corrected by giving corticosteroids.

Some forms of over-activity are cured by removing a tumour, which may be in the adrenal cortex and secreting corticosteroids, or in the pituitary and secreting ACTH. Others can be suppressed by X-ray treatment of the pituitary. As a last resort it may be necessary to remove the adrenals and then treat the resulting Addison's disease in the usual way.

adrenaline (known in the US as **epinephrine.** 'Adrenalin' is a registered name). The first ◊ *hormone* to be discovered (Schäfer and Oliver; University College, London; 1894). An extract of adrenal gland caused a dog's blood pressure to rise. Adrenaline was isolated from these extracts and, in 1901, synthesized. It reproduced many of the effects of stimulating ◊ *sympathetic* nerves, and for a time these nerves were thought to act simply by releasing adrenaline. In fact, a closely related substance *nor*adrenaline is released from most sympathetic nerve-endings, together with smaller amounts of adrenaline and probably of other similar substances.

Adrenaline stimulates the heart action and raises the blood pressure, releases glucose and increases its consumption, increases the circulation of blood in the muscles, relaxes the air passages and stimulates breathing, and produces a sense of excitement. In short, it prepares the body for physical action. At the same time it inhibits digestion and excretion, and reduces blood flow except in the muscles and heart.

Noradrenaline (arterenol) behaves a little differently. Whereas adrenaline causes some structures to contract and others (e.g. blood vessels in muscles) to relax, noradrenaline is almost entirely concerned with contraction. Broadly speaking, noradrenaline does the routine jobs such as maintaining an even blood pressure (by adjusting the resistance of the small arteries) and adrenaline deals with emergencies, when it can be released in large amounts from the adrenal glands.

These and similar substances are active in the ◊ *brain*, where they appear to determine mood and emotion.

Adrenaline is a valuable drug in certain emergencies such as severe ◊ *allergy*. It gives rapid relief from bronchial asthma. Since it is destroyed in the stomach it has to be injected, and its action is short-lived. It has to be given with great care, because an injection of adrenaline disturbs many organs other than the one that is being treated. For instance, while relieving asthma it causes disagreeable or even dangerous over-activity of the heart. Drugs with similar but fewer actions can often be used instead (◊ *sympathetic*).

Aëdes. A genus of mosquito able to transmit several tropical virus diseases, including yellow fever.

aerobic. Living or taking place in the presence of air or oxygen; e.g. aerobic bacteria need air, whereas anaerobic bacteria thrive without it and may actually die in its presence. Similarly, in human muscle, energy is normally provided by the combustion of glucose with oxygen (aerobic), but for a short time the muscle can do without oxygen (anaerobic). ◊ *muscle* (1).

aerophagy. Air-swallowing; a mildly neurotic habit which commonly causes discomfort from flatulence.

aetiology. The branch of pathology that deals with the causes of disease.

affect. The state of mind produced by an emotion. The emotion itself is here regarded as a process; affect as its effect. For instance fear is an emotion with certain physical manifestations; its effect is usually but not necessarily unpleasant, for some fear is exhilarating. In mentally normal people, emotion and affect are related in more or less appropriate ways, but in some types of mental disorder they are not. Among serious disorders, *schizophrenia* is characterized by extreme poverty of affect, i.e. the patient evinces little or no response to his own emotions. On the other hand the patient with *affective* (manic-depressive) psychosis is carried away by his emotions; at different times he may be wildly elated or utterly dejected.

afterbirth = ◊ *placenta*.

after-pains. A symptom that troubles some women after the end of labour. Labour pains are due to contraction of the muscle of the uterus. Rhythmic contractions of this muscle continue when labour is over; this ensures that all bleeding stops, and begins the process of involution by which the uterus regains its non-pregnant shape and size. After-pains are an unpleasant awareness of this necessary function. The uterus cannot safely be discouraged from contracting, but the painful sensation can be relieved with analgesics.

ageing. There is no apparent reason why cells should not live indefinitely if they are provided with enough water and oxygen and a few simple nutrients such as glucose, amino acids and salts. When a living cell reaches a certain stage of maturity it splits into two new young cells. In a sense, the cells of all creatures now living have been alive for a few hundred million years, for they are the products of repeated splitting of the first living cells.

In the laboratory, portions of tissue or even whole organs can be kept alive beyond the life-span of the animal from which they were taken. A heart, for instance, seems able to go on beating for as long as an adequate circulation of essential nutrients is maintained in its vessels, and waste products are removed. Yet the life of a complete animal is limited. A man who manages to escape every sort of illness or injury is still very unlikely to live beyond a hundred.

A substance that seems bound to degenerate is *collagen*, which forms the scaffolding between the cells of the body. Its slender fibres gradually lose their strength, and the accompanying elastic fibres harden.

In the nervous system, worn-out cells are not replaced when they die, because unlike other cells they cannot reproduce themselves. If only for this reason an old brain is less efficient than a young one.

In the arteries, a kind of degeneration (◊ *atheroma*) probably begins in childhood and ultimately causes the arteries to harden. On its own, atheroma may not be very harmful but when it is combined with civilized habits such as lack of exercise and overeating it becomes the leading cause of ill health and death in middle and old age.

The joints stiffen partly because of changes in the fibrous tissue and partly because the wear and tear of a lifetime inevitably causes some ◊ *osteoarthritis*. Old bones begin to lose their substance (◊ *osteoporosis*), but this process may not be as inevitable as it has seemed.

Finally, there is the statistical truism that the longer one lives the greater the chance that something will go seriously wrong.
◊ *senility*.

agglutination. Clumping together of bacteria (an effect of some ◊ *antibodies* which inactivate bacteria in this way) or of red blood cells (a similar effect is seen when bloods of different groups are mixed; this is different from clotting, which is solidification of the fluid part of blood).

agranulocytosis. Lack of white blood cells (◊ *blood* (3)).

ague. Violent shivering (*rigor*) at the beginning of a fever; malaria (tertian ague – malaria with shivering on first and third days; quartan ague – on first and fourth days).

air. A mixture of nitrogen (about 78 per cent), oxygen (21 per cent), small amounts of carbon dioxide and other gases, and a variable amount of water vapour.
Nitrogen has no biological action, but the

human body is adapted to live in diluted oxygen and functions better in air than in pure oxygen. (But nitrogen under pressure has some importance: see ◊ *compressed-air sickness*.)

Oxygen is essential to all forms of life except certain (anaerobic) bacteria. All activity depends on a source of energy, and the usual source is combustion, i.e. combination with oxygen of fuels such as fat and sugar. Oxygen is taken up in the lungs by the blood, and for this to take place satisfactorily a sufficient *pressure* of oxygen is needed. At sea level the pressure of the oxygen in the air is about 150 mm. of mercury – 3 lb. per square inch – which provides all the oxygen that the blood can carry. At the top of a mountain the air still contains 21 per cent of oxygen but at a lower pressure. A reduction of pressure by about a third is fairly well tolerated but below this the shortage begins to be serious. At an altitude of 3 miles the pressure is only half that at sea level and the blood is able to take up much less than the required amount of oxygen, and conditions are distressing. Many alpine resorts are a mile or more above sea level. A visitor may notice the reduced pressure of oxygen if he exerts himself, but he soon becomes acclimatized. Shortage of oxygen is a real hazard only at very high altitudes and in confined spaces (where accumulation of carbon dioxide is an even more pressing danger). It is not the essential objection to poor ventilation (◊ 'Fresh Air', below).

Carbon dioxide forms a very small proportion of the air. Plants are able to use it as a food, combining it with water to form carbohydrates and oxygen. Animals convert these products back to carbon dioxide and water, which they exhale. A man breathes out a volume of carbon dioxide equal to about 80 per cent of the volume of oxygen he takes in. In a confined space with no sort of ventilation, a poisonous concentration (6 per cent) of carbon dioxide is reached before the oxygen falls to a dangerous level.

1. Fresh Air

Enough air to support life (some 15 cu. ft per hour) will leak into the worst ventilated of rooms; but this is far short of adequate ventilation. For comfort, the air in a room needs to be replaced once or twice an hour, depending on the size of the room and the number of occupants. The unpleasantness of an ill-ventilated room arises from lack of air movement and excessive water vapour, both of which impede the evaporation of sweat; from disagreeable smells; and often from irritant smoke. These may look like minor annoyances, but it is on just such apparent trifles that health (as against absence of obvious disease) depends. That their effect may be psychological is beside the point, for psychological influences profoundly affect physical health.

Good ventilation greatly reduces the risk of air-borne infection. The outside air is exposed to the strongly antiseptic action of ultraviolet radiation from the sun. For this reason the air in sickrooms and hospitals needs to change rapidly: the official recommendation is 10 times per hour.

Central heating without ventilation removes too much water from the air and causes the mucous membranes of the nose to dry out. In very cold climates where windows have to be tightly closed some form of humidifier is needed.

Defective gas-taps and inefficient oil or gas burners provide a grave hazard, because small amounts of carbon monoxide are lethal unless ventilation is good. Every year there are several hundred deaths from accidental carbon monoxide poisoning in Britain, mostly among old people who feel the cold and seal off every possible source of fresh air. ◊ *dampness*.

2. Town and Country

The air of most towns is unfit for human consumption. Soot cuts out sunlight; this effect coupled with poor diet was responsible for the rickets of industrial England in the 19th century. Loss of sunlight causes more than rickets. It increases the chances of bacteria at the expense of humanity and, perhaps worst of all, it makes life less pleasant and therefore less healthy.

The danger of air-pollution by smoke was recognized in the 13th century, and a half-hearted law was passed against the use of coal in London. Since there was no other means of keeping warm, the law was never observed. The recent Clean Air Act has been more successful, but it deals with smoke only in terms of soot. Probably the most harmful component of smoke is sulphur dioxide, which is invisible. This gas is an even worse irritant than soot, and is probably the main reason why chronic bronchitis is many times more common in large towns than in the country.

Air-pollution comes next to cigarette

smoking as a cause of lung cancer. Coal smoke and oil and petrol fumes contain various substances known to cause cancer.

The virtue of clean air away from towns is simply that it is clean. It has no positive health-giving properties, but it puts no obstacles in the way of health. There is no evidence that sea air or mountain air have special merits except that one or the other may be free of something to which a particular person is allergic. A 'change of air' brings change of occupation, company, diet, and scenery, any or all of which may be beneficial. The value of a holiday is not measured by analysing the atmosphere.

air embolism. Blockage of a blood vessel by an air bubble. Air entering a vein is carried to the heart and pumped into the arteries. Small quantities have no effect, but a large quantity can form an air-lock and stop the circulation in a vital area such as brain or heart muscle. The danger of air embolism arises with wounds of the neck, where the negative (less than atmospheric) pressure in the veins may suck in air, causing sudden death. The risk of air embolism from hypodermic syringes is a myth, because the quantity is too small.

air sickness ◊ *travel sickness.*

air-swallowing = ◊ *aerophagy.*

alastrim (variola minor). A mild form of ◊ *smallpox.*

albino. Person in whom normal body-pigment is not formed. Albinos lack an enzyme needed for the synthesis of the brown pigment *melanin*, normally found in the hair, skin, and eyes. They have white hair, bright pink skin (strictly, dead white skin that does not modify the colour of the blood flowing through it), and pink instead of blue or brown eyes. Lacking protective pigment, their skin is very sensitive to sunlight – it cannot develop a tan – and their vision is impaired by over-illumination and, in many cases, a flickering movement of the eyes (*nystagmus*). Albinism is inherited as a recessive character (◊ *genetics* (2)).

albumen. White of egg.

albumin. The most abundant of the proteins dissolved in blood, the principal factor in maintaining the osmotic pressure of blood (◊ *osmosis*).

alcohol. Any of a large group of organic hydroxides; only two need be considered here – ethyl alcohol and methyl alcohol.

1. ETHYL ALCOHOL

Ethyl alcohol (ethanol, C_2H_5OH) is a colourless, almost tasteless liquid formed during the fermentation of sugar by yeast, known simply as *alcohol*. In medicine it has been widely used as a solvent (a *tincture* is an alcoholic solution of a drug) and as an antiseptic. Pure alcohol is an inefficient antiseptic; a 70 per cent solution in water is better.

The effects of alcoholic drinks can be considered as *acute* (immediate) and *chronic* (effects of habitual drinking).
Acute effects. Alcohol reaches the bloodstream rapidly. It can be absorbed from the mouth, and in the stomach it quickly passes through the mucous membrane to the blood. On the way through, it irritates the mucous membrane and sets up inflammation; the increased flow of blood accelerates absorption. Dilute alcohol, e.g. beer or light wine, is less irritating and less rapidly absorbed than spirits. Food in the stomach further reduces irritation and rate of absorption. A mealtime drink may improve appetite and digestion by irritating the stomach and so promoting the flow of gastric juice, and by suppressing the anxiety that so often impairs appetite; on the other hand neither alcohol nor anything else improves a perfectly healthy appetite. The habitual appetizer sets up a conditioned reflex, and then appetite fails without a drink.

After absorption, alcohol depresses the function of all living cells. The brain is more sensitive than other organs, and at every stage from the first drink to unconsciousness the effect of alcohol on the brain is to lessen activity. A few drugs have a double action, first stimulating, then depressing; but alcohol is not one of them. First to last, it is an anaesthetic like chloroform.

The most refined faculties are the first to suffer: judgement, concentration, self-control. Moderate drinking is mistaken for a stimulant because it deadens anxiety and self-criticism. It enlivens conversation by relieving shyness. The subject often thinks that manual skills, such as handling the controls of a car, are improved; but all objective tests show that this an illusion. Reactions are slowed and muscular co-ordination is impaired, but alcohol makes a man less critical of his own performance.

The amount needed to produce a given effect depends mainly on the size of the person. Alcohol spreads rapidly through the body fluids, which account for some 70 per cent of the body weight, or in an average man to 40 litres of water. 32 grammes of alcohol in 40 litres gives 0·8 grams per litre or 80 mg. per cent, which is the legal limit for drivers in Britain. This corresponds to about 3 oz. of whisky. An experienced drinker can behave himself perfectly at this level; socially speaking he is sober. But his reactions are demonstrably slowed. Most people become dead drunk at a concentration somewhere between 250 and 350 mg. per cent, and the lethal dose is not much greater. Death from acute alcoholic poisoning is rare because vomiting and unconsciousness set limits to drinking.

Alcohol is eliminated at a constant rate which reduces the level in the blood by 15–20 mg. per cent per hour, regardless of the amount drunk. Some is excreted unchanged in urine, breath, and sweat, but most is broken down in the liver. To eliminate half a bottle of whisky takes about 12 hours. Hence a man who goes to bed drunk may not be quite sober in the morning, and on the other hand a chronic alcoholic who drinks steadily round the clock may keep pace and stay more or less sober.

Chronic effects. Everything absorbed from the stomach passes first to the liver by way of the portal vein, and the liver bears the brunt of habitual drinking. After some years of continuous low-grade inflammation the lining of the stomach and the whole of the liver are gradually converted to fibrous scar tissue (this is the end-result of sustained inflammation of all kinds anywhere in the body). In clinical terms, the chronic alcoholic has chronic gastritis and cirrhosis of the liver. In time the kidneys and heart muscle are also affected, the heart by deposition of fat in place of muscle.

Vitamin deficiency (mainly vitamin B_1) is common, partly because alcoholics neither attend to their diet nor digest properly what they do eat, and partly because alcohol makes special demands on the supply of vitamin B_1. Because alcohol supplies ready energy and takes precedence over normal fuel, fat and carbohydrate are stored instead of being burnt and the drinker puts on weight.

The chronic effects on the brain are serious. Alcohol is not a true drug of ◊ *addiction.* The lethal dose is no higher for a habitual drunkard than for an abstainer (whereas an opium addict may be able to take enough opium to kill a score of ordinary people), and the drinker is not physically ill if he is made to stop. A dipsomaniac usually alternates between gross excess and total abstention; this is quite unlike drug addiction. A habitual heavy drinker is a victim of emotional stresses that he cannot face without alcohol. If his emotional climate improves he can usually stop drinking. But an insidious effect of alcohol is to lessen the will-power that is needed to stop.

In time all higher mental faculties are impaired, and alcohol can lead to undoubted insanity. *Delirium tremens* is a state of extreme agitation with hallucinations, seen in chronic alcoholics (also sleeping-pill addicts) with injuries or acute infection. (Delirium tremens was thought to be an ◊ *abstinence syndrome* due to sudden withdrawal of alcohol, but it now seems that this is not so; sick alcoholics are brought to hospital where drink is not supplied but that is not the cause of the trouble.)

Medical problems. Alcohol poses more social than medical problems. Heavy drinking is a symptom of the social misfit. Much thoughtless drinking (e.g. before driving) arises from a social convention that has survived from an age when only horses needed to stay sober.

The diagnosis of mild intoxication can be very difficult unless clinical evidence is confirmed by laboratory tests. Chronic alcoholism can also be hard to recognize, because the symptoms and signs are vague until the condition is advanced, and the patient's own account is seldom reliable; in fact evasion and lying are among the leading symptoms. Treatment is almost bound to fail unless the patient wishes to overcome the habit, and prolonged psychotherapy may be needed to establish or reinforce the wish and overcome the emotional disorder underlying the habit. Cutting down drink is useless; it has to be cut out. The drug *disulfiram* causes acetaldehyde to accumulate in the blood-stream if the patient drinks, with most unpleasant effects (nausea, headache, faintness). This treatment is dangerous unless the patient is supervised, and inapplicable unless he co-operates. *Alcoholics Anonymous* gives patients a chance to meet and talk with others who have tackled the same problems, and for many this has proved the most successful of all forms of treatment.

The *medicinal value* of alcohol is rather limited. As a 'stimulant' after injury or exposure it is disastrous because it is the reverse of a stimulant, and it further depresses a blood pressure that is already too low.

Nor can alcohol be taken seriously as a food, for although it provides energy it does so at the expense of more natural processes. Apart from calories, drink contributes nothing to the diet. But it may, as already stated, improve appetite and digestion.

Where alcohol does help is in allaying anxiety. It is not as safe as the latest tranquillizers, but many people find it pleasanter. The objection is that alcohol so readily gives cause for new anxieties while doing nothing for the causes of the old ones.

Alcohol is often said to reduce the risk of angina by dilating the coronary arteries. It certainly dilates the arteries of the skin, but any improvement of angina is probably due to relief of worry, decreased perception of pain, and lowered blood pressure. And in many cases drinking has contributed to the arterial disease that causes the angina.

This is no place to discuss the social merits of alcohol, except to indicate the lack of evidence that emotionally stable people do themselves any harm by occasional drinking.

2. METHYL ALCOHOL

Methyl alcohol (methanol, wood spirit, CH_3OH) is a highly poisonous substance found in badly distilled liquor. Its boiling point is 14° lower than that of ethyl alcohol, and an inefficient still or wrong technique does not completely separate the two. Methyl alcohol produces stupor and unconsciousness without elation. The lethal dose is only one tenth as large as that of ethyl alcohol. It has a special affinity for the optic nerves, and a single bout of drinking can cause temporary or permanent blindness.

alderman's nerve. An anatomical absurdity: it is a small twig of the ◊ *vagus nerve* to the skin of the ear. A more important branch of the vagus nerve controls the stomach, and a drop of cold wine behind the ear is said to stimulate the stomach by reflex action and help the alderman to digest his share of the banquet.

aldosterone. A hormone of the ◊ *adrenal cortex* responsible for regulating the excretion of salt by the kidney.

alimentary canal. The digestive tract: mouth, pharynx, oesophagus, stomach, and intestine.

alkaloid. An organic substance with certain chemical properties of an alkali, and medicinal or poisonous effects. Many drugs obtained from plants are alkaloids, e.g. atropine (nightshade), morphine (poppy), quinine (cinchona).

alkalosis. A shift in the ratio of acid to alkali in the blood and tissue fluid towards an excess of alkali (cf ◊ *acidosis*). It can be caused by loss of acid from the stomach through vomiting, overdosage of alkalis such as sodium bicarbonate (or both when the one is treated with the other), or excessive elimination of carbon dioxide (carbonic acid) by overbreathing. The most important symptom is exaggerated reactivity of the muscles, which may go into cramp-like spasm (◊ *tetany*).

Alkalosis is treated by eliminating its cause. Antacids such as magnesium trisilicate or aluminium hydroxide are as effective as sodium bicarbonate in the stomach without altering the alkalinity of the blood. Overbreathing is usually a neurotic symptom.

allergen. A substance capable of provoking allergy.

allergy. Allergy is biological tilting at windmills. It is a misuse of ◊ *immunity*, a defence against infection, in times of no danger. Healthy people develop immunity to infectious diseases by forming antidotes (◊ *antibodies*) that inactivate the infecting microbes and their poisons. Since unopposed infection would be lethal, unpleasant symptoms due to the action of the antibodies are acceptable. Allergic people have similar or worse symptoms to no purpose because they form antibodies against, for example, articles of food or clothing; they react to innocent chemical intruders as normal people react to dangerous invaders.

An antibody is a protein (a *globulin*) made in the blood-forming tissues in response to contamination with a substance known as an *antigen*. It inactivates the antigen by combining chemically with it, forming an inert compound. As a rule an antibody will react only with the antigen responsible for its formation. Hence the antibodies that confer immunity to, say, the virus of measles are useless against any other kind of infection; they react with measles virus and with nothing else. Similarly, a person with abnormal antibodies against egg-white may have symptoms of allergy whenever he eats an egg, but other foods will not upset him unless he develops other abnormal antibodies.

1. SENSITIZATION AND REACTION

As regards immunity, an antigen is a protein belonging to a microbe and different from any of the body's own proteins. Infection for the first time with a particular microbe introduces new antigens, which evoke new antibodies after a week or 10 days. The body has then been immunized to that infection; in future it will be able to bring appropriate antibodies into action at once if it meets the same kind of infection. The antibodies circulate in the blood.

Allergy was first described by von Pirquet (1905) as an abnormal reaction to foreign proteins. In fact, the antigens of allergy (*allergens*) are not all proteins. They include drugs and other chemicals, and even chemical elements have been known to cause allergic responses. These simpler substances – *haptens* – are thought to combine accidentally with a protein in the body to form a new 'foreign' protein which evokes antibodies to itself. There is no adverse reaction to the first encounter with an allergen, except that by a similar process to immunization the body becomes *sensitized*, i.e. it produces antibodies. In future, the antibodies will react with the allergen whenever it reappears and cause symptoms.

The antibodies of allergy tend to link themselves to particular tissues, and the symptoms depend on the tissue involved. For instance, if allergens meet corresponding antibodies in the nose they cause hay fever; if in the skin, they cause urticaria or eczema.

Histamine. This is a substance released by damaged tissues. It sets up ◊ *inflammation* by causing minute blood vessels to expand, thus increasing the amount of blood in the damaged area, and causing fluid to leak from the blood into the tissues. Inflammation is a defensive mechanism and also the first step toward repairing damaged tissue.

Many symptoms of allergy are apparently due to histamine released from tissues slightly injured by the reaction between antibodies linked to them and allergens. The most obvious is *urticaria* or nettle-rash: the symptoms (redness and itching followed by weals) are identical with those that follow

injection of histamine into healthy skin of superficial injuries, except that with injury pain masks itching. The inflamed mucous membranes of hay fever represent a similar reaction. Histamine also causes tightening of the air passages in the lungs (asthma) and over-activity of the stomach and intestine. Other active substances in varying amounts are released as well as histamine, so that allergy can take many forms.

It has been shown that normal components of the body can become allergens and evoke antibodies against themselves, a serious matter because the allergen is permanently to hand and the reaction is continuous (◊ *autoimmunity*).

A few diseases such as rheumatic fever have many features of a sustained allergic response, yet no allergy can be proved. Since they regularly follow bacterial infection, as a rule with streptococci, it seems possible that antibodies against streptococci may also react with the body's own connective tissue.

2. ANAPHYLAXIS

The symptoms of allergic reactions are more obvious than those of immune reactions against bacteria because allergic antibodies are linked to the tissues instead of circulating in the blood, and for the same reason allergy is confined to particular organs or tissues. In some animals, particularly guinea-pigs, an allergic reaction is likely to involve the whole body at once. The air passages are tightly constricted, the blood pressure falls abruptly, and often the animal dies. This condition is called *anaphylaxis*.

Anaphylaxis is very rare in man, but cases have followed large doses of horse serum in people previously sensitized by receiving horse serum and forming antibodies against it. Anaphylaxis has also been known to follow severe stinging by bees and wasps and the use of some drugs. Now that horse serum has largely given way to antibiotics in the treatment of infection, anaphylaxis is a very rare accident, but the slight risk makes it important that people sensitive to, say, penicillin should be given some other drug.

Serum sickness is an allergic reaction without previous sensitization. After a very large dose of serum there may still be enough in the circulation 10 days after the injection to react with the antibodies that have then had time to appear. It is unpleasant but not very dangerous.

3. TYPES OF ALLERGY

Greatly as allergic diseases differ from one another, they are all symptoms of the same fundamental defect. The common ones have already been mentioned. They fall into three groups. Firstly, the response to the offending allergen may be immediate, with symptoms almost certainly due to histamine. This group includes ◊ *hay fever*, ◊ *urticaria*, some cases of ◊ *asthma*, and some digestive disturbances. These last are distinct from true food poisoning although the symptoms may be the same: with allergy the trouble lies in the patient, but with food poisoning the food is at fault, usually through contamination with bacteria. Allergens may be inhaled as dust particles, or swallowed in food, or they may get into the skin. One might expect the symptoms to arise at the site of entry: hay fever and asthma from inhaled allergens; stomach ache, vomiting, diarrhoea, constipation from food allergens; urticaria from allergens entering the skin. This is often true, but there are many exceptions. Antibodies can attach themselves to the wrong tissue, so that, for example, food allergy causes a reaction in the skin or lungs. Some people have more than one type of symptom at the same time, e.g. hay fever with urticaria.

Secondly, the response may be delayed until a few days after contact with the allergen. The ensuing inflammation is less violent but more protracted than with the immediate type of response, and histamine is not involved. The immediate cause of the damage is unknown. With this type of allergy, antigens and antibodies appear to react inside the cells of the affected tissue. The commonest example is contact ◊ *dermatitis* (eczema), a grumbling inflammation of the skin clearly different from the transient eruption of urticaria. Allergic reactions to bacteria (as opposed to the defensive reaction of immunity) are of the delayed type. They account for some of the symptoms of prolonged infectious diseases such as tuberculosis, and perhaps also for diseases such as rheumatic fever which come on after an acute infection has subsided.

Thirdly, there are conditions where some kind of allergy appears to be involved but only as one of several factors, and the changes are not altogether like either of the two types of reaction described above. Some disorders of this kind are discussed under ◊ *autoimmunity*.

4. CONTRIBUTORY FACTORS

Most people go through life without developing allergies, although they form all the antibodies they need against infectious diseases. The tendency to form antibodies against harmless substances (or perhaps it is a tendency for such antibodies to become linked to vulnerable tissues) has a strong hereditary basis; that is as much as can be said of it. Particular allergies are not inherited. If someone has an itchy rash from eating strawberries his children will not be especially liable to the same trouble, but they will run more than an average risk of some kind of allergy, perhaps asthma from chrysanthemums or upset stomach from shellfish.

Infection plays two parts. Damaged tissue, whatever the cause, is vulnerable to microbes, and various kinds of allergy may be complicated by infection. With asthma, mucus trapped in the lungs by the narrowed air passages provides a breeding ground for bacteria. Allergic skin diseases itch, and scratching increases the damage and introduces infection. But infection can also cause allergy because one can be allergic to bacteria.

In people with an allergic tendency, symptoms identical with those of true allergy may have purely *physical* causes. A light scratch on allergic skin may look like a whiplash or sunlight may cause an unsightly and irritating rash. No satisfactory explanation has been found. These physical 'allergies' differ only in degree from normal responses: some allergic people react to trivial stimulation as normal people react to a real whiplash or a real burn. Similarly, cold air can set off attacks identical with allergic asthma or hay fever (whereas it does not cause the common cold, which is a virus infection). The hair-trigger responses of certain tissues and organs in allergic subjects give ground for some interesting speculation about the nature of allergy in general, but for the present it can be no more than speculation.

From physical causes of allergic disease it is a short step to psychological causes. Emotion has obvious effects on blood vessels, (blushing, blanching, altered blood pressure), heart (rapid pulse), involuntary muscle in the intestine and urinary bladder, and most if not all other organs. Since these effects, brought about by impulses in nerves and the release of chemical stimulants from nerve-endings, alter the state of tissues quite as much as a minor physical injury, it need be no surprise that they too can set off allergic responses in susceptible people. And in fact all allergic diseases can be aggravated by emotional disturbances, and some, notoriously asthma, can reach a point where emotion is the principal factor. ◊ *psychosomatic disease.*

5. CONTROL OF ALLERGY

The fundamental defect is unknown, and at present nothing can be done about it: particular allergies can be treated and often cured, but the tendency remains.

Treatment becomes easier if the allergen can be identified. Sometimes the patient finds out by experience what causes his attacks. In other cases, possible allergens (e.g. various pollens with hay fever) are applied to the skin and a reaction indicates the culprit. The history of the attacks generally suggests the sort of things to investigate e.g. cosmetics, clothes, food.

If the allergen is one that can be avoided, such as a particular face-powder, fabric, or food, the problem is solved.

If the allergen can be identified but not avoided it may be possible to *desensitize* the patient. A dose small enough to cause no ill effects is injected, and at intervals gradually increasing doses of the allergen are given. By the end of the course, the patient can tolerate a dose that would previously have caused severe symptoms. The small doses appear to evoke antibodies in the blood, like normal antibodies against bacteria, which can inactivate the allergen and prevent it from reacting with the antibodies in the sensitive tissues. Sometimes an allergy disappears on its own, and one can suppose that desensitization has occurred naturally. Unfortunately, desensitization does not always work. It is most often successful with hay fever. Failure may be due to other, unidentified allergens. Sodium cromoglycate disarms allergic reactions by blocking the release of substances such as histamine, which are the direct cause of symptoms.

Sometimes a change of home or job cures an allergy. A move is clearly indicated if it takes the patient away from a known allergen such as an industrial chemical or a particular type of pollen. Change also has psychological effects: the patient may recover because he is happier in new surroundings.

There are various effective ways of treating actual attacks. Where the symptoms are mainly or wholly due to histamine, the many *antihistamine* drugs work well. They are generally successful with hay fever and urticaria but not with asthma or eczema.

Adrenaline and various related drugs are most useful for treating attacks of ◊ *asthma,* and several other types of drug also relax the constricted air passages.

Corticosteroids arrest all kinds of inflammation, and will put a stop to almost any allergic symptom. As ointments they are useful for allergic skin disorders. Given internally for more than a short time their disadvantages outweigh their value in the treatment of most forms of allergy. But for dealing quickly with dangerous conditions, such as the rare cases of asthma that do not respond to simpler treatment, they are invaluable.

Obviously enough, associated troubles such as infection are treated at the same time as the allergic symptoms.

Finally, there is no group of diseases in which emotional factors are more important. Emotional disturbances help to cause allergic symptoms, which in turn engender emotional disturbances. Sedative drugs are sometimes added to the more direct remedies. The patient may need anything from a word of explanation to full-scale psychotherapy.

allopathy. Treatment of disease with drugs having opposite effects to the symptoms; a term coined by Hahnemann to describe orthodox medicine as against his own system ◊ *homoeopathy.*

allopurinol. A drug used for treating ◊ *gout,* a condition arising from an excess of uric acid in the blood. Allopurinol closely resembles a natural precursor of uric acid. The enzyme responsible for forming uric acid from the precursor occupies itself with allopurinol instead, so that less uric acid can be formed. With this treatment, gout can be almost completely suppressed.

aloes. Subtropical plants, some of which yield laxatives of the same type as senna and cascara.

alopecia. Loss of hair. ◊ *baldness.*

alveolus. Small cavity or socket: toothsocket: air-pocket in the lung where oxygen diffuses into the blood and carbon dioxide escapes.

21

amanita. A genus of ◊ *mushroom* (toadstool) of which several species are poisonous.

ambivalence. Conflicting emotions as a source of neurosis. ('Mixed feelings' is the same thing but without the suggestion of unresolved conflict and turmoil.)

amblyopia. Loss of vision – partial or complete, temporary or permanent – without apparent disorder of the eyes themselves; e.g. as a result of a stroke. Several forms of chronic poisoning can cause *toxic amblyopia*. The poisons include lead, arsenic, and benzene; the commonest are alcohol and tobacco.

amenorrhoea. Absence of menstrual periods. Literally, the term includes the state of girls before puberty and women after the menopause, but it is more sensibly confined to women of childbearing age who do not menstruate. *Primary* amenorrhoea means that menstruation has never begun: perhaps the most important point here is that some girls start late; but each case needs full investigation because some defect of structure or hormone balance may need attention.

Secondary amenorrhoea means that the patient who has previously had periods has stopped having them. The obvious and usual reasons are pregnancy and the menopause (which can be unexpectedly early). Otherwise the condition can be a symptom of all kinds of illness, including emotional upsets.

Amenorrhoea is not an illness but a symptom, and it is harmful in itself only because the feeling that she is not behaving normally disturbs the patient.

amentia. A word formerly used in psychiatry as a counterpart to *dementia*, to signify inborn mental defect as opposed to deterioration of a mind that was once healthy.

amidopyrine. An ◊ *analgesic* drug. Because of early reports of damage to blood cells it has never been popular in Britain, but it is widely used in some other countries.

amino-acids. Chemically simple substances of which ◊ *proteins* are composed. Hundreds of amino-acid molecules are linked together (◊ *polypeptide*) to form a single molecule of a protein. Human proteins contain about 22 different kinds of amino-acid. Nine of these, the 'essential' amino-

acids, cannot be synthesized by the liver and must be provided ready-made in the proteins of the diet. Animal proteins (meat, milk, eggs etc.) contain all the essential amino-acids, and are known as first-class proteins. Any good mixed diet contains enough of them to supply all the amino-acids that are needed. But in many poor parts of the world, the standard diet lacks not only protein in general, but first-class protein in particular. Children are especially vulnerable, and the malignant form of malnutrition ◊ *kwashiorkor* is common where the miserable ration that they get is not even of good quality.

Lack of the amino-acid tryptophan is a factor in *pellagra*, a kind of malnutrition among people who live on maize.

Unwanted amino-acids are broken down by enzymes in the liver to sugars, which are consumed for energy, and nitrogenous waste, which is excreted by the kidneys. Patients whose kidneys are not working can be given a diet in which protein is replaced by measured quantities of the right amino-acids, so that there will be no surplus waste to burden the kidneys or to accumulate in poisonous amounts because the kidneys cannot excrete them.

◊ *Phenylketonuria* is a hereditary disorder in which the enzyme for breaking down the amino-acid phenylalanine is lacking.

aminophylline. Theophylline-ethylene-diamine; a synthetic compound of the natural alkaloid theophylline, used to dilate blood vessels (e.g. with angina) and to relieve asthma.

amnesia. Loss of memory. The term is not applied to forgetfulness or the gradual deterioration of memory as one grows older, but to sudden and complete loss of memory over a particular time or particular events. Only two types are at all common: 'found wandering, suffering from loss of memory' is nearly always a kind of acute neurosis; the patient may forget his name, where he lives and so on, but in fact his memory is suppressed, not lost. A severe emotional shock, more than he can bear to remember, is a likely cause. Investigation and psychotherapy are needed. The second type is *retrograde amnesia* after an injury to the head. Here, the patient has no memory of events leading up to the injury, and in this case the loss is real and permanent. It has been suggested that some time must elapse before memories are put into storage, and concussion during this time interrupts the process – so these 'lost' memories were never stored, never reached the stage of being true memories. Concussion does not affect earlier memories.

amniocentesis. Taking a specimen of amniotic fluid, to be examined as a guide to the condition of an unborn baby. Towards the end of pregnancy, the specimen can be taken from below, through the cervix of the uterus. Chemical and microscopical examination may indicate, for example, that the baby is undernourished and should be brought into the world as soon as possible for treatment before irreparable damage is done. Amniocentesis can also be carried out early in pregnancy if the family history suggests a strong possibility of serious congenital disease, which may be indicated by defects in the cells shed from the baby's skin into the fluid. At this stage the specimen may be taken through the abdominal wall. The needle is guided with the help of an ultrasonic echo device, on the principle of a marine depth-sounder, which indicates the position of the baby in relation to the needle. If the examination shows that the baby is certain to be grossly abnormal, there is no need to let the pregnancy go any further. At present only a few congenital diseases can be recognized in this way, and the technique is not yet ready for general use. But there is every hope that in future many couples who would have avoided pregnancy because the risk of a serious congenital defect was too high will be able to have children of their own, knowing that they can be told whether the foetus is affected or healthy at an early enough stage for an abortion to be easy and safe. ◊ *genetics*

amnion. Membranous bag containing amniotic fluid, a watery liquid in which a baby floats in the uterus until birth.

amoeba. A very simple animal; a kind of ◊ *protozoon.* The species *Entamoeba histolytica* causes amoebic dysentery.

amphetamine. A drug related to adrenaline; it has been used to relieve nasal congestion, for slimming (by suppressing appetite) and to combat lethargy and depression. There are safer ways of doing all these things. Amphetamine, which has taken the place of

cocaine among drugs of addiction, can injure the heart and cause serious mental derangement if taken habitually.

Amphetamine first became popular in the 1930s, mainly in the form of an inhaler for relieving congestion in the nose. It was not very efficient because, although it gave instant relief, when the effect wore off the congestion became worse than it had been before. Tablets of this or one of the related drugs were also widely used as a mental stimulant or pick-me-up, and later for suppressing appetite. The tablets were subjected to restrictions in the same way as sulphonamides and other drugs thought to be potentially harmful but not liable to deliberate abuse. Drug addicts seem to have noticed before most doctors that the effect of amphetamine drugs on the brain is like that of cocaine. In Britain, thanks largely to the initiative of the Pharmaceutical Society, these drugs are now as strictly controlled as heroin and cocaine, and they are seldom prescribed.

ampicillin. A synthetic derivative of penicillin, effective against a wider range of infections than the natural penicillins, and fully active when taken by mouth.

amputation. Surgical removal or accidental loss of a limb. Until the discovery of anaesthetics and antiseptics in the second half of the 19th century amputation was probably the commonest surgical operation. It was dangerous but offered the only hope of preventing fatal gangrene after major injuries to limbs. As recently as the First World War amputation was the routine treatment for compound fractures (those where the broken bone was exposed in a wound and infected).

With the advance of plastic surgery, including the repair of severed blood vessels, and the use of antibiotics to overcome infection, amputation is now much less often needed; and although it remains the surgeon's last resort it has been made less deplorable than it was by the ingenuity of modern artificial-limb makers.

The usual purpose of amputation is to save life, but in some cases where there is no immediate danger to life a limited amputation done soon may save a more extensive operation later: for instance, gangrenous toes cannot be restored, but removing them may save the rest of the limb.

amyl nitrite. A drug used for treating ◊ *angina.*

amyloid disease (amyloid degeneration, amyloidosis, lardaceous disease). A gradual change in living cells, usually a result of severe and long-standing infection elsewhere in the body, and presumably a sort of slow poisoning. Affected organs have a pale, waxy (lardaceous) appearance. The name *amyloid* (starch-like) was given because affected tissue forms a dark stain with iodine, as does starch. The function of such organs (liver, kidneys, heart) gradually deteriorates. The usual causes are tuberculosis, chronic lung disease, and chronic infection of bone. But since these diseases have to be active for a long time before amyloidosis sets in, and they can now be controlled with antibiotic drugs, amyloidosis is no longer the common condition that it used to be.

Amyloidosis cannot be treated directly, but it may be arrested or even reversed when the underlying infection is cured.

anabolism. Chemical synthesis of new substances in the body.

anaemia. Literally, anaemia means lack of blood, but in fact it is shortage of ◊ *haemoglobin*, the oxygen-carrying pigment of the red blood cells (◊ *blood* (2)). The effects of anaemia are due to shortage of oxygen throughout the body.

Symptoms are vague (though very real) unless the anaemia is severe and the concentration of haemoglobin is reduced to, say, half the normal value. Acceleration of the heart beat keeps the available haemoglobin circulating more quickly and to some extent compensates for the deficiency; in time, untreated anaemia can overtax the heart. The patient feels weary and inefficient, looks pale, and may suffer headache, slight fever, and physical weakness. But anaemia is itself only a symptom and not a disease in its own right, and symptoms ascribed to anaemia are often due to the underlying disorder which is causing the anaemia.

Anaemia may be due either to abnormal loss of haemoglobin or defective production. The types to be considered are:
A. Abnormal loss, due to
  1. bleeding;
  2. excessive destruction of red cells
B. Defective production due to
  1. iron deficiency;

  2. vitamin deficiency (including pernicious anaemia);
  3. other causes

A. EXCESSIVE LOSS OF HAEMOGLOBIN

1. *Bleeding.* The danger of severe and rapid bleeding is not anaemia but death from ◊ *shock.* If someone suddenly loses a quarter of his blood he still has 75 per cent of his haemoglobin, which is more than enough to keep him going, but the loss of a quart from the total volume of a gallon may reduce his blood pressure to a dangerously low level. Blood transfusion is needed after a sudden haemorrhage to combat decreased volume of blood rather than anaemia.

The first response to bleeding (apart from purely local effects such as clotting) is reflex constriction of blood vessels in the less vital parts of the body such as the skin, which reduces the space to be filled with blood and so maintains the pressure. In the next few hours the remaining blood is diluted with water from the tissues to restore the volume, and in the next few weeks the lost red cells and haemoglobin are restored. If the bleeding is spread over, say, 24 hours, so that the volume of blood can be maintained by dilution, a man will survive the loss of half of his blood. He will be severely anaemic for a time, and he will be all the better for a blood transfusion, but his case will not be desperate.

Continuous slow bleeding, or repeated losses of small amounts of blood, deplete the body's reserves of iron until the lost haemoglobin can no longer be replaced (◊ B.1, below).

2. *Excessive destruction.* Healthy red cells live about 4 months. When they die they are treated as foreign bodies and digested in the same way as bacteria, by white cells in the spleen, liver and elsewhere. They are replaced by new cells from the bone marrow, which has no difficulty in meeting reasonable demands. But if the destruction of red cells (*haemolysis*) increases beyond about six times the normal rate, the marrow cannot keep pace; demand exceeds supply and a *haemolytic anaemia* develops.

When haemoglobin is broken down by haemolysis, its iron is stored for future use, leaving a yellow pigment, *bilirubin*, which passes through the liver into the bile to be excreted by way of the intestine. If there is too much haemolysis, bilirubin accumulates, and the complexion is tinted yellow.

Thus ◊ *jaundice* is often seen with haemolytic anaemias.

Haemolytic anaemia can be due to an abnormality that makes the red cells unduly fragile. Two such abnormalities – sickle-cell anaemia and Cooley's anaemia – are described under ◊ *haemoglobin*. In pernicious anaemia (◊ B.2, below), not enough red cells are formed, and those that are formed are liable to early haemolysis; so this is a case of deficiency anaemia with haemolytic anaemia added.

Many poisons damage red cells and cause haemolytic anaemia. They include lead, various derivatives of benzene, and some kinds of snake venom. Some people become sensitized to a drug that would otherwise be harmless, and may develop haemolytic anaemia if they take the drug again. In people whose red cells lack the enzyme G–6–P D, numerous drugs and also some foods (fava beans) cause severe haemolysis. This defect is commonest around the Mediterranean, or in people with Mediterranean ancestors.

Much the commonest cause of haemolytic anaemia around the world is ◊ *malaria*, because malaria parasites enter and destroy red blood cells.

Outside the tropics, most cases of haemolytic anaemia are due to ◊ *autoimmunity*: the body treats its own red cells as foreign matter and destroys them in the way that it destroys bacteria. A variant of this kind of anaemia occurs in unborn babies whose blood is incompatible with the mother's (◊ *rhesus factor*).

Only severe episodes of haemolytic anaemia call for treatment other than the treatment of the cause when it is known (e.g. treating malaria, avoiding an offending drug). With the more obscure types, haemolysis tends to come in waves, when for a time the patient becomes very anaemic, and needs transfusions of healthy blood. A curious complication of the disease and its treatment is overloading with iron, because haemolysis involves no loss of iron from the body, and repeated transfusions put more and more in. After scores of transfusions enough may be stored to be harmful; the excess can, however, be removed chemically (◊ *iron*).

B. DEFECTIVE PRODUCTION

1. *Iron deficiency.* The complication just described arises because the body hoards iron regardless of need, presumably because iron is difficult to absorb and the diet seldom contains an excess. When red cells break down after a normal life of 3 or 4 months, their iron is stored for use in new cells. The diet has only to replace small amounts lost in cells shed from the skin and intestine (◊ *iron*).

The average man's 5 litres of blood contain 2·5 grammes of iron, and the reserve, stored mainly in the liver, is about half this amount. If he bleeds, the bone marrow replaces the lost blood cells quite quickly, but the cells can be given their full complement of haemoglobin only while the stores of iron last. Iron lost by slow bleeding can be replaced in the diet only at a rate corresponding to a few c.c. of blood daily. Even slight losses of blood from, say, piles or a duodenal ulcer will cause anaemia if the bleeding continues long enough.

One of the commonest causes of unsuspected anaemia is bleeding into the stomach from abuse of aspirin (◊ analgesic). Women are much more vulnerable than men. An average Western diet barely keeps pace with even an average monthly loss, and if the loss is excessive, or other bleeding is added to it, a woman is liable to become anaemic. The 'normal' percentage of haemoglobin in the blood is often said to be lower in women than men, but here 'normal' may be confused with 'average', which is not the same. It has been shown in some large surveys that about a sixth of the adult women in Britain are anaemic, and a further third (making 50 per cent in all) have virtually no iron in reserve to meet emergencies.

There is a special risk of iron deficiency at certain times. During the years of growth a child needs iron not only to maintain the blood but to increase it and this leaves little chance of building up any reserves. When a girl reaches puberty she may have no stored iron, and with the onset of menstruation she becomes anaemic. The underfed factory girls of the 19th century developed a gross iron-deficiency anaemia known as *chlorosis* (from the yellowish complexion).

During pregnancy and while feeding a baby a woman has to provide for the baby's needs from her own iron stores, but the fact that she is not menstruating compensates to some extent for this loss. However, the milk provided by the mother contains no more than just enough iron for the baby's needs. When weaning begins, cereal foods provide a better source.

Symptoms are apt to be more severe with iron deficiency than with the same degree of anaemia from some other cause. This is because small amounts of iron are needed by many tissues other than blood. Cracked lips and deformed finger nails are caused by shortage of iron-containing enzymes, and some part of the general unfitness may arise in the same way.

Iron deficiency is usually due to bleeding. Poor diet is seldom the sole cause, but inability to absorb iron from the food may be, particularly after major operations on the stomach and small intestine.

The best sources of iron are meat, eggs, cereals and leguminous vegetables such as beans. Vitamin C, in fresh fruit and vegetables, is needed for iron to be assimilated from the food. A good mixed diet meets the normal demands. But when the stored iron has been depleted, a medicinal supplement is needed. Ferrous sulphate is the most widely used, but many other iron salts are suitable. Only a small amount can be assimilated at a time, and if the case is urgent (e.g. at the end of pregnancy) the iron can be given by injection instead of by mouth.

The symptoms of iron deficiency improve almost as soon as treatment is begun, and the patient, feeling better, often stops taking the preparation. In fact, she may need several months of treatment to build up adequate reserves. Sydenham, the first person to use iron systematically, treated his anaemic patients for as long as a year.

2. *Vitamin deficiency and pernicious anaemia.* Anaemia can be a symptom of most forms of malnutrition, because most of the components of a good diet play some part in the formation of blood. Two vitamins are especially involved: vitamin B_{12}, and folic acid. Although they are chemically unrelated, deficiency of either has the same effect on the blood: the development of red cells is arrested. Too few cells are formed, and those that are formed are misshapen and fragile, so that a haemolytic anaemia is added to the primary disorder. Lack of folic acid causes only the anaemia, but lack of vitamin B_{12} affects other tissues, in particular the nervous system. Severe and prolonged B_{12} deficiency can lead to partial paralysis of the limbs.

Folic acid deficiency can be due to lack of vegetables, to poor absorption in states of chronic diarrhoea (e.g. ◊ *sprue*), or to increased demand (e.g. in pregnancy).

Vitamin B_{12} deficiency is nearly always due to failure to absorb the vitamin. To be absorbed it has first to be combined with *intrinsic factor*, a protein formed in the stomach. After very drastic operations on the stomach there is sometimes a shortage of intrinsic factor and therefore defective absorption of vitamin B_{12}.

But much the most important disease of this class is *pernicious (Addisonian) anaemia.* It was first described in 1849 by Addison, of Guy's Hospital, London, as 'a very remarkable form of general anaemia, occurring without any discoverable cause whatever'; it was invariably fatal. In 1872 Biermer of Zürich called it 'pernicious anaemia'; in some countries it is now known as Biermer's anaemia. It remained hopelessly untreatable until 1926, when G. R. Minot and W. P. Murphy, following work on dogs by G. H. Whipple, showed that raw liver cured the disease. These three American physicians shared a Nobel Prize in 1934. The curative factor, vitamin B_{12}, was isolated in 1948, and its structure was established in 1955. Pernicious anaemia is now treated with regular doses of the vitamin, which completely control it.

The fundamental disorder in pernicious anaemia is in the stomach and not the blood. Why the lining of the stomach should stop producing the intrinsic factor (and, incidentally, acid) is not known; an autoimmune process has been suggested (◊ *autoimmunity*).

3. *Other causes.* All chronic infection (tuberculosis etc.) leads to some degree of anaemia; nobody knows why, or how to treat the anaemia apart from curing the infection. Similarly, there is usually anaemia with cancer, more than can be explained by bleeding: indeed, some cancers do not bleed at all, yet cause anaemia.

Advanced kidney disease causes anaemia, perhaps because the hormone erythropoietin, which promotes red-cell formation, is secreted by the kidneys, and diseased kidneys fail to secrete it.

Certain poisons affect the bone marrow. Suppression of all blood-cell formation leads to *aplastic anaemia*, an uncommon but highly dangerous state; one can only keep the patient alive with blood transfusions, and hope that the marrow will recover in time. The causes of aplastic anaemia are the same as those of lack of white cells (leucopenia) – ◊ *blood* (3).

anaerobic. Living without air (oxygen). ◊ *aerobic.*

anaesthesia. Absence of sensation, either in the whole body (general anaesthesia) or in a part (local anaesthesia). Anaesthesia may be induced by drugs or other means (◊ *anaesthetics*), or it may be a symptom of a defect in the nervous system.

Sensation means awareness in the brain of change elsewhere in the body. Impulses are conveyed along nerves to the spinal cord and then by several relays to the higher centres of the brain and consciousness. Different kinds of sensation are conveyed separately and are not necessarily all lost together. When a nerve is compressed the sense of touch is lost before that of pain, whereas local anaesthetic drugs abolish pain first. Sensation is abolished or diminished by obstructing the impulse at any point on its path. Since nerves contain sensory fibres carrying impulses to the brain and motor fibres carrying impulses to muscles from the brain, damage to a nerve impairs movement as well as sensation. Typical causes are wounds, infection (a notorious example is leprosy), and compression (as when a foot 'goes to sleep' from pressure on the sciatic nerve by the edge of a chair). An impulse in a nerve is a small electrical charge resulting from movement of potassium out of the nerve fibre and sodium into it; the original balance is restored as soon as the impulse has passed on. Local anaesthetics prevent sodium from entering the fibre, 'blocking' the nerve by making it unable to hold an electrical charge.

In the spinal cord and brain, sensory and motor nerve fibres are in separate bundles, and one may be impaired while the other is intact, or only a particular type of sensation may be lost. It has even been possible to relieve pain that responded to no other treatment by operating on the spinal cord to interrupt pain fibres from the affected region without disturbing others.

General anaesthesia follows blockage of impulses in the brain. It is seen in all forms of coma (injuries, epilepsy, stroke, intoxication etc.). How anaesthetic drugs work in the brain is not known. Some drugs (e.g. morphine in small doses) appear to affect the attitude to pain rather than prevent the impulses from reaching consciousness –

pain is perceived but the subject does not mind. Whether pain that does not hurt can still be called pain is a question of philosophy rather than physiology. It is an important question, because in some cases of hysteria there is total anaesthesia of part of the body without any apparent disorder of conduction in nerve fibres. A hypnotist can abolish pain by suggestion, and most people have experienced injuries that ought to have hurt but did not because they were preoccupied. In other words, awareness of pain can sometimes be suppressed in the same way as awareness of the ticking of a clock, or awareness of the touch of clothing.

anaesthetics (◊ *anaesthesia*). Anaesthetic drugs abolish sensation either in a restricted area (local anaesthetics) or in the whole body (general anaesthetics).

1. LOCAL ANAESTHETICS

The cola plant (*Erythroxylon*) is a traditional drug of addiction among Peruvian Indians. In 1860 Niemann isolated the active principle *cocaine* from cola leaves, and in 1884 Koller used the drug for painless surgery of the eye. Cocaine is rapidly absorbed by the mucous membranes around the eye, in the nose and mouth and elsewhere, producing complete numbness. It was also given by injection. But cocaine has many undesirable effects and in 1905 it was largely superseded by a synthetic drug, *procaine*, that could safely be injected into the area of an operation. Numerous drugs related to procaine are now in use. They can be injected into the immediate area of operation, or around nerves carrying impulses from the area, e.g. inside the angle of the jaw to anaesthetize the lower teeth. For some operations on the lower half of the body a local anaesthetic is injected around the spinal cord in the small of the back.

2. GENERAL ANAESTHETICS

From very early times surgeons have used drugs to lessen pain during operations. Substances extracted from two of the oldest pain-killers (morphine from poppies, hyoscyamine from henbane) are still used to prepare patients for general anaesthesia, but not for anaesthesia itself. Such drugs dull both perception and memory of pain, but doses large enough to abolish pain are apt to be lethal. The same applies to alcohol. One could do painless surgery on a man who was dead drunk, but one could not predict the appropriate dose (even if it did not make him vomit). The time-lag while alcohol takes effect adds to the danger, for there is no way to tell how much more effect is still to come and no way of keeping the effect within the bounds of safety.

Many good anaesthetics act like alcohol but with a different time-scale. They are very quickly absorbed by inhalation of their vapour, and since they act within seconds their effect can be held up at any stage by giving no more. Anaesthesia is rapidly induced and then kept at the desired level with a mere trickle of vapour. Recovery begins as soon as the anaesthetic is stopped. *Ether* (diethyl ether) is a drug of this type. It was used for the first operation under general anaesthesia by an American surgeon, C. W. Long, in 1842, and became generally accepted after demonstrations in 1846 by W. T. G. Morton in Boston, Mass., and Robert Liston in London.

A year later (Sir) James Young Simpson, an Edinburgh gynaecologist, showed that *chloroform* was easier to use and less unpleasant for the patient. It caused less agitation in the preliminary stage of anaesthesia, less coughing, and less nausea. For many years chloroform was the most widely used general anaesthetic, but in the end it became clear that ether, for all its disadvantages, was a safer drug for long operations. Chloroform held its place for very short operations.

Nitrous oxide ('laughing gas') was first used by an American dentist. Horace Wells, in 1844. It is still the safest and easiest means of inducing light anaesthesia for small operations such as dental extraction, and for major operations it can be mixed with more powerful agents.

Many drugs related to ether or chloroform have been tried; so far the most successful has been *halothane*. Even this, though safer and more reliable than other drugs of its class, shares with them the disadvantage that it occasionally damages the liver, especially if used repeatedly on the same patient.

Some important anaesthetics are injected into a vein. These are mostly *barbiturates*, closely related to drugs used to promote sleep but with a much more rapid and transient effect. The patient slips into unconsciousness in a few seconds, without preliminary agitation. The first of these drugs, *hexobarbitone*, was introduced in Germany in 1933. The most widely used has been *thiopentone*. Recently some short-acting anaesthetics given by injection have come into use, e.g. *propanidid*, which has the advantage that it leaves no hangover, and *ketamine*, used mainly with children because adults sometimes behave strangely after taking it.

3. Supplementary Methods

Anaesthetics are safer and better if the patient has been prepared. A drug to calm the patient beforehand prevents the early stages of anaesthesia from being stormy – until this was known, patients had to be strapped down – and prevents dangerous stimulation of the heart by the combined effects of anxiety and certain anaesthetic drugs, notably chloroform, which reinforce the action of adrenaline. Since anaesthetics abolish coughing the patient has to be protected against inhaling saliva by a drug to inhibit the salivary glands such as *atropine* or *hyoscine* (= *scopolamine*), which also diminish the fluid secreted within the lungs.

Except for minor anaesthetics the old method of dripping the drug on a pad in front of the patient's face ('rag-and-bottle') has given way to adding the vapour to a mixture of oxygen and nitrous oxide which is delivered to the patient through a fitted mask. The dose can be exactly regulated, and at any moment the anaesthetist can switch over to pure oxygen.

Controlled respiration, or rhythmic inflation of the lungs without the patient's help, has made anaesthesia safer and greatly extended the scope of surgery. Given a simple apparatus it no longer matters if the patient ceases to breathe of his own accord, and the chest can be as safely opened as the abdomen.

The practice of controlled respiration made possible the most significant advance in anaesthesia of this century: the use of *curare*. The action of this drug, which prevents muscles from responding to their motor nerves, was described by Claude Bernard in 1856, but curare was not used with anaesthetics until 1946. For many operations the surgeon needs the patient's muscles to be relaxed. He generally has to work in a gap between muscles, and he cannot see what he is doing unless the muscles are lax enough to be separated. The more powerful anaesthetics cause muscles to relax, but only at an advanced stage of anaesthesia. If curare has been given, only enough anaesthetic to abolish sensation is needed, and this means a very much smaller and safer dose. With effective methods of inflating the lungs artificially the action of curare on the muscles of the chest does not matter.

analeptic. (Drug) used to stimulate the nervous system or some part of the system. *Strychnine*, now practically obsolete, is one of the oldest. *Caffeine* is sometimes given to counteract the soporific action of pain-killing drugs. Other drugs, perhaps the only real analeptics, are used to stimulate respiration in certain cases of collapse. For instance, *nikethamide* and similar drugs have been given to all manner of patients who looked as if they might stop breathing, almost regardless of the cause of their trouble. In England, at least, this was partly because some coroners thought it negligent to let a patient die without giving him an analeptic first. On the other hand, drugs such as *bemegride* appear to be genuine antidotes to respiratory failure from barbiturate poisoning.

A new and fruitful offshoot is a kind of stimulant used to brighten the patient's mood, in other words to combat depression. These drugs are now known as antidepressants or thymoleptics. (◊ *depression*).

analgesia. Absence of the sense of pain, as opposed to *anaesthesia*, absence of all sensation.

analgesic (analgetic). (1) lacking the sense of pain. (2) relieving pain; drug used to relieve pain.

Many drugs have analgesic effects, including all ◊ *anaesthetics* and ◊ *narcotics*, which were formerly the only effective drugs for relieving pain (e.g. alcohol; opium), at the cost of stupefying the patient. Tranquillizers and hypnotics, taken in the usual doses, relieve mental turmoil or promote sleep but have little direct effect on pain except, perhaps, to make the patient more able to bear it. But all these classes of drugs overlap: thus the barbiturates are primarily hypnotics, but very small doses calm the patient without putting him to sleep and large doses are anaesthetic. Some drugs act at the source of a pain: for instance, *atropine* relieves intestinal colic by relaxing the painful

spasm of the intestinal muscles. But analgesia is taken to mean blunting the conscious perception of pain. The drugs to be considered here, sometimes called simple analgesics, are used to relieve pain regardless of its source, without impairing other faculties. These drugs are nearly all related to one of three substances discovered in Germany in the 19th century, namely *salicylic acid* (1874), *phenazone* (1883), and *phenacetin* (1887). In addition to dulling pain they are all antipyretic, i.e. they lower raised body temperature, and they reduce inflammation. None of these effects has been explained. The actions on pain and temperature take place in the brain. There is no effect on a normal temperature, but if the temperature is high the drugs act on a centre in the brain which controls sweating. The action on inflammation is most noticeable with rheumatic diseases. According to the use to which they are put, these drugs are known as analgesic, antipyretic, or antirheumatic.

Salicylic acid irritates the stomach too much to be given by mouth (though it is a useful ingredient of various ointments). Its salt *sodium salicylate* has a good antirheumatic effect, but by far the most widely used derivative is *acetylsalicylic acid* (= *aspirin*). The proper uses of aspirin include the relief of minor aches and pains and the suppression of rheumatic inflammation – its effect on rheumatic fever is as remarkable as it is mysterious, but then the disease itself is something of a mystery. The more usual chronic rheumatic diseases do not respond quite so readily, but their symptoms are generally alleviated. The value of aspirin with common colds and the like is in relieving headache and other discomfort. Lowering the temperature is incidental and probably not useful. Only very high temperatures are harmful in themselves, and analgesic drugs do not affect them.

Aspirin is also put to various improper uses. It does nothing to relieve worry or depression – to calm the nerves – and it does not promote sleep, except by relieving a pain that keeps the person awake. Yet these are the commonest grounds for habitual use of the drug. If it seems to work in these ways that is only because it is a medicine; anything else that the patient expected to work would do as well. But aspirin is not harmless. Very large doses cause a severe and sometimes lethal acidosis.

The usual symptoms of mild poisoning are giddiness and buzzing in the ears.

Regular doses as small as two or three aspirin tablets a day can cause bleeding in the stomach. The daily loss of as little as a teaspoonful of blood is enough to cause anaemia in time, and in many countries the aspirin habit is a major cause of anaemia. The risk may be less with soluble compounds of aspirin, but it is not overcome.

Phenazone and *aminophenazone* (*amidopyrine*) are used in exactly the same way as salicylates. They have never been popular in Britain because they occasionally poison the bone marrow, suppressing the formation of white blood cells. But this is a rare event, and in some countries amidopyrine is considered safer than aspirin. A much newer drug, *phenylbutazone*, is related to phenazone. It is especially valuable with certain rheumatic disorders but has to be used more cautiously than other analgesics. It is not a suitable household remedy for minor aches and pains.

Phenacetin is a good analgesic but has little antirheumatic action. Taken over long periods, phenacetin is poisonous to the kidneys. This delayed effect has only recently been recognized, but there is no doubt that many people have died from it. The harmful effects of phenacetin are largely due to a by-product, para-phenetidin, formed from it in the body. Most of a dose of phenacetin is converted to *paracetamol*, and the medicinal effect of phenacetin is due to this substance. Paracetamol is now widely used instead of phenacetin in the hope of getting the same analgesic action with less risk.

Indomethacin, ibuprofen and several other drugs unrelated to the earlier analgesics are alternatives to phenylbutazone for treating rheumatic diseases.

Codeine, an opium alkaloid closely related to morphine, has little narcotic action and in small doses can be counted as a simple analgesic; in Britain various preparations containing small amounts of codeine are exempt from the strict controls applied to narcotics in general. Another drug on the border between simple analgesics and narcotics is *pentazocine*.

No analgesic drug can do more than suppress particular symptoms; these drugs do not cure diseases.

analogous. Having similar function but different origin (of anatomical structures);

e.g. lungs and gills, as opposed to *homologous* organs with different function but similar origin, e.g. arms and wings.

anamnesis. Account of previous illnesses, an aid to the diagnosis of the present condition. (The word is more often used in other languages; 'case history' is commoner in English.)

anaplasia. A tendency of cancer cells to resemble the cells of an embryo rather than adult types. Whether this represents a survival of embryonic cell types into adult life or a reversion of adult cells to an earlier type is not known.

anastomosis. 1 (anat.). Direct communication between two arteries, or between an artery and a vein without an intervening capillary network. Most arteries communicate with other arteries, and if one is obstructed others can take over its work. An *end artery* is one without anastomoses. If it is blocked, e.g. by a blood-clot, the tissue beyond it is likely to die. Many of the terminal branches of the arteries in the brain, kidney, and intestine are end arteries, and the coronary arteries of the heart do not have enough effective anastomoses to deal with a sudden blockage. Arterio-venous anastomoses are between very small branches, e.g. those of the ◊ *renal* artery in the kidney.

2 (surg.). Artificial opening between two tubular structures; operation to establish this. The commonest surgical anastomoses are between the cut ends of stomach or intestine when a part has been removed.

anatomy. The primary discipline of scientific medicine. It is essentially a descriptive science, dealing with the form and arrangement of the parts of the body. Surgery is applied anatomy. General medicine is applied physiology, and physiology – the science of how the parts of the body work – is an extension of anatomy.

The first real anatomist seems to have been Herophilus of Alexandria, around 300 B.C. He described what he saw in dissections of bodies, not what prevailing theories said he ought to see. In this respect he had no known predecessors and not many successors. Herophilus described the nervous system and brain and their function, most of the abdominal organs, and the major blood vessels. He distinguished arteries from veins and insisted, contrary to current opinion, that the arteries contained blood and not air.

The greatest anatomist of antiquity was Galen in the 2nd century A.D., who was to be the last for many centuries. He described the structure of the body in great detail but with two kinds of mistake: much of his human anatomy was inferred from his

scholars. When learning at last revived in Europe, Avicenna's Arabic translation of Galen became a standard text. Even then, professors of anatomy were still content to teach by intoning ancient doctrines; the few dissections were done by menials to whose work scholars paid little attention – if the facts shown in the body disagreed with approved authority then the body must be

(Left) *Illustration to a text-book from which Vesalius was expected to learn anatomy in 1530, based entirely on superstition.* (Right) *Illustration to Vesalius's* Fabrica *(1543); it is correct in every detail.*

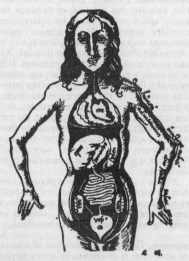

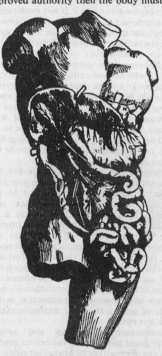

study of animals; and if facts did not fit theories then the facts had to suffer. Galen's mistakes would not have mattered if they had not been enshrined for the next twelve centuries and more. The Church approved of Galen and Aristotle. Their Stoic philosophy with its suggestion of divine planning was easily adapted to Christian teaching (also to Jewish and Moslem teaching). Because the Church approved, nobody dared to question Galen's authority – besides, theology was the one true science and nobody thought the human body worth studying.

Even Galen's work would have been lost if it had not been nurtured by Moslem

wrong. The first exception was Mondino, professor at Bologna, whose *Anatomia* (1316) was at least partly based on his own observations. His example was not followed until two centuries later when the artists took a hand. Leonardo's drawings of his own dissections are without equal. But his concern was beauty of design, not medical progress, and his many discoveries did not reach the doctors of the time. It was left to Vesalius, a generation later, to establish anatomy as a science.

Vesalius published *De humani corporis fabrica* in 1543. He was then 29 years old, and had held the chair of anatomy and surgery at Padua for six years. This work is the beginning of modern medicine. It is a precise record of observed facts, where all earlier authors had recorded opinion and speculation.

Before Vesalius, doctrines had been judged by the personal authority of the teacher. What Aristotle or Galen or Avicenna had said was taken for revealed truth, not to be questioned. Vesalius asked nobody to believe anything simply because he had said so; he asked them to look for themselves. Therefore his errors and omissions were not perpetuated. The great anatomists who followed him at Padua had only to make further dissections to complete the work that Vesalius had so brilliantly started, and by 1600, when Harvey was a student at Padua, anatomy had progressed almost as far as the naked eye could take it. By discovering the circulation of the blood Harvey founded modern physiology – the study of how the body works based on the knowledge of how it is constructed.

In the 17th century the focus moved from Italy to Holland. The University of Leyden, under the influence of Boerhaave, took the lead from Padua, and the next great advance in anatomy – the use of a microscope – was introduced by the Italian Malpighi and developed by Leeuwenhoek and numerous other Dutchmen. *Histology*, the microscopical study of tissues, became even more important to physiologists than to anatomists; and in the 19th century, under the influence of Virchow, was the basis of a completely new approach to the study of disease. The microscope also revolutionized *embryology*.

Ancylostoma (Ankylostoma). Hookworm (◊ *worms*).

androgen. Any substance acting as a male *sex hormone*.

androsterone. One of the male sex hormones.

anencephaly. Failure of the brain to grow in an embryo, a rare and lethal defect.

aneurin = ◊ *vitamin B₁* (thiamine).

aneurysm. A bulge at a weak spot in the wall of an artery. Arteries carry blood at a considerable pressure, and their walls need to be tough.

An aneurysm need not cause any trouble

unless it is large enough to interfere with neighbouring organs; but there is a danger that the bulge may give way and lead to serious internal bleeding.

The commonest cause of aneurysm used to be *syphilis*, which usually affected the upper part of the aorta. At present *atheroma* is a more usual cause; it most often affects the lower part of the aorta. Considering that most of us develop atheroma in time, these aneurysms are not very common. A few aneurysms are due to a congenital weakness in the wall of the aorta. Other possible causes are injuries to blood vessels (especially if they create a short-circuit between an artery and a vein) and bacterial infection.

Small but dangerous aneurysms occur in the arteries at the base of the brain. The defect is probably present at birth, but there is seldom trouble in early life. These aneurysms may cause symptoms by compressing nerves, or they may bleed and cause a stroke.

Only surgical treatment has any effect on aneurysms. John Hunter (1728–93) was, as in so much else, the pioneer. If an aneurysm is shaped like a balloon (saccular aneurysm) it may be possible to tie a thread round its neck and remove it. If, as is more likely, the bulge extends along an artery, the artery itself must be sealed above and below the aneurysm. With a small artery, neighbouring vessels can supply blood to the region, but with a main artery the flow has to be restored. In the past the problem has sometimes been solved by leaving the aneurysm and reinforcing its walls with fibrous tissue taken from another part of the body, but the method is not reliable. Arteries could be grafted in the same way as skin, but the patient has no large arteries to spare. Veins are expendable and can be used as grafts, and in time the transplanted vein takes on the structure of an artery. Another method is to insert a tube of synthetic fabric. Even a defective length of aorta can be replaced in this way. A smooth plastic tube does not work as well as a finely woven fabric which can become impregnated with the patient's own living tissue.

angina. 1. A sense of suffocation. 2. Acute infection in the throat or mouth such as a *quinsy* (abscess around a tonsil), or *Vincent's angina* (trench mouth). 3. *Angina pectoris*, a severe pain due to shortage of oxygen in the heart-muscle, which is the subject of this account.

Like any other muscle, the heart needs a

supply of oxygen in proportion to the work it is doing, and the supply depends on the rate of flow in the arteries. The blood pumped through the heart is useless to the muscle because the chambers of the heart have waterproof linings. Two small branches of the aorta, the *coronary arteries*, distribute oxygenated blood to the heart muscle. If the work of the heart increases, more fuel (fat and sugar) is burnt: more oxygen is taken up and more carbon dioxide is formed in exchange. The increased concentration of carbon dioxide makes the coronary arteries relax and admit more blood. In healthy people the flow of blood to the heart muscle keeps pace with the demand.

If the demand for oxygen is greater than the supply the heart cannot work efficiently, but it does not necessarily fail at once. The combustion is incomplete, i.e. the conversion of fat and sugar to carbon dioxide and water stops at an intermediate stage, and some intermediate product irritates nerve-endings in the heart and causes violent pain. (A familiar example of incomplete combustion is a domestic coal fire, pouring out smoke that a blast furnace would consume.)

The pain of angina serves some purpose. It stops the patient in his tracks and promptly reduces the amount of work that his heart is asked to do, so adjusting demand to supply.

Healthy young arteries are flexible enough to maintain an adequate flow in any ordinary circumstances. Angina means that the coronary arteries are not healthy. The predisposing disorder is *atheroma*, a degeneration of the lining of arteries with loss of elasticity, which appears to be a penalty of our civilization. (Possible causes are discussed under ◊ *atheroma*.)

Even with atheromatous coronary arteries the heart works normally within a limited range of activity, but if the range is exceeded the arteries cannot expand enough to provide the additional oxygen that is needed, and the patient has an attack of angina. The immediate cause of angina is thus physical effort (a patient may learn exactly how far he can walk or how many steps he can climb without trouble), excitement, or a heavy meal: in short, whatever makes the heart beat faster.

The capacity for useful work is further reduced by shortage of oxygen in the air (high altitude), or by anaemia, which diminishes the amount of oxygen carried

in the blood. Smoking has the same effect, because carbon monoxide in tobacco smoke replaces some of the oxygen in the blood. (Smoking also contributes to the underlying arterial disease.) In these conditions the heart must work harder to provide a given amount of oxygen. Excessive fat is a useless burden to the heart. Flabby untrained muscles are inefficient and waste oxygen.

Angina is mainly a disease of middle-aged men and old people of either sex. It can often be recognized by the characteristic sequence of exertion, pain in the centre of the chest (perhaps spreading to the neck, midriff, or arms), rest, relief. But pain about the heart is a misleading symptom, due as often as not to trouble in the stomach or elsewhere.

The course of angina is almost unpredictable. It can lead to early heart failure, or the patient may remain well for twenty years and more. People with angina are predisposed to ◊ *coronary thrombosis* because both conditions arise from the same disorder of the coronary arteries.

At present nothing can be done to restore the elasticity of atheromatous arteries, though the condition may perhaps be prevented (◊ *atheroma*).

Angina, however, can be treated in several ways. There are two principles: to keep the work of the heart within the limits of its blood supply, and to increase the amount of work that can be tolerated.

Obviously the patient's activity is limited to what he can do without symptoms, and here excitement is equivalent to exercise. Diet is restricted because a heavy meal can cause an attack, and because if the patient loses unwanted weight he can make better use of a given amount of effort. ◊ *atheroma*.

A lower limit to exertion is almost as important as an upper limit. Angina is its own warning, and the patient gains nothing by exerting himself only half as much as he might. Some exercise is needed to avoid putting on weight. The state of the coronary arteries may well deteriorate further if no demands are made on them. Muscles that are used are more efficient than those that are idle: they do more work with a given amount of energy. The heart is apparently no exception. Scandinavian cardiologists have shown that carefully controlled physical training, with some dietary restrictions and a strict ban on smoking, improve the patient's condition and reduce the risk of dangerous complications.

Drugs given to expand the coronary arteries include *glyceryl trinitrate* (trinitrin, nitroglycerin) and related drugs taken by mouth, and *amyl nitrite*, inhaled as vapour. Many patients know in advance what is likely to cause an attack, and avert it by taking the drug before the exertion. (Although these drugs dilate healthy coronary arteries, it seems that diseased arteries do not respond, and that the real effect is to dilate arteries elsewhere, diminishing the resistance to the blood-stream and the load on the heart.) *Practolol* and ◊ *propranolol* prevent the heart muscle from responding to adrenaline, which amounts to imposing a speed limit. Exercise and emotion stimulate the heart by causing adrenaline to be released; with this stimulus blocked, the heart is not made to over-exert itself.

Apart from drugs for the angina itself, others are often needed for associated disorders, such as high blood pressure, that aggravate the angina.

Several operations have been devised for improving the blood supply to the heart by diverting arteries from the chest wall and elsewhere, and an isolated blockage in a coronary artery can sometimes be bridged over by grafting a blood vessel, taken from some other part of the body to the coronary artery, across the blockage.

angiography. A technique for showing defects in blood vessels by means of X-rays: an iodine compound which casts a shadow is injected into the suspected artery or vein immediately before the film is exposed.

angioma. A tumour composed of blood vessels: a *naevus*. Angiomata are generally harmless, and most are congenital malformations of blood vessels rather than true tumours. An angioma inside the skull may interfere with the surface of the brain and have to be removed. ◊ *birth-mark*.

angiotensin. A polypeptide circulating in the blood. If the flow of blood through the kidneys decreases, the kidneys secrete *renin*. Renin reacts with angiotensin to make a substance that raises the blood pressure to restore the flow. ◊ *circulation* (1).

aniline. A poisonous coal-tar derivative, the basis of most synthetic dyes and of a few drugs. It poisons by inactivating

haemoglobin, the blood-pigment responsible for the transport of oxygen. The dye methylene blue is an antidote, but with severe aniline poisoning transfusions of healthy blood may be needed. Children are highly susceptible to aniline, and may not tolerate phenacetin, a drug derived from it.

ankle. The ankle is a simpler joint than the wrist. Only one bone of the foot, the *talus*, takes part, and movement is only in one plane.

The talus rises above the other bones of the foot. Its summit is shaped like half a drum. The under surface of the tibia is arched to roll over the talus, and the two *malleoli*, the knobs at either side of the ankle, clasp the faces of the drum. The inner malleolus is an extension of the tibia, and the outer is the lower end of the fibula. Thus the talus is clasped in a square mortice. Strong ligaments radiating from the malleoli to the bones of the foot support the joint on each side.

The only possible movements of this joint are to straighten, i.e. to point the foot (plantar flexion) and to draw it up towards the shin (dorsiflexion). The side-to-side movements of the foot are made at the tarsal joints (◊ *foot*). The feet are turned in and out from the *hip*.

Plantar flexion is a very powerful movement for pushing away from the ground in walking or jumping, and the calf (gastrocnemius) muscles are large. Dorsiflexion is much less important, and the extensor (tibial) muscles beside the shin are accordingly weaker.

A *sprain* of the ankle is among the commonest of all injuries. Usually the anterior fibres of the ligament at the outer side are torn; a sprain at the inner side is unusual. Few sprains are serious, but there is no clear line between a sprain and a tear large enough to make the joint unstable. A very extensive tear may need surgical repair, but such injuries are nearly always associated with a fracture.

Because the talus is held in a mortice, dislocation is hardly possible without fracture of one or both of the leg bones. Fracture-dislocation of the ankle is known as ◊ *Pott*'s fracture.

ankylosing spondylitis ◊ *spondylitis*.

ankylosis. Loss of movement in a joint, usually from severe arthritis or injury, especially fractures involving joint surfaces. With complete ankylosis the moving parts 'heal' together in the same way as the broken ends of a healed fracture. Prolonged immobility can lead to ankylosis of a joint from shrinkage of the surrounding tissues; when a limb is out of use, good nursing includes keeping the joints supple. ◊ *arthrodesis*.

Ankylostoma. Hookworm (◊ *worms*).

Anopheles. A genus of mosquito, responsible for transmitting malaria.

anorexia. Loss of appetite. *Anorexia nervosa* is a neurosis of young women. The patient eats no more than enough, and sometimes not quite enough, to keep her alive, yet as a rule she persuades herself that she eats well. If food is forced on her she may make matters worse by vomiting. It is a dangerous condition, for although the patient seldom literally dies of starvation she becomes severely under-nourished and may succumb to what should be trivial infection.

The sexual conflict, which Freud insisted was a factor in all neuroses, is unusually obvious in this one. The rejection of food seems to be a symbolic rejection of adult sexuality, an inability to accept the meaning of puberty.

Anorexia nervosa was commoner in the 19th century than now, firstly because convention repressed female sexuality, and secondly because the pattern of neuroses tends to follow fashion, and the neurotic of the 20th century has a much wider choice than her grandmother had. It has become easier for a young woman to accept the fact that she is designed for childbearing; and if she still cannot come to terms with it, various patterns of neurotic behaviour that were once taboo are now open to her (e.g. drugs, drink, perhaps even promiscuity).

As a rule the patient's family is too much involved in the conflict to be able to help her, but the condition responds well to psychotherapy.

anoxia. Shortage of oxygen in the body, from breathing deficient air (e.g. at high altitudes), from failure to transport enough oxygen from the lungs (e.g. anaemia), or failure to assimilate oxygen in the tissues (e.g. cyanide poisoning). It differs from *asphyxia* (suffocation): with asphyxia, carbon dioxide accumulates in the blood and stimulates deeper breathing. Pure anoxia, lacking this defensive stimulus, is more dangerous than asphyxia; the victim is unaware of anything wrong and quietly passes out.

antacid. A drug given to counteract excessive acid in the stomach for treating gastritis and peptic (gastric or duodenal) ulcer. Loosely, the term means the same as 'alkali', but not all antacids are alkalis in a strict chemical sense. *Sodium bicarbonate* is the most popular, but it causes uncomfortable distension by releasing carbon dioxide, and some of it is absorbed from the stomach and disturbs the acid/alkali balance of the blood. Preparations which have neither of these disadvantages can be had, e.g. *aluminium hydroxide* or *magnesium trisilicate*.

antenatal care. Over recent years the medical care of expectant mothers and their unborn children has come to be regarded as the most important part of obstetric practice. Whereas obstetricians used to pride themselves on their conduct of actual confinements, they now concentrate on sending mothers into delivery rooms in the best possible condition for uneventful parturition, resulting in unscathed mothers and mentally and physically healthy babies.

Antenatal care should begin as soon as pregnancy is suspected. The fact of the pregnancy and the date of conception must be established. Once the obstetrician knows when the pregnancy has begun he can monitor the foetus's growth, comparing it, at every stage, with what he expects of a normal foetus, and therefore quickly noticing any major deviation from that norm. In the last stages of pregnancy the date at which it began becomes even more critical. It is on the basis of this date that the obstetrician may have to decide whether a baby that seems very small or very large is likely to be in difficulties. ◊ *prematurity*; *postmaturity*.

The mother's general health needs careful attention throughout pregnancy as even minor disorders can become a serious threat either to her or to her child. Problems such as poor nutrition, abnormal blood pressure, subclinical urinary infections and latent diabetes are watched for from the beginning. Supplementary vitamins and iron will probably be prescribed, and the mother will be advised on how to feed her unborn child adequately without laying down layers of unwanted fat herself.

These regular medical checks, together, perhaps, with the mother's previous obstetric history, may suggest that special care will be needed. Trouble that is foreseen can always be better dealt with than trouble that presents itself as an emergency. This is why a Caesarean section may be suggested in advance, rather than being carried out as an emergency operation, and why bed rest may be suggested at the first signs of a ◊ toxaemia of pregnancy, without waiting for the disorder to become serious.

Even with expert antenatal care, and a problem-free pregnancy, a confinement makes heavy physical and emotional demands on a woman. A programme of antenatal training, designed to prepare both the muscles and the mind, can do much to promote easier childbirth.

antepartum. Before childbirth. *Antepartum haemorrhage*: bleeding from the uterus before delivery of the child, commonly because the placenta lies below the baby and becomes dislodged at the beginning instead of the end of labour.

anthracosis. Deposition of coal-dust in the lungs. ◊ *pneumoconiosis*.

anthrax. An infectious disease of farm animals occasionally transmitted to man, either as a severe localized inflammation of the skin (*malignant pustule*) or as a fulminating pneumonia (*woolsorter's disease*). Without treatment, the former is dangerous and the latter nearly always fatal. Serum treatment, for many years the only hope, often failed, but penicillin and other antibiotics are effective.

The anthrax bacillus was the first bacterium to be identified (F. A. Pollender, 1849), and in 1881 Pasteur successfully vaccinated sheep against the disease. Anthrax is now rare in W. Europe and N. America, and imports of potential sources of infection such as hides are controlled.

antibiotic. A class of drug used to treat infection. Biologists of the 19th century knew that one type of microbe might oppose the growth of another. This antagonism was called *antibiosis*.

In 1928 (Sir) Alexander Fleming noticed that bacteria would not grow on a culture-medium accidentally contaminated with a mould, *Penicillium notatum*. Evidently the mould produced something poisonous to bacteria, which Fleming called *penicillin*. An antibiotic is either a substance such as penicillin, produced by one mould or bacterium to destroy others, or a synthetic analogue.

Fleming's discovery could not be used in medicine until penicillin had been isolated and tested by Florey and Chain at Oxford. The first patients were treated in 1941, and the three men shared a Nobel Prize in 1945.

A few people become sensitive to penicillin and may have severe allergic reactions, but otherwise penicillin is a very safe drug. It destroys various common and dangerous bacteria, including streptococci, staphylococci, and the spirochaetes of syphilis and other diseases. It has no effect on tuberculosis or virus infections, except by overcoming the secondary bacterial infection which often complicates virus diseases – e.g. pneumonia with measles.

Many different penicillins, all members of the same chemical family, have been prepared. Some can be taken by mouth, others work only by injection. Some act quickly, others slowly but for much longer. Some of the newer penicillins act against a wider range of bacteria than the original preparations.

Since 1941 antibiotics have been prepared from many other moulds (fungi). Some are effective against diseases which penicillins do not cure. They include streptomycin (tuberculosis), chloramphenicol (typhoid), and tetracycline (a very wide range of infections).

Antibiotics act by obstructing a chemical reaction vital to the bacterium, i.e. by interfering with an enzyme. Penicillin prevents the formation of the protective cell walls of bacteria, and streptomycin that of the inner lining. Chloramphenicol and tetracycline disturb the formation of proteins within the bacteria. Clearly a useful antibiotic must not obstruct a reaction that human cells also need, at least not in the doses used against infection. One of the earliest, actinomycin-D, was rejected because it did damage human cells, but was later used in the treatment of certain cancers, more susceptible to it than healthy tissue.

Streptomycin can cause deafness by injuring the auditory nerve if it is given over long periods (and with severe tuberculosis it may be needed for many months). Chloramphenicol has been known to suppress the formation of blood cells in the bone marrow. Tetracycline may cause defective growth of the teeth in infancy, or before birth if the mother has large doses. Except for the occasional cases of allergy, ordinary doses of penicillin have given no trouble. The point is, of course, that these are life-saving drugs, and the risk of injury has to be weighed against the risk of not giving them.

Laboratory tests show which antibiotics are likely to work in a given case, and the safest can then be chosen.

1. RESISTANCE TO ANTIBIOTICS

On the whole, antibiotics have lived up to the hopes aroused when penicillin first appeared. The one great disappointment is that more and more bacteria have come to the fore which can resist them. In the early days penicillin nearly always worked against staphylococci (the commonest cause of blood-poisoning) and against gonorrhoea. Now, three quarters of the staphylococci in some hospitals, and more than half the cases of gonorrhoea in large towns, cannot be cured with penicillin. Natural selection has favoured the few resistant strains, once an insignificant minority, at the expense of the others.

Resistance is most likely to develop when antibiotics are given indiscriminately and when, in individual cases, not enough is given. Often the symptoms of infection are rapidly controlled; if treatment is then stopped a few bacteria will survive. A later infection with these survivors may not respond to the antibiotic, and another, usually of a different type attacking a different part of the bacterium, has to be used. For instance, penicillin-resistant gonorrhoea responds to tetracycline, and the sulphonamide drugs, which were rather neglected in the early days of penicillin, may come to the rescue.

Sometimes an antibiotic is too effective. The healthy lungs and intestines contain many harmless bacteria. Some are even useful: they synthesize vitamins such as B_{12} and K. A powerful antibiotic can destroy these along with the germs under attack, leaving the way clear for microbes which had never before had a chance of causing disease. The new infection is sometimes more serious than the old. This 'superinfection' is fortunately rare, but it is a distressing development.

antibody. A protein (gamma-globulin, molecular weight *c.* 200,000) formed in the spleen or lymph nodes in response to the presence in the tissues of an *antigen*. An antigen is a protein different from the body's own proteins. An antibody combines with the antigen that provoked its formation and inactivates it. By combining with the proteins of bacteria, antibodies are an important defence against infection. But antibodies are also formed against innocent 'foreign' proteins, and this is the basis of ◊ *allergy.*

An antibody is effective only against the particular antigen that caused it to be formed; thus antibodies against measles virus have no effect on chickenpox. It takes a week or more to form antibodies against a new antigen, but the knack persists, and if the same antigen reappears it can be dealt with at once; an attack of measles confers lasting immunity to the measles virus.

Two current theories of the origin of antibodies are: (1) that an antigen in some way determines the synthesis of a new antibody; (2) that we are born with samples of all the antibodies we shall ever be able to form, in individual cells, and that an antigen causes the appropriate type of cell to multiply.

◊ *autoimmunity; immunity.*

anticoagulant. (Drug) that impedes the clotting of blood. Clotting is a complex process, the result of a chain of chemical reactions involving a dozen or more reagents (◊ *blood* (4)). Interference at any stage prevents blood from clotting, but of the many methods of keeping blood liquid in a test-tube only a few are safe in the living body.

Heparin is found in various tissues, especially liver, lung, and peritoneum. It inhibits several of the intermediate stages of clotting.

Coumarin, found in sweet clover, is the basis of several compounds that prevent clotting by displacing vitamin K (one of the essential reagents). Their action was discovered by studying animals poisoned by spoiled clover.

These drugs are used in conditions where blood clots in veins or arteries (phlebitis, coronary thrombosis, certain types of stroke). Heparin acts promptly; coumarin compounds have a slower but more prolonged effect. Close supervision is needed to avoid abnormal bleeding. Heparin can be neutralized with protamine, a substance derived from fish, and the other drugs with vitamin K.

To what extent continuous treatment with anticoagulants prevents further attacks in people who have recovered from a thrombosis is still in doubt.

antidepressant. Any of the drugs used in psychiatry for relieving ◊ *depression.*

antidote ◊ *poison.*

antigen. A protein against which an ◊ *antibody* is formed. Many substances that are not proteins behave as antigens by modifying a protein in the tissues to form a new 'foreign' protein; thus one can develop allergy to them.

antihistamine. Acting against histamine. Histamine, one of the poisons of nettles and insect stings, is also formed in damaged human tissue. Its effects include stimulation of the stomach and intestine, contraction of the bronchi (asthma), and widening of small blood vessels with leakage of fluid into the tissues (nettle-rash, inflammation). Many symptoms of ◊ *allergy* are apparently due to histamine.

Antihistamine drugs are chemically related to histamine but lack its biological effects, and sensitive tissues react harmlessly with the drug instead of harmfully with histamine. These drugs are often effective in hay fever and urticaria but seldom in asthma. Some of them relieve travel sickness, and also cause drowsiness – a hazard to motorists who use them.

antimony (stibium). An element with chemical properties and poisonous effects similar to those of arsenic. It has been used medicinally since early Egyptian times. Many of its compounds cause vomiting (e.g. *tartar emetic*), and since vomiting was considered a good way to get rid of disease antimony was an esteemed remedy until quite recently. Compounds of antimony still find some use against certain tropical parasites (bilharzia, leishmania).

antipyretic. Reducing fever, i.e. lowering a raised body temperature. The antipyretic drugs chance to be the same as those commonly used for relieving pain: ◊ *analgesic.*

antiseptic. Chemical used to destroy microbes. The terms *antiseptic* and *disinfectant* both describe this sort of chemical, with the difference that antiseptics can be more or less safely applied to the body whereas dis-

infectants cannot. The distinction is often vague. The first antiseptic, phenol, is too poisonous to be anything but a disinfectant, and safe modern antiseptics are excellent as disinfectants in all but price.

An ideal antiseptic would kill all types of bacteria without damaging human tissues; it would work in the presence of blood, pus etc.; and it would be convenient to handle. No such substance exists, but a suitable one can usually be found for a particular purpose. Hundreds of antiseptics have been used. A few examples of different types can be given.

Phenol (carbolic) is of historical importance, because it enabled Lister to introduce modern surgery. It was soon discarded because it is almost as poisonous to man as to microbes. By present standards it is not even an efficient disinfectant.

Simple modifications greatly enhance the efficiency of phenol without making it more poisonous; these modified compounds still work when they are sufficiently diluted to be harmless, and many of them are less poisonous than phenol eve n before dilution.

The older compounds of this type include *cresol* (methyl-phenol), *thymol* (isopropyl-methyl-phenol, and *xylenol* (dimethyl-phenol.) Chlorination of these substances to *chlorocresol* etc. provides more powerful but safer antiseptics. *Hexachlorophene*, an effective skin cleanser, is a recent example. It is about 100 times more potent than phenol. This is not considered a safe antiseptic for babies, with whom there is some risk of toxic effects from absorption through the skin.

Chlorine gas is used for destroying bacteria in water. Concentrations below one part per million are effective. *Iodine* is equally powerful. For many years it was used in wounds, but it injures exposed tissues and is itself inactivated by blood. It is still used to prepare the intact skin before surgical operations.

All oxidizing agents are antiseptic. *Potassium permanganate* is effective but messy. *Hydrogen peroxide* is *activated* by blood and tissues generally, and in dirty wounds the bubbles of oxygen help to dislodge debris.

Soap is among the most convenient if not the most powerful antiseptics, and some detergents, such as *cetrimide*, are especially suited to the cleansing of minor wounds and of the skin around major ones. They are almost completely non-poisonous. But they

are easily inactivated, e.g. by pus. House-hold detergents are not suitable antiseptics.
Alcohol is a poor antiseptic. A 70 per cent solution in water is better than pure alcohol. It is, however, a good fat solvent. It physically removes bacteria from the skin by removing the layer of grease in which they are embedded.

Many *dyes* are effective and fairly harmless antiseptics. Brilliant green and crystal violet are also effective against some types of ringworm, and acridine dyes such as acriflavine are widely used for wounds.

The list might be continued almost indefinitely. Scores of antiseptics have particular uses, and none is suitable for all occasions. There are times when special antiseptics are much needed, but for most ordinary domestic purposes soap and sunlight seem as good as any.

antiserum. Serum extracted from the blood of a person or animal immune to a particular infection, therefore containing antibodies against that infection. Antisera are used in the laboratory for identifying bacteria and in clinical practice for treating certain types of infection. Serum can provoke severe allergic reactions, and antisera directed against bacteria have given way to antibiotic drugs. But sera against bacterial and some other poisons are still used (◊ *antitoxin*; *antivenene*).

antitoxin. Antidote to bacterial poisons, formed naturally in the body. Most harmful bacteria directly injure tissues in their own vicinity, but a few cause disease by releasing poisons (*toxins*) into the blood-stream. The bacteria of tetanus and diphtheria do little if any local damage, but their toxins are highly poisonous to nerve cells; diphtheria toxin also damages the heart. These toxins are *antigens*, and in time *antibodies* are formed against them. Serum containing such antibodies or antitoxins is used in the treatment of these diseases.

antivenene (antivenin). Serum containing antitoxins against animal poison, e.g. snake, scorpion, or spider venom.

antrum. A natural cavity in the body, especially the *maxillary antrum* (*sinus*), the cavity of the upper jaw, a hollow space between the floor of the orbit and the roof of the mouth, with a narrow opening into the side of the nose.

anus. The last inch of the intestine. It is closed by a system of muscular rings under partly voluntary and partly reflex control. It is lined with mucous membrane above and ordinary skin below. The upper part is sensitive to distension, and the lower part to the usual sensations of skin. The network of veins under the lining is liable to become engorged or varicose, a condition known as *internal piles* (◊ *haemorrhoids*).

Two common and painful disorders are *fissure*, a small crack in the skin of the anus; and *external piles*, a blood blister at the outer margin of the anus. Both are caused by straining, and are among the very few troubles that can be ascribed to constipation.

Itching (*pruritus ani*) is a distressing symptom. It can be due to minor disorders of the anal skin, but more often it is a kind of neurosis. Scratching does enough damage to give the itch an obvious physical cause.

anxiety. In a biological sense, anxiety is the same as fear. It is the normal response of the body to recognized danger. Numerous reflexes are involved, and they have presumably evolved with the species by the usual process of natural selection.

An animal survives physical hazards either by fighting or by fleeing. The same preparation is needed in either case: the body is geared to athletic performance at the expense of all other functions.

The supply of blood to the muscles is greatly increased, partly because the heart beats more rapidly and strongly, and partly because the blood vessels of the muscles dilate while those of many other organs constrict, diverting the flow to where it is most needed. The muscles themselves are tensed. Breathing is deeper and more rapid. The mind becomes more alert. The pupils dilate, admitting more light to the eyes. Some of the reflexes may serve to frighten an adversary, such as baring the teeth and raising the hairs by small muscles in the skin.

There are also negative components. At the start the bladder and rectum may be emptied, but then excretion and digestive functions are suppressed. Fear removes appetite.

In the wild, all these reflexes enhance an animal's fitness for survival, just as much as protective colouring, powerful claws, or an efficient brain.

Modern man has inherited the response to danger that served his wild ancestors so well. On rare occasions when he must fight or flee for his life it still serves its old purpose. In more ordinary circumstances anxiety is still useful. An athlete who feels 'the needle' – nervousness before a contest – is more likely to win than one who is quite unconcerned, and a touch of stage-fright animates an actor. Anxiety, whether fear of criticism or of dismissal or of self-reproach, is a necessary motive for good work, and also makes good work possible by keeping a man alert and improving his mechanical performance.

Though in sum the reflexes of fear act as a useful spur, individually many of them can be a nuisance. Increased alertness helps a man during an alarming interview, but muscular tension and rapid breathing do not. The hair reflex, shown as goose-flesh, lost its purpose thousands of generations ago.

1. ANXIETY AS AN ILLNESS

The effects of anxiety are like any other reflexes: they are automatic, inherited responses to a particular stimulus. They can be modified by conscious effort, but only to a limited extent. Fundamentally, they are beyond the control of the will. The stimulus is awareness of danger. The response is appropriate to *physical* danger. But at the unconscious level where these reflexes are determined, there is no distinction between physical and other hazards. Therefore the processes designed for meeting physical danger are indiscriminately applied to social, financial, or marital 'dangers', to which they are largely inappropriate.

Nor can there be any distinction at this level between genuine dangers and purely imaginary ones. A man who is really about to be dismissed and one who mistakenly believes that his employer wants to get rid of him are equally apt to lose their appetites or their sleep.

Fear or anxiety is for dealing with emergencies, which seldom last long. But many of the hazards of modern life – real or imagined – are persistent; in general the further removed they are from the tooth-and-claw emergencies of wild life the more they are likely to be prolonged. An imaginary danger will nearly always outlast a real one, for a real danger usually has a climax – it strikes or is overcome – while an imaginary danger simply persists. The man who

rightly thinks he may lose his job either does lose it or improves his work; in either case the particular danger is over. But for the man who wrongly thinks the same thing there is no reason why the supposed danger should ever pass. Now, the body is not designed for this kind of treatment. It is all very well for the blood to race through the muscles and for digestion to stop while one is running from a lion or dealing with burglars, provided that the normal balance is restored fairly soon. But if the body is kept in a state of emergency for weeks or months on end it is bound to suffer.

The physical effects of natural fear can become established instead of transient, and in time they may even lead to structural changes like those of illnesses with obvious physical causes. The life-saving reactions to physical dangers are translated into digestive disorders, headache or backache from muscle spasm, continuous high blood pressure and many other troubles. Sexual function is obviously suppressed by fear, and impotence and frigidity are common symptoms of sustained anxiety.

All these symptoms are as 'real' as those of any other illness. The cause may be in the mind, but the effects are very much in the body, and they have a definite physical basis.

Anxiety and its symptoms easily form a vicious circle, for the patient becomes anxious about the symptoms themselves. If, as often happens, he is told there is nothing the matter with him, his troubles increase because he then thinks that his disease must be a very obscure one. Perhaps he has a pain in his chest. X-rays and other tests show that his heart and lungs are perfectly healthy, but he is not in the least reassured by being told so. He still has his pain, now reinforced by the belief that nobody knows what is causing it. The only reassurance that will help him is an explanation of his symptom: that it is due to tension of his chest muscles, an unconscious defensive action.

2. SOURCES OF ANXIETY

Every reflex has three components: a stimulus, a response, and a definite pathway of nerves between the organ which receives the stimulus and the organ which carries out the response. With the reflexes of anxiety the pathways and responses are part of our hereditary make-up; they are much the same for everyone. But the stimulus – awareness of danger – depends on what the

individual unconsciously regards as dangerous, which in turn depends on his previous
experience. This means that anxiety is a
conditioned reflex.

In the classic experiment, Pavlov showed
that an inborn reflex, salivation in response
to food, could be modified or *conditioned* by
ringing a bell at each meal; his dogs then
salivated in response to the bell even
without food.

Fear can become similarly conditioned in
humans, usually in childhood. An object or
situation which is not in itself alarming is
associated with, and replaces, one which is.
In this way completely irrational fears can
arise. The process is of course unconscious.
The patient does not know why he is thrown
into a state of panic by the sight of a cat or
the prospect of a journey. He probably does
know that his fear (if he recognizes it as fear)
is irrational; but the symptoms are automatic reflexes over which he has no conscious control.

A *phobia*, which is morbid fear aroused
by a specific stimulus, is almost certainly a
conditioned reflex of this kind. Other types
of anxiety, where the patient seems to be
afraid of life in general, may well arise in the
same way, and at least they begin to make
sense if they are regarded as conditioned
reflexes.

3. MODIFIED RESPONSES
Even with severe anxiety states the patient
seldom shows all the signs of natural fear.
Usually one or two symptoms predominate:
sweating, perhaps, or painful spasm of a
particular group of muscles.

Sometimes the response is the very opposite to what it should be. Instead of being
inhibited, the stomach and intestine
become over-active, or instead of breathing
more deeply the patient has an attack of
asthma and cannot take in enough air. This
can be regarded as a reaction of despair:
the patient sees no escape from his fears and
simply puts up the shutters.

A *hysterical* response is usually centred on
a single part of the body in some way associated with the source of anxiety. In this way
a limb can become apparently numb or
paralysed.

In *obsessional* or *compulsive* states the
response takes the form of a more or less
absurd repetitive action, or sometimes only
a strong urge to perform it. The action is
supposed to symbolize, or perhaps expiate,
a repugnant deed which the patient is

unconsciously afraid of committing. Lady
Macbeth's hand-washing is an example.

4. TREATMENT OF ANXIETY
Some anxiety is healthy and indeed necessary. There can be no clear distinction
between what is normal and what is abnormal. Anxiety does not call for any
treatment unless it is a nuisance, and even
then the object of treatment is to keep it
within reasonable bounds rather than to
suppress it entirely. A patient relieved of all
anxiety is unlikely to hold down his job.

The people who most need attention are
those whose fears have ceased to serve any
useful function and make them ill without
enhancing their efficiency. Continued
anxiety upsets the balance between the
various bodily functions, which is harmful,
and it actually impairs efficiency because
the patient's concentration becomes centred on the fears themselves, with which he
cannot deal because they are not under
conscious control, instead of on their
original object.

The most important step is for the
patient to understand why he has his
symptoms. Even if they persist, they are
more tolerable when he knows that they
have a rational explanation.

Psychotherapy may be needed. This is a
very wide term. Sometimes intelligent
reassurance is enough (and this is a form of
psychotherapy). Certain types of anxiety
have been cured by behaviour therapy. In
essence, this means that the patient is
helped to unlearn his troublesome conditioned reflex. The original process by which
he learned it is put into reverse. The unconscious stimulus to fear is brought to
consciousness, and the patient acquires a
new habit of accepting it without disagreeable effects.

Drugs are very useful for suppressing
the symptoms of anxiety. Hypnotic drugs,
given in doses too small to send the patient
to sleep, will do this, but they tend to lower
the patient's whole efficiency. But the
milder of the modern tranquillizers relieve
anxiety without making the patient sleepy.
They also cause tense muscles to relax, thus
directly relieving one of the commonest
symptoms. Thanks to these drugs many
people who would otherwise be semi-
invalids can lead fairly normal lives; yet
drugs are not and never can be the whole
answer to anxiety. Good drugs are a priceless adjunct to other forms of treatment, but

the anxious patient is cured only by learning to redirect his fears in more profitable directions.

aorta. The principal ◊ *artery*: a muscular tube about an inch in diameter. Blood from the lungs enters the left atrium of the heart, passes to the left ventricle, and is pumped into the aorta to be distributed. The aortic valve at the origin of the aorta is discussed under ◊ *heart*. As it leaves the heart the aorta points upwards. It curves back in a hairpin bend, the *aortic arch*, and runs straight down, directly in front of the backbone, to the 4th lumbar vertebra. It then divides into the two common ◊ *iliac* arteries, which supply the pelvis and lower limbs.

The two ◊ *coronary arteries* leave the aorta just above its origin and spread themselves over the heart. Three large branches from the summit of the arch supply the head and upper limbs. These are the ◊ *innominate* artery, which divides into the right ◊ *carotid* and ◊ *subclavian*, and the left carotid and subclavian arteries. The branches in the thorax include the ◊ *intercostal* and ◊ *bronchial* arteries and several vessels to the oesophagus. The abdominal branches include the ◊ *coeliac* and mesenteric (◊ *mesentery*) arteries to the digestive organs, the ◊ *renal* arteries to the kidneys, separate arteries to the adrenal and reproductive glands, and branches to the abdominal muscles.

The veins corresponding with the aorta are the superior ◊ *vena cava* above, the ◊ *azygos vein* in the middle, and the inferior vena cava below.

1. DISORDERS

Coarctation is a congenital narrowing of a section of the aorta beyond the origins of the carotid and subclavian branches. The blood pressure is high in the head and arms and low in the rest of the body, sometimes too low to maintain adequate circulation. The narrow section can be removed surgically.

Atherosclerosis (◊ *atheroma*) is the commonest disease of the aorta. Other arteries, e.g. coronary, are often involved. ◊ *Aneurysm*, a bulge at a weakened part of the vessel, may compress neighbouring structures (veins, nerves, trachea, oesophagus). Syphilis used to be the commonest cause of aortic aneurysm, but the aneurysms seen today are mostly due to atherosclero-

sis. The affected part can sometimes be replaced with an artificial tube.

Cases are described of an ill-defined 'aortitis', with narrowing of the aorta, and sometimes of its branches, and defective circulation in the afflicted region. The condition may be related to the connective-tissue diseases.

aperient = ◊ *purgative*.

apomorphine. Emetic drug from opium, chemically similar to morphine. Whereas morphine occasionally causes vomiting, apomorphine invariably does so. Like other emetics, it is now seldom used.

apoplexy = ◊ *stroke*.

apothecary. Pharmacist or druggist, a person who prepares and supplies medicines. In England, the Society of Apothecaries was an offshoot of the Grocers' Company. Until the 19th century nobody distinguished drugs from spices. The few doctors of medicine in the Middle Ages left surgery to the barbers and drugs to the apothecaries; they concerned themselves mainly with theories and fees. The apothecaries came to know more about the realities of medical practice than the physicians. Since 1815 the Society of Apothecaries has conferred medical diplomas, which like all medical qualifications are now supervised by the General Medical Council.

appendicectomy. Surgical removal of the appendix. (Most American writers prefer 'appendectomy'.)

appendicitis. Acute inflammation of the appendix; the commonest emergency in abdominal surgery. It is extremely dangerous, because the appendix may burst and cause a fatal spread of infection (*peritonitis*); though there is a fair chance that in the early stages the inflamed peritoneum around the appendix will stick together and limit the infection to a localized abscess. Even this is bad enough, but it is much better than widespread infection in the abdomen.

The appendix is part of the intestine, and all intestinal pain is ◊ *referred* vaguely to the middle of the abdomen. The first symptom is thus an indeterminate bellyache. Some nausea is usual, and vomiting not uncommon; it is a reflex response to stretching of the intestine (in this case by inflammatory swelling). As with any infection, the temperature is likely to rise, and the number of white blood cells to increase. If the appendix happens to lie anywhere near the wall of the abdomen, then in due course the inflammation will irritate the lining of the wall; and this pain is felt directly over its origin, below the level of the navel on the right side. It is generally severe enough to obscure the pain from the appendix itself; hence the pain is said to shift from the mid-line to the right side. If peritonitis follows, the pain may shift back to the mid-line.

The diagnosis is easy if the symptoms follow this pattern. From the earliest stage light pressure on the appendix is painful. But the appendix is a mobile organ, and its inflamed tip may be far from its text-book position. If it lies behind several loops of intestine there may be no local pain; if it hangs down into the pelvis the characteristic tenderness can be shown only by examining the rectum. The diagnosis may be in doubt until the appendix is inspected at operation.

The standard treatment of appendicitis is early operation. The appendix is easily removed, and even a healthy appendix is useless. The alternative is to nurse the patient in a half sitting position so that if an abscess forms it will gravitate to the pelvis where it can do least harm, withhold food, and give antibiotics; but this is done only when surgery is impossible or, rarely, if it is certain that an abscess has already formed, when it may be easier to operate later. Uncertainty of diagnosis is not generally considered a good reason for delay, because several of the alternative diagnoses also need operation, and it is very much safer to remove a healthy appendix than to leave an inflamed one even for a few hours.

It is easy to say that appendicitis is caused by infection. The appendix is full of bacteria – but so is the whole of the large intestine, and no other part of it suffers in this way. But the appendix is a slender tube with a rather precarious blood supply. It may be that inflammation mild enough to pass unnoticed elsewhere is enough to block the tube and prevent mucus from escaping (much as a cold in the nose can cause trouble by blocking the sinuses); and that the increased pressure obstructs the flow of blood. This would damage the lining and give bacteria a foothold in the tissues of the appendix. Quite commonly the appendix is found to be blocked by a small hard fragment of faeces (or traditionally, but in fact very rarely, a grape-pip). This sort of obstruction could cause inflammation, or it could be an effect – inflammation inhibiting the muscle of the appendix and preventing it from emptying itself.

Nobody knows why appendicitis suddenly became a common disease at the end of the 19th century. There are earlier descriptions, e.g. by Celsus in the 1st century, Fernel in the 16th and Addison in the 19th, but they are very few. Even Rokitansky, who meticulously described 30,000 postmortem examinations between 1827 and 1866, gave no account of it. The first successful appendicectomy was done in 1887, and within 20 years the operation was commonplace. This was not simply a new fashion. Acute appendicitis is unmistakable at operation or postmortem examination, and in a large hospital it is almost a daily occurrence. Yet a century ago it was practically unknown, and it is hardly possible that the many observant pathologists of the time would have failed to notice it, unless it was in fact rare.

Chronic appendicitis – the 'grumbling appendix' – is another matter. There is not much evidence that such a disease exists, or, if it does exist, that it causes trouble. As a fashion it was at its height around 1930. Whether reality or myth, it has served a useful purpose. When persistent abdominal symptoms cannot be explained an exploratory operation may be needed to ensure that nothing serious is overlooked. A provisional diagnosis reassures both patient and surgeon. In many cases the reassurance probably does more good than the loss of the appendix.

appendix (vermiform appendix). A worm-like protrusion of the large intestine. It opens off the *caecum*, and is closed at its far end like the finger of a glove. It is usually about 3 ins. long. Any purpose that it may have served in some remote ancestor has vanished in the course of evolution.

It is important only as the site of appendicitis.

appetite. Appetite is a conditioned reflex – a learned response to sensations or thoughts associated with food. The physical effects are secretion of saliva and of digestive juice in the stomach; the sensation is agreeable. It is not the same as hunger, which is an inborn response to variations in the concentration of sugar in the blood. The main effect of hunger is rhythmic contraction of the stomach, which is not necessarily a pleasant sensation.

arachnoid (arachnoid mater). A gossamer-like membrane covering the brain and spinal cord, the innermost of the ◊ *meninges.*

arcus senilis. Opaque ring seen round the iris in elderly eyes.

areola. Pigmented skin around the nipple.

areolar tissue. Kind of ◊ *connective tissue.*

Aristotle (384–322 B.C.) was the son of a Macedonian physician. The impetus he gave to scientific thought, especially by his treatise on logic and by his insistence that theory must be based on observation, still endures. The scientific renaissance a thousand years later was inspired more by Aristotle than by any other classical writer: partly because his work was congenial to Christianity and so survived the Dark Ages, but mainly because if anyone 'invented' the scientific method it was he. This, rather than any particular discovery, is his great importance to medicine. He made detailed studies of the anatomy of animals, though not of man, and his classification of animals is only a short step from a theory of evolution. His account of ◊ *embryology* leads in the same direction, for he showed in chick embryos that the organs are formed successively in the order of their importance to life. The first organ to be distinguishable is the heart, which Aristotle therefore supposed to be the seat of the mind (soul?) and of life itself. This fallacy was soon dispelled by ◊ *Herophilus.* It remained for others to describe the anatomy of the human body, but Aristotle had paved the way to an understanding of what anatomy means.
◊◊ *teleology.*

arm. In descriptive anatomy the arm extends only from the shoulder to the elbow, beyond which is the *forearm.*
The skeleton of the arm is the ◊ *humerus.* Three muscles make the contours: ◊

deltoid over the shoulder, ◊*triceps* behind, and ◊ *biceps* in front. The nerves are all branches of the ◊ *brachial* plexus. The main artery is the ◊ *brachial,* but most of the blood to the arm comes from a branch of this, the *profunda brachii.* Veins accompany the arteries, and in addition two large veins lie under the skin – the *basilic* vein on the inner side and the *cephalic* on the outer side.
Movements are described under ◊ *shoulder;* ◊◊ *skeleton.*

arrhythmia. Any disturbance of the natural rhythm of the ◊ *heart.* The word is inaccurate, for it means absence of any rhythm, and with most arrhythmias the heart still has a rhythm, though not the right one. 'Dysrhythmia' would be better.
Sinus arrhythmia is no disturbance, but the natural variation of the heart rate caused by breathing. The heart beats faster during inspiration and slower during expiration, with an effect like *tempo rubato* in music. In some children the difference is great enough to suggest a real abnormality, but it has no significance.
The second commonest arrhythmia is the *extrasystole* (ectopic beat; dropped beat). A contraction wave starts in some area of heart muscle other than the natural pacemaker. The beat is premature and ineffective. When the next normal impulse arrives the muscle is still recovering from the extrasystole and does not respond. The sensation of a missed beat may be disagreeable or even alarming, but in an otherwise normal heart extrasystoles are unimportant. Smoking appears to be one of the causes. This arrhythmia is similar to *syncopation* in music.
Heart-block is a failure of the conducting fibres which carry the impulse from the atria to the ventricles. In a normal heart, when the contraction wave has spread through the receiving chambers (atria) it stimulates the conducting fibres (bundle of His) which convey the impulse to the pumping chambers, the ventricles. By this means the ventricles are ready to contract just when they have been filled by the atria. Conduction in the bundle of His takes about 1/6 second. There is no other path for the impulse, because the muscle fibres of the atria and ventricles do not communicate. Degeneration of the conducting fibres impairs or prevents conduction, and some or all of the impulses fail to reach the ventricles. Various degrees are possible.

An occasional missed beat resembles extrasystole. Sometimes only 3 beats in every 4, or 1 in 2 reach the ventricle (4:3 or 2:1 heart-block). If conduction fails entirely the atrium beats at the proper rate, while the ventricle takes up its own rhythm, about 30 beats per minute. This may not be enough to maintain efficient circulation, and the patient is liable to fits of unconsciousness (Stokes–Adams attacks) which may be fatal. An artificial pacemaker, giving regular electric pulses at the rate of a healthy heart, can be implanted in the ventricle if adrenaline and similar drugs fail.

Paroxysmal tachycardia is a sudden acceleration of the heart to a rate between 150 and 250 beats per minute. The paroxysm may last anything from a few minutes to several days. The rapid rhythm usually arises from some over-irritable area of heart muscle other than the natural pacemaker in the right atrium. A paroxysm may sometimes be shortened by simple measures such as holding the breath, pressure on a carotid sinus, or vomiting, presumably by stimulating the vagus nerve which in turn inhibits the heart muscle.

Flutter is akin to paroxysmal tachycardia with partial heart-block. The abnormal rhythm of the atrium is so rapid that even with an intact conducting mechanism the ventricle cannot keep pace; consequently only every second or third impulse is effective.

Fibrillation is a state of continuous and unco-ordinated activity of the heart muscle: instead of beating, it quivers, and ceases to act as a pump. Contraction of the atria is not essential to life, because filling of the ventricles is largely passive. The blood simply flows in as the ventricles relax between beats. But with atrial fibrillation the effective impulses reaching the ventricles are haphazard, and the response is irregular both in time and in intensity. Fibrillation is the only true arrhythmia. It may occur in the course of most kinds of heart disease, and it precipitates ◊ *heart failure* because the rapid irregular contraction of the ventricle is extremely inefficient. The effect of the drug ◊ *digitalis* is to slow the ventricle so that it has time to fill between beats. The fibrillation remains, but the heart becomes reasonably efficient. In some cases, ◊ *quinidine* restores normal heart action. Fibrillation of the ventricles is rapidly fatal because the circulation stops. Immediate cardiac massage or, better,

stimulation of the ventricle by an electrical 'defibrillator' can be life-saving.

arsenic. A metallic element found in many minerals, used from early times as medicine and poison. Mithridates of Pontus (c. 100 B.C.) protected himself against poisoning by taking regular small doses.

Compounds of arsenic poison all living cells. In many the primary damage is to capillary blood vessels, which are so weakened that blood simply distends them and stagnates instead of flowing through; thus the affected tissue is deprived of a free circulation and is poisoned by its own waste products. Plasma leaks from the damaged vessels and the blood in them becomes more viscous. The first tissue to be affected is nearly always the lining of the stomach and intestine. The symptoms – violent diarrhoea and vomiting, dehydration, circulatory failure – are like those of a fulminating bacterial infection such as cholera. The symptoms do not start soon enough for the diarrhoea to eliminate much of a dose. If the victim survives this stage he may still die from widespread effects on the nervous system.

Like lead and other heavy metals, arsenic remains in the body for a long time; it is only gradually eliminated in shed skin, hair, and nails. A small regular intake, e.g. from industrial exposure to arsenic, adds up in time to a poisonous amount. The tissues become tolerant to arsenic (as with Mithridates, above), but this only means that a larger dose is needed to poison an habitué than a newcomer to arsenic. An early sign of slow poisoning is thickening and darkening of the skin. This tanned, weatherbeaten appearance must account for the use of arsenic as a tonic until very recent times.

Ehrlich's discovery in 1910 of *arsphenamine* (Salvarsan; 606) was a turning-point in the history of drug-treatment, for it was the first drug to be manufactured as a specific remedy for a particular disease. It was a compound in which arsenic was rendered comparatively harmless to man but remained poisonous to the germs of syphilis. It was not quite harmless enough, and in 1914 Ehrlich replaced it with neoarsphenamine, which was the standard treatment of syphilis until the advent of penicillin.

The treatment of arsenical poisoning was very unsatisfactory until the discovery of B A L (British Anti-Lewisite; dimercaprol),

45

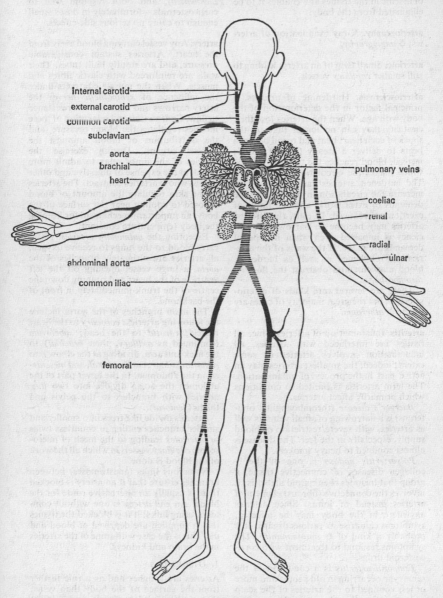

internal carotid
external carotid
common carotid
subclavian
aorta
brachial
heart
pulmonary veins
coeliac
renal
radial
ulnar
abdominal aorta
common iliac
femoral

Arrangement of principal arteries.

which obstructs the chemical combination of arsenic in the tissues and enables it to be eliminated from the body.

arteriography. X-ray examination of arteries; ◊ *angiography*.

arteriole. Small twig of an artery, leading to still smaller *capillary* vessels.

arteriosclerosis. Hardening of arteries, a principal factor in the deterioration of the body with age. When the arteries lose their elasticity they can no longer take up the shock of each heart beat and recoil between beats to deliver a steady flow of blood; instead, blood reaches the tissues in spurts which makes the circulation less efficient. The hardened arteries cannot expand to increase the circulation in response to the demands of extra work, and the limits of exertion are reduced. In time, the affected arteries may become so narrow that efficiency is impaired even when no special demands are made. If the walls of the arteries are roughened as well as hardened, blood may clot and obstruct the flow (◊ *thrombosis*).

There are several rare kinds of arteriosclerosis, but the great majority of cases are due to ◊ *atheroma*.

arteritis. Inflammation of arteries. Since all tissues are interlaced with arteries, all inflammation involves arteries to some extent; indeed, the smallest arteries play an active part in the process of inflammation. The term arteritis is limited to conditions which primarily affect arteries.

Buerger's disease (thromboangiitis obliterans) is a narrowing of small veins as well as arteries, with severe restriction of blood supply, especially in the feet. The disease is almost confined to heavy smokers.

Polyarteritis nodosa is one of the ◊ collagen diseases of connective tissue, a group that includes rheumatoid arthritis; it involves the connective (fibrous) element of arteries instead of joints. Since arteries anywhere in the body may be affected, symptoms can arise in various organs. It is probably a kind of ◊ *autoimmunity*. The symptoms respond to treatment with corticosteroid drugs.

Temporal arteritis is a condition of the same type occurring in old people and more or less confined to the arteries of the scalp and, occasionally, the eyes. It is often associated with muscular pains (*polymyalgia rheumatica*), and both respond well to corticosteroids – fortunately in doses small enough to cause no serious side-effects.

artery. Any vessel carrying blood away from the heart. Arteries sustain considerable pressure, and are stoutly built tubes. Their walls are reinforced with elastic fibres and muscle. When the muscle contracts under the influence of *sympathetic nerves* the artery narrows and increases the resistance to flow. Contraction and relaxation of these muscles regulates the blood pressure, and the distribution of blood amongst the various organs. During exercise the arteries of the limbs relax to admit more blood, at the expense of digestive and other organs whose arteries contract. The arteries of the skin regulate the amount of blood exposed to cooling near the surface of the body, an important mechanism for keeping the body temperature constant.

Excepting the *pulmonary arteries*, which carry blood to the lungs to receive oxygen, all arteries are ultimately branches of the *aorta*, a huge vessel opening off the left ventricle of the heart and running down the centre of the trunk immediately in front of the backbone.

The main branches of the aorta include the following arteries: *coronary* to the heart muscle; *carotid* to the head; *subclavian* (continued as *axillary*, then *brachial*) to the neck and arm, dividing at the elbow into *radial* and *ulnar*; *coeliac*, *renal*, and *mesenteric* in the abdomen. In the lower part of the abdomen the aorta divides into two *iliac* arteries with branches to the pelvis and thighs (*femoral*).

Arteries divide like trees into smaller and smaller branches ending in countless twigs or *arterioles* leading to the mesh of microscopic *capillary* vessels in which all the work of the blood is done.

Numerous links (anastomoses) between branches ensure that if an artery is blocked there is usually an alternative route for the blood. An *end artery* is one without communicating links; if it is blocked the tissues that it supplied are deprived of blood and die. This is the case with some of the arteries in the brain and kidneys.

1. DISORDERS

Arteries are tougher and as a rule further from the surface of the body than veins; they are therefore less often wounded. A cut artery is recognized by the bright colour of the blood and the force with which it is ejected. The jet pulsates with the heart beat. When an artery is cut through, its muscle contracts tightly, and the bleeding is much less than from an incompletely severed vessel, where the muscle tends to hold the wound open. Bleeding can always be stopped by direct pressure over the cut ends of the artery. Most of the bleeding is from the end nearer the heart, but where there are efficient links with other arteries it can be brisk from both sides of the wound, e.g. in the scalp and the palm of the hand. Most small arteries are expendable and can safely be sealed with a ligature after injury. Where there are not enough other arteries to take over the work, cut arteries can be repaired, or even replaced with synthetic tubes.

An artery is the life-line of a tissue. About a third of all deaths in Britain are due to failure of an artery either in the brain (*stroke*) or the heart muscle (*coronary thrombosis*). Disease can weaken an artery and cause a bulge (*aneurysm*) or bleeding; or it can lead to narrowing (*stenosis*) or complete blockage. An artery can be blocked by stagnation and clotting of blood (*thrombosis*) or by a solid fragment, e.g. of a clot elsewhere, carried in the blood-stream (*embolism*).

Diseases as totally different as *diabetes* and *syphilis* cause most of their chronic effects by damaging small arteries and so jeopardizing the blood supply of tissues.

Raynaud's disease is over-sensitivity of small arteries, or of the nerves that control their muscles. The natural contraction of these vessels in response to cold is greatly exaggerated, especially in the fingers. Other stimuli, such as emotional upsets, can also cause arterial spasm in these cases.

Arteritis (inflammation of arteries) is considered in the preceding entry.

↷ *arteriosclerosis*; *atheroma*.

arthritis. Inflammation of a joint. The term has been applied to many types of joint disease, not always correctly because with some types there is no real inflammation. The common factors are pain – ranging from an occasional dull ache with osteoarthritis to the sharp stab of gout – and restriction of movement.

The common cause of inflammation in most parts of the body, infection, is no longer among the leading causes of arthritis, since the two infections most likely to settle

in joints, tuberculosis and gonorrhoea, are prevented from doing so by treatment with antibiotics. Similarly rheumatic fever, where arthritis follows infection though not directly caused by it, has become rare since the discovery that streptococcal sore throats were quickly cured by penicillin.

The three common types of arthritis, ↷ *rheumatoid arthritis, osteoarthritis,* and ↷ *gout,* are discussed under their own headings.

arthrodesis. Surgical operation to fix a joint in one position. If the moving surfaces of a joint are stripped of their smooth coating of cartilage, the exposed ends of bone join in the same way as a broken bone; e.g. if the knee is treated in this way the femur and tibia join to form a single bone from hip to ankle. The operation is a valuable last resort for painful joints that do not respond to less drastic measures. A rigid joint is painless and is not disturbed by movement at other joints. The effect of successful arthrodesis is to make the limb as a whole more mobile than before, because the patient is no longer afraid to move neighbouring joints, and the affected joint had already lost any useful movement.

arthroplasty. Surgical reconstruction of a joint – the opposite to arthrodesis. An old method depends on the fact that if a broken bone is not splinted the broken ends become hard and smooth and a false joint is eventually established. If a joint has become completely fixed by injury or disease it may be possible to cut through the bone and keep some movement between the cut ends. A more satisfactory method is to implant an artificial joint of material that is not corroded by body fluids.

artificial respiration. Any method of getting air into the lungs when natural breathing is suspended. In the widest sense, the term covers mechanical aids ranging from the elaborate respirators ('iron lungs') to a simple hand insufflator that is no more than a modified bellows. In principle, a large respirator is a box in which the patient lies with his head on the outside through an airtight collar. The pressure inside the box fluctuates: when it falls below atmospheric pressure, air is drawn into the patient's lungs, and when it rises air is driven out. But in the more usual sense, artificial respiration is a first-aid procedure needing no equipment.

The oldest, most obvious, and easiest method is also the most efficient. This is the mouth-to-mouth technique mentioned in II Kings, iv, 34.

The patient is laid on his back.

The head is tilted back by drawing the chin upwards and forwards to keep the tongue away from the back of the throat.

The helper looks inside the mouth and runs a finger round the back of the tongue to ensure that there is no obstruction to the airway by food, weeds, false teeth etc.

He pinches the patient's nose so that the air will not leak, takes a deep breath, and blows steadily into the patient's mouth. The chest is seen to rise as the air flows in.

The helper raises his head and watches the patient's chest fall as the air is passively expelled.

These breaths are repeated every 5 or 6 seconds.

If the method is to be used with a baby the quantity and pressure of air have to be much reduced. This can be done by inflating the cheeks and puffing air in by the mouthful. The helper's mouth covers the baby's mouth and nose together. The rate of breathing should be rather fast, about a puff every two seconds.

Although expired air contains less oxygen than atmospheric air, it provides enough for the patient's needs.

Many other methods have been used. With Schaefer's method the patient is laid on his face with the head turned to one side, and the helper kneels beside or astride him and rhythmically presses the lower ribs with the flat of his hands. It is tiring and not very efficient. With the Holger Nielson method, the patient is in the same position but with the head resting on the hands. The helper kneels at the head and draws air into the lungs by raising the patient's elbows, then expels it by pressing the lower ribs. Lastly, Eve's method is to lay the patient on an improvised see-saw and tilt him up and down, so that the weight of the abdominal organs provides a piston-like action. These methods are no longer recommended.

If artificial respiration is needed at all it is needed at once. A person who stops breathing has only three or four minutes to live unless something is done about it.

Three common situations where lives are saved by prompt action are drowning, gas (carbon monoxide) poisoning, and electrocution.

With drowning, trying to get the water out of the lungs is a waste of precious seconds. As in other situations the mouth has to be cleared of obstructions, then mouth-to-mouth respiration begins at once.

With gassing, fresh air is needed, or artificial respiration will be useless and the helper will become another casualty.

With electrocution, helpers have lost their own lives by forgetting to switch off the current before touching the patient, or at least to drag him clear with a stick, an article of clothing or any non-conductor.

asbestosis. Chronic disease of the lungs from inhaling asbestos dust; a kind of ◊ *pneumoconiosis.*

ascaris. Roundworm; the species *Ascaris lumbricoides* is a parasite of man in many parts of the world. ◊ *worms.*

Aschheim-Zondek test. A test for ◊ *pregnancy.*

ascorbic acid = ◊ *vitamin C.*

asepsis. Exclusion of bacteria from the site of surgical operations, injections, wound dressings etc.

The technique was evolved soon after Lister's discovery that surgery could be freed from the danger of infection by using a carbolic spray to kill germs in the air, and applying carbolic dressings to wounds. It soon became clear that there was no need for the carbolic if everything that was to come into contact with the patient's tissues was first disinfected, and Lister's antiseptic surgery gave way to the present practice of aseptic surgery.

◊ *Lister; surgery.*

aspergillus. A common fungus; one species is the familiar and harmless mould which grows on jam. Another species sometimes causes asthma. What appear to be cases of severe infection (*aspergillosis*) are sometimes found; a few may be genuine, but most are probably other diseases (e.g. virus pneumonia) with aspergillus incidentally, and harmlessly, in the lungs, Aspergillosis is common and dangerous in birds, including poultry, but rare in man.

asphyxia. Suffocation; interference with *respiration* so that tissues neither receive enough oxygen nor get rid of carbon dioxide. It is rather less dangerous than simple lack of oxygen (*anoxia*) because accumulation of carbon dioxide provokes compensatory responses: it deepens breathing, and dilates blood vessels to improve the supply of oxygen to deprived tissues. General asphyxia is due to obstruction of the air-passages, e.g. by strangulation or disease of the lungs. Local asphyxia is due to impaired circulation, which may be widespread as with heart failure, or restricted as with blockage of a blood vessel.

aspirin. ◊ *analgesic.*

asthenia. Weakness.

asthma.

1. BRONCHIAL ASTHMA

The original meaning of asthma is heavy or difficult breathing, but now the word is taken to mean a particular kind of difficulty arising from spasm of involuntary muscle around the small branches of the air-tubes (*bronchi*) in the lungs. As these muscle fibres contract they squeeze the tubes and impede the flow of air. The effect is partly counteracted by breathing in, because expanding the chest creates a partial vacuum and tends to widen the tubes; but breathing out raises the pressure around them and increases the constriction. Therefore the prime symptom of asthma is difficulty in breathing out, and it is then that the characteristic wheeze or whistling sound of asthmatic breathing is loudest. During an attack the asthmatic uses the muscles of his shoulders to help him to force air out of his lungs (◊ *respiration* (1)). The spasm makes it difficult to cough away mucus, which collects in the small bronchi and further impedes breathing. The mucus itself is abnormally tenacious. It takes on almost the consistency of a contact adhesive, and the little that the patient manages to cough up during an attack is often in the form of beaded threads, still keeping the form of the bronchi in which they were lodged. Sometimes asthma is precipitated by bronchitis. Then the mucus is infected, i.e. contaminated with pus, from the start. In other cases, the clear mucus trapped in the bronchi by persistent asthma is an ideal incubator for bacteria, and then bronchitis is an effect instead of a cause of asthma. The irritation of bacterial infection causes further spasm of the bronchial muscles, and a vicious circle is set up. With all attacks of asthma, and especially those complicated by bronchitis, the mucous membrane lining the bronchi is congested and swollen, like the lining of the nose with hay fever or a common cold.

Thus three factors contribute to difficult breathing: muscle spasm, blockage by mucus, and narrowing of the bronchi by their swollen lining.

Causes of asthma. Asthmatic attacks are ascribed to three main causes: allergy, infection, and emotional disturbance.

With some patients, the attacks are as obviously allergic as *hay fever* or *urticaria.* They follow exposure to something such as a pollen or a food to which the patient is sensitive, and they respond to the same kind of treatment as other allergic reactions. For many years, 'house-dust' has been regarded as a common cause of asthma. But allergy is highly specific, and 'dust' is all-embracing. In a given case of asthma, no more than one or two of the hundreds of ingredients of house-dust is likely to cause trouble, perhaps fluff from a feather pillow or spores from a mould on a damp wall. The commonest of these culprits appears to be a mite, a spider-like creature about the size of a full-stop on this page, known as Dermatophagoides pteronyssinus. With many if not most asthmatics it is impossible to prove that the attacks are allergic. Nevertheless, some highly competent authorities regard all asthma as a form of allergy.

This view does not conflict with the known association between infection and asthma. As already explained, infection is often a direct complication of an asthmatic attack that could well have begun as a purely allergic reaction. Or, if the infection comes first, as in the familiar sequence common cold–bronchitis–asthma, then the asthma could in some way be an allergic response to the infection: perhaps the inflamed bronchi are unusually susceptible to the agents of allergy.

The third factor, emotional disturbance, is the most controversial. With many, though by no means all, asthmatics there is an obvious association between ◊ *anxiety* and the attacks. This is especially common in children, who sometimes appear to use their asthma as a means of getting their own way. And in some adults, frustration, worry or even reminders of past worries are enough to set off a severe attack. The type of neurosis seen with asthma is often shared by the whole family and may reach a stage where the patient seems more balanced than anyone else in the house. It is then easy to blame a child's asthma on parents (or an adult's on a spouse) who suffocate him with too much affection or overwhelm him by expecting too much. As if to prove the point, the patient may be instantly relieved by taking him from this tense environment into e.g. a boarding school or a hospital. So asthma is sometimes described as a ◊ *psychosomatic* disorder. The main objection to this is that cause and effect are not easily distinguished. An asthmatic child fighting for his breath is very frightened, and so is anyone who happens to be watching. Both may well develop anxiety neuroses as an effect rather than a cause of asthma. In time, the association of asthmatic attacks with anxiety may establish a conditioned reflex, so that a state of anxiety is enough to provoke the asthma.

In fact, the primary cause of asthma is still unknown. Simple but carefully conducted experiments have shown that in some people there is a paradoxical response of the bronchi to stress. The expected and normal response is the widening of the bronchi to admit more air, more oxygen, to meet a special demand. But if an affected person is subjected to stress, e.g. violent physical exertion, the muscles around the bronchi contract instead of relaxing. The reason is unknown, but it is the people who have this anomaly who are liable to asthma. In people who do not have it neither allergy nor infection nor anxiety can ever, it seems, lead to asthma. In the unfortunate minority whose bronchi react abnormally, any of these factors might trigger off an attack, as can sudden exposure to cold, unaccustomed exertion and other stresses. This is still a vague concept, but for the time being it makes some sense of a disease with too many alleged causes.

Course and Treatment. The general tendency of asthma is to improve with time. It can be called incurable only in the sense that the underlying anomaly is not understood and cannot be corrected. But most patients are healthy between attacks. If they cease to have attacks, it is difficult to see in what sense they are not cured. Many affected children simply grow out of having attacks, and with most adult asthmatics ways can be found of dealing with the factors that trigger off the attacks, and of mitigating the attacks when they do occur.

An untreated attack can last minutes, hours, or even days. If an immediate cause such as bronchitis is not treated, the asthma may last as long as the bronchitis.

Bronchodilators are drugs that relax the bronchial muscles. The prototype is *adrenaline*, a hormone formed in the body which meets physical demands by increasing the output of the heart, and the circulation of blood, especially to the muscles, inhibiting organs that are not concerned with meeting emergencies, such as the digestive and urinary systems, and providing more oxygen for the blood by dilating the bronchi. Bronchodilators are the first line of treatment of asthma because spasm of the bronchi is the original symptom, and if it can be dealt with in time other symptoms have no chance to become a nuisance.

The use of adrenaline itself is limited: it has no effect unless it is injected, and its action on the heart is dangerous unless the drug is given cautiously. But it works very quickly and will often stop even a severe attack. *Ephedrine* is closely related. It can be taken orally; it acts slowly and for some hours. It is useful for preventing attacks. *Isoprenaline* works quickly if a tablet is placed under the tongue; it can also be inhaled as a spray. *Orciprenaline, salbutamol,* and *terbutaline* are drugs of the same class with a more selective action on the bronchi and less effect on the heart. They are taken by mouth to ward off attacks, or inhaled if an attack has begun. Though they are safer than adrenaline, they are still dangerous in excess. If the recommended dose does not stop an attack, a larger dose (more puffs from the spray) must *not* be tried under any circumstances. It is time for some other form of treatment to be used.

Sometimes a different type of bronchodilator such as *aminophylline* works when others fail. This drug can be taken by mouth, injected, or given as a suppository (which acts almost as quickly as an injection). And the simplest of remedies, a hot drink, sometimes relieves quite a severe attack. In any case the patient needs to drink plenty, because if the attack lasts long he will become thirsty, and when it is difficult for him to breathe it will also be difficult to drink. With the thirst the mucus in the bronchi becomes drier and even more difficult to cough up.

All the drugs so far mentioned help to clear mucus from the bronchi, if only because widening the bronchi makes coughing more effective. If these drugs fail to ease the patient's breathing, the usual reason is that he still cannot clear the mucus that is blocking the air-passages. It is worth repeating that an overdose cannot help because the drug has already done its best: it can only be a danger.

The value of cough mixtures is limited. It is probably more helpful to moisten the air that the patient breathes. The old-fashioned steam kettle is better than nothing, but if the patient sits right over the steam with the time-honoured towel over his head, while the moisture loosens the mucus, the heat aggravates the third factor, the swelling of the mucous membranes. A better solution is a humidifier in the room to spread a cool mist of water droplets.

A physiotherapist can teach the patient to cough effectively and train his chest muscles in the art of breathing. She can also do a great deal for the patient's confidence, which is often in a poor state.

If the mucus or sputum is infected, as it is from the start if asthma is triggered by bronchitis, and as it always is if a series of attacks has lasted more than a few days, an *antibiotic* such as penicillin is called for.

In extreme cases of blockage by mucus, the bronchi can be literally washed clear by means of a tube passed down the trachea.

All the bronchodilator drugs related to adrenaline also shrink the swollen mucous membranes. Occasionally, though, the combined effects of spasm, mucus and swelling, each seeming to perpetuate the others, are such that the patient does not come out of the attack: this is *status asthmaticus*. Then, treatment with ◊ *corticosteroids* is invaluable. These drugs suppress all allergic reactions. In particular, they cause the swelling to subside. In addition, supplementary oxygen eases the work of breathing at the height of the attack, and in very rare cases mechanically aided respiration may be needed for a time.

Emergencies apart, corticosteroids are also used over longer periods in the few cases that do not respond to other treatment. Formerly the drug had to be given by mouth or by injection, with undesirable effects on the rest of the body and a risk of dependence. There are now inhalers which take the drug straight to the bronchi. This is similar to the use of corticosteroid ointments for skin diseases, and much reduces the risks of the treatment.

Instead of treating the attacks, one can sometimes forestall them. If an allergen can be identified, it may be worth trying to ◊ *desensitize* the patient. *Sodium* ◊ *cromoglycate* stops certain toxic substances from being released in response to allergic and other reactions. Inhaled regularly as a powder, this drug prevents or mitigates attacks in 75 per cent of cases known to be allergic, and in some 30 per cent of other asthmatics.

As to avoiding attacks associated with infection, the suggestions given under chronic ◊ *bronchitis* also apply to asthma.

Emotional or psychological factors are the hardest to diagnose and treat. One problem has been mentioned: that the state of anxiety often affects the entire household, and the doctor may wonder whose neurosis he should be treating. Another is that many asthmatics seem to resent and resist attempts to help them. And a third is that an apparent neurosis may be no more than a symptom of the asthma itself, relieved like the other symptoms when the attacks are controlled by physical means. Many asthmatics need a specialist's advice at times, and a few (e.g. with status asthmaticus) urgently need treatment in a well-equipped hospital. For the rest, there is no better example of the continuing need, in an age of specialization, for the all-round family doctor.

2. CARDIAC ASTHMA

A condition with symptoms resembling those of ordinary bronchial asthma but quite unrelated to it: cardiac asthma is a symptom of inadequate performance by the heart (◊ *heart failure*).

astigmatism. A common defect of vision: the transparent *cornea* at the front of the eye should be a section of a perfect sphere, but with astigmatism it is a section of a spheroid, i.e. the radius is greater in one plane than another, and when a line is seen in focus another line at right angles is blurred. Astigmatism is corrected by a lens in which a similar fault is set at right angles to that of the cornea.

astragalus = ◊ *talus*.

astringent. (Ointment, lotion etc.) causing shrinkage and drying of surface membranes; e.g. silver nitrate, aluminium salts, hamamelis (witch-hazel), tannin.

ataxia. Failure to co-ordinate the actions of the various muscles involved in performing a movement. The conscious brain directs the result of a movement (I will pick up a pin; I will place my foot there), but the choice of muscles and the balance of their actions depends on unconscious reflexes. Ataxia is a disturbance of these reflexes. There are several rare hereditary forms.

   Locomotor ataxia = ◊ *tabes dorsalis* (syphilis of the spinal cord).

atelectasis. Incomplete expansion of (part of) a lung. A lung is a spongy structure and should contain a good deal of air even after breathing out as much as possible. Until birth there is no air in the lungs, but after the new-born infant's first breath his lungs should contain air for the rest of his life. Breathing varies the amount of air in the lungs but does not exhaust them.

   Atelectasis may be present from birth, when the infant fails to breathe and the lungs have no chance to expand, or it may arise after birth if the lungs, having expanded, promptly shrink and lose their air (◊ *hyaline-membrane disease*).

   After infancy, atelectasis is generally due to blockage of an air-passage, e.g. by an inhaled foreign body, a plug of mucus, or a tumour. The air in the part of the lung beyond the block is absorbed into the bloodstream and cannot be replaced. Alternatively, air in the pleural cavity, between the lung and the chest wall (*pneumothorax*), or fluid (*pleural effusion*) will cause a lung to deflate.

   Many medical writers restrict the term atelectasis to the infantile types and describe the others as *collapse of lung*.

   Atelectasis due to failure to breathe is treated by artificial ventilation of the lungs through a tube passed down the windpipe. With other types, the lung expands when the cause is removed.

atheroma; atherosclerosis. *Atheroma* is a deposit of greasy material, mainly cholesterol, in the lining of an artery. *Atherosclerosis* is thickening and hardening of the walls of arteries (i.e. arteriosclerosis) associated with atheroma. This is the only common type of arteriosclerosis.

   The earliest beginnings of atheroma can be seen before puberty with fatty streaks in the lining of the aorta, but there are seldom any ill effects before middle age.

   The principal effects are narrowing of the channel of the affected artery, with impaired circulation beyond; loss of the smooth 'duck's back' lining, with a tendency for blood to stick to the vessel wall and clot there (*thrombosis*); loss of elasticity of the vessel (◊ *arteriosclerosis*); and weakening of the vessel with a tendency to bleeding.

   The common symptoms arising from these changes are thrombosis of arteries supplying vital organs such as the heart (coronary thrombosis) and brain (stroke); loss of efficiency in heart (angina), brain, muscles, kidneys etc. from deficient blood supply – in short, many of the symptoms generally ascribed to growing older. If the blood supply of the kidneys is threatened the blood pressure rises to compensate, and this sets up a vicious circle where high blood pressure aggravates atheroma.

   Despite its grave complications, atheroma on its own is a comparatively harmless condition. The danger arises when it is combined with other factors, considered with causes below.

1. CAUSES OF ATHEROMA

Much statistical and other research has shown numerous factors associated with atheroma and its complications, but no primary cause has come to light. Some degree of atheroma is so common that one is tempted to dismiss it as the normal state of arteries after a certain age.

   The likeliest culprit is an excess of *beta-lipoprotein* in the blood. This is a protein linked to cholesterol and other fatty substances found in atheromatous deposits. The statistical evidence that people with atheromatous diseases such as angina tend to have an excess of the chemical ingredients of atheroma in their blood does not prove anything but it is highly suggestive. Several factors associated with a tendency to angina and the like have direct or indirect effects on the amount of beta-lipoproteins and cholesterol ('fats') in the blood. *Diabetes* and *thyroid deficiency* greatly increase the risk of these complications unless they are adequately treated; both increase circulating fats. *Overeating* also has both effects, especially if the diet contains a preponderance of animal fat. Vegetable oils have a protective action. Some authorities hold that *refined sugar* is an even greater danger; it appears to have adverse effects on the disposal of fat in the body. *Lack of exercise* also increases the danger from atheroma, and not only because sedentary people put on weight. Exercise protects the heart regardless of body weight. *High blood pressure* increases the risk of complications and also

53

AUENBRUGGER

directly aggravates the underlying atheroma. Constant *emotional stress* probably acts mainly by keeping the blood pressure high. *Tobacco* apparently increases the risk of thrombosis.

The evidence against all these factors is largely statistical, and a statistical association is not proof of cause and effect. Some factors are inter-related – e.g. overweight and lack of exercise; overeating and diabetes; emotion, heavy smoking, and blood pressure; lack of exercise (recreation) and sustained stress. Some factors are associated with life in an affluent urban society. One could produce other statistics to suggest that owning a television set or a refrigerator increases the danger of atheroma. It is quite clear that something in this civilization is the cause of the trouble, but statistics alone do not show precisely what. All the factors in the previous paragraph, however, are also suspect for purely chemical reasons. The practical problem is made easier by the knowledge that these factors all contribute to ill health in other ways, and would be worth eliminating even if further research should prove that they do not really cause or aggravate atheroma. The diseases mentioned can be treated, and the other factors are all involved in the undefined but well recognized business of keeping fit.

As regards the treatment of established atheroma, as opposed to prevention, drugs that reduce the amount of cholesterol in the blood ought at least to slow the process down, but their value is disputed. Anticoagulant drugs, which discourage blood from clotting, are given to reduce the risk of further thrombosis in patients who have had an attack, but here again opinion is divided, especially about the long-term value of such treatment. Some very successful surgery has been done to replace or repair severely affected arteries.

athetosis. Uncontrolled, purposeless movements, seen in one type of congenital ◊ *spastic paralysis.*

athlete's foot. Ringworm of the feet; infection of the skin, especially between the outer toes, with a microscopical fungus. The only association with athletics is that the changing rooms of schools and sports clubs are likely places for the infection to be passed on. ◊ *ringworm.*

atlas. First cervical ◊ *vertebra*, the upper-most segment of the backbone, on which the skull rests.

atopy. Allergy; allergic reaction in a part of the body other than the point of entry of the irritant. For instance, two forms of skin allergy are *contact* eczema, a reaction confined to the area of skin in contact with the irritant, and *atopic* eczema, a reaction to irritants applied elsewhere – perhaps swallowed.

ATP. Adenosine triphosphate, a substance essential to the storage and transfer of ◊ *energy* in living cells.

atrium. Antechamber of the ◊ *heart*: the left atrium receives blood from the lungs; the right atrium from the rest of the body.

atrophy. Shrinkage, wasting of an organ or tissue. Atrophy may be due to undernutrition (the literal meaning), especially if the blood supply is impaired by disease; or it may be a result of disuse – e.g. the wasting of muscle in a limb that has been splinted because of a fracture.

atropine. Alkaloid extracted from belladonna (deadly nightshade); this drug abolishes most actions of the parasympathetic nerves by chemically obstructing *acetyl choline*, the substance released at the ends of these nerves. When the parasympathetic nerves are put out of action, the sympathetic nerves are left unopposed; thus atropine mimics some actions of sympathetic nerves and of adrenaline. In this way it causes acceleration of the heart, and also the effect from which belladonna gets its name – widening of the pupils. Its most useful action is the relief of colic (painful over-activity of the muscles of the intestine and other abdominal organs) by preventing stimulation of the intestine by acetyl choline. Given before an anaesthetic, it inhibits the secretion of mucus in the lungs, and of saliva, which the anaesthetized patient cannot cough up.

Although large doses can be lethal, atropine is less dangerous than many alkaloid drugs. Drugs such as eserine, which reinforce acetyl choline, serve as antidotes to atropine.

ATS. Anti-tetanus serum; ◊ *tetanus.*

Auenbrugger, Leopold (1722–1809). Viennese physician, the inventor of diagnosis by

◊ *percussion* of the chest – assessing the texture of underlying organs from the resonance when the surface is lightly tapped. Auenbrugger showed how to plot the outlines of the heart and lungs by percussion and recognize diseased areas of lung, repeatedly confirming his opinions by post-mortem examination. His booklet, published in 1761, seems to be the first ever devoted entirely to diagnosis, and the method it describes was the first objective sign of disease (as opposed to subjective symptoms, coloured by the feelings of patient and doctor).

Nobody paid much attention until Corvisart (1755–1821) adopted Auenbrugger's method in Paris and passed it on to his students.

aura. Sensation at the beginning of an attack of illness such as epilepsy or migraine, before more definite symptoms set in. An epileptic attack is a wave of abnormal electrical activity spreading over the brain. If the spread is rapid the patient loses consciousness with little warning, but if the wave spreads more slowly from a part of the brain concerned with a sensation, then the patient feels that particular sensation as a sort of premonition. The aura can warn the patient to lie down and put a pad between his teeth to avoid hurting himself in the coming attack; some people say that they can abort the main attack by keeping perfectly quiet from the moment when the sensation begins.

The aura of migraine is visual, often an illusion of flickering light. It is not a constant symptom.

aural. Of the ear.

auricle. 1. The visible part of the ear. **2.** A pocket protruding from either ◊ *atrium* of the heart. **3.** The atrium itself.

auscultation. Diagnosis by listening, e.g. to heart or breath sounds. *Immediate auscultation* is by putting an ear to the patient's body; *mediate auscultation* is by means of a ◊ *stethoscope*.

autism. A very strange disorder of the mind, beginning in childhood and (unless treated) persisting into adult life. The child seems cut off from the rest of the world. Sensation is normal, but there is little perception. Because he hears without listening the child

may not learn to speak; nor has he any evident wish to communicate. Some autistic children are wrongly thought to be deaf, others blind. The *potential* intelligence is generally high, but it is not used. The child is often preoccupied with some apparently meaningless repetitive action. An occasional outburst of rage may be the only sign of emotion.

The cause of this uncommon condition is not known. It was not recognized until 1943, and for some time the outlook seemed hopeless. But with expert and patient management many autistic children now do extremely well.

autogenous vaccine. A vaccine prepared from bacteria with which a patient is afflicted and given to immunize the patient against their effects. If the patient has not developed immunity to the living bacteria it is not obvious that the dead bacteria in the vaccine will help, and the evidence that they in fact do so is rather thin.

autoimmunity. An abnormal injurious reaction by the body to one of its own tissues. An important part of the body's natural defences against infection by microbes is the development of ◊ *immunity*. The body forms a specific antidote – an ◊ *antibody* – which combines chemically with the invader and puts it out of action. The antibody is tailormade to deal with a particular foreign substance, some part of the microbe, known as an *antigen*. The reaction between antigen and antibody not only kills the microbe; it also does some damage to the body itself. Some of the symptoms of infection are due not to the infecting microbes but to the *immune response*, the effects of the patient's own antibodies. It is a fair price for overcoming the infection. One does not complain if the fire brigade has to break down a few doors to save the house.

The immune response is indiscriminate. Apart from microbes, other substances foreign to the body can be antigens, and evoke antibodies that will combine with them. This is the basis of ◊ *allergy*. Some people form antibodies against pollen, for instance, and if they inhale a few grains of this innocent matter they react as healthy people would react to bacteria, paying the same price to no purpose.

In recent years it has been shown that certain diseases are caused by antibodies formed against some normal component of the patient's own tissues. Here the antigen is not a foreign substance at all but part of the body. Such antigens are called *auto-antigens*. The antibodies formed against them are *auto-antibodies*, and the harmful reaction between them is *autoimmunity*.

The response to infection is like what happens when a wasp invades a bee-hive. The wasp is stung to death, but an unlucky bee damages or kills herself in the process. It is apparently worth a few casualties to keep the hive free of invaders. But if a bee killed herself stinging a petal blown into the hive, that would be a futile sacrifice like allergy. Autoimmunity is like civil war, with bees stinging other members of the hive.

Since nobody knows how the healthy body distinguishes between its own chemical components and foreign substances, ignoring the one and attacking the other, there is no clear explanation of autoimmunity. Some substances are normally confined to one organ, and have no contact with antibody-forming tissue. If the organ is damaged and the substance leaks into the circulation it might be treated as an antigen and evoke antibodies. But when autoimmune responses damage, say, red blood cells or connective tissue, found all over the body, then either the affected cells have started producing a new, unfamiliar substance to act as an antigen, or the unknown mechanism for sparing the body's own components (immune tolerance) has broken down.

Auto-antibodies against various tissues have been found in a number of diseases. It cannot always be proved that they are the cause and not an effect of the disease, but the evidence for their being the cause is growing. The characteristic of all these diseases is inflammation or gradual destruction of a particular type of tissue in the absence of infection or other known cause.

Diseases possibly or probably due to autoimmunity include more than one kind of goitre (damage to thyroid gland), pernicious anaemia (damage to stomach lining with failure to absorb factors needed by blood cells), a kind of haemolytic anaemia (direct damage to red blood cells), nephritis (kidney), ulcerative colitis (lining of intestine), and rheumatoid arthritis (connective tissue). Some are easy to treat, e.g. thyroid deficiency by giving thyroid hormone, or pernicious anaemia by injecting the missing factor, vitamin B_{12}. Others are more difficult, and may have to be treated by suppressing symptoms as they arise. Attempts to suppress the actual process of autoimmunity are still in the experimental stages. This research is hand in hand with attempts to suppress the immune reactions that interfere with transplanting organs.

Autoimmunity ('exemption from oneself') is an unfortunate term. 'Autoallergy' expresses the idea better.

autonomic. Outside conscious control. The *autonomic nervous system* regulates bodily functions other than voluntary movement and conscious sensation, by ◊ *reflex* action. The autonomic system embodies two distinct sets of nerves: *sympathetic* and *parasympathetic*. Many organs receive nerves from both sets, and are regulated by the balance of their opposed actions.

Sympathetic nerves originate throughout the length of the spinal cord. Impulses in them generally cause adrenaline and noradrenaline to be released at their endings.

Parasympathetic nerves are in two groups. One, of which the most important is the *vagus* nerve, arises from the base of the brain; the other arises from the lower end of the spinal cord. They act by releasing acetyl choline.

The actions of these nerves are discussed further under ◊ *sympathetic* and ◊ *parasympathetic*. In short, sympathetic nerves stimulate the heart, suppress digestive activity, and enhance physical activity; parasympathetic nerves have the opposite effects.

The autonomic nerves also convey sensation from the organs to the brain. Much of it does not reach consciousness but stimulates reflex effects. For instance, raised blood pressure is reported to the brain by these nerves, and this causes impulses to be sent by the vagus nerves to decrease the activity of the heart.

Avicenna (Ibn Sina) (980–1037). Persian physician and philosopher. He was born at Bokhara, and practised and taught at Bagdad. He was the most celebrated of the Moslem physicians, the only practitioners of rational medicine in an age when Europe had rejected all learning except theology. These men kept alive the spirit of inquiry that had died in Europe at the end of the 2nd century with Galen, and they preserved and translated the great medical books of antiquity.

Avicenna's *Canon* was for centuries the

standard if not the only accepted text-book of general medicine. Much of it was derived from classical Greek sources, of which even the worst were better than anything that the Europe of the time had to offer. But Avicenna was no mere compiler; he was a doctor in the tradition of Hippocrates, learning from his patients and recording what he observed.

Until the 16th century and later, the physicians of Europe idolized Avicenna, placing him second only to Galen – not, sadly, for his clinical wisdom but for his loyalty to the approved doctrines of Galen and Aristotle.

axilla. Armpit: space between the upper part of the arm and the side-wall of the chest, enclosed by the pectoral muscles in front and the latissimus dorsi muscle behind.

The *axillary* artery, accompanied by the axillary vein and the nerves of the arm, enters the axilla through an opening bounded by the first rib, the clavicle, and the scapula. The artery is the continuation of the *subclavian* artery, and its continuation in the arm is the *brachial* artery.

The axilla contains an important group of lymph nodes.

axillary nerve = ◊ *circumflex* nerve.

azygos (Gk = unpaired) **vein.** Galen's name for a vein on the front of the thoracic vertebrae. It receives blood from the right side of the chest wall. On the left side two *hemiazygos* veins serve the same purpose; they drain into the azygos vein, itself a tributary of the superior *vena cava*.

B

bacillus. A rod-shaped ◊ *bacterium*. The many diseases caused by bacilli include ◊ *anthrax*, ◊ *diphtheria*, a kind of ◊ *dysentery*, gas ◊ *gangrene*, ◊ *tetanus*, ◊ *tuberculosis*, and ◊ *typhoid*.

backache. Pain in the back is among the commonest of symptoms. The possible causes are very numerous. Most of them are not dangerous, but since backache occasionally indicates serious trouble the cause needs to be ascertained. As a rule, when backache is a symptom of disease elsewhere there are other indications to be found; but some cases can be very puzzling.

The likeliest source of a backache is the back itself, and the likeliest cause is mechanical strain. Sometimes the effect of strain can be exactly defined, e.g. a slipped disc (◊ *vertebra* (1)) or a crack in a vertebra. More often the precise effect of strain, the exact cause of pain, is obscure: one can say that through faulty posture a ligament has probably been stretched or that the smaller joints of the back are carrying an unfair load, but the details are open to discussion. What matters is that training in correct posture relieves the symptom. Much the commonest fault is illustrated by someone tucking in the sheets on the far side of a bed. The muscles and ligaments of the human back support it best in the upright position; they are not designed for a quadruped. When the body is suspended, cantilever-fashion, at right angles to the thighs there is a severe shearing strain on the joints of the back. ◊ *vertebra* (1).

Pain in the small of the back and around the shoulder blades often seems to arise in the muscles and is called fibrositis; but there is evidence that this pain is ◊ *referred* from the region of the backbone, where the nerves destined for the painful muscles are being pinched as they pass between the vertebrae.

Purely mechanical faults are a commoner cause of backache than actual disease of the backbone. The pain may also be referred from further afield, e.g. from various organs in the abdomen and pelvis. Pain from the uterus – menstrual or labour pain – commonly includes some backache but is not usually confined to the back.

A good deal of nonsense has been talked about 'psychogenic' backache, i.e. backache that is really all in the mind. The mind can certainly play a part. Anxiety can cause muscular tension and faulty posture, and misery can cause a slouched and equally faulty posture. The resultant backache is in the back, not the mind. Mental attitudes may well determine the degree of pain, and a particular kind of backache may well seem much worse to someone worrying about compensation for an injury or about his doctor's apparent lack of concern than to someone else with no worries.

Backache is a favourite symptom of malingerers, perhaps because it is difficult to disprove (or because some 'malingerers' have real backaches of which the cause is not known?).

backbone. The vertebral column or spine. ◊ *skeleton* (4); *vertebra*.

bacterium. A living creature too small to be seen without a microscope is a micro-organism or *microbe*. The microbes of medical importance include various kinds of minute animal (◊ *protozoon*), e.g. the parasite of malaria; and some simple forms of plant or vegetable life (◊ *fungus*), e.g. the moulds which cause 'ringworm'. Bacteria are smaller than either, and they hold an intermediate position between animal and vegetable microbes. A still smaller form of life, the ◊ *virus*, is on the border between living and non-living matter.

1. STRUCTURE

A large bacterium is about 1/100 mm. by 1/1000 mm.; a small one is about 1/1000 mm. each way. A group of bacteria big enough to be seen with the naked eye contains millions of individual microbes.

Under an ordinary microscope a bacterium does not appear to have any structural elements (nucleus etc.). It is simply a speck of living matter. With the much greater magnification of the electron microscope a certain amount of cell-architecture can be seen. Every bacterium has a strong cell-wall, a protective shell to prevent it from becoming waterlogged and bursting. A few species have fine motile hairs (flagella) by which they are able to swim. The corkscrew-shaped *spirochaetes* can move quite briskly. But most species of bacteria are static.

Apart from the spirochaetes, bacteria are either rod-shaped (*bacillus*) or spherical (*coccus*). Bacilli can be slender, e.g. tubercle bacillus, which causes tuberculosis, or short, more or less oval, e.g. *Haemophilus influenzae*, which does not cause influenza. Cocci include *streptococci*, growing in chains, and *staphylococci*, growing in clumps.

2. FUNCTION

The chemical components of bacteria are like those of other living creatures – protein, fat, carbohydrate etc. At one end of the scale are bacteria that can synthesize these substances from inorganic, 'mineral' sources in the manner of plants. Those of the genus *Rhizobium*, which live in the roots of leguminous plants (clover, beans etc.), can use the nitrogen of the air as a food, providing the plant with essential compounds which it could not synthesize for itself. Leguminous plants can be used, thanks to these bacteria, to replace nitrogen compounds in soil impoverished by other plants, an important factor in crop rotation. They are also, of course, valuable foods.

Other bacteria have a similar economy to animals, living off organic foods synthesized by other creatures. All the bacteria involved in human disease are of this type; they are parasites living off human hosts.

Not all parasitic bacteria cause disease; in fact it is against the interests of a parasite to do so, because if the host dies the parasite must either find another host or die itself. The skin and the various openings of the body teem with harmless bacteria which prevent the growth of harmful species, and some of the bacteria of the intestine synthesize vitamins. Hence drugs which destroy bacteria indiscriminately can be a mixed blessing (◊ *antibiotic*, last paragraph).

Bacteria reproduce simply by growing until they are large enough to split into two. Under ideal conditions of humidity and temperature, and given unlimited supplies of food, they can do this at an almost incredible rate. Some species are ready to split again within half an hour of reproduction. If the number is doubled every half hour a single bacterium will have increased to over a thousand in five hours and a million in ten hours. Even in the laboratory this rate cannot be kept up for more than a few hours, and in the body it is slowed or stopped by natural defences (◊ *immunity*). But the body can succumb very rapidly to an infection to which it has no resistance. The accounts of medieval plagues in which people died within a few hours of falling sick were not exaggerated.

Like all other living creatures, bacteria produce numerous ◊ *enzymes*. These are substances which promote the various chemical changes necessary for sustaining life. Some of the effects of infectious disease are due to enzymes which promote changes unfavourable to the host. Enzymes from various types of bacteria and microscopic fungi (yeasts and moulds) are responsible for all kinds of decay and putrefaction. Frozen food stays fresh because bacteria cannot multiply at low temperatures. Boiled milk will not turn sour if it is protected from further contamination, because boiling destroys bacteria. Creosote preserves wood by killing the moulds that would cause it to rot. Over a century before bacteria were first seen, and three centuries before their role in disease was recognized, Fracastorius said that contagion and putrefaction were the same thing (◊ *infection*).

3. IDENTIFICATION

Bacteria are classified in the same way as other creatures, but the distinctions between different groups are very unsure and the classification is constantly having to be revised. With so little known of their detailed structure and behaviour it is all too easy to make the sort of mistake that would include bats among birds or whales among fish. The characteristics to be studied include shape and size, ability to take up various dyes, presence of particular enzymes, e.g. those that will ferment one or other of a selection of sugars, and patterns of growth under various conditions in the laboratory. A few can be identified by their ability to cause a known disease, e.g. tuberculosis, in laboratory animals. Exact identification usually depends on the fact that a person or animal infected with bacteria forms protective antibodies (◊ *immunity*) which will inactivate that species but no other. The antibodies can be isolated and kept, and bacteria can be identified by the antibodies which react with them.

As a rule, rough identification by simple tests gives enough information for diagnosis and treatment of an infected patient. For instance, if a patient with diarrhoea is found to be passing bacilli of the genus *Shigella*, then he has bacillary dysentery and suitable treatment can be prescribed. But in order to identify the source of his infection and control an outbreak of dysentery, much more precise information is needed. There are four species of *Shigella* and over two dozen sub-species, and the public health officer needs to know exactly which one he is looking for.

In practice, the bacteriologist does not have to go through the whole gamut of tests. He knows from the clinical history what types of bacteria he is likely to find, and he provides an appropriate medium for their growth (some species will grow in one medium, others in another). If a sufficiently dilute suspension from the specimen (blood, urine, pus, sputum etc.) is spread over a solid medium such as agar jelly, small colonies will grow from single bacteria, and the type of colony gives useful information about the species.

Bacteria are stained before being examined under the microscope. The original reason was to make them easier to see, but it was soon found that different species had affinities for particular dyes. Gram's method, using two dyes, divides bacteria into two classes – Gram-positive, stained purple, and Gram-negative, stained pink. Together with the general appearance of the bacteria this stain sometimes gives all the information that is needed. Another technique, the Ziehl-Neelsen stain, uses the red dye fuchsin. The dye is washed out of the stained specimen with acid and alcohol, but the bacilli of tuberculosis and leprosy hold the colour and stand out as crimson rods against a neutral background. It is important to have a selective stain for these two closely related species, because it is very difficult to grow tubercle bacilli in an artificial medium and impossible to grow leprosy bacilli. Most other bacteria will form colonies in a suitable medium, and the colonies can then be identified by chemical and other tests.

4. BACTERIA AND DISEASE (◊ *infection*)

Bacteria can be found almost anywhere – in the soil, in the air, on healthy skin. They are very abundant on warm moist surfaces such as the linings of the nose and mouth and of the large intestine. In common-sense terms intestinal bacteria are inside the body, but the digestive tract is a corridor through the body; bacteria in it are walled off from the body proper almost to the same extent as those on the skin.

Only a few of the many species of bacteria are *pathogens*, i.e. can cause disease. Those which do must first penetrate the surface of the skin or mucous membrane. Any kind of wound allows them to do so; an invisible scratch may suffice. A few species seem able to cross an intact mucous membrane, and some others force an entry by damaging a mucous membrane. They may be able to attack one type of mucous membrane but not another. Typhoid bacilli regularly enter the body by way of the small intestine, gonococci (gonorrhoea) by way of the eyes and reproductive organs, but not elsewhere, and many bacteria by way of the pharynx. The harmless bacteria of a healthy intestine, which breed there throughout life without ever crossing the mucous membrane, cause serious trouble if they contaminate the lining of the urinary system.

Having entered the body, a pathogen must be able to meet the next line of defence, the white blood cells. Harmless bacteria which find their way in by chance are promptly engulfed by white cells and destroyed. Pathogens either resist destruction or actually destroy the white cells.

The symptoms of infection arise mainly in two ways. Firstly, bacteria produce *toxins*, highly poisonous substances. Some toxins (endotoxins) are an integral part of the bacterium and are released into the surrounding tissues when the bacterium is destroyed. Others (exotoxins) are much more dangerous; they are released by living bacteria and diffuse into the circulation, producing their effects far beyond the site of infection. Diphtheria bacilli in the throat can release toxins which injure the nervous system, and tetanus bacilli in a wound have a similar and even more dangerous effect. With certain types of bacterial ◊ *food poisoning* there is no actual infection – the bacteria themselves do not invade the body, but they release toxins into the contaminated food.

Secondly, symptoms are caused by the body's own defences. Fever and its accompaniments are part of the body's response to infection – anyone with pneumonia but no fever is in a bad way, and debilitated old people may die of an infection without ever feeling ill. The process of ◊ *immunity* is akin to ◊ *allergy*, and with chronic (i.e.

prolonged) infectious diseases such as tuberculosis the symptoms produced in this way can be as bad as those produced directly by the infecting bacteria. Certain diseases are associated with infection but are not direct results of it. Rheumatic fever, for instance, is regularly preceded by a streptococcal infection such as tonsillitis, but does not come until after the infection has subsided. It is possible that antibodies formed to destroy the streptococci also damage the body's own tissues, but there is still a good deal of mystery about it.

5. CONTROL OF BACTERIA

If all bacteria were to be destroyed, many if not most other forms of life would disappear because in the course of evolution so many essential jobs have become delegated to microbes. Bacterial decomposition of dead organisms is essential to fertile soil. Herbivorous animals, on which carnivores feed, rely on bacteria in their digestive organs to break down the cellulose of plants into digestible sugars – man, lacking any such bacteria, cannot live on grass. Thus bacteria must not be destroyed wholesale. On the other hand, selective destruction is often necessary to health.

Polluted water can be made fit to drink by filtration.

Most bacteria are killed by ultraviolet radiation, either artificial or from direct sunlight. All bacteria are destroyed by heat. Boiling water quickly kills nearly all of them, but certain spores can survive prolonged boiling. A spore is a sort of hibernating form adopted by a few species under unfavourable conditions. In hospitals, surgical dressings and instruments are completely freed of bacteria, including spores, with compressed steam in an *autoclave*.

Refrigeration prevents bacteria from multiplying but does not usually kill those that are already present.

Chemicals which kill bacteria are roughly divided into *disinfectants*, noxious to any living matter, and *antiseptics*, which kill bacteria without greatly damaging human tissues. But these categories overlap and are hardly worth distinguishing; one needs to know the exact purpose of the substance. An antiseptic that would be quite safe on intact skin may be harmful to an open wound, or it may be inactivated by blood. There is no satisfactory all-purpose substance for killing bacteria.

The discovery of drugs that kill or inactivate bacteria in the body must be counted the most important medical advance of the present century. They include ◊ *sulphonamides* and ◊ *antibiotics*.

◊ historical note under *microbe* (1).

Baer, Karl Ernst von (1792–1876). German biologist; the greatest modern embryologist (◊ *embryology*).

Von Baer's law, the biogenetic law, only confirms what earlier embryologists (e.g. Harvey) had suggested: that the embryos of widely different species resemble one another. It is an important argument in favour of evolution. The law is sometimes restated: the development of the individual recapitulates the development of the species. But this presupposes evolution, of which von Baer knew nothing, and is not quite true. A human embryo never resembles a fish, but only a fish's embryo.

Baghdad button = ◊ *oriental sore*.

BAL. British Anti-Lewisite; dimercaprol. It was evolved as an antidote to the arsenical war-gas lewisite. BAL prevents arsenic from becoming chemically bound in the tissues and so enables it to be eliminated from the body. It is also effective against lead and other poisonous metals which otherwise become fixed in the tissues.

balantidium. A parasitic ◊ *protozoon*, one of the rarer causes of dysentery.

baldness (alopecia). Most other mammals shed hair seasonally, but human hair moults throughout the year. An average rate might be 100 hairs a day. The rate increases in various types of symptomatic baldness (see below), and these are likely to recover as the rate of moulting returns to normal. But much the commonest kind of baldness arises not from shedding hair, but from a change in its character. The adult hair follicles regress and instead of producing normal hair they produce a kind of *vellus* or baby hair, which gives the usual type of bald pate a velvety look in a cross light. As far as anyone knows at present, the change is irreversible. The tendency is hereditary. The loss of normal hair, spreading from the temples and crown, often starts to affect males very early in adult life. A similar condition in women usually starts later and seldom goes beyond thinning rather than extensive loss of hair. In women, this or a similar condition can arise from defective function of the ovaries, e.g. at the menopause, and such cases may respond to hormone treatment. Otherwise, common baldness is a normal condition.

If most baldness is a natural process that has nothing to do with health, loss of hair can on occasion be a symptom of illness. Treatment of symptomatic baldness is almost as futile as treatment of natural baldness, with the difference that symptomatic baldness commonly recovers of its own accord. *Alopecia areata* is a sudden, patchy loss of hair without obvious physical cause; it may follow severe mental strain. As a rule the hair returns as mysteriously as it was lost. Some loss of hair is a regular symptom of thyroid or pituitary gland deficiency, and is corrected along with the other symptoms by suitable hormone treatment. Rarely, some drugs and other chemicals cause temporary baldness. Some affections of the skin, notably ringworm, damage the hair. Generalized infections such as scarlet fever occasionally cause some loss of hair, and the fashion of wearing wigs in the 17th century is said to have been adopted to hide patches of baldness due to syphilis.

bandage. Bandages have several uses: (1) covering wounds to exclude contamination; the bandage holds a clean or antiseptic dressing in place; (2) stopping wounds from bleeding; the bandage is not a tourniquet to prevent blood from reaching the wound but simply keeps the dressing still enough to provide a scaffolding for a firm blood clot; (3) splinting injured tissues, which hurt and will not heal if they are constantly moving; (4) supporting weak structures such as varicose veins.

The gauze roller-bandage is the most widely used but it needs considerable skill. If it is too loose it falls off, and if it is too tight it does more harm than good. In non-expert hands, sticking plaster is a better means of holding a dressing, and if the plaster goes only halfway round a limb it cannot obstruct the circulation. Unfortunately some people's skin does not tolerate sticking plaster.

Crêpe bandages give excellent support. They are easily put on too tightly, especially if elegant figure-of-eight turns are used.

Any bandage that feels too tight probably is too tight. Swelling below a bandage is a warning to loosen it at once.

For anyone without special training, by far the most useful bandage is the triangular bandage, which can be adapted to almost any purpose. The standard first-aid manuals describe its use in detail.

Banti's disease. (G. Banti (1853–1925), Italian physician.) Splenic anaemia; not a specific ailment but simply enlargement of the spleen as a result of back-pressure in its vein from constriction of the *portal vein*, of which the splenic vein is a tributary. The usual cause is cirrhosis of the liver.

barber's itch (barber's rash). Bacterial infection around the roots of the beard. Antibiotic treatment usually clears it up and prevents it from becoming chronic and producing unsightly scars. Growing a beard or changing to an electric razor often cures it.

barbitone (barbital). Diethyl barbituric acid; a ◊ *hypnotic* drug.

barbiturates. A large group of ◊ *hypnotic* drugs derived from barbituric acid. They are much pleasanter to take than older hypnotics such as chloral, but they are habit-forming and may cause true addiction.

In addition to their main use in promoting sleep, some barbiturates (those with a very rapid and short-lived effect, e.g. thiopentone) are given as anaesthetics. Slow-acting barbiturates such as phenobarbitone are used as day-time sedatives, and for controlling attacks of epilepsy.

Barbiturate poisoning is common. It may be chronic or acute. Chronic (slow, cumulative) barbiturate poisoning affects either people who have started taking the drug for insomnia and have developed an addiction, or people who take drugs as part of their way of life. The symptoms are like those of heavy drinking. Expert attention is needed, because sudden withdrawal of the drug can have serious physical effects (◊ *addiction*). Acute poisoning, by a single heavy overdose, is a widespread form of attempted suicide and can also occur by accident. The drug usually kills by paralysing the respiratory centre in the brain, thus switching off the mechanism of breathing. The immediate danger is of suffocation by the back of the patient's own tongue, and the first-aid is exactly the same as that described under ◊

head injury. If the patient can be brought alive to a hospital, the chances of recovery are excellent.

barium sulphate. A substance opaque to X-rays; since it is not absorbed from the intestine it can safely be given by mouth (*barium meal*) or by the rectum (*barium enema*) to outline the digestive tract under X-rays.

barotrauma. Injury by change of pressure (e.g. explosion; diving) illustrated by painful ears in aircraft. Any part of the body can suffer, but ear-drums, sinuses and lungs are the most vulnerable. The fall in pressure as a shock-wave passes by or a diver surfaces, leaving compressed air in the body, is as harmful as the previous rise. Torn ear-drums can lead to infection and deafness, and burst lungs to fatal ◊ *air embolism*. (◊◊ *compressed-air sickness*.)

basal ganglia (basal nuclei). The core of grey matter (nerve cells) at the centre of the cerebral hemispheres. The basal ganglia serve movement in the same way as the *thalamus* serves sensation, i.e. they are a relay station immediately below the level of consciousness.

Various types of purposeless involuntary movement are due to disease of the basal ganglia, of which by far the commonest is ◊ *parkinsonism* (shaking palsy; paralysis agitans).

basal metabolism. Chemical turnover in the body at complete rest; it represents the chemical energy provided for vital processes such as breathing, circulation and digestion. It is assessed from the rate at which oxygen is consumed when the subject is warm and still, in bed. The result can be expressed as energy produced in a given time; for an average man basal metabolism (basal metabolic rate; BMR) is about 1,700 Calories in 24 hours. Or it can be expressed as a percentage of the calculated normal rate for the subject's height and weight.

The rate is regulated mainly by the thyroid gland. With an over-active thyroid (toxic goitre) it is above normal; with a defective thyroid (cretinism, myxoedema) it is below.

Basedow's disease (toxic goitre; Graves' disease). ◊ *thyroid* (2). Karl von Basedow (1799–1854), a German physician, described the condition in 1840, five years after Graves's account, which was not known to him. In fact, neither was the first, but Basedow's was the first really detailed description.

baths. The main value of bathing is aesthetic rather than medical. People who wash are pleasanter to know and more comfortable than people who do not, but except that they are less liable to be infested with lice etc. it is doubtful whether they are much healthier.

A skilful bed-bath works wonders for the morale and comfort of anyone confined to bed.

Very hot baths raise the body temperature and can be dangerous. Cold baths are doubtless a moral tonic, but are not known to do any physical good.

Certain diseases affecting large areas of skin can be treated with medicated baths.

The success of spa treatment depends at least as much on the regimen of controlled diet, exercise and relaxation as on the special virtues of the water. But baths have a special place in the treatment of rheumatic disease, and of all disorders involving stiff or painful joints or weak muscles. Buoyancy allows movement that would be impossible in air, and the warmth of the water may ease pain. Gentle exercise under water is among the best ways of re-educating limbs that have been out of action.

BCG (bacille Calmette-Guérin). A vaccine against ◊ *tuberculosis* (4), prepared from a strain of bacilli that have lost their virulence after years of growth in an artificial medium. It was first prepared at the Pasteur Institute in Paris in 1906 by Léon Calmette and Camille Guérin and used to prevent tuberculosis. In France it has been used for human vaccination since 1922, but in Britain its value and safety have only recently been accepted.

beat elbow (beat knee; beat hand). Chronic, often severe inflammation from continuous pressure on a small area of skin, sometimes with *bursitis*; a scheduled industrial disease of miners and some other workers.

Bedsonia. Kinds of microbe formerly regarded as viruses. The diseases they cause include *lymphogranuloma venereum, ornithosis*, and *trachoma*, all of which respond to treatment with antibiotics. These microbes are also able to synthesize their own proteins. This ability, and the response to antibiotics, distinguish them from true viruses. They are probably small bacteria.

bed-sore (decubitus). Damage to skin and underlying tissue by constant pressure which prevents blood from circulating and deprives the area of its oxygen supply. Any sustained pressure, e.g. from a badly fitting plaster cast, can destroy skin; and since pressure also interferes with conduction in nerves the patient may be unaware of what is happening. Bed-sores arise in areas where skin is compressed against bone when a patient lies still in bed (buttocks, hips, ankles, heels). They are most likely to affect paralysed or debilitated people who do not move in bed, and are promoted by slight injury or infection of the skin. The first warning sign is a reddened area of skin; unless pressure is relieved this rapidly forms an ulcer that can be difficult to heal. Bed-sores are almost entirely prevented by good nursing. This includes regular changes of the patient's position, cushioning of pressure points, and scrupulous hygiene of the skin.

bed-wetting (enuresis). Some children continue to pass urine in their sleep after the third year (by which time most children are dry) because of physical irritation, e.g. inflammation in the urinary passages; but in most cases there is no obvious cause and the condition is thought to be emotional. Training has to be based on encouragement; scolding makes matters worse. Aids to training include various drugs, and an electric alarm that wakes the child when the first drops of urine close the circuit.

bee sting. Bees, wasps, and hornets inject venom which, like viper venom, interferes with the clotting of blood; but the amount is too small to be significant when they sting man. The only danger is to a few people who are allergic to the stings and may react violently (◊ *allergy*). Bee-handlers become immune to bee stings, and allergic people can be immunized (desensitized).

Alkaline solutions such as sodium bicarbonate or dilute ammonia help to neutralize the venom, and antihistamine drugs relieve most of the symptoms.

Bees often leave their stings in the skin. If the sting can be seen it needs to be gently removed.

behaviour therapy. A form of psychotherapy for treating neuroses and oddities of behaviour thought to represent abnormal conditioned reflexes. A conditioned reflex is a *learned* response that has become automatic or unconscious (as opposed to an inborn reflex that does not have to be learned). A flow of saliva while actually eating is an inborn reflex, but salivation at the sight of food is conditioned – one has first to learn what food looks like and associate it with the act of eating. The response (salivation) is then transferred from the inborn stimulus (taste) to the learned stimulus (sight). But the process can be put into reverse. If a child tries to eat an addled egg he may afterwards be sickened by the sight of an egg. More subtly, if he associates a particular dish with unhappiness he may become unable to stomach it. Thus a conditioned reflex can be unlearned.

It has been suggested that many disorders such as symptoms of irrational anxiety and abnormal or defective sexual responses are conditioned reflexes that can be unlearned, either by giving them disagreeable associations or by establishing pleasant associations with more normal responses. Behaviour therapy, in short, is a refinement and rationalization of two ancient teaching aids: the stick and the carrot. The 'stick' principle is exemplified by *aversion therapy*, which builds up unpleasant associations with a habit that the patient wishes to break such as alcohol or an anomalous sexual urge. Thus an alcoholic may be given a drug to make him vomit when he drinks, in the hope of establishing a conditioned reflex that makes alcohol nauseating to him.

A more amiable form of behaviour therapy has been named *desensitization* because it is like desensitizing a patient to an allergy by getting him to tolerate gradually increasing doses of the offending substance. Here, a well-defined anxiety is treated by getting the patient to relive, in fact or in imagination, the kind of situation that troubles him, starting with mildly alarming scenes and building up over a series of treatment sessions to situations that would formerly have terrified him.

bejel ◊ *yaws.*

belladonna. Extract of deadly nightshade; used internally to correct over-activity of the stomach and to relieve spasm of involuntary muscle in the bronchi and digestive tract, and externally, as belladonna plaster, without any apparent effect. Its active principles are the alkaloids *atropine* and *hyoscyamine.*

Bell's palsy. Paralysis of the facial nerve, described in 1828 by Sir Charles Bell (1774–1842), a Scottish surgeon.

The facial nerve is unusual in that it carries no conscious sensation; it only activates the muscles of the face. (The sensory nerve of the face is the trigeminal.) Therefore disorders of this nerve, unlike those of any other nerve, affect movement not sensation. The lop-sided appearance of the face is unmistakable.

Bell's palsy might arise from any kind of damage to the nerve – head injury, infection, stroke, etc. – but the term is often restricted to paralysis with no obvious cause and a tendency to recover spontaneously. The nerve passes through a long and narrow tunnel in the base of the skull, around the inner ear, and may be compressed by slight inflammation in this area. An abnormal response to cold is sometimes blamed. In a few cases the pressure on the nerve can be relieved surgically.

bemegride. An analeptic drug (stimulant of the central nervous system) used in the treatment of barbiturate poisoning.

bends ◊ *compressed-air sickness.*

benign. A term applied to various diseases to distinguish a relatively mild form from a *malignant* or dangerous form. A benign tumour does not disseminate itself to other parts of the body, whereas a malignant tumour or cancer does. *Benign tertian* fever is the form of *malaria* caused by *Plasmodium vivax.* It does not have the lethal complications of malignant *tertian* fever, caused by *P. falciparum.*

benzyl benzoate. An oily fluid used to treat ◊ *scabies.*

beriberi. A form of malnutrition seen mainly in the Far East, due to deficiency of vitamin B_1 (thiamine). Outbreaks have been traced to eating polished rice (from which the husks are removed) in a diet with no other source of thiamine than rice husks. The principal symptoms are *neuritis*, with disturbed sensation and loss of muscle power, and *heart failure.*

Bernard, Claude (1813–78). Professor of physiology at the Sorbonne and of medicine at the Collège de France; the greatest of all physiologists. His sole aim, he said, was to establish scientific method as the basis of medicine. He dismissed as sentimental nonsense the idea of a 'vital spirit' directing the affairs of living bodies according to its own laws, and insisted that living bodies are bound by the same natural laws as inanimate matter. Like Descartes before him, he took nothing for granted, but trusted logical conclusions drawn from proven facts. Unlike Descartes, he pursued an argument no further than could be confirmed by experiment. That is, he would draw conclusions from the result of an experiment, and then devise new experiments to test the conclusions; these in turn became the basis of fresh conclusions and experiments.

His first practical contribution was to show that animals, like plants, could synthesize new material and were not confined to breaking down vegetable products. He later discovered several functions of the liver; the digestive action of the pancreas; the control of blood vessels by nerves; the carriage of oxygen by red blood cells and the abolition of this function by carbon monoxide; the nature of curare poisoning and its implications as regards the control of muscles by nerves; new facts about the brain and spinal cord and the behaviour of secreting glands and of the kidneys. If Nobel Prizes had existed, Bernard could hardly have won fewer than four.

Even more important than Bernard's many particular discoveries was his concept of internal environment (*milieu intérieur*). The external environment – the world around us – constantly changes; but the delicately balanced mechanisms of our bodies are not affected, although all natural processes are extremely sensitive to change of any kind. Bernard realized that a highly developed organism such as the human body is not a unit continually adapting itself to a changing environment, but a community of living cells in an unchanging environment – the blood and tissue fluid in which each cell lives as an aquatic creature. Most bodily functions are directed to keeping this *milieu intérieur* stable in the face of external change – to keeping constant the amount of water, temperature, oxygen supply, pressure, and chemical composition. For instance, in hot weather, the skin flushes and then sweats, preventing the temperature of the blood from rising. Or if muscular work threatens to deplete the blood of glucose, the liver puts more into the circulation. Physiology is largely the study of how each organ helps to maintain a constant environment for all the others, and medicine of how the process goes wrong.

Much of Bernard's experimental work was done with animals. He had an almost unerring sense of how far the results applied to man, and of when human experiment was necessary and justified. He insisted that morals did not forbid doing experiments on people, but only doing people harm.

Bernard's *Introduction à l'étude de la médecine expérimentale* is nothing less than a charter for 20th-century medicine. It is incidentally among the most readable of medical classics, and a smattering of general science is enough to keep abreast of the argument. An English translation has been published.

biceps. Two-headed: strictly speaking the word is an adjective to describe a Y-shaped muscle formed of two muscles that remain separate in their upper parts but are fused in their lower parts, so that the muscle is attached to the skeleton by two tendons above and a single tendon below. Thus *musculus biceps brachii* = the two-headed muscle of the arm. In practice, the word has become a singular noun.

Biceps brachii is the large muscle at the front of the upper arm, attached by two tendons to the scapula and one to the radius. It flexes the elbow and shoulder because it passes in front of both joints, and rotates the forearm (◊ *radius*; *shoulder*).

Biceps femoris is one of the hamstring muscles at the back of the thigh. Its two 'heads' are attached to the pelvis and the back of the femur, and its 'tail' to the fibula.

Bichat, Marie-François-Xavier (1771–1802). French physician and scientist, the founder of ◊ *histology* – the study of *tissues*, which he was the first to describe. Working without a microscope, an instrument which he apparently despised, Bichat showed by dissection and the use of chemical solvents that the organs of the body were composed of various kinds of fabric (*tissu*). Diseases, he maintained, attacked not whole organs but particular tissues. This idea set pathology in a completely new light, and led directly to the study of the constituent cells of tissues which is the basis of modern pathology (◊ *Virchow*).

bile (gall). The secretion of the liver, a viscous yellow-brown fluid with rather the appearance of motor oil. The daily output of the liver is about a litre of fluid, but the effective volume of bile is less because it becomes concentrated in the ◊ *gall* bladder, where much of its water is returned to the blood. Bile accumulates in the gall bladder until after a meal. Fats and the like stimulate contraction of the gall bladder, which injects bile into the duodenum, the first part of the intestine.

The active functions of bile depend on the *bile salts*, formed in the liver from *cholesterol*. These salts enable fat to be digested by making an emulsion of it; unemulsified fat simply passes down the intestine. The fat-soluble vitamins A, D, and K are also poorly assimilated in the absence of bile salts. In addition, bile salts activate certain digestive enzymes.

Bile is also a vehicle for excreting waste products from the liver, such as *bile pigments*, excess cholesterol, and various drugs. The bile pigments are derived from the haemoglobin of destroyed red blood cells; they are what remains when the protein fraction has been put back into circulation and the iron has been stored. ◊ *jaundice; liver*.

bilharzia (schistosoma). A small fluke (flatworm, trematode), parasitic during one phase of its life-cycle to water-snails and during another to man. Three species cause human disease. *Schistosoma haematobium* is found in most of Africa and in parts of Spain and the Middle East; *S. mansoni* in Africa and South America; *S. japonicum* in the Far East.

The eggs hatch in fresh water, and the emerging embryos or *miracidia* invade the bodies of snails; there they grow into larvae or *cercariae* and return to the water. Cercariae penetrate intact human skin, enter the circulation, and grow in the veins of the liver. The adult worms settle in the veins of the urinary bladder (*S. Haematobium*) or the intestine (*S. mansoni, S. japonicum*). Their eggs, each armed with a sharp spike, set up irritation in the affected organ, and leave the body in the urine or stools. If these contaminate water in which there are snails the cycle begins again, and anyone who enters the water can become infected.

Soon after infection, while the cercariae are circulating, there is a transient fever and skin rash (snail-fever). There are no symptoms for some weeks or even months; then symptoms arise from the site of the adult worms – bleeding into the urine, or dysentery. Eggs may be carried to the liver from the intestinal veins or to the lungs from the bladder. In whatever tissue they are embedded the eggs provoke a mild but relentless inflammation, and normal structures are gradually (over many years) replaced by scar tissue. Thus the bladder becomes rigid and shrunken, and cirrhosis of the liver may develop, in turn causing enlargement of the spleen. By no means all cases go so far; the disease can burn itself out before any serious permanent damage is done. But it is still a serious problem in many hot countries, affecting whole populations with anaemia, discomfort, and general ill health. Often the same people are affected with malaria and other infections.

For many years the only treatment was with compounds of *antimony*, which have unpleasant effects and may have to be given for a long time. *Lucanthone* does not contain antimony but it, too, causes vomiting and is not always effective. Several newer drugs are getting favourable reports.

In theory, bilharzial disease can be eradicated in several ways: (1) successful treatment of every case, for which there are neither the drugs nor the means of administering them; (2) adequate sanitation and education in its use, so that water would not be contaminated; (3) eradication of snails by clearing river banks of the vegetation where they breed, or chemical treatment of the water, or the use of sluices to keep changing the water level and dislodge the snails from their breeding places. In practice, the expense and difficulty are very great.

bilirubin; biliverdin. Two closely related pigments, one orange, one green, found in bile. ◊ *jaundice.*

Billroth, Theodor (1829–94). Professor of surgery in Zürich, later Vienna; one of the first surgeons to recognize the full significance of Lister's discovery that infection after operations could be prevented, and to venture into parts of the body that had previously been too dangerous to touch, particularly the abdomen, where the old methods would inevitably have caused a fatal peritonitis. Many of today's standard operations on the stomach, intestine, and thyroid gland were devised by Billroth.

biochemistry. The chemistry of living processes, a young but already very extensive science.

Biochemical reactions follow the same laws as other chemical reactions, but they are nearly always activated by biological catalysts – *enzymes.* A few important reactions are briefly mentioned under ◊ *energy,* ◊ *enzyme,* ◊ *fat,* ◊ *carbohydrate,* ◊ *protein,* ◊ *vitamin.*

biopsy. Diagnosis by removing a portion of living tissue for examination.

birth. The process is considered from the mother's point of view under ◊ *labour.*

Until birth, the *foetus* (unborn infant) has only one task – growth. The work of maintaining a constant environment (*milieu intérieur:* ◊ *Bernard, Claude*) is done by the mother by way of the placenta and umbilical cord. Almost the only contribution the foetus has to make is to maintain a circulation of its own blood for the distribution of supplies and the return of waste products to the mother's circulation.

The newborn infant suddenly finds itself in a completely strange environment to which its organs must adapt. Some, such as the liver, kidneys and endocrine glands, need little adaptation. They have gradually begun to work in the womb, in conjunction with the mother's glands. The digestive apparatus has no work to do until after birth, when it has to begin to deal with food, in particular milk. At this stage the stomach forms no acid, and in place of the protein-digesting enzyme *pepsin,* the baby has *rennin,* which starts the digestion of milk protein without the help of acid. The muscular system is well developed at birth but its function is very limited because it depends on the nervous system, which is, comparatively speaking, still rudimentary: it is capable of no more than reflex actions, such as sucking and grasping. Many functions that we regard as inborn and automatic are in fact learnt after birth. Some of the nerve fibres in the brain and spinal cord have not yet acquired their insulating myelin sheaths and are therefore not in working order. As a result, functions that will appear later are still dormant, and some of a baby's reflexes differ from those that will develop later as fresh nerve-pathways come into action. The reflexes of a newborn baby vividly suggest a need to clutch at branches in an emergency; this is one of the many pieces of evidence that our early ancestors lived in the trees. The long, arduous apprenticeship of the human child before it becomes independent of its elders is arguably a reason for the intellectual superiority over other animals that it will finally achieve.

But certain functions have to be established at once if the infant is to survive: provision of oxygen and of warmth.

Two processes are needed to supply oxygen: breathing to get oxygen into the lungs, and circulation of blood to distribute the oxygen to the rest of the body. The movements of breathing begin in a small way before birth and draw water into the lungs; this is added to fluid actually produced by the lungs. During birth the baby's chest is firmly squeezed – wrung out – and if he is born in the usual way, head first, the recoil draws some air in. More important, the impact of cold air causes the baby to gasp. This first gasp apparently brings in enough oxygen to activate the respiratory centre at the root of the brain and start automatic rhythmical breathing.

The lung fluid has an unexpected but vital function. If the inside of the lungs were moistened with pure water, the surface tension around the thousands of tiny air-pockets would empty the lungs of air as effectively (and by the same mechanism) as pricking a bubble. But the lung fluid contains a substance which lowers the surface tension to a point where the lungs easily hold air. With a *premature birth* this property may not have developed and the infant cannot then breathe (◊ *hyaline-membrane disease*).

The circulation of the foetus is arranged to transport oxygen from the placenta, and the lungs, having no function, are by-passed. At birth, blood is diverted to the lungs by changes described under ◊ *heart* (1).

The urgency of starting to breathe is rather less than it might be, firstly because converting glycogen to lactic acid provides energy without oxygen for some minutes, and the infant has a large store of glycogen; secondly, because the haemoglobin (the blood-pigment that conveys oxygen) in an infant is different from adult haemoglobin and works at a lower concentration of oxygen. But premature babies have little stored glycogen and therefore less time to spare.

Next to oxygen, the infant's most urgent need is warmth. At all times a baby has to work harder than an adult to keep warm. Roughly speaking, a body loses heat in proportion to its surface area and can create heat in proportion to its mass or volume. Thus a body twice as tall as another can lose heat at $2^2 = 4$ times the rate, but can generate heat at $2^3 = 8$ times the rate of the other. But although a baby loses much more heat in proportion to its size than an older child, a healthy newborn baby emerges from its natural incubator the uterus and maintains its body temperature without even shivering. It does so by virtue of a large store of fat, mostly in the neck and down the front of the backbone, in a special form (◊ *brown fat*) that is rapidly burnt. Premature babies, on the other hand, have little fat of any kind.

birth-mark. A congenital blemish of the skin, of which there are several types. Birth-marks include the *pigmented naevus* or mole, which is a conglomeration of pigment cells resembling those scattered throughout the skin, and several types of *vascular naevus* composed of small blood vessels. The commonest vascular naevus is the *strawberry mark*, bright red and slightly raised, with a tendency to grow larger before shrinking and finally vanishing. The *port-wine stain*, seen most often on the neck, does not change. An unusual type is the *cavernous haemangioma*, composed of much larger vessels but also harmless, though it may be a clue to a similar collection inside the skull and needing removal.

Unless there are very strong cosmetic reasons for interfering most birth-marks are best left alone. Strawberry marks in any case disappear in time, and no treatment of port-wine stains obliterates them without the risk of an equally disfiguring scar.

bismuth. A heavy metal, formerly much used

in the treatment of syphilis. Some of its compounds are insoluble and biologically inert, and can be applied to body surfaces as a protective barrier.

Black Death. Bubonic plague, so called either from the dark bruises of spontaneous bleeding into the skin or from the blue-grey complexion of patients with the pneumonic form of the disease. ◊ *plague.*

blackhead (comedo) ◊ *acne.*

blackout. Momentary loss of consciousness, especially when due to rapid acceleration, which propels blood away from the head and leaves the brain without enough oxygen.

blackwater fever. A rare complication of ◊ *malaria*: red blood cells are rapidly destroyed. The liberated pigment passes through the filters of the kidneys (which are much too fine to let intact cells through) and, in an altered form, blackens the urine. It may block the fine tubes of the kidney and stop the flow of urine. It occurs only in *subtertian* malaria, and seems to be brought on by quinine.

bladder. Several receptacles in the body are called bladders; the two important ones are the ◊ *gall* bladder attached to the liver, and the *urinary* bladder, generally known simply as the bladder and described below.

The bladder is a flexible muscular bag. It receives a continuous dribble of urine from the kidneys, which gradually stretches its walls. But this is not like inflating a rubber bladder in which the pressure steadily increases. The muscle fibres of the bladder remain at rest through a considerable range of distension. They simply adapt themselves to the volume of stored urine, and show signs of stretch only when this volume is considerable. They then begin to resist, and the sensation of needing to pass urine is felt. In an infant, this sets off reflex emptying of the bladder. After training the reflex can be suppressed; the muscle relaxes and the bladder can be further distended before giving a further signal. The cycle can be repeated several times before reflex emptying supersedes voluntary control. An average bladder will hold at least a pint without serious discomfort. Emptying is usually complete: if the muscle is allowed to contract it does so until the bladder is empty.

The bladder is in the ◊ *pelvis,* immediately behind the pubic bones. As it fills, it protrudes into the lower abdomen.

The two *ureters,* carrying urine from the kidneys, enter the back of the bladder. Their openings are guarded by valves which prevent urine from flowing back towards the kidneys when the bladder is full. Failure of these valves is probably a cause (but possibly an effect) of bacterial infection ascending to the kidneys from the bladder.

The *urethra,* by which the bladder empties, opens from the lowest point. It is guarded by a tight ring of muscle (a *sphincter*) which relaxes when the main muscle of the bladder is allowed to contract. The female urethra is little more than an inch long and is not a very efficient barrier to bacteria from outside, whereas the male urethra passes through the *prostate* gland and then runs the length of the penis.

1. DISORDERS

Because the bladder lies on the bone it may be torn when the pelvis is fractured; an empty bladder is seldom injured in any other way, but a full bladder can be ruptured by a blow on the abdomen. According to the site of injury, urine is spilt into the peritoneal cavity and causes peritonitis, or between the layers of the abdominal wall where it also causes dangerous inflammation. In either case, surgical repair is imperative. The bladder heals surprisingly well when it is stitched up, considering that urine prevents healing in other tissues.

Injuries to the spinal cord commonly paralyse the bladder. If nervous pathways below the injury are intact, though no longer controlled by the brain, a simple reflex automatically empties the bladder as soon as the pressure of urine begins to rise, and the patient only needs a receptacle. But if reflex emptying fails, the bladder has to be regularly emptied with a tube (*catheter*) passed up the urethra, in order to prevent stagnation and infection of the urine.

Obstruction to the outlet causes *retention of urine.* If the obstruction is sudden and complete the patient is acutely distressed. Passing a catheter brings prompt relief. Acute retention of urine due to spasm of the sphincter muscle is not uncommon after surgical operations – not necessarily those involving the bladder. Or the outlet can be blocked by a ◊ *calculus* (stone). Small stones may pass on but larger ones need surgical removal.

In middle-aged and older men the urethra may be blocked by enlargement of the ◊ *prostate gland.* Narrowing of the urethra used to be a common complication of gonorrhoea before the days of antibiotic treatment.

Cystitis – inflammation of the bladder – is very much commoner in women than men because the urethra is so much shorter and therefore less of a barrier to bacteria. Stone in the bladder is often associated with cystitis; one is not always sure which came first.

Tumours of the bladder generally make their presence known by bleeding into the urine. They need prompt attention because they are generally curable if taken early but tend to do badly if neglected. Some bladder tumours are known to be caused by exposure to *naphthylamine* and other chemicals in the dyestuff and rubber industries. A very high incidence of bladder cancer in Egypt suggests that *bilharzia* may be another cause.

The bladder can be directly examined with a *cystoscope*, an optical instrument passed up the urethra.

For surgical operations the bladder is easily approached by way of the lower abdomen. Until the time of Lister the abdomen could not be opened without courting a fatal peritonitis, and the very ancient operation of lithotomy (cutting for stone) was done by opening the bladder from below, through the perineum.

blastomycosis. A group of rare and dangerous fevers caused by infection with fungi of the genus *Blastomyces*, confined to North and South America. Blastomycosis was generally fatal until the discovery of the antibiotic *amphotericin-B.*

blastula. A hollow cluster of cells, representing a very early stage in the development of an embryo.

bleeding (haemorrhage). Blood is essentially a means of transporting oxygen and other raw materials around the body. When it leaves the network of blood vessels it is as useless as a derailed train. Bleeding is loss of blood from the circuit of tubular vessels – arteries, capillaries, veins. Whether it actually escapes from the body does not matter. A quart of blood between the muscles around a broken thigh-bone is as much lost as a quart of blood from a cut throat. One can bleed to death from a blow over the

spleen without appearing to lose a drop of blood.

The effects of bleeding are described elsewhere. Rapid profuse bleeding causes ◊ *shock.* Slow sustained bleeding causes ◊ *anaemia* (A.1).

Slight loss of blood has no ill effects, though the associated injuries may. But 'slight' is relative. A person in reasonable health can lose 15 per cent of his blood with impunity. In a grown man, this means 15 per cent of a gallon; in a 10-year-old, of half a gallon; in a 3-year-old, of a quart; in a 1-year-old, of a pint.

Bleeding reduces the total volume of blood, but after 'slight' bleeding the vessels automatically contract enough to maintain the blood pressure. It is this, and not sudden anaemia, that causes the pale skin after bleeding.

The normal volume of blood is restored within a few hours of bleeding by dilution with water from the tissue spaces, and the lost plasma proteins (◊ *blood* (1)) are restored in a few days. It takes several weeks to replace the blood cells.

The natural mechanisms to stop bleeding include reflex shrinking of cut blood vessels, and clotting of blood (◊ *blood* (4)). These processes can be helped by firm pressure over the wound, such as that of a padded dressing. The pressure reduces the flow of blood, and the dressing provides a scaffolding for the clot.

Blood from a cut artery is bright scarlet, and comes in spurts like water from a stirrup pump. It can sometimes be stopped by pressure on a 'pressure point', where the artery runs near enough to a bone to be flattened against it. The pressure point must obviously be between the heart and the wound.

Blood from a vein is much darker, and it flows smoothly. There is no positive pressure in veins at or above the level of the heart. Bleeding from a vein in a limb stops when the limb is raised, and increases if the limb is allowed to hang. The effect can be seen in the veins at the back of the hand: they empty when the hand is raised and fill when it is lowered.

bleeding disorders. The bleeding or haemorrhagic disorders form a small group. They do not include the hundreds of diseases in which bleeding from damaged tissues is a symptom. They are abnormalities – most of them rare – of bleeding itself. Either bleeding starts too readily, or it does not stop as quickly as it should. They are defects of one or more of the mechanisms by which bleeding is normally stopped, described under ◊ *blood* (4). Three categories are described: defects of the small blood vessels, defects of blood platelets (particles in the blood which block breaches in vessels), and defects of clotting.

The symptoms of all bleeding disorders are similar. Wounds bleed for too long, and spontaneous bleeding can occur anywhere – under the skin, into joints, from the kidneys into the urine.

Purpura, a usual symptom, is bleeding under the skin or mucous membranes, giving scattered unprovoked bruises. Pinpoints of bleeding from capillaries are called *petechiae*.

1. BLOOD-VESSEL DEFECTS

Some infectious fevers can cause purpura. The rashes of severe forms of typhus and epidemic meningitis (spotted fever) are of this type. The bleeding is mainly due to bacterial poisoning of the capillaries, but platelets may be affected too. (◊ *Black Death*.)

An uncommon type of *allergy* weakens the capillaries and causes purpura with bleeding into the intestine. It was first described by the Berlin paediatrician E. H. Henoch in 1874. The patients are mostly young. Henoch's purpura nearly always clears up in a few weeks.

Vitamin C is necessary to the health of all connective tissue. Lack of vitamin C (◊ *scurvy*) shows mainly as weakness of the bonds between the cells of capillary blood vessels, which become very fragile and bleed with the least provocation.

2. PLATELET DEFECTS

Anything that suppresses the formation of white blood cells (◊ *blood* (3)) can also suppress platelets. Thus radiation, poisoning of the bone marrow, and diseases such as leukaemia can cause abnormal bleeding.

In some cases the number of platelets falls for no apparent reason, while the other blood cells remain normal. Surgical removal of the spleen sometimes cures the trouble, also for no apparent reason.

3. CLOTTING DEFECTS

The clotting of blood is a complex reaction (◊ *blood* (4)). It involves about a dozen reagents or 'factors'. If one is absent, clotting is delayed.

Vitamin K is needed for the synthesis of certain clotting factors. This vitamin cannot be absorbed from the intestine in the absence of bile. When the flow of bile is obstructed, in some types of ◊ *jaundice*, vitamin K is not absorbed and clotting is impaired. The danger is greatest in jaundiced new-born babies, and in adults who need an operation for obstructive jaundice but would bleed excessively if the operation were done. In either case the vitamin can be injected.

The best known of all bleeding disorders is ◊ *haemophilia*, due to congenital absence of one of the factors. It is a rare disease, but one of great interest to historians because of the people who have suffered from it, and to biologists because of its peculiar mode of inheritance. A number of similar and even rarer diseases, due to absence of different clotting factors, have been described.

blennorrhoea. 1. Excessive secretion of mucus. **2.** = ◊ *gonorrhoea*.

blephar(o)-. Prefix = 'of the eyelids'; e.g. *blepharitis*, inflammation of the eyelids, bacterial or allergic.

blindness. Total blindness – absence of any sensation of light – is uncommon apart from actual loss of the eyes or their nerves through injury. In practice, blindness means absence of useful sight.

About two thirds of the 100,000 blind people in England and Wales are aged over 65; most of them have some form of degenerative disease associated with ageing. Among younger adults the commonest causes of blindness are *diabetes*, *glaucoma*, and various little-understood disorders of the retina. Of about 3,000 blind children, most have congenital defects of the eyes. The venereal diseases gonorrhoea and syphilis can both cause blindness from birth, but with present methods of treatment and proper antenatal care such cases are no longer common.

In some hot countries, *trachoma* causes much blindness.

blood. A grown man has about a gallon of blood. More precisely, the blood makes up one fourteenth of the body weight, i.e. 5 litres for an average man. The blood is contained in a closed system of tubes or blood vessels: arteries, capillaries, and veins. The arteries and veins are waterproof, but the capillaries, the minute vessels by which blood crosses from arteries to veins, allow water and other small molecules to leak into the tissues. Since water leaks into the capillaries as fast as it leaks out (◊ *osmosis*), the total volume of the blood remains constant.

Like bone or muscle, blood is a ◊ *tissue*, and like other tissues it is composed of living cells set in unformed ground-substance. The peculiarity of blood is that its ground-substance is liquid, and more abundant than that of most tissues. Blood consists of *red cells* and *white cells* floating in a pale yellow, clear fluid, *plasma*. The cells occupy about 45 per cent of the volume, so that in 5 litres of blood we have rather less than 3 litres of plasma. The plasma and the two kinds of cell are best regarded as three separate organs, each with its own function and each with its ailments.

1. PLASMA

Plasma is a sticky, pale amber liquid with a faint sickly smell. It is a solution in water of proteins (7 per cent), salt (0·9 per cent), glucose (0·1 per cent), and various substances in transit from one part of the body to another. Plasma is a vehicle for all the raw materials of the tissues: water, oxygen, glucose etc., and for removing waste products.

The molecules of protein are too big to pass through the walls of the capillaries, but the other constituents of plasma are free to do so. Their tendency to escape into the tissues under the pressure of the heart's pumping action is counteracted by the osmotic pressure of the protein molecules, which cannot escape; this is the first function of the plasma proteins.

Plasma proteins (albumin, globulin, and fibrinogen) are all formed in the liver from digested amino-acids, except gamma-globulin, which is formed in the lymphoid tissue of the spleen, lymph-nodes and elsewhere. Gamma-globulin carries immunity to infectious diseases, some of which is inherited and some acquired as a result of infection. Hence gamma-globulin from someone known to have had a particular infection can often be used to immunize others against that disease.

Plasma proteins, especially albumin, may be deficient because of liver disease (not enough formed), kidney disease (loss of albumin in the urine), or starvation. If the amount in the plasma falls below a critical level the osmotic pressure is too low to prevent an excess of water from leaking into the tissues (◊ *oedema*).

Fibrinogen is responsible for the clotting of blood (◊ 'Platelets and Clotting', below).

Serum is not quite the same as plasma. It is the fluid which separates from clotted blood, namely plasma without fibrinogen and other components of clot.

2. RED CELLS (ERYTHROCYTES)

A red blood cell is a parcel of the pigment ◊*haemoglobin*, which conveys oxygen from the lungs to the rest of the body. Its diameter is about 7·2 microns (1/3000 in.) and its greatest thickness is 2 microns. A cubic millimetre of blood (not much larger than a pin's head) contains 5 million red cells, and the whole 5 litres of blood contains 25 million million.

Since haemoglobin represents about a third of the mass of the red cells, which make up 45 per cent of the blood, the normal concentration of haemoglobin in the blood is about 15 per cent. The actual concentration indicates the capacity of the blood for oxygen (i.e. the presence or absence of anaemia). Most of the tests in routine use measure the shade of red of the blood against a standard, and the result is given either in grammes per 100 c.c. or as a percentage of an arbitrary 'normal'.

Red cells are derived from unspecialized cells which may also be the precursors of white blood cells. These primitive blood cells can multiply very rapidly. In the process of development, cells destined to become red cells lose their nuclei and with them their ability to reproduce themselves, and they acquire their load of haemoglobin. Haemoglobin cannot be formed without a supply of iron, and the red cells cannot mature without vitamin B_{12} and certain other factors. The rate at which red cells are formed is governed by a hormone, erythropoietin, derived from the kidneys. If the body is short of oxygen, for instance through living at a high altitude or with defects of the lungs, the number of red cells is increased. The life-span of a red cell is 4 months.

An abnormal excess of red cells is a fairly rare disorder known as ◊ *polycythaemia*.

Deficiencies of the red cells, of which there are many types, are known collectively as ◊ *anaemia*. (◊ *haemoglobin*.)

3. WHITE CELLS (LEUKOCYTES)

The 'white' blood cells are colourless

bodies, larger than red cells. There are normally about 10,000 of them in a cubic millimetre of blood during childhood, and rather fewer in adult life.

When a thin film of blood is stained with a standard mixture of dyes and examined under a microscope, several types of white cell can be identified. All have darkly stained nuclei. In about 70 per cent, small granules are scattered throughout the cell; these cells are *granulocytes*. Because its nucleus is segmented like a string of sausages or a map of the Great Lakes, a granulocyte is sometimes called a polymorphonuclear leukocyte or polymorph. There are three types of granulocyte: *neutrophil*, the commonest, with faintly stained granules; *eosinophil*, with granules stained red by the acidic dye eosin; and *basophil*, with granules stained by the basic (alkaline) dye methylene blue.

Most of the remaining white cells are *lymphocytes*. A mature lymphocyte is only the size of a red cell; it is nearly all nucleus. The *monocytes* are large round cells with about three times the diameter of red cells.

In addition to the true cells, the blood contains small particles, *blood platelets*, described in the next section.

The functions of the white blood cells are not known in any detail. They are all able to insinuate themselves out of the capillary blood vessels into the surrounding tissues, unlike the red cells which cannot get out of intact blood vessels. In fact, the white cells probably do all their work outside the vessels, and use the blood-stream only as a means of transport.

The granulocytes can engulf and destroy bacteria and other invaders. Neutrophil granulocytes seem to be especially concerned with combating bacterial infection, and eosinophils are involved in allergy and in the response to certain parasites. Lymphocytes are concerned with ◊ *immunity* to infection; they form the antibodies (gamma-globulins, see above) which neutralize bacterial poisons and poison the bacteria. The lymphocytes circulating in the blood are only a small fraction of those in the whole body. They are scattered through all the tissues except the brain, and are most concentrated in the spleen, lymph nodes, and thymus.

Granulocytes are ready for instant action. They congregate rapidly at a site of infection or injury, and their number in the blood is increased. Since they are easily counted, this increase is a useful pointer to a diagnosis of acute infection: for instance, with an ill-defined belly-ache an abnormally large number of white cells in the blood would suggest appendicitis rather than green apples. Lymphocytes, on the other hand, respond slowly, and they are associated more with chronic or prolonged infection

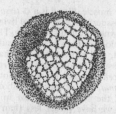

lymphocyte

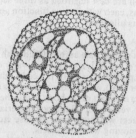

granulocyte

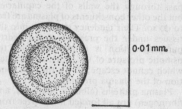

0·01mm

red corpuscle

Blood cells.

such as tuberculosis. Many viruses provoke a response from lymphocytes but not from granulocytes, e.g. the virus of ◊ *glandular fever*.

White cells are formed alongside red cells, in the bone marrow. Lymphocytes are also formed in the thymus, spleen, and lymph nodes. Hormones of the adrenal cortex suppress lymphocytes and eosinophils. The factors which stimulate the formation of white cells are unknown.

Proliferation of white cells is a healthy

response to infection. During an acute bacterial infection their number in the blood may increase three- or four-fold.

Like the cells of other tissues, the white cells occasionally multiply regardless of the body's needs. This produces a cancer-like disorder, ◊ *leukaemia.* The lymphocytes are involved in a somewhat similar disorder known as ◊ *Hodgkin's disease.*

Bone marrow is the most sensitive of all tissues to agents such as radiation and poisons which hinder the reproduction of cells. In aplastic ◊ *anaemia* (B.3) the formation of all types of blood cell is suppressed. More often the white cells are more affected than the red. Shortage of white cells is *leukopenia.* Complete absence of granulocytes is *agranulocytosis.* A few poisons regularly cause leukopenia, as does an excess of radiation. Others, including a number of widely used drugs, affect a few unfortunate people who are sensitive to them. Leukopenia is serious, because it leaves the patient without his first line of defence, and he may succumb to what would ordinarily be the most trivial infection. Before the discovery of antibiotics, severe leukopenia was usually fatal. With antibiotics and strict precautions to avoid chance infection, most patients can now be tided over while the bone marrow recovers.

4. PLATELETS AND CLOTTING

Bleeding, or *haemorrhage,* means loss of blood from the circulation; the blood need not escape from the body. The general effects of rapid bleeding are discussed under ◊ *shock,* and those of sustained bleeding under ◊ *anaemia* (A.1).

The natural course is for bleeding to stop, and this involves several mechanisms (◊ *bleeding*).

The *blood platelets* (thrombocytes) have various effects on bleeding. The platelets are small particles – much smaller than red cells – extruded by large bone-marrow cells. A cubic millimetre of normal blood contains about a quarter of a million of them. When a vessel is damaged, platelets stick to each other and to the site of injury and plug the breach. This is one of the ways in which unhealthy arteries, of which the walls are no longer smooth, become blocked (◊ *thrombosis*).

Shed blood tends to clot. Clotting is primarily a chemical change in one of the plasma proteins, *fibrinogen.* Fibrinogen is dissolved in the plasma, but after bleeding it is converted into threads of an insoluble protein, *fibrin.* The threads enmesh the blood cells to form a semi-solid mass. The fibrin mesh then contracts, squeezing out a clear yellow fluid, *serum,* and leaving a firm clot.

A dozen or more factors are concerned in the conversion of fibrinogen to fibrin. Most of them are present in circulating blood, but they are ineffective until acted on by other factors released from injured tissue, especially from the platelets when they stick to each other.

Platelets also release a hormone, ◊ *serotonin,* which encourages blood vessels to contract.

For disorders of clotting etc., ◊ *bleeding disorders.*

5. BLOOD GROUPS

A red blood cell has a thin shell, of which the chemical structure differs slightly in different people. Several components of the shell vary. A component and its variants form a *system.* People whose red cells have the same variant belong to the same blood group as regards that particular system.

At least 14 systems have been described. Since they are independent of each other there are many possible combinations. Although blood groups cannot yet be used like finger-prints for positive identification, they can often prove that two samples of blood are not from the same person. And since they are inherited, they may prove that someone is not the child of particular parents. They are sometimes a valuable tool for research into other supposedly inherited states: for instance, an association of duodenal ulcer with a particular blood group would strongly suggest a hereditary factor behind duodenal ulcer. The prevalence of blood groups in different populations has been used to study such matters as early migrations.

The great importance of blood groups in medicine is that chemical compounds different from those of an individual are treated as 'foreign' by his body defences. If red cells of a foreign group enter his blood, they are liable to be destroyed as though they were infecting bacteria.

The most important of the blood-group systems, the A B O system, was discovered in 1900 by Karl Landsteiner, in Vienna. 'Blood group' normally means the A B O group (A, B, A B, or O). Until Landsteiner's discovery, blood transfusion was most hazardous, because if a patient is given blood of the wrong ABO group his own blood may destroy its cells, and in the process he becomes dangerously ill.

Another system of blood groups (◊ *rhesus factor*) was discovered in 1940, again by Landsteiner, who had had a Nobel Prize in 1930. Some dangerous illnesses of new-born babies are due to their belonging to a different rhesus group from their mothers.

The other known blood groups have much less significance. ◊ *transfusion*.

blood count. Number of cells per cubic millimetre of blood.

blood group ◊ *blood* (5).

blood-letting. A very ancient method of treating disease, probably based on the idea that ill health is due to imbalance of the four humours (blood, yellow bile, black bile, phlegm). Many symptoms were ascribed to surfeit of blood or *plethora*.

Blood-letting still has a place in the treatment of *polycythaemia*, a condition in which blood cells are formed too profusely, and the blood does not flow as freely as it should. In some types of heart failure blood-letting may give temporary relief by reducing the load on the circulation.

blood-poisoning. A non-technical term used to describe at least three conditions: (1) *toxaemia* (the literal sense of blood-poisoning), the spread of poisons formed by bacteria such as the toxin of *tetanus*, which affects the whole nervous system although the actual bacteria are confined to the region of a wound; (2) *cellulitis*, the spread of bacteria (usually streptococci) from a wound into neighbouring tissues; (3) *septicaemia*, dissemination of bacteria by the blood-stream.

blood pressure (BP). The pressure at which the heart pumps blood into the major arteries. Subject to some individual variation, a normal BP fluctuates with the heart beat between about 120 mm. of mercury, or 2·4 lb. per sq. in. (systolic pressure), and 80 mm. (diastolic pressure). The main arteries are wide enough not to impede the flow significantly, so that the pressure in the brachial artery of the arm, where BP is normally measured, is nearly the same as at the outlet from the heart. But the small branches of arteries (arterioles) are narrow enough to exert considerable resistance, and the blood loses much of its pressure in flowing through them. When blood reaches the capillaries the pressure has fallen to about 32 mm., which is enough to oppose back-pressure from the tissue fluid (◊ *osmosis*) and carry the blood through to the veins. On the return journey to the heart, the BP in the veins is so low that the blood has to be helped on its way by neighbouring muscles.

Elaborate nervous and chemical controls adjust the circulation to the demands of the moment. The total flow is determined by the volume and rate of the heart beats. The flow to a particular organ, e.g. the leg muscles during exercise, or the stomach after a meal, is increased by widening its arteries, with compensatory narrowing of arteries elsewhere. But the demands of the brain do not vary. At work or idle it needs about 750 c.c. of fresh blood per minute. The function of the blood pressure is to maintain this constant flow of blood to the brain. Anyone who has ever fainted knows what happens if the pressure is momentarily lowered.

While insufficient pressure deprives the brain of its supplies, excessive pressure overtaxes the heart and blood vessels. Therefore the BP has to be kept within narrow limits.

Pressure is determined by rate of flow and resistance to flow. But the rate of flow is adapted to the constantly varying demand, between 5 litres per minute at rest and 30 or 40 litres in an athlete at full stretch. Therefore the BP must be kept constant by adapting resistance to rate of flow.

Resistance has two components: the *viscosity* of the blood, which does not normally change, and the size of the vessels – in effect, of the arterioles, of which the diameter is varied by contraction and relaxation of their muscular walls. At constant pressure, the flow in a pipe varies with the fourth power of the diameter; thus doubling the diameter of the pipe increases the flow sixteen-fold. Only small changes in the arterioles are needed for large effects. With a 6:1 increase of blood flow, the average diameter of the arterioles has to increase by only 3:2 in order to keep the BP steady.

If the arterioles fail to expand, then either the flow must decrease or the pressure must rise. But the heart is geared to maintain an adequate flow for as long as possible, and if the resistance to flow is increased it simply works harder; the flow is maintained and the pressure rises.

The regulation of blood pressure by the

sympathetic nervous system and by a hormone (renin) from the kidneys is discussed under ◊ *circulation*.

Blood pressure is measured with a *sphygmomanometer*, invented in 1896 by the Italian physician Riva-Rocci (who is commemorated in some countries by the symbol R-R for blood pressure). The instrument is a column of mercury supported by the air pressure in an inflatable cuff. The cuff is wrapped round a limb. When the pressure in it is just enough to obliterate the pulse, the height of the column of mercury indicates the systolic BP. When the pressure in the cuff is reduced to the diastolic BP a characteristic slapping sound is heard over the artery beyond the cuff.

1. HIGH BLOOD PRESSURE

It is normal for the systolic BP to rise in response to exertion or emotion, but it does not vary by more than about 50 per cent even when the rate of flow increases by 300 per cent or more. The diastolic pressure, between beats, hardly changes. After exertion the BP quickly returns to its resting level.

The normal blood pressure is said to increase with age. It may do so to some extent, but what increases greatly is the *average* BP in the population, which is not the same thing. People with perfectly healthy blood vessels show little if any increase of BP as the years go by; but in civilized communities they are a minority. The unhealthy majority puts up the average.

Most diseases of the kidneys can cause hypertension, by interfering with the blood-flow through the kidneys and so causing the hormone *renin* to be released; this in turn promotes the formation of *angiotensin*, which stimulates contraction of arterioles.

A very rare tumour of the adrenal glands, phaeochromocytoma, secretes noradrenaline, with the same effect as stimulation of sympathetic nerves – contraction of arterioles, increased resistance, raised BP.

Excess of blood cells (polycythaemia) increases the viscosity of the blood, and therefore the resistance and the pressure.

But most high blood pressure has no recognized cause, and is known as primary or *essential* hypertension. This condition cannot be properly defined because there is no clear division between the ranges of normal and abnormal pressures. Essential hypertension probably includes various unidentified disorders. It need not cause any symptoms at all, in which case one cannot

really describe it as a disorder. But a blood pressure that is persistently higher than would be expected is a warning; the records of insurance companies show that it lessens the chance of living to an old age.

The symptoms – if there are any – are vague and might or might not be really due to hypertension: fatigue, dizziness, headache and the like. With severe hypertension the heart first enlarges to meet the added demands, as does any hard-worked muscle, but may later be overtaxed and fail to keep up an adequate circulation (◊ *heart failure*). Very high blood pressure injures the kidneys, and a late stage of hypertension, with impairment of the kidneys as an effect, is indistinguishable from a late stage of chronic kidney disease with hypertension as a symptom. This is a vicious circle, since kidney disease causes high BP and vice versa.

Hypertension aggravates other disorders arising from unhealthy arteries. It increases *atheroma* (the underlying defect with most arteriosclerosis) and the likelihood of suffering coronary thrombosis or a stroke. Many other factors are involved; some are discussed under ◊ *atheroma*.

The rational treatment of any symptom is to tackle its cause, but this can be done in only a minority of cases of hypertension. The cause of essential hypertension is still unknown, and the symptom itself has to be treated as though it were the actual disease. It is at least possible that in the early stages the BP is raised by spasm of arterioles due to over-activity of sympathetic nerves, and that in time a high BP causes structural damage to the arterioles, which are then permanently narrowed. This is a strong argument for trying to lower the BP in all cases. A contrary view is that many people with high BP come to no harm without treatment. But there is still no way of telling which patients are likely to develop serious complications, and the present trend is towards early treatment.

Hypertension is probably less common and certainly less dangerous in people who are otherwise fit than in the unfit; some of the factors involved are mentioned under ◊ *atheroma*.

Until quite recently there was no safe and reliable way of lowering the blood pressure. Since 1947, numerous *ganglion-blocking* drugs have been discovered. They prevent the relay of impulses in sympathetic nerves, and so prevent arterioles from being stimulated to contract. But these drugs act indiscriminately on the sympathetic and parasympathetic nervous systems, with many unwanted effects. Some of the newer drugs suppress the action of sympathetic nerves without other effects, mostly by interfering with noradrenaline, the substance released by sympathetic nerves to constrict arterioles. For example, *guanethidine* (1960) prevents noradrenaline from being released; *methyldopa* (1963) interferes with its synthesis; and *rauwolfia* (1953) removes it from nerve-endings. The *thiazide* (1953) drugs promote elimination of salt and water by the kidneys and may lower blood pressure by reducing the volume of fluid in the circulation. They reinforce the action of the other drugs mentioned.

None of the effective drugs is entirely without undesirable effects, but when more than one drug is used at a time each can be given in small enough doses to minimize these effects.

The great improvement in the treatment of hypertension is among the most significant products of recent medical research; but essential hypertension is itself very largely a product of modern civilization.

2. Low Blood Pressure

Apart from rare disorders such as Addison's disease, with which the patient has more serious worries, it is very doubtful whether people really suffer from persistently low BP, though the diagnosis is quite popular in some countries, perhaps as a change from 'neurasthenia'.

Some people feel dizzy if they suddenly stand up from a chair or when they get out of bed. This is simply because the reflexes that adjust the BP to the standing posture do not act at once, and gravity carries blood away from the head before the blood vessels of the lower half of the body have time to contract enough to oppose gravity. A faint is a similar event produced by sudden relaxation of these vessels.

◊ *Shock* is a dangerous state following severe injury etc., with the blood pressure so low that the circulation may fail.

blood tests. Hundreds of different blood tests are occasionally used in diagnosis; scores of them are matters of routine in any medical laboratory. There are three main groups.

1. *Haematology*. Tests of the state of the blood itself for the diagnosis of anaemias

etc., e.g. number and condition of blood cells, amount of haemoglobin; blood group; clot formation.

2. *Blood chemistry*. Tests reflecting chemical functions elsewhere in the body, e.g. various enzymes (bone, liver, muscle); sugar (pancreas); urea (kidney disease); uric acid (gout).

3. *Microbiology*. Detection of actual microbes (e.g. malaria, typhoid); detection of immunity (antibodies) as evidence of past or present infection – many types of infection can be recognized in this way.

blood vessel. Tube – ◊ *artery*, ◊ *capillary*, or ◊ *vein* – carrying blood (◊ *circulation*).

blue baby. New-born infant in whom the blue complexion of partial asphyxia shows that a congenital defect of the heart is depriving the blood of its full supply of oxygen. ◊ *heart* (4).

BMR ◊ *basal metabolism.*

Boerhaave, Hermann (1668–1738). Dutch physician; the most celebrated medical teacher of modern times. More than anyone else, Boerhaave established the method of learning from actual patients rather than from lectures and texts. Under his influence, Leyden became the leading medical school of the day. Several other schools owe their greatness to pupils of Boerhaave: Edinburgh (Alexander Monro), Vienna (Gerard van Swieten), Berne (Albrecht von Haller).

boil. Small abscess around the root of a hair, or in a sweat gland. Single boils are painful for a day or two but as a rule take care of themselves; they extrude a core of dead tissue and heal. The process is accelerated by warm applications (poultices). Occasionally a boil has to be opened surgically, but otherwise physical interference is more likely to spread the infection than cure it. Squeezing boils is unhelpful and can be dangerous. Antiseptics are useful for discouraging infection of neighbouring sweat glands.

Boils on the face need more care than others because infection can be carried by the veins into the skull. They may call for treatment with antibiotic drugs.

bone.

1. Structure

The adult skeleton is made almost entirely

of a hard, rigid tissue, bone, which consists like other tissues of living cells suspended in an inert ground-substance. But in bone the cells are scanty. The ground-substance gives bone its characteristic properties. It is a network of protein fibres with insoluble mineral salts, mostly phosphates of calcium, deposited among them. The fibres confer resilience and the salts hardness. If the fibres are destroyed, e.g. by bacterial action after death, the remaining bone is brittle; if the salts are dissolved with acid the bone becomes rubbery.

All bones have a hard, dense shell of *compact bone* traversed only by very fine channels, the *Haversian* canals. Inside this shell the bone is porous (cancellous), or hollowed out and replaced with soft blood-forming tissue, ◊ *marrow*. There is a hole in the shell (usually only one) for the passage of blood vessels, of which small branches reach the periphery by the Haversian canals. A fibrous membrane, the periosteum, tightly surrounds the bone. It has a network of nerves and blood vessels, which penetrate only the outermost layer of the bone. *Sensation* from bone is really from the periosteum; bone itself is insensitive.

2. Development and Growth

Bone, like muscle, connective tissue, and blood, is formed in the embryo from ◊ *mesoderm*. With a few exceptions, prototypes of the bones appear as a modification of the mesoderm to cartilage. Towards the end of the 2nd month of pregnancy *ossification* begins: an island of true bone is formed in each unit and spreads until all the cartilage has been replaced. The process is not complete at birth. Some small bones of the hands and feet are still entirely cartilaginous. At the ends of the 'long' bones (◊ 'Anatomical Classification', below), at various protrusions where powerful muscles are attached, and at the sites of certain atavistic bones, *epiphyses* are formed. An epiphysis is a part added to a bone in which ossification begins late. Of about 100 epiphyses in the body only those at the knee contain bone at birth. The others remain cartilaginous until a time, roughly predictable for each, between birth and adolescence. After ossification the epiphyses are attached by cartilage which is not converted to bone until the bones reach their adult length.

The exceptions mentioned are the clavicle and most of the skull, which start as bone without first being formed in cartilage.

The stage of ossification indicates the age of a skeleton, and may be a useful guide in identifying human remains.

Bone grows by the activity of *osteoblasts*. These cells produce an enzyme which causes insoluble calcium phosphate to be precipitated from the soluble phosphates in the blood. They are active only under the periosteum and at the ends of bones where the epiphyses join them. Thus bones grow thicker by the addition of new tissue at the outside, and longer by addition at the ends. Injury to the end of a young bone may interfere with its growth.

Simultaneously, the core of a growing bone is eroded; there, *osteoclasts* produce an enzyme with the opposite action to that of the osteoblasts.

The general shape of a bone is determined by hereditary factors, but its details are modified by the pull of muscles, which stimulates bone formation.

Growth is stimulated by the growth hormone of the ◊ *pituitary*, and by the ◊ *sex hormones*, which also promote the fusion of the epiphyses with the rest of the bone. Since growth stops when this fusion is complete, the sex hormones may also be said to inhibit growth. Thus although sex hormones may be given to undersized children, they defeat their own object unless the dose is carefully regulated, because although they accelerate growth they may stop it too soon.

The ◊ *parathyroid* glands are indirectly concerned with bone growth, because they regulate the amount of calcium in the blood. If the level falls, calcium is drawn from the bones by the action of parathyroid hormone.

Healthy growth of any tissue needs a proper diet. Any reasonable diet includes the essential elements of bone, but there may be a defect of vitamin D and consequent ◊ *rickets*. Vitamin D was formerly thought to stimulate the actual formation of bone, but it now appears to act only indirectly, by increasing the absorption of calcium from the food into the blood and perhaps by decreasing loss of calcium from the kidneys: if enough calcium is available to them, the osteoblasts will do their work.

3. Anatomical Classification

Bones are described as *long*, *short*, or *flat*. *Long bones* are cylindrical or prismatic, usually hollow, with a knob at each end. *Short bones* are simple blocks of cancellous (spongy) bone with a thin compact shell. *Flat bones* consist of two parallel sheets of compact bone with a spongy layer between.

The *carpal* and *tarsal* bones in the hand and foot are 'short'; all the other limb bones including those of the digits, are 'long'. The vault of the skull, the sternum, the scapula, and part of the pelvis are 'flat'. The end of a rib joined to the spine is 'long', but the rest is flat. The body of a vertebra is a compressed long bone. A few irregular bones in the base of the skull and elsewhere remain unclassified.

Sesamoid bones are not really parts of the skeleton. They are imbedded in tendons subject to excessive friction, and are usually very small. Only one is important: the *patella*, in the tendon at the front of the knee.

Supernumerary bones are usually epiphyses which have failed to join their principal bones. They often correspond with bones which are normally separate in other animals.

4. DISORDERS

Bone is subject to the same kinds of trouble as any other tissue, but its physical peculiarities modify the effects of disease.

Bone is very strong, but also rigid. If it yields at all it does so completely (◊ *fracture*). And whereas in most other tissues an ◊ *abscess* can close once the pus is released, the rigid walls of an abscess in bone cannot fall together; thus the infection persists. Nor can bone expand to make room for inflammation (◊ *osteitis*). The increased pressure in an inflamed or injured bone may interfere with the circulation and kill part of the bone. Dead bone, being largely insoluble, is not readily broken down and absorbed as are other dead tissues. It therefore remains, cut off from the defensive elements of the blood, as a focus of infection where microbes can breed without hindrance.

The arteries in bone do not communicate freely with each other: if one is blocked the area it feeds may have no alternative supply. Where an epiphysis joins a bone there is no communication across the line of fusion, which is therefore a bulkhead against the spread of disease.

Sensation is confined to the periosteum, so that unless this outer membrane is involved disorders of bone are painless. But pain is severe if the periosteum is even slightly stretched, e.g. by inflammation or bleeding.

Except at the ends of young bones, growth of new bone depends on the osteoblasts in the periosteum. If the periosteum is destroyed an injured bone does not heal.

Various kinds of tumour (◊ *osteoma*) arise in bone. Cancer of bone is discussed at ◊ *sarcoma*.

◊ *cartilage; skeleton.*

booster dose. Supplementary dose of a vaccine to meet a special emergency, such as entering the area of an epidemic, or to reinforce the effect of an earlier vaccination as this begins to wear off. ◊ *immunization.*

boracic (boric) acid. H_3BO_3; a mild antiseptic used as a dusting powder, and in various solutions for treating infections of skin and mucous membranes.

Borellia. A kind of spiral bacterium or spirochaete. *B. vincentii* is a normal inhabitant of the mouth; very rarely it provokes severe inflammation of the mouth and throat (Vincent's angina). Several species of Borellia can cause *relapsing fever.*

Bornholm disease (epidemic myalgia; epidemic pleurisy; devil's grip; pleurodynia). A virus infection with fever and pain in the muscles of the ribs and abdomen. The disease was first observed in the island of Bornholm, but there have been outbreaks in many parts of the world. An attack lasts a day or two and is sometimes repeated a few days later. Complications are extremely rare.

bothryocephalus (Diphyllobothrium). A kind of tapeworm found mostly in Finland and Japan, causing severe anaemia (◊ *worms*).

botulism. A rare but exceedingly dangerous type of ◊ *food poisoning*, caused by a toxin formed by the bacterium *Clostridium botulinum*. This common microbe does not infect man, but it may contaminate badly preserved food. It multiplies only in the complete absence of air, as in a preserving can. Minute doses of the toxin paralyse the nervous system and are commonly fatal.

Most reported outbreaks have been in the United States, where home-canning is (or has been) popular. Factory-canned foods are safe because the high temperatures destroy any bacteria.

Cooking destroys the toxin; so does the acid of uncooked fruit. Home-canned vegetables have been the greatest hazard.

bowel = ◊ *intestine.*

brachial. Of the arm (usually in the strict anatomical sense of upper arm).

The *brachial artery* is the main blood vessel of the upper limb, a continuation of the *axillary* artery. It runs down the inner side of the humerus, where its pulsation can be felt in the groove between biceps and triceps muscles, and where it can be compressed to stop bleeding lower down. In front of the elbow the artery divides into the *radial* and *ulnar* arteries of the forearm,

The *brachial plexus* is a leash of nerves with various intercommunications, arising from the spinal nerves in the lower part of the neck. Its branches provide the nerves of the shoulder-girdle and upper limb. The plexus is sometimes injured during birth, and this causes a temporary paralysis of the arm. In adult life the nerves of this plexus may be subject to irritation or pressure from disorders of the neck such as arthritis of the vertebrae or a slipped disc. ◊ *vertebra* (1).

brain. The part of the central nervous system enclosed by the skull. Like its continuation the spinal cord, the brain starts life as a simple tube. But whereas the spinal cord retains this form throughout life, the brain grows into a complex system of bulges and folds.

At an early stage of embryonic life, three bulbous swellings appear at the front end of the tube that is to form the central nervous system, and these develop into the three main divisions of the brain: the *hindbrain*, the *midbrain*, and the *forebrain*.

The original tube is still recognizable in the adult brain as the *brain-stem*, seen as an extension into the skull of the spinal cord, It is a central core from which the larger portions of the brain (cerebellum and cerebrum) grow.

Very roughly speaking, the further from the spinal cord the more advanced the function, progressing from reflexes for maintaining vital functions such as the circulation of blood and breathing in the lower part of the hindbrain to the processes of intelligent behaviour in the outer layers of the forebrain. But structure and function are only loosely related, for the whole nervous system works as an integrated unit.

1. HINDBRAIN

The spinal cord continues into the skull as the *medulla oblongata*. In the cord, the nerve cells form a fluted rod (grey matter) surrounded by nerve fibres (white matter). In the medulla the grey matter is gathered into more or less distinct groups of cells or *nuclei*; this tendency increases further up the brain. These nuclei include the cells of

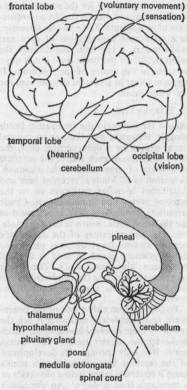

Parts of the brain: (above) *left side,* (below) *mid-line.*

several cranial nerves and also the *vital centres* which regulate fundamental activities such as the heart beat.

Above the medulla oblongata is a large, rounded, backward projection, the *cerebellum*. It fills the posterior fossa of the skull, i.e. the part immediately above the nape of the neck. The cerebellum governs many reflex actions such as balance and posture. At the same level, the *pons* is a broad band across the front of the brain-stem, like a strap to hold the cerebellum in place.

2. MIDBRAIN

Above the pons the brain-stem resumes its primitive tubular structure. The midbrain is a short cylinder from which the stalks of the two cerebral hemispheres (forebrain) arise. It contains the cells of some cranial nerves, relay stations for the senses of sight and hearing, and centres for the co-ordination of movements. The *reticular formation* is a criss-cross arrangement of grey and white matter. It can be traced through the whole length of the brain-stem but is most obvious in the centre of the midbrain. It appears to act as a central switchboard for the whole brain.

3. FOREBRAIN

Above the midbrain the brain-stem bends sharply forwards, and the narrow central canal widens to a deep vertical cleft, the third ventricle. At each side of the ventricle is a mass of grey matter, the *thalamus*. Sensation of all kinds is received here and distributed to reflex pathways or to the cerebral cortex and consciousness. Crude sensation, particularly pain, is perceived in the thalamus itself. Below is the *hypothalamus*, the highest centre of the autonomic nervous system, from which is suspended the ◊ *pituitary* gland. Behind is a small protrusion, the *pineal body*. The whole complex, representing the headward end of the brain-stem, is sometimes called the tween-brain.

Projecting from either side of the tween-brain and completely enclosing it are the relatively huge *cerebral hemispheres*, which make up the greater part of the human brain. It is only through the development of the cerebral hemispheres that a man's brain is relatively larger than a monkey's or a monkey's than a dog's. (An elephant's brain is about four times as large as man's, but in relation to the size of the animal it is much smaller.)

The central cavity of a cerebral hemisphere, the lateral ventricle, opens by a narrow isthmus (foramen of Monro) into the third ventricle. It is surrounded by masses of grey matter, the *basal ganglia*, which are concerned with muscle action immediately below the level of consciousness. Disorders of the basal ganglia cause *parkinsonism* – shaking palsy. The surface of the hemispheres is covered with a layer of grey matter, the *cerebral cortex*. Between the cortex and the underlying basal ganglia

and thalamus is a broad zone of white matter, composed of nerve fibres to and from the cells of the cortex.

Definite functions can be ascribed to certain areas of the cerebral cortex. The areas for voluntary movement and for most types of sensation have been plotted in detail, but no particular area can be allotted to such functions as reason or memory.

4. SUPPORTING STRUCTURES

Nervous tissue needs a large and constant supply of oxygen and glucose, waking or sleeping, thinking or idling. It ceases to work after a few seconds if the supply is cut off, and irreparable damage is done in a few minutes. The rate of circulation in other organs varies widely but the brain receives about 750 c.c. of blood per minute, by the carotid and vertebral arteries, regardless of what is going on elsewhere. The complicated mechanisms for maintaining the blood pressure serve mainly to keep up this supply.

The brain is enclosed by fibrous membranes, the ◊ *meninges*, and by the ◊ *cerebrospinal fluid*.

The behaviour of nervous tissue, of which the brain is composed, is discussed under ◊ *nervous system*.

More detailed descriptions are given under the names of the various parts of the brain.

brain-stem. The direct upward extension of the spinal cord into the skull, composed of *medulla oblongata*, *pons*, and *midbrain*. The major portions of the brain, *cerebellum* and *cerebral hemispheres*, project from it.

breast. The breasts (mammary glands) develop in the fatty tissue under the skin as columns of cells radiating from the nipples; these columns later become ten or twenty tubes or *ducts*. Thus far, their development is the same in either sex. In a girl (and in a few perfectly normal boys) the ducts branch out at puberty, under the influence of sex hormones from the ovaries (or testes), and a very variable amount of fat is deposited. The size of the breasts depends on this fat and is therefore not related to their efficiency: small flat breasts are as likely to feed twins – and their owners to bear twins – as 'well-developed' breasts and their owners.

During pregnancy the breasts change rapidly under the influence of hormones from the placenta. The ducts proliferate and milk-forming tissue grows around their ends. Towards the end of pregnancy hormones from the pituitary gland stimulate the secretion of milk.

Suckling stimulates the nipple, and this, by an unknown mechanism, causes the release from the pituitary of a hormone, *oxytocin*, which acts on the breast to eject milk and form more milk. Oxytocin also stimulates the uterus to contract and regain its resting size and shape after pregnancy (it does so without this stimulus, but suckling probably accelerates the process). When the baby is weaned the stimulus of suckling is withdrawn and milk soon ceases to be formed. Thyroid hormone is also required for milk production.

The adult female breast is comma-shaped: in addition to the obvious dome of tissue over the pectoral muscles it has a tail-like extension towards the armpit.

Rudimentary breasts may develop anywhere along a line from the armpit to the middle of the groin. They have no significance except as evolutionary curiosities.

1. DISORDERS

Serious deficiencies of the breast are unusual. Complete inability to form milk is very rare, because the breasts develop with the other reproductive organs, and if a woman is capable of having a child at all she is likely to be able to feed it at least for a time. Inadequate (as opposed to absent) milk supply has many causes, including almost any kind of ill health after childbirth. It is the quantity rather than the quality of the milk that suffers. The influence of suckling on the pituitary gland can be disturbed by emotional factors, of which not wishing to feed the infant is among the most important. The commonest physical cause of poor milk supply is a sore or cracked nipple, which destroys the pleasure of suckling and inhibits the formation of milk. Much of this kind of trouble is avoided by antenatal care of the nipples.

Mastitis – inflammation of the breast – is generally due to bacterial infection from a cracked nipple. Antibiotic drugs usually clear it up quickly, but sometimes an abscess forms and has to be relieved surgically. Such complications nearly always mean that breast-feeding has to be interrupted, and often it cannot be successfully resumed.

Cancer of the breast is the commonest form of cancer in women, and also one of the easiest to recognize and treat. The earliest sign is nearly always a painless lump in the breast, which the woman can easily feel for herself. The best time to examine the breasts is shortly after a menstrual period (before a period they may be congested and difficult to examine). Eighty per cent or more of cases treated when a lump first appears are completely cured. The longer treatment is delayed, the greater the risk of relapse.

A few cases of breast cancer show themselves in other ways, e.g. fluid from the nipple or discomfort; any change in the breast after the age of 30 or 35 is suspect.

Several harmless conditions imitate breast cancer. Many lumps turn out to be innocent tumours (fibroma, papilloma), but their innocence has to be proved before they can be dismissed. An effective technique is to have a microscopical examination of the tumour done during an operation. If the tumour is harmless the surgeon need do no more than remove it; but if it shows signs of cancer he must extend the operation. There is still no satisfactory alternative to removing the whole of the affected breast; any smaller operation invites relapse. X-ray treatment and drugs also have a place in the treatment of breast cancer, but it is secondary to that of radical surgery.

The commonest affection of the breast used to be called chronic mastitis – a misnomer, for there is no inflammation. It is better called *cystic disease*, or simply *adenosis* (which means no more than 'glandular condition', an apt summary of present knowledge). The texture of the breast becomes lumpy, and there may be discomfort. It is in some way associated with the hormones of the ovary. Its only importance is that it must be carefully distinguished from cancer. Adenosis has often been said to lead to cancer. Both are so common that they must often affect the same person by chance. There is no good evidence of cause and effect. Similarly, injuries often *precede* cancer because they are so common, but they do not cause cancer.

breath-holding. Breathing is essentially a reflex action, but unlike other reflexes it can be transferred for a while to conscious control. When the breath is deliberately held, carbon dioxide accumulates in the blood, stimulating the respiratory centre in the brain until reflex action overrides volition and a breath must be taken.

Small children sometimes acquire the trick of breath-holding to get attention; they can actually lose consciousness for a second or two, giving a fair imitation of epilepsy.

breathing ◊ *respiration*.

breech. = buttocks; *breech delivery* is the birth of a baby buttocks first instead of the usual head first. It adds to the difficulties of both mother and child, and is usually avoided by turning the baby to a head-down position before confinement. When breech delivery cannot be avoided, it is facilitated by bringing the baby's feet down so that his legs are born straight and not bunched in front of his belly.

Bright, Richard (1789–1858). Physician at Guy's Hospital, London, and a member of one of the most brilliant groups in the history of medicine, led by the surgeon Sir Astley Cooper, and including another physician, Thomas Addison, and a pathologist, Thomas Hodgkin. All these names are household words in the language of medicine.

Although mainly concerned with the living, Bright paid great attention to post-mortem examination of patients who died in the hospital, and the relation of structural changes seen after death to the symptoms of the patient in life.

Bright's *Reports of Medical Cases* include accurate accounts of abdominal tumours, diseases of the liver, and many other conditions, several of which he was the first to describe. He made a special study of dropsy (◊ *oedema*), which he showed to be not a disease in its own right, but a symptom of various kinds of disease. Dropsy associated with abnormal kidneys could be distinguished from other types by examining the urine, which with kidney disease was 'coagulable'. (Damaged kidneys allow protein to leak from the blood into the urine, which therefore curdles when heated.) Bright pointed out that the kidney disease which now bears his name might be the cause of the dropsy or only a consequence of some other disease – a kind of scientific caution that is all too rare.

Bright's disease. Any disorder of the kidney associated with retention of water in the body (◊ *oedema*) and loss of protein in the urine could properly be called Bright's disease, but the term is generally restricted to inflammation of the kidneys (◊ *nephritis*) not directly due to bacterial infection. It is probably not a single disease but a reaction in the kidney which can be provoked in various ways.

bromide. Any salt of hydrobromic acid. The bromides of sodium and potassium were very widely used as ◊ *hypnotic* (sleep-inducing) drugs, and in smaller doses as day-time sedatives and for the control of epileptic attacks. They have various unpleasant effects such as mental sluggishness, skin rashes, and digestive disturbances, and are no longer much prescribed. More modern hypnotics such as the barbiturates are not more toxic or habit-forming than bromides and they have fewer unwanted effects. For the day-time treatment of emotional disorders bromides have given way to tranquillizers, which allay symptoms of anxiety without dulling the mind. Epilepsy is treated with phenobarbitone, phenytoin and other drugs.

bronchial. Of the *bronchi*, the air-tubes of the lung.
Bronchial artery and vein. The lungs receive the whole of the circulating blood and return it, oxygenated, to the heart, by the *pulmonary* arteries and veins. The pulmonary circulation takes no account of the needs of the lungs themselves; this blood is like money through a banker's hands, which he cannot spend. The lungs are supplied with blood for their own needs by the bronchial arteries, branches of the aorta. The corresponding veins drain into the azygos veins.

bronchiectasis. A chronic disease of bronchi: severe infection such as a prolonged attack of whooping cough in childhood weakens the bronchi, which then stretch and lose their elasticity and their ability to clear themselves of secretion. Affected bronchi offer a permanent base for infecting bacteria. Any severe sustained infection can cause bronchiectasis, which in turn leads to indefinitely prolonged infection. This disease has become much less common since the discovery of antibiotics, which usually clear up the initial infection before lasting damage is done. Antibiotics have also much improved the treatment of established bronchiectasis.

Other useful measures are physiotherapy to help bring up infected sputum, and in cases where the defect is severe but confined to one zone of a lung the affected zone can be removed surgically.

bronchiole. A very small branch of a bronchus.

bronchiolitis. A pneumonia-like affection of infants caused by the ◊ *respiratory syncytial virus*.

bronchitis. Inflammation of the air-passages in the lungs, either acute or chronic.

1. ACUTE BRONCHITIS

Most cases are due to spread of a virus infection from the nose and throat – 'a cold settling on the chest'. Bacterial infection usually follows. The bronchi are much more vulnerable to infection when they are irritated by smoke, noxious fumes or, in susceptible people, cold air.

Most attacks are mild and last only a few days. Characteristically a dry, uncomfortable cough develops after a cold in the nose or a sore throat, and the patient feels feverish and unwell. The inflammation causes rapid secretion of mucus from the lining of the bronchi; this gives the patient something to cough up and makes coughing much less of a burden. A cough may persist for some time after an attack, especially in winter.

The virus infection runs its course regardless of treatment, but much can be done to keep the patient comfortable and to minimize secondary infection by bacteria. For both these reasons cold air, smoke, and exertion are avoided. Steam warms and moistens the inspired air and is especially comforting in the early stage when the cough is dry and painful. Menthol, friar's balsam etc. add a reassuring medicinal smell. Various ◊ *cough medicines* relieve the main symptom. Medications rubbed into the chest redden the skin but do not affect the bronchi. Antibiotic drugs deal effectively with bacterial infection, shortening the attack and preventing serious damage to the bronchi.

2. CHRONIC BRONCHITIS

Chronic bronchitis has become the new 'English disease' (the old one was rickets). It accounts for well over 20,000 deaths per year, a much higher rate than in other countries. Exact comparisons are impossible because there is no international agreement about what chronic bronchitis means; but the death rate from what in Britain is called chronic bronchitis is higher than the rate from all related diseases anywhere else.

The characteristic symptom is a regular cough with sputum. The smoker's morning cough is an example; bringing up a little phlegm in the morning is not, as he thinks, normal but evidence of inflammation. It is due in the first place to over-production of mucus; later the lining of the bronchi loses its ability to keep mucus on the move because the *cilia* – hair-like structures that normally maintain a wave motion – are smoothed over. In healthy bronchi the cilia sweep the small amount of mucus up to the throat, where it is swallowed with the saliva. With bronchitis there is more mucus, and it is moved only by coughing.

A simple classification has been adopted in Britain: (1) *simple chronic bronchitis* with sputum of clear mucus; (2) *mucopurulent bronchitis* with muco-pus rendering the sputum opaque and as a rule yellowish, either from time to time or continuously; (3) *obstructive bronchitis* with narrowing of the air-passages and impairment of breathing.

Grade (1) is due to mild but persistent irritation of any kind; (2) to bacterial infection of already inflamed and vulnerable bronchi; (3) to structural damage done by persistent infection, irritation, and coughing. The damage is of several kinds. The bronchi are narrowed by thickening and scarring of their lining membrane. The functional lung tissue for exchange of oxygen and carbon dioxide is reduced and the lungs lose their elasticity, so that breathing involves more work for less effect. If the damage is severe the heart is overtaxed by trying to keep up an efficient circulation in the lungs.

The reason for the very high death rate from bronchitis in Britain is not just that bronchitis is very common. The English disease is grade (3), obstructive bronchitis. The milder grades are common abroad; it is severe, complicated chronic bronchitis that is so much commoner in Britain than anywhere else. A research team has done comparable surveys in Britain and the United States: *simple* bronchitis is not much commoner in Britain, but the severer forms are several times commoner.

The known causes include air-pollution, fog, and smoking. The air of all industrial towns is heavily polluted. Soot and sulphur dioxide are the main irritants, and coal smoke is a rich source of both. The recent Clean Air Act deals with soot but not sulphur dioxide. Fog tends to keep these contaminants at ground level, and cold damp air is itself an added source of irritation. Two British institutions might have been designed to cause bronchitis: the domestic coal fire – which heavily pollutes the air and also provides one over-heated focus in an otherwise cold house – and the cold draughty British bedroom.

The individual has little if any control over some of the factors predisposing to bronchitis. He can seldom move to a warmer or less smoky climate. But if some factors are eliminated others lose most of their effect. Even in the worst towns non-smokers do not have much bronchitis, and in most cases the most effective treatment is not to smoke. Fog can be kept at bay by shutting windows. Episodes of acute bronchitis on top of chronic bronchitis are particularly harmful; they drag on because the chronic bronchitic has a residue of sputum that he does not cough up, and after each acute attack the chronic state tends to be a little worse than before. Antibiotics, e.g. tetracycline, deal with these attacks and greatly improve the health and prospects of bronchitics. Influenza vaccine protects against an important source of acute episodes.

bronchodilator. Drug used to relax spasm of the bronchi in the treatment of asthma and bronchitis. The muscles of the bronchi are constricted by parasympathetic nerves and relaxed by sympathetic nerves. Bronchodilators are of two types: drugs that suppress parasympathetic action, such as belladonna and the derivatives of atropine, and drugs that enhance or imitate sympathetic action, such as adrenaline, ephedrine and isoprenaline. These drugs have the disadvantage that they stimulate the heart, sometimes dangerously. Some of the newer bronchodilators, such as orciprenaline and salbutamol are much safer in this respect.

bronchopneumonia ◊ *pneumonia.*

bronchoscope. Lighted tube passed down the trachea for direct examination of the main bronchi.

bronchus. Air-passage in the lungs: the ◊ *trachea* divides above the heart into left and right main bronchi, forming an inverted Y. The main bronchi are divided and sub-divided into smaller branches, first to the lobes, next to the segments (◊ *lung* (1)), and ultimately into minute bronchioles opening into the air sacs.

The bronchi and all but their smallest branches are held open by incomplete rings of cartilage in their walls. The rings are completed by involuntary muscle, which contracts under the influence of the ◊ *vagus nerves*, reducing the volume of *dead space* during shallow breathing. Over-activity of these muscles narrows the bronchi, an important factor in ◊ *asthma.*

The lining membrane of the bronchi resembles that of the trachea.

Some common disorders of the bronchi are listed under ◊ *lung* (5).

bronzed diabetes ◊ *iron* (2).

brown fat (brown adipose tissue). This tissue looks like the layer of fatty tissue under the skin, but under the microscope the fat is scattered through the cells in tiny droplets instead of forming a single large drop in each cell. 'Brown' refers to the supporting tissue, not to the fat itself. The cells are equipped for immediate combustion of the fat to provide heat (whereas ordinary fatty tissue releases fat into the circulation to be used in the liver as a source of chemical energy). In hibernating animals, brown fat is used to raise the body temperature after hibernation. In man, it is the new-born baby's source of heat. The recent discovery of deposits of brown fat around the backbone answers the question: how does a baby suddenly exposed to the air keep warm without shivering? A *premature* baby has little fat of any kind, and unless it is artificially kept warm its temperature quickly falls to a dangerous level.

Brucella. A genus of bacteria, causing contagious abortion in cattle, sheep, and pigs; in man these bacteria cause ◊ *undulant fever.*

brucellosis. Infection with ◊ *brucella.*

bruise (contusion). Bleeding into injured skin. The spilt blood is gradually decomposed and absorbed; in the process the red pigment haemoglobin turns blue as it loses its oxygen, and is later broken down to green and yellow bile pigments. Bruises seldom need treatment. A large collection of blood (*haematoma*) may have to be drawn off with a needle. Expert technique is needed because any contamination of stagnant blood – an ideal environment for bacteria – can lead to serious infection.

bubo. A swelling in the groin due to inflamed lymph nodes.

bubonic plague. The usual type of ◊ *plague* with enlarged lymph nodes.

Buerger's disease (thromboangiitis obliterans). Narrowing of arteries and veins, especially in the legs, with a tendency for vessels to be obstructed by blood clot. It causes symptoms of inadequate blood supply: muscular pain on exertion, cold skin, poor healing. Symptoms usually start before the age of 40, and the patients are men who smoke heavily. The outlook depends mainly on whether the patient gives up smoking: if he does, the circulation can be expected to improve; if he does not, he may need an amputation in time. The blood flow can sometimes be improved by drugs to dilate the vessels.

bunion. A deformity of the joint at the base of the big toe with a tender ◊ *bursa* over the protruding 'knuckle'; due solely to wearing unsuitable shoes. Chiropody, splinting, and a change of shoes may suffice, but a severely deformed joint may need a surgical operation to straighten it.

burn. True burns need not be distinguished from many other kinds of injury that are called burns though they have nothing to do with fire. Protein, the chief material of living tissue, is unstable. Quite small changes in its environment alter its properties by changing the shape of its molecules. This process, *denaturation*, hardly affects the chemical properties of a protein but abolishes its biological properties – in other words, kills it. Raw white of egg is a solution of a protein in its natural state. Hot water completely changes its character. Curdling of milk is another example of denaturation. The type of injury called a burn is denaturation of tissue proteins. Boiling water – which cannot literally burn anything – works as well as a naked flame, as do electric currents, and acids, alkalis and other corrosive poisons.

In addition to the immediate damage to burnt tissue, burns cause blood vessels to leak *plasma*, the fluid part of blood. The blood cells remain in the vessels. With small burns the only effect of the leakage is swelling or blistering in the area, but with extensive burns the volume of blood is reduced enough to impair the circulation, while the proportion of solid to liquid in the blood increases enough to slow down the flow still further. Failure to keep up an adequate circulation is the basis of ◊ *shock*, and this is a much more serious matter than the loss of burnt tissue. The amount of fluid that leaks from the blood into the tissues, and hence the severity of shock and the immediate danger to life, depend on the area and not the depth of the burn. Burns involving 15 per cent of the skin area in an adult or 10 per cent in a child are likely to cause shock severe enough to need hospital treatment. The leakage is not necessarily rapid, so that shock can develop over some hours. The essential part of treatment is to restore and maintain the volume of the blood (◊ *shock*).

The treatment of the damaged tissue – of the burn itself – depends on the depth of the burn. Very complex classifications were devised in the 19th century, with as many as seven degrees of burn. They have no practical value, and surgeons now recognize three degrees, as suggested by Fabricius Hildanus in about 1600.

First-degree burns damage only the inert surface of the skin, which in any case is due to be shed and replaced. The burn itself needs no special attention, though the patient may need treatment for shock.

Second-degree burns destroy living tissue, but leave enough of the growing layer of the skin for the surface to be fully restored provided that no further damage is done, e.g. by infection.

Third-degree burns involve the whole thickness of the skin. New skin can only grow from the edges of the burn, unless the defect is covered by skin-grafting. Some scarring is inevitable. Skin-grafting hastens recovery, reduces the risk of infection, and prevents deformity from shrinkage of scar tissue. It also improves the final appearance; this was the original object of skin-grafting, but the experience of two World Wars taught that skin-grafts had even more important uses.

All burns are painful, and pain contributes to shock; drugs to mitigate pain and distress contribute to safety as well as comfort. The loss of nerve-endings in the deeper layers of the skin often makes 3rd-degree burns less painful than 1st- or 2nd-degree.

The best way to dress burns is still disputed. Only 1st-degree burns present no problem: they can be left to their own devices. Applications that form a crust, such as tannin and some antiseptic dyes, delay healing and prevent any assessment of the damage; they are now seldom used. Plain, sterile gauze would be ideal if it were not apt to stick, and non-adherent (petrolatum) gauze is more often used. Since the object is to interfere with healing as little as possible, some surgeons use no dressings at all, but leave the burns exposed. This method is especially suitable for burns of the head and neck, but is also used for other parts of the body. It needs a specially ventilated and equipped hospital unit.

With corrosive burns, the area should be flushed with cold water at once. There is no point in trying to neutralize the substance, e.g. by bathing an acid burn with a weak alkali, for the interaction of the two generates heat and could make matters worse. The corrosive needs to be washed away, preferably under a running tap.

Immediate bathing in cold water is also good first-aid for true burns and scalds. The tissues retain heat, causing the damage to spread for some little while after the actual injury has taken place. This delayed damage is prevented by immediate cooling, which also helps to relieve the pain.

Apart from the direct consequences of the injury, the main risk with any burn is infection, because the damaged tissue is a perfect incubator for bacteria. Closed blisters are free from infection. It is highly dangerous to puncture them except under strict surgical *asepsis*, which in practical terms means that a burn-blister is best left alone until the patient is in trained hands. The best first-aid dressing is a simple pad of sterile gauze. A sterile adhesive dressing is suitable for small burns. For a larger area, the inner surface of a freshly laundered and ironed handkerchief is as sterile as anything in an average household. No dressing at all is better than a contaminated one.

Except with really trivial burns and scalds it is a wise precaution to get professional advice early, because the appearance does not always indicate the severity. Electric burns are especially misleading: they are nearly always worse than they look because the damage extends for some depth below the skin.

bursa. A pocket of fibrous tissue lined in the same way as a joint with a slippery synovial membrane. Bursae reduce friction, for example where tendons or ligaments move over bones. Some bursae are standard anatomical structures. Others develop in response to unusual pressure and friction.

bursitis. Inflammation of a bursa; sometimes bacterial, sometimes rheumatic, but usually a result of repeated pressure, friction or other injury. Bursitis is often due to wear and tear arising from a particular trade, e.g. housemaid's or clergyman's knee, dustman's shoulder, miner's elbow, weaver's bottom.

buttock ◊ *thigh.*

byssinosis. Chronic disease of the lungs from cotton dust, a form of ◊ *pneumoconiosis.* In the early stages the symptoms are troublesome only after a day or two without exposure to cotton, and the disease is known as 'Monday fever'.

C

cachexia. Loss of weight and general bodily deterioration from chronic disease.

caecum. First part of the large intestine, situated low down on the right side of the abdomen. The *appendix* opens off it. ⟡ *intestine* (1).

Caesarean section. Surgical operation : at a late stage of pregnancy the abdominal wall is opened and the incision is carried through the front of the uterus; the baby is lifted out, and the layers of the incision are stitched. Caesarean section is used when the birth-passage is too narrow for the baby, or when the placenta lies across the passage from the uterus and would be liable to bleed danger-ously during natural labour, or in any situ-ation where the health of mother or infant requires immediate delivery.

Legend has it that Julius Caesar was born in this way, but the operation may be named from an ancient law, restated by Caesar, that a woman dying in labour must be cut open in the hope of saving the child.

caffeine. Alkaloid drug extracted from cof-fee, identical with *theine* from tea. It has numerous effects, not unlike those of adren-aline. Caffeine increases alertness for a time if the subject is drowsy beforehand, but not if he is already wide awake; it also interferes with normal sleep. It dilates blood vessels and stimulates the heart. It increases the flow of urine. It relaxes the bronchi.

Caffeine is not a particularly efficient drug in any of these respects, and if it is given for the sake of one effect the other effects are a nuisance.

Cal. (abbreviation) = ⟡ *Calorie.*

calamine. Zinc carbonate or zinc oxide coloured pink with ferric oxide, used on the skin to allay itching and as a mild astringent.

calcaneum. The bone of the heel. ⟡ *foot.*

calcitonin. Hormone antagonistic to the action of *parathyroid* glands, formed by the thyroid gland.

calcium. Metallic element: its compounds are very widely distributed in mineral (e.g. chalk) deposits and in animals and plants.

In man, calcium salts resembling the mineral apatite (a compound containing calcium, fluorine, and phosphorus) form the hard framework of bones and teeth.

The blood carries about 0·01 per cent of calcium in solution, and this small amount is essential to life. Deficiency or excess of calcium in the blood seriously disturbs the function of nerve cells and muscle fibres. The correct concentration is maintained by the action of hormones (⟡ *parathyroid*).

Calcium is also necessary to the clotting of blood.

If the hormones are working properly, the vital calcium of the blood is kept constant by adjustments to the very large quantity stored in the skeleton. If there is a deficiency of calcium in the body the blood remains normal but the bones are weakened (⟡ *rickets*; *osteoporosis*). In the much less com-mon event of a surplus, e.g. with a grossly excessive intake of vitamin D, calcium may be deposited in tissues other than bone.

Calcium salts are sometimes deposited in tissues affected by injury or disease, e.g. in the walls of ageing arteries, or in scars where healing has been unduly slow. X-rays commonly show small calcified scars in the lungs, evidence that at some time in his life the patient was infected with tuberculosis and recovered – often with little or no obvi-ous illness.

Insoluble compounds such as calcium phosphate may form stones in hollow organs (⟡ *calculus*).

An average person needs about 1 gramme of calcium in his daily diet; growing child-ren, pregnant women and nursing mothers need rather more. Milk is the best source, but any good mixed diet contains enough calcium. Old people who live alone and lose interest in their diet are apt to be short of calcium; a pint of milk daily would supply their needs.

calculus. 1. Chalky deposit ('tartar') on teeth, mainly precipitated from saliva. 2. Hard insoluble mass ('stone') in any hollow organ. The common sites for stones are the urinary tract (kidneys, bladder) and the biliary system (gall bladder, bile ducts). The stones are made of substances normally dissolved in the fluid contents of the organ, which for some reason form a precipitate like the fur in a kettle.

Urinary stones are commonly of calcium phosphate or calcium oxalate. They are often associated with infection of the kidney or bladder. Infection may help to cause them, though it is difficult to see how; and the presence of a foreign body such as a stone helps to keep infection going. The only easily explained stones are of substances passed through the kidneys in greater quantities than can be dissolved, such as uric acid in people with gout.

Gall stones are of cholesterol, bile pigment, or both together with calcium salts. They, too, are often associated with infection, but they have not been satisfactorily explained.

Stones can also form in other places, such as the salivary glands.

Stones that cause symptoms generally have to be removed surgically. Small ones may find their own way out. Attempts at dissolving stones have had little if any success.

callosity. Thickening and hardening of the outermost layer of the skin in response to pressure or friction.

callus. 1. = ◊ *callosity.* **2.** Hard tissue formed at the site of a broken bone, gradually converted into new bone (◊ *fracture*).

calomel. Mercurous chloride; subchloride of mercury; HgCl. In the past it was widely used as a purgative and for the treatment of syphilis. It is less poisonous than mercuric chloride (corrosive sublimate; $HgCl_2$), but like all compounds of mercury is far from harmless.

Calorie. Unit of energy: the amount of heat required to warm a kilogram of water by 1° C. (It is spelt with capital C and known as *large calorie*; it is 1,000 ordinary calories with small c, in fact a kilocalorie.) The calorie value of food is the number of Calories it would yield if it were completely burnt. ◊ *diet*; *energy*.

camphor. A crystalline substance obtained from the camphor tree or from turpentine, formerly used to promote coughing and sweating and to stimulate vital centres in the brain; it survives as an ingredient of *paregoric* (camphorated tincture of opium) and of *camphorated oil.*

camphorated oil. A solution of camphor in cotton-seed oil used as a liniment. ◊ *counter-irritation.*

cancellous bone. Porous, spongy bone inside the solid casing of *compact* bone.

cancer. A disorder of cell growth. The millions of cells of the body are all derived from a single cell, the fertilized ovum, by a process of duplication and reduplication. All cells (except perhaps those of nerve and voluntary muscle) are capable throughout life of reproducing themselves by splitting into two.

At first, an embryo is a cluster of identical cells, of which the number is repeatedly doubled. Any one of these cells could grow into a complete organism. As growth proceeds, cells become less versatile: they are *differentiated* or specialized for the functions of particular tissues or organs. In general a differentiated cell can do three things: (1) perform a special task – e.g. one kind of cell lays down bone, another stores fat, another makes saliva; (2) look after its own nutrition; (3) replace exhausted cells by dividing to form two new cells.

At birth the nervous system has its full complement of cells, and they are so highly differentiated that they have lost the ability to replace themselves and they rely on supporting (glial) cells for their nutrition. They have to last for a lifetime. The cells of voluntary muscle do not as a rule reproduce themselves. A muscle grows by increasing the size, not the number, of its cells.

All other types of cell continue to multiply. The rate gradually slows; when growth is complete it just keeps pace with the continuous degeneration and loss of cells (in old age or times of illness it may not keep pace). How this rate is adjusted is unknown. In most organs it can be increased to meet added demands, so that lost tissue is at least partly replaced.

Cancer begins in a group of cells, or perhaps a single cell, that divides regardless of need. Although some cancer cells keep the special function of their cell-type, most tend to lose it; in fact they regress towards an embryonic type with less differentiation. The rare cancers of infancy may well arise from cells that have failed to outgrow the embryonic state, but this is no longer thought to explain adult cancer. For convenience, cancers are often classified according to the embryonic tissue they resemble, but this is no more than a useful convention. It seems clear that cancer cells arise from normal, differentiated adult cells that have changed their nature. The change is fixed: it persists in the descendants of the affected cells.

In effect, a cancer is a parasite formed from the patient's own tissues. It is a family or tribe of cells that has become alienated from its neighbours; it no longer serves as part of the integrated community of cells that is a healthy body; it is not subject to the normal control of nerves and hormones; it draws on the general supply of nutrients and contributes nothing in return.

Because they are subject to no control, and because they have nothing to do but reproduce themselves, cancer cells in time outnumber the healthy cells in their neighbourhood. They tend to spread beyond the limits of their original organ, and groups of cells may be carried in lymph vessels or veins to other parts of the body where they form *metastases*.

It is very rare for a cancer to replace so much of a vital organ that life becomes impossible, except that any kind of intruder in the brain can be fatal (a blood clot or an abscess can do harm out of all proportion to its size). It is also unusual for cancer to kill by invading a major blood vessel and causing fatal bleeding, or indeed to do anything obviously lethal. In the great majority of cases, the progressive loss of health is a complete mystery. True, the cancer competes with working tissues for food and oxygen, but its demands should not be enough to cause serious deprivation elsewhere; yet this is the ultimate effect unless the cancer can be treated.

1. Causes of Cancer

Cancer is probably no more a specific disease with a single defined cause than, say, bleeding or heart failure. It is an alteration in the behaviour of cells in response to various harmful factors, some known, many unknown; often different factors work together (rather as overeating, anxiety and lack of exercise may together cause heart disease when none of them would do so alone).

Inherited constitution plays some part:

people with a family history of cancer are rather more liable to the disease than others; but only in a few types of cancer is the hereditary factor the most important. Hereditary factors may predispose to cancer, but they are seldom if ever the sole cause.

Repeated simple injury – 'chronic irritation' – has been invoked more than any other factor; it has even been called the sole cause of cancer. But the evidence is very poor, and it is now doubtful whether cancer ever arises in this way. On the other hand, many special types of injury can certainly cause cancer. If they have anything in common, it is that they can all *prevent* cells from dividing if the dose is large enough. It is as if some critical dose interfered with the process of cell division just enough to take the brake off. Presumably they alter the genetic make-up of a cell – cause *mutation* – so that not only the reproductive behaviour of the cell is disturbed but also that of its progeny. The altered cell breeds true.

The known physical and chemical agents of cancer include *ionizing radiation*, and many chemical poisons.

Many of the pioneers of X-ray work developed cancer in exposed skin. Prolonged exposure to tropical sunlight can also cause skin cancer, and strict precautions are needed in industries that use radioactive substances. The atom bombs in Japan caused an outbreak of leukaemia (blood cancer) among the survivors.

A chemical cause of cancer was first recognized by the London surgeon Pott in 1775; he showed that soot caused cancer in chimney-sweeps. Many substances able to cause cancer (*carcinogens*) have been extracted from coal, and some lubricating oils have also been incriminated. Other carcinogens are arsenic and some intermediate products in the synthesis of dyes. None of these poisons causes cancer by occasional contamination; the trouble comes from daily exposure, month after month.

By far the most significant chemical carcinogen is ◊ *tobacco* smoke.

Several types of cancer in animals are caused by infection with viruses. A virus is little more than a parcel of genetic material, and it would not be remarkable for some of this material to become incorporated with the cell's own material and cause the kind of mutation that would lead to cancer. No virus infection has been positively identified in human cancer, but there is evidence that Burkitt's sarcoma, a cancer seen in Africa, may be due to a virus transmitted by mosquitoes.

International statistics show that wholly unsuspected causes must still await discovery. Cancer of the rectum is twice as common in Denmark as in Norway. Finland has one of the highest rates of stomach cancer yet one of the lowest of cancer of the intestine. When facts such as these are explained more will be known about causes, and therefore about what to avoid in order to prevent cancer.

2. MANAGEMENT OF CANCER

One cannot exaggerate the size of the problem. In Britain and many other countries, one death in five is from cancer. Even the best treatment is destructive. Taken reasonably early, some 80 per cent of breast cancers can be cured, but at the cost of a breast. It is the same with many other types of cancer: the best chance of permanent cure is complete removal of the cancer and any neighbouring tissue that might be involved. As long as this remains the best chance there is no sense in haggling, but nobody can pretend that wholesale removal is the ideal treatment of a disease. And there remain the inaccessible cancers and the cases recognized too late for even drastic surgery to cure.

X-rays and radioactive material are used in several ways. They completely cure some surface cancers, where the radiation can be directly applied without passing through healthy tissue. They are a valuable adjunct to surgery: irradiation may pick off stray cancer cells that the knife has missed, or at least retard the progress of disease that is no longer curable. The results of irradiating accessible cancers show that this treatment can cure; but if the cancer is deep or widespread the patient may be unable to tolerate a large enough dose. Techniques are evolving for confining the rays to their target with less damage to healthy tissue. Some cancers can be made more susceptible to radiation by increasing their supply of oxygen.

Many drugs that suppress division of cells have been used against cancer. Some are derived from the mustard gas of the First World War. A common plant, the periwinkle (*Vinca*), contains alkaloids able to retard some forms of cancer. Antibiotics are primarily drugs for treating bacterial infection. They prevent bacteria from multiplying; and a few, e.g. actinomycin, mithramycin, have a similar effect on cancer cells.

Drugs are most used in the treatment of cancers of the lymphatic system (Hodgkin's disease) and blood (leukaemia).

Both radiation and these drugs suppress cell division in general. They work because cancer cells are much more actively engaged in reproducing themselves than normal cells. The appearance and behaviour of cancer cells are distinctive, but no chemical difference from normal cells is yet known. When one is found it should be possible to attack cancer cells specifically.

Some cancers of sex organs (e.g. breast, prostate) are influenced by sex hormones and are sometimes successfully treated with a hormone of the opposite sex.

Since cancer cells differ from normal cells, they are foreign to the rest of the body, and one would expect them to provoke the same kind of response as any other foreign living matter. They should act as ◇ *antigens*, stimulate the production of ◇ *antibodies*, and so cause their own destruction by the reactions of ◇ *immunity*. This possibility has opened up a promising field of research. It has already been shown that many cancers do in fact form antigens, even though the resistance they provoke is not enough to destroy them. Once an antigen is known, it can be identified in the laboratory, so in future it may become possible to diagnose cancer by simple blood tests in the same way as an infection such as typhoid fever. And beyond this, given the presence of antigens it becomes logical to seek ways of increasing the body's response to them or immunizing the patient. This research is still only at an early stage of guarded optimism.

Treatment, then, offers much hope; cancer is by no means the incurable disease that many people think it. The picture looks gloomier than it is because one does not hear much of the many cures. When a surgeon is fairly sure that he has cured a cancer he may decide that to tell the patient the diagnosis would be pointless cruelty, because few people, knowing that they have had a cancer removed, can simply forget it. Nor do people who know necessarily wish to talk about it.

Prevention is mainly of two kinds. The first is to avoid known causes: smoking is far the most important. The second is to recognize cancer early enough for it to be cured. Screening tests for routine checking of large numbers of people are now quite extensively used. Health education may be

more important than mass examination. The Metropolitan Life Insurance Company of New York has widely publicized seven 'warning signals' that people should have investigated as soon as they appear:
1. any sore that does not heal;
2. a lump or thickening in the breast or elsewhere;
3. unusual bleeding or discharge;
4. any change in a wart or mole;
5. persistent indigestion or difficulty in swallowing;
6. persistent hoarseness or cough;
7. any change in normal bowel habits.

cancrum oris ⟡ noma.

Candida (Monilia). A fungus related to the yeasts, a normal inhabitant of the mucous membrane of the mouth and intestine which occasionally sets up infection with characteristic white patches known as thrush. As a rule, simple mouth washes clear up thrush, but in obstinate cases antibiotics (nystatin, amphotericin) may be needed. The vagina can also be affected.

Bacteria normally suppress Candida; it is apt to proliferate when bacteria are eliminated by intensive treatment of infection with the more versatile antibiotics; a further antibiotic is then needed to control the Candida until the normal bacteria of the body are re-established.

cannabis (hashish etc.) ⟡ hemp.

cantharides. An irritant of no medical value, extracted from a small beetle, the Spanish fly. Its reputation as an aphrodisiac depends on irritation of the whole urinary system, which has been known to cause failure of the kidneys and death.

canthus. Either corner of the eye.

capillary. Smallest blood vessel: blood leaves the heart in arteries and returns in veins, crossing from arteries to veins in minute vessels, the capillaries, with a diameter of about 1/100 mm. Thus capillaries are at once the least twigs of the arteries and the least tributaries of the veins.

There are many more capillaries than can be filled with blood at one time. The amount of blood circulating through an organ is adapted to the demand for oxygen and for removal of carbon dioxide by opening the entrances to an appropriate number of capillaries. The skin is exceptional; here the flow is adapted to ⟡ temperature. A capillary is opened or closed by a minute ring of muscle in the wall of the parent arteriole. There is no muscle in the capillary itself, yet it seems that capillaries are able to contract to some extent.

The small arteries (arterioles) and veins (venules) are impermeable. Exchange of materials between the blood and the tissues takes place entirely across the walls of the capillaries, which allow free passage to small molecules such as water, salts, glucose, and amino-acids, but not to proteins (⟡ tissue fluid). Solid particles, including blood cells, have been shown by electron microscopy to pass through the cells of the capillary walls.

capsule. Fibrous sheath enclosing an organ; especially the tough, flexible casing of a joint, strengthened with fibrous bands (ligaments) and lined with a slippery synovial membrane.

caput succedaneum. Fluid swelling in the scalp of a new-born baby caused by pressure during birth; often a source of anxiety to a woman with her first child unless she has seen other new-born babies. The swelling disappears in a few days.

carbachol. Synthetic drug related to acetyl choline; it has similar effects to acetyl choline but is more slowly destroyed in the body. It is used to stimulate the intestine, bladder and other organs normally activated by acetyl choline.

carbohydrate intolerance. It sometimes happens that an enzyme needed for converting a disaccharide to monosaccharides is missing from the intestine. The enzyme is most often lactose, which converts milk sugar to glucose and galactose, but failure to break down maltose and sucrose also occurs. The deficiency may be congenital or it may arise in adult life.

Disaccharides are not adequately absorbed from the intestine. If they cannot be converted to absorbable monosaccharides they remain in the intestine and attract water by osmosis, which causes diarrhoea; in fact unabsorbable carbohydrates can be used as purgatives. If one has no lactase, a glass of milk acts as a dose of salts. Bacterial fermentation of unabsorbed sugar in the large intestine causes flatulence and discomfort.

Carbohydrate intolerance has only lately been recognized. It may be a much commoner cause of digestive trouble than at present appears. It is cured by avoiding the offending sugar.

carbohydrates. A large class of compounds of carbon, hydrogen, and oxygen, including sugars and starches. They are found in all living cells; the ultimate source is green plants which synthesize them from carbon dioxide and water under the influence of sunlight; ◊ *energy*.

The simplest form of carbohydrate is a *monosaccharide* – a simple sugar. There are two groups of these in human chemistry: the *pentoses* with the general formula $(CH_2O)_5$ and the *hexoses* $(CH_2O)_6$. Much the most important pentose is *ribose*, a component of *nucleic acids* (DNA and RNA), which are the chemical basis of life itself.

Apart from ribose, the carbohydrates of the body are either hexoses (*glucose, fructose, galactose*), or compounds of two or more hexoses. Two hexoses form a *disaccharide*. A chain of disaccharides forms a *polysaccharide*.

The three disaccharides of the diet are *maltose* (glucose + glucose), *sucrose* or cane sugar (glucose + fructose), and *lactose* or milk sugar (glucose + galactose).

The only important polysaccharide in the human diet is *starch*. Its molecules are long branched chains of maltose; it is converted to maltose by enzymes in saliva and pancreatic juice. A very similar compound to starch, widely distributed in plants (e.g. grass) is *cellulose*, which is useless as human food because man has no enzyme for converting cellulose to maltose. (Nor has a cow, but a cow's stomach contains bacteria that break down cellulose.)

All the 'human' carbohydrates can be converted by enzymes to glucose.

Carbohydrate is broken down to monosaccharides in the intestine before it can be assimilated into the blood-stream. It passes to the liver, where most of it is stored as a polysaccharide, *glycogen* (animal starch). Muscle also contains a store of glycogen. As glucose is used up in the tissues to provide energy, the concentration of glucose in the blood (about 0·1 per cent) tends to fall. This stimulates the breakdown of enough glycogen to restore the level.

The ultimate fate of carbohydrate is combustion of carbon dioxide and water with release of energy (a reversal of the photosynthesis by which plants make carbohydrate). One gramme of carbohydrate yields 4·1 Calories. With very few exceptions (e.g. Eskimos) carbohydrates provide most of the energy of a diet, but a mixture of different classes of food is essential to health (◊ *diet*). The simplest way to reduce is to cut down carbohydrate and leave other foods to look after themselves.

Since all carbohydrates end as glucose, the choice ought not to matter. Yet there is evidence that refined sugar (sucrose) contributes to disease of the arteries (◊ *atheroma*), whereas other carbohydrates do not.

carbon dioxide. Colourless gas, a component of air (0·03 per cent), assimilated by plants for the synthesis of carbohydrates, and given off by all living organisms (animal and plant) as the end-product of respiration.

Carbon dioxide is formed throughout the body and carried by the veins to the lungs. Some is dissolved in the plasma but most is carried in the red blood cells. In the lungs, carbon dioxide is released from the blood. Inspired air contains only 0·03 per cent, but expired air contains about 4 per cent.

The concentration of carbon dioxide in the blood is the main stimulus to breathing. The excess formed during exertion reinforces the reflexes controlling rate and depth of breathing, so that carbon dioxide is eliminated more quickly. This has the effect of supplying more oxygen, which is needed because oxygen uptake and carbon dioxide output are exactly balanced. An excess of carbon dioxide in a tissue also increases the flow of blood.

Carbon dioxide (about 5 per cent in air or oxygen) is sometimes used to stimulate breathing.

Although not as deadly as carbon monoxide, carbon dioxide is poisonous in concentrations over about 6 per cent. It leads to over-stimulation of the heart, depression of reflexes, and finally unconsciousness and death. But except in case of asphyxia, carbon dioxide poisoning is unusual because it tends to right itself by increased breathing. Slight symptoms of poisoning are common with severe chronic disease of the lungs, e.g. chronic bronchitis, because breathing is impaired to the point of slight asphyxia. The patient may get used to a high concentration of carbon dioxide and no longer respond by breathing more deeply.

carbon monoxide. A poisonous component of coal gas, exhaust fumes, and most smoke.

It combines with the haemoglobin of the blood in exactly the same way as oxygen; but it does so 300 times as readily as oxygen. From a mixture of 300 parts oxygen to 1 carbon monoxide the blood will take up equal quantities. Air contains only 1 part in 5 of oxygen; therefore a 1:1500 concentration of carbon monoxide will displace half the oxygen of the blood. The effect is worse than losing half the blood, because the oxygen that remains is not given up in the tissues to be used. So a concentration of 1:1500 is likely to be lethal, and very much lower concentrations cause severe illness.

Carbon monoxide poisoning differs from ordinary asphyxia in the patient's bright pink complexion, instead of the blue of asphyxia. It is treated by giving pure oxygen if possible, or otherwise fresh air, which gradually displaces the carbon monoxide from the blood. ◊ *Artificial respiration* may be needed.

carbuncle. Bacterial infection (usually by staphylococci) in the skin, of the same kind as a boil but larger and deeper; a carbuncle can be regarded as several boils run together. The back of the neck, where the hair roots are especially liable to infection, is the commonest site. The principles of treatment are the same as with a ◊ *boil*, except that surgery and antibiotics are more often needed.

carcinogen. Any substance liable to cause ◊ *cancer* (1).

carcinoma. Literally = cancer; generally applied to one group of cancers, the commoner, arising in covering and lining membranes (as opposed to *sarcoma*, cancer arising in bone, connective tissue, muscle etc.).

cardiac. Of the heart (also: of the part of the stomach nearest the heart).

Cardiac massage has become an important method of resuscitation, as an adjunct to *artificial respiration*, in cases where breathing and heart beat have stopped. Firm pressure on the lower half of the sternum is applied with the heel of the palm once a second. In an adult the sternum is depressed about an inch by leaning on both hands. In children light pressure with two fingers is enough, and the rate is rather faster. Because cardiac massage has been known to break ribs of people who did not need resuscitation there has been some opposition to teaching it to otherwise untrained people, but against this view is the fact that if cardiac massage is needed at all it is needed at once. If the heart is out of action for more than a very few minutes there is no chance of survival.

cardiology. Branch of physiology and medicine concerned with the heart.

caries. **1.** Dental decay; ◊ *teeth* (3). **2.** Tuberculosis of bone.

carminative. Drug alleged to relieve flatulence, e.g. cardamom, coriander and other spices, gentian and other bitters. Carminatives tempt appetite and thus set up reflex activity of the stomach and intestine: they belong to imaginative catering rather than to medicine.

carotene. Orange pigment of carrots and many other vegetables, also found in egg yolk and milk; converted in the body to vitamin A.

carotid artery. Main artery of the head. The two common carotid arteries run straight up the neck at either side of the trachea, under cover of the sternomastoid muscles. Above the level of the Adam's apple the common carotid divides into external and internal carotid arteries.

The external carotid sends branches to the neck, face and scalp. Only one small branch, the middle meningeal artery, enters the skull. It lies in a deep groove on the inner surface of the side of the skull, and is readily torn if the bone is fractured. Bleeding from this vessel is one of the most important hazards of head injuries. It requires prompt surgery.

The internal carotid arteries pass through the floor of the skull to the brain, of which they supply the top and front with blood. The rest of the brain is supplied by the ◊ *vertebral* arteries. Although all these arteries meet at the ◊ *circle of Willis* to provide an alternative supply if one is blocked, this is not an efficient system and the brain can be injured by interference with any one of its arteries. Partial blockage of a carotid artery by ◊ *atheroma* is a common precursor of a ◊ *stroke*. Sometimes the blockage can be cleared surgically.

carotid body. Small gland in the angle between the external and internal carotid arteries. It is sensitive to changes in the concentrations of oxygen and carbon dioxide in the blood, and responds by releasing hormones that act on the parts of the brain controlling respiration.

carotid sinus. Bulge in the wall of the carotid artery at its division into external and internal branches. It contains nerve endings sensitive to changes of pressure, and is concerned in maintaining a steady pressure of blood, above all to the brain. If the sinuses are squeezed, e.g. by a judo stranglehold, the blood pressure falls by reflex action and the victim may lose consciousness.

carpal tunnel. A fibrous bridge, the *flexor retinaculum*, spans the small bones at the base of the palm of the hand. The carpal tunnel is the opening between the flexor retinaculum and the bones. The flexor tendons to the fingers pass through this tunnel, enclosed in slippery synovial sheaths which prevent friction in this narrow space. Between the tendons is the ◊ *median* nerve.

The *carpal tunnel syndrome* arises from compression of the median nerve in the tunnel. In the hand, the median nerve carries motor fibres to the muscles of the ball of the thumb and sensory fibres from the thumb and the index, middle, and ring fingers. Pressure on the nerve causes pins-and-needles, numbness, or pain in this area, and sometimes weakness of the thumb. Arthritis or injury of the wrist may produce this syndrome, but usually there is no obvious reason for it. The fact that it is commonest in middle-aged women and during pregnancy suggests a glandular disturbance. The symptoms are often worst after lying down. Some cases respond to splinting the wrist at night. Injection of hydrocortisone usually gives at least temporary relief. If these simple measures fail, the condition is often cured by cutting the constricting fibres of the retinaculum.

carpus. Base of the ◊ *hand*; of its eight small carpal bones three articulate with the forearm to form the wrist-joint.

carrier. Person who harbours an infectious microbe without ill effects. About 10 per cent of healthy people carry dangerous streptococci in their noses, and as many as 50 per cent carry staphylococci; unless they take precautions such as wearing a mask when treating patients with open wounds they may convey serious infection.

Some people recover from infection without completely eliminating the bacteria: they establish a sort of truce, by which they and the bacteria tolerate each other, but at any time they may infect others who have not yet had the disease. Diphtheria and typhoid fever can be carried in this way.

Subclinical infection is like a temporary carrier state. One may actually have a disease without any obvious symptoms; for instance most people with poliomyelitis suffer no more than a mild stomach upset but during the attack – which passes unrecognized – others can contract the serious form of the disease with paralysis from them.

cartilage. Gristle; the tough, smooth, milk-white tissue which coats the moving surfaces of the joints; called *hyaline* cartilage to distinguish it from fibrocartilage and elastic cartilage (see below).

Apart from the clavicles and most of the skull the whole skeleton of the embryo is formed in cartilage which is gradually replaced by bone. At birth the shafts of the principal bones are of real bone but the expanded ends are still cartilaginous. When growth is complete only thin sheets of cartilage remain.

Unlike bone, cartilage has no blood vessels. It therefore lacks many of the properties of other living tissues. It cannot become inflamed, and cannot heal if it is cut or broken. It has few diseases, but those few tend to be irreversible. ◊ *Achondroplasia* is a hereditary defect of embryonic cartilage: all the bones that are preformed in cartilage remain underdeveloped. In ◊ *rickets* the replacement of cartilage by bone fails.

In the two most important diseases of joints, ◊ *osteoarthritis* and ◊ *rheumatoid arthritis*, the cartilages at the ends of the bones are eroded and roughened.

The living cartilage cells, embedded in their plastic ground-substance (◊ *tissue*), can form a tumour – a *chondroma* – which is usually slow-growing and harmless apart from the mechanical nuisance of any abnormal lump in a tissue.

Fibrocartilage is not so much cartilage as exceedingly dense and tough fibrous tissue. It is the material of the intervertebral discs between the ◊ *vertebrae* – the shock-absorbers of the backbone – and of the pads, like washers, between the bones of certain joints such as the *knee*. *Elastic cartilage* is the rubbery tissue of the ear.

cascara sagrada. Dried bark of *Rhamnus purshiana*, an American tree; it contains various anthracene compounds that act as laxatives by irritating the large intestine.

castor oil. = Ricinus oil; extracted from the seeds of a subtropical bush, *Ricinus communis*. Castor oil as such is so completely inert that it is safely used to protect the very sensitive membrane covering the eye. But the digestion of castor oil in the stomach releases *ricinoleic acid,* which irritates the small intestine. The fluid contents of the intestine are propelled so rapidly that they reach the rectum before most of the water has had time to be absorbed: thus castor oil is a quick-acting laxative.

catabolism. Chemical breakdown in the body of complex substances to simple ones (e.g. proteins to amino-acids); the reverse process is *anabolism.*

catalepsy. A kind of hysterical or self-induced trance, in which the patient remains fixed in even the unlikeliest position, as in the children's game 'statues'.

catalyst ◊ *enzyme.*

cataplasm = ◊ *poultice.*

cataract. Opacity of the lens of the eye, causing dimness of vision; if the cataract progresses, useful vision is completely lost, though light and dark can be distinguished. The defect is confined to the lens; when this is removed vision returns and only the ability to focus is lost. The front of the eye is a powerful compound lens of which the 'lens' itself is only a minor component for altering the focus. Most of the strength of the compound lens is provided by the curved front of the eye, which is not affected by cataract and remains after the lens has been removed. Restoration of sight by this comparatively simple operation is one of the most dramatic and rewarding events in the whole practice of medicine.

Most cataracts are a result of ageing, but some are a result of injury and some, occurring in infancy, are due to faulty development of the lens.

catarrh. Any inflammation of a mucous membrane with excessive formation of mucus. As a technical term, catarrh is almost obsolete, but it is still in general use for inflammation of the mucous membrane of the nose – *rhinitis* (◊ *nose* (1)).

catatonia. A severe form of schizophrenia: during an attack the patient seems wholly out of touch with his surroundings. He may show purposeless excitement, or pass into a kind of trance when he is as still as a wax dummy. Between attacks he may behave normally. A similar condition can be seen in a deep hypnotic trance.

catgut. Surgical catgut is similar to that used for stringed musical instruments. It is the fibrous layer of sheep's intestine, toughened with chromic acid. Catgut ligatures are easy to handle, and they are slowly digested in the tissues, finally disappearing without trace.

catharsis. Cleansing; purging – either of the intestine by *cathartic* drugs (◊ *purgative*) or of the emotions by psychoanalysis, when a suppressed memory, the hidden cause of emotional conflict and illness, is brought into the open. In principle this is similar to the catharsis that Aristotle said was the purpose of the theatre.

cat-scratch fever. Virus infection transmitted by cats: a small abscess appears at the site of the scratch after an interval of a week; there is some fever, and lymph nodes are enlarged all over the body (neck, armpits, groins). The original sore may take some time to heal, but otherwise recovery is rapid and complete.

cauliflower ear. Deformity of the ear due to bleeding or infection between the supporting cartilage and its covering membrane; this separates the cartilage from its blood vessels and causes it to degenerate, while an irregular mass of fibrous (scar) tissue is formed as a result of persistent inflammation.

cautery. The branding-iron or cautery is a very ancient tool for the treatment of disease. It was used in ancient Egypt to stop bleeding, and Hippocrates advised treatment by fire as a last resort when medicine and surgery had failed.

The medieval use of cautery to burn out such conditions as epilepsy was pure superstition, but cautery to treat wounds, ulcers and cancers was rational if cruel. It stops bleeding and kills bacteria along with the patient's tissues. But the burnt tissue is an ideal haven for the next bacteria to arrive; in it they can breed without interference from the natural defences of living tissue, and in the long run a cauterized wound is worse infected than a wound left to itself. As long as pus was considered 'laudable' surgeons positively sought infection, and the cautery was not seriously challenged until the 16th century when Ambroise Paré showed that wounds did better without it.

A kind of electric cautery is used in modern surgery. It produces an almost microscopically small burn. It coagulates bleeding points too small to be closed with ligatures, and used as an electric knife it cuts delicate tissue bloodlessly, sealing the cut edge as it goes. Sometimes the light-sensitive membrane of the eye (*retina*) becomes detached from the inside wall of the eye, and a form of cautery is used to stick it in place. A laser beam – a concentrated form of light – serves this purpose well, and lasers are likely to find many other applications in surgery. Extreme cold, e.g. from liquid nitrogen, also 'burns' tissue and can be used as a cautery.

c.c. Cubic centimetre. In many contexts, millilitre (ml.) is the more exact term, but the difference is very small indeed. In this book 'c.c.', the more familiar term, is used for both.

CDH. Congenital dislocation of the ⟡ *hip*.

cell. The smallest unit of the body that is capable of independent life. The whole body is a community of individual cells of which the primary function is to maintain a suitable environment for themselves and for each other. Physiology – the study of normal function – shows how each type of cell contributes to the task of preserving constant conditions within the body in the face of constant change outside it. Pathology – the study of disease – shows what happens when the balance is disturbed.

A cell is a blob of jelly, the *cytoplasm*, mainly a solution of protein, in a fine but strong container, the *cell membrane*. Most cells have a dense kernel, the *nucleus*, which directs the activity of the rest of the cell, and various *organelles* that can be discerned only with an electron microscope. Even these tiny structures have enclosing membranes, which can hardly be more than a molecule thick. Among the organelles found in all cells are *mitochondria*, where combustion takes place to provide energy for the cell's activities, and *ribosomes* for the synthesis of proteins. With few exceptions cells can reproduce themselves by dividing into two cells, each an exact replica of the original one. (In an embryo, successive generations of cells are not identical: they are modified to form different tissues and organs.)

In a suitable environment, a cell remains alive on its own; but the conditions have to be exactly right. Isolated cells from every part of the human body have been kept alive in tissue cultures, under carefully regulated conditions of temperature and chemical supplies, and most kinds of cell have been persuaded to multiply. But tissue culture is a most laborious business. Slight changes in the environment are enough to kill the cells.

Robert Hooke recognized the cellular structure of plants in 1665, but it was not until 1839 that Theodor Schwann showed that the structure of plants and animals was fundamentally the same. Schwann thought that cells arose spontaneously in a formless ground-substance, but within the next twenty years it was shown that the ground-substance was formed by cells, and that every cell was the offspring of a cell. Each of the millions of cells in the body has arisen by division and subdivision from the single cell formed at conception.

The largest cell of the human body – the *ovum* – is just visible to the naked eye. Most human cells are much smaller, about 0·01 mm. in diameter.

cellular pathology. The doctrine that the processes of disease are to be studied in the changes undergone by individual cells. It is the title of Rudolf ⟡ *Virchow's* great masterpiece, published in 1858.

cellular tissue. Loosely woven connective tissue, allowing movement between adjacent structures, e.g. the tissue beneath the skin, which allows a good deal of play between the skin and the underlying bundles of muscle.

cellulitis. Inflammation of cellular tissue, commonly due to infection by streptococci from contaminated wounds. The open structure of cellular tissue allows the infection to spread, and cellulitis was always very dangerous until the discovery of drugs (sulphonamides; penicillin) that effectively control streptococcal infection.

Celsus, Aulus Cornelius (1st century A.D.). Author of the earliest Latin medical treatise (and also of books now lost on veterinary medicine, agriculture, and philosophy). The eight surviving volumes are a survey of medical history and practice. They represent all that was best in Graeco-Roman medicine. Celsus advocated sensible and humane treatment in the manner of Hippocrates. He described surgical operations of remarkable difficulty, including one for removing a goitre.

He is particularly remembered for his account of the signs of inflammation: redness and swelling, with heat and pain. Celsus's books were neglected during the Middle Ages, but with the Renaissance they became the first medical works to be printed (Florence, 1478).

cephaloridine. An antibiotic, chemically related to penicillin.

cerebellum. Part of the brain occupying the hindmost part of the floor of the skull. Its surface, like that of the cerebral hemispheres, is covered with grey matter and thrown into folds or *convolutions*, but the folds are much narrower. The cerebellum is mainly concerned with the reflex adjustment of voluntary movements, with muscle tone, and with balance.

A voluntary movement (turning a screw-driver) is described under ◊ *muscle* (2). The kind of movement to be made is 'decided' by cells in the cerebral cortex, but the technical details such as which muscles are to contract and which to relax are left to the cerebellum. If the cerebellum is injured the muscles lose their normal tone (i.e. they become flabby) and all movement becomes inaccurate in both force and direction. The gait is unbalanced and all deliberate movements are shaky instead of smooth. The gaze cannot be fixed: it wanders and has to be repeatedly brought back. This oscillation of the eyes is called *nystagmus*. Even the muscles of the larynx are affected so that each syllable has to be spoken as a separate word. The whole picture is reminiscent of drunkenness.

cerebral cortex ◊ *cerebrum.*

cerebral hemisphere ◊ *cerebrum.*

cerebral palsy = ◊ *spastic paralysis.*

cerebrospinal fever. Epidemic meningitis, a bacterial infection due to the *meningococcus*, a microbe that many healthy people carry in their throats. Outbreaks of illness seldom occur unless people are over-crowded, e.g. in barracks or at sea.

There are three grades of infection. 1. Most people get rid of meningococci without serious symptoms, or they simply harbour them without suffering infection (◊ *carrier*). 2. Infection spreads from the nose and throat to the blood-stream, causing fever with a characteristic rash (*spotted fever*). 3. In the most serious form, infection lodges in the *meninges* – the membranes covering the brain and spinal cord. This is the real cerebrospinal fever.

Meningococci are very sensitive to sulphonamide and antibiotic drugs, and what used to be a most dangerous disease can now almost always be rapidly controlled.

◊ *meningitis.*

cerebrospinal fluid (CSF). A watery fluid surrounding the brain and spinal cord, filling the space between two layers of the ◊ *meninges* and also the ventricles of the brain and the narrow central canal of the spinal cord. CSF is derived from the blood in the *choroid plexuses*, networks of small blood vessels protruding into the ventricles of the brain. It circulates through the ventricles, which communicate with the space between the meninges by small openings in the fourth ventricle, between the cerebellum and the brain-stem. It is reabsorbed into the veins of the skull and backbone. The formation and absorption of CSF are balanced to maintain a constant pressure.

The CSF serves the brain and cord as a shock-absorber.

The passages between the ventricles and from the ventricles to the meninges are narrow. If one is congenitally defective or blocked by inflammation the pressure of fluid inside the brain rises. In infants the skull, which is still plastic, may become greatly enlarged (◊ *hydrocephalus*). With a rigid adult skull increased pressure is a surgical emergency.

Examination of the CSF is important in the diagnosis of disorders of the brain and meninges. Normal CSF is a clear solution mainly of glucose and salts. Blood-stained fluid indicates bleeding, and pus cells and bacteria indicate infection. Minor changes in the chemical composition may be equally important clues.

◊ *lumbar puncture.*

cerebrum. The largest and most highly evolved part of the brain. It consists of two large outgrowths from the forward or upper end of the brain-stem, the *cerebral hemispheres*. Each hemisphere has a central cavity (ventricle) filled with cerebro-spinal fluid. Around the cavity are clusters of nerve cells or grey matter, the *thalamus* and *basal ganglia*, concerned with more or less instinctive behaviour. These are connected by a zone of nerve fibres or white matter with an outer coating of grey matter, the *cerebral cortex.*

The cortex forms most of the surface of the brain. The area is large because the whole surface is thrown into folds (a fold is a *gyrus*; a cleft between gyri is a *sulcus*). The nerve cells of the cortex are concerned with the conscious and intelligent activities of the nervous system.

Neither voluntary movement nor conscious sensation depends wholly on the cortex. Semi-automatic actions such as walking, once they have been thoroughly learnt, seem to be delegated from the cortex to lower centres; the cortex is then needed only to direct them. Skilled, dexterous movements do, however, depend largely on the cortex. Nor does damage to the cortex lead to anaesthesia of the corresponding part of the body; rather it dulls sensation and makes it impossible to interpret what is felt. Hearing, though impaired, is not entirely lost if the auditory area of the cortex is destroyed. On the other hand destruction of the visual area does cause total blindness. Briefly, the cortex plays an important part in consciousness but not the only part. Consciousness itself depends on the reticular formation in the brain-stem; the emotions are largely a function of the hypothalamus; movement and sensation are both possible without the cortex. Its function seems to be to refine the activities of the lower centres, which is as much a matter of suppressing activities as of initiating them.

Willis, in 1664, suggested that the cerebrum might be concerned with voluntary, the cerebellum with involuntary actions. This was confirmed experimentally by Rolando in 1809. At the end of the 18th century Gall made important studies of the location in the brain of different functions but then allowed himself to be diverted into the absurdities of phrenology. A century later Hughlings Jackson identified the area of the cortex concerned with movements. Considerable areas have now been plotted, thanks largely to the work of Penfield. Adjacent to each of the clearly defined areas (vision, general sensation, particular movements etc.) is an *association area*, in which the specific function is co-ordinated with others. One such area is especially important: the speech centre next to the area for movements of the mouth and throat, usually on the left side. In general, one side of the cortex (and of the whole brain) is concerned with the opposite side of the body, but many functions are represented on both sides. This often allows some return of lost function after damage to the cortex, e.g. from bleeding; the opposite side of the brain learns to deputize.

cervical. 1. Of the neck. **2.** Of the *cervix uteri.*

Cervical screening is microscopical examination of cells shed from the *cervix uteri*; by this means the earliest stage of cancer of the cervix can be detected and eradicated before it has any chance to spread.

cervix uteri. Neck of the womb; the part of the ◊ *uterus* that projects into the upper part of the vagina. It is a powerful ring of muscle, closed at most times but able to expand widely during childbirth.

Cesalpinus (Andrea Cesalpino) (1524–1603). Pupil of ◊ *Columbus*; physician; professor of botany at Pisa. He is said by some historians to have anticipated Harvey's discovery of the circulation of blood, but the claim is not well founded. Cesalpino had learnt from Columbus that blood circulated through the lungs, and from his own observations that blood in the veins flowed towards the heart. But he did not recognize that the heart was a pump, or that the blood flowed continuously. In fact he thought it flowed outwards in the arteries by day and back in the veins by night as a result of cooling.

Cesalpino's undisputed claim to immortality is as the founder of systematic botany.

cetrimide. An ◊ *antiseptic* of the detergent type, suitable for cleansing the skin.

Chagas' disease. South American variety of *trypanosomiasis* (◊ *trypanosome*).

chancre. Localized inflammation at the point of entry of an infection that later produces its main effects in other parts of the body; the earliest sign of ◊ *syphilis*. The syphilitic chancre is a small painless lump that may pass unnoticed unless it forms an ulcer. It usually recovers quickly, and for some time the patient has no symptoms at all; but in due course the signs of widespread infection appear.

Some other infectious diseases are heralded by a chancre, e.g. sleeping sickness.

chancroid (soft sore). A venereal disease, less common than gonorrhoea or syphilis, caused by Ducrey's bacillus. The usual symptom is a painful and persistent ulcer, often with swelling of lymph nodes in the groins. The infection responds well to sulphonamide drugs.

charcoal. Activated charcoal holds to its surface (adsorbs) many substances including some poisons. It is therefore commonly given as an antidote. It is also used for the relief of flatulence.

Chauliac, Guy de (*c.* 1300–1370). Physician and surgeon at the papal court in Avignon. His account of the treatment of wounds and fractures became the standard text. He recognized the need to cleanse wounds, bring the edges together and hold them in place, and protect them from further damage; but like most of his contemporaries he thought that pus was to be encouraged. He gave narcotic drugs before operating on patients.

Guy de Chauliac wrote classic accounts of the plague (he survived an attack of the Black Death) and of leprosy.

chaulmoogra. The seed of an Indian tree, *Hydnocarpus*; formerly the standard treatment of leprosy but now supplanted by sulphones and other synthetic drugs.

chelating agent. Substance of which the molecules can engulf molecules of a metal. Synthetic chelating agents are used to treat poisoning by metals such as lead.

cheloid ◊ *keloid*.

chemotheraphy. Treatment of infection with drugs (originally synthetic, but now including natural antibiotics) that poison the infecting microbes without serious harm to the patient.

chest ◊ *thorax*.

Cheyne-Stokes respiration. (John Cheyne (1777–1836) and William Stokes (1804–78), physicians in Dublin.) A pattern of breathing common in severe illness: instead of the normal rhythm, successive breaths are deeper, then shallower until breathing seems to stop; then the cycle is repeated. Some 23 centuries before Cheyne and Stokes, Hippocrates perfectly described it as like a person 'remembering to breathe'.

chickenpox (varicella). The most infectious and one of the commonest of virus diseases. Since an attack generally confers life-long immunity, chickenpox is seen mostly in children. After an incubation period of a fortnight, the temperature rises and an itchy rash appears almost at once. It consists of small raised spots, later turning to inflamed blisters. Fresh spots develop for several days, first on the trunk, later on the face and limbs. Scarring is unusual. The patient recovers in a few days, but is considered infectious until the last spot has formed a scab and flaked off.

The same virus causes ◊ *herpes* zoster or shingles.

chigger. 1. *Sand-flea*, a small insect common in hot countries; it burrows into the skin and causes severe itching. **2.** *Harvest mite*, another small insect with an itchy bite.

chilblain. An exaggerated response to cold. In everyone, the flow of blood through the skin decreases when the skin is chilled; in this way the body is protected from losing too much heat. In people whose skin is abnormally sensitive to cold, the blood vessels of the skin contract so much that the skin is deprived of blood and oxygen. This causes swelling, itching, and a characteristic burning sensation, usually confined to the fingers and toes but sometimes affecting the ears and other parts. Prevention, by keeping the sensitive areas warm, is much more effective than treatment. Smoking further reduces the circulation of blood in the skin; alcohol improves it.

childbirth. ⟡ *labour* as regards the mother, and ⟡ *birth* as regards the baby.

chill. Shivering attack (*rigor*) due to illness (nearly always infection): the immediate cause of raised body-temperature.

Chinese medicine. The traditional medical practices of China are very ancient: they have persisted almost unchanged for five millennia. Only a few broad generalizations can be made here, for the whole concept of Chinese medicine is alien to Western thought. It is based on philosophical speculation, in which neither observed events nor deductions play any part. To discuss it in the terms of Western science or even, perhaps, in a European language is like trying to explain poetry by algebra.

The body, like everything else, is governed by the two essences Yin and Yang, which are at once opposed and complementary. Health is a perfect balance of the two. Yin is female. It dominates earth, moon, winter, water. Yang is male and dominates heaven, sun, summer, and fire.

There are five elements (wood, fire, earth, metal, and water) and likewise five of many other things. Five solid Yin organs correspond with five hollow Yang organs, and each pair responds to a tissue. The triads are as follows. Lungs (Yin) and large intestine (Yang) respond to skin; heart and small intestine to arteries, liver and gall bladder to ligaments, spleen and stomach to muscle, kidney and bladder to bone or hair.

Yin and Yang are stored in three receptacles called burning spaces, from which they are conveyed through the body by twelve meridians. Neither the burning spaces nor the meridians actually exist in any physical sense, but since Yin and Yang are invisible essences they do not need visible structures for their storage and transport.

Disease is a disturbance of the balance between Yin and Yang by influences such as emotion and weather. The diagnosis is made by examination of the pulse at both wrists. Each organ has its characteristic effect on the pulse, and the examination may take a long time. Its object is to determine the exact site of the harmful excess of Yin or Yang.

Two methods of treating such an excess are well enough known to have been used beyond China. These are *moxibustion* and *acupuncture*.

Moxibustion is setting fire to a small heap of dried mugwort on the skin over the affected meridian.

Acupuncture is the insertion of needles at precisely determined points on the meridians, to allow the harmful accumulations to escape. This encourages the blood to circulate, moistens the bones and ligaments, and lubricates the joints.

There are several points of resemblance to Western beliefs, past or present. Three of the four Greek elements (earth, fire, and water) are among the Chinese five, and there is a clear resemblance between the Greek ⟡ *humours* and Chinese theory. In all Romance languages earth, moon, and water are feminine, and sky, sun, and fire are masculine nouns. But nothing in the foregoing account has ever been verified; indeed none of it is open to verification. It must be taken on trust, or rejected.

If the almost mystical theories of Chinese medicine cannot be reconciled with Western scientific method, there is still much to be learnt from the practice. The most revered physician in the history of Europe, Hippocrates, based his practice on wrong ideas of bodily functions, yet nobody doubts his professional competence.

Chinese doctors practised inoculation against smallpox centuries before anyone else. They saw the importance of cleanliness (which is by no means obvious) and the therapeutic value of bathing. Their extensive materia medica includes drugs later adopted by Western medicine. The most important of these is *ma huang* or ephedrine.

Certain principles of Chinese medicine deserve close study everywhere. Its first object is the prevention rather than the cure of disease — ensured by paying the doctor only while his patient remains well. Its underlying theories emphasize the dependence of one part of the body on the rest, and of the patient on his surroundings. Scientific medicine, by analysing the whole into its parts and by encouraging the specialist, is apt to lose sight of these things.

In modern Chinese hospitals students have to learn traditional as well as scientific medicine, and practitioners of both kinds work side by side, each studying the other's methods. By all accounts the system works well.

chiropractic. A system of treatment mainly by manipulation of the backbone, said to relieve pressure on nerves to allow them to function freely so that the body can restore itself to health. Chiropractic is one of several systems that appeared in the United States during the 19th century. It was invented by D. D. Palmer who had no formal scientific training but had considered the problems of ill-health for some years before this idea came to him. Superficially the methods resemble those of ◊ *osteopathy*, but the theory is quite distinct. ◊ *manipulation*.

chloral hydrate. Synthetic drug for promoting sleep; introduced in the 19th century as an alternative to bromides, it was generally supplanted in the 20th by the barbiturate hypnotics. It has a very disagreeable bitter taste, but it is safer than most hypnotics, especially for children, and has never completely lost favour.

chloramine-T. An effective and safe antiseptic, used for disinfecting wounds.

chloramphenicol. An antibiotic, originally extracted from the fungus *Streptomyces venezuelae* but now synthesized. It is effective against a wide range of infections, including typhoid and typhus fevers and whooping cough.

chlorine. Chlorine gas is a corrosive poison. Inhalation (e.g. by troops gassed in the First World War) causes a violent bronchitis which may be rapidly lethal or may leave permanent damage to the lungs by replacement of normal lung tissue with useless scar tissue. Strong solutions are poisonous when swallowed, e.g. as bleaching powder. It injures or destroys the mucous membranes of the mouth, throat and stomach. Sodium thiosulphate (photographer's hypo) is to some extent an antidote.

Chlorine is a valuable antiseptic, especially for making water safe for drinking.

chloroform (trichlormethane). $CHCl_3$; discovered in 1831 and first used as an ◊ *anaesthetic* in 1847.

chloroquine. Antimalarial drug, introduced in 1946 as an alternative to quinacrine. It cures attacks of malaria, and taken weekly it suppresses attacks. It is also effective against amoebic infection of the liver (◊ *dysentery* (1)).

Chloroquine sometimes suppresses symptoms of rheumatoid arthritis and some skin diseases. The mechanism is not known.

chlorosis. Very severe anaemia with yellow or greenish pallor, formerly common among young women, due to lack of iron. ◊ *anaemia* (B.1).

chlorpromazine. A powerful drug used as a ◊ *tranquillizer*: introduced in 1954, it is the prototype of the *phenothiazine* group.

chol(e)-. Prefix = 'of the ◊ *bile*'.

cholecyst(o)-. Prefix = 'of the ◊ *gall* bladder'.

cholera. An acute infection caused by *Vibrio cholerae*, a short, curved bacterium ('comma bacillus'); contracted from food or drinking water contaminated by human faeces. The disease is transmitted by people with cholera or about to develop symptoms or very recently recovered. There are no unaffected carriers of these bacteria (as there are, for instance, of typhoid bacilli).

After a short incubation period (1–6 days) during which the bacteria multiply rapidly in the duodenum, violent diarrhoea sets in. Within hours of the onset the patient is so thoroughly purged that his motions are no more than water with dissolved salts and flakes of shed mucous membrane. In an extreme case the amount of water passed from the intestine in 24 hours may be a quarter of the total body weight. Loss of alkali (bicarbonate) causes ◊ *acidosis*, and loss of potassium salts disturbs the conduction of electrical impulses, especially in the heart. Any of these three effects – dehydration, acidosis, loss of potassium – can be rapidly lethal. The mortality of untreated cholera is over 50 per cent.

The infection never spreads beyond the intestine, and it has no important effect other than diarrhoea. Cholera, more than any other serious illness, is a disease of one symptom. If the losses of water, alkali and potassium are made good then complete recovery is the rule. Early in this century Sir Leonard Rogers reduced the mortality among his patients in India from 50 per cent to 5 per cent simply by replacing salt and water.

Antibiotics probably hasten recovery but they are of secondary importance; it is by maintaining the chemical balance of the body fluids that lives are saved.

Vaccination against cholera is effective for a shorter time than other kinds of vaccination: people continually exposed to a risk of infection are revaccinated twice a year.

Cholera is overcome by prevention rather than treatment, and since human excrement is the only source of infection, adequate sanitation eradicates the disease: if nobody with the infection contaminates food or drinking water, cholera cannot spread. This was first recognized in 1849, by John Snow. Snow was a London doctor, a pioneer of anaesthesia. Five years later, Snow showed that all the victims of an outbreak in London had drunk water from the same pump in Broad Street, and he inferred that the pump had been contaminated with sewage. The pump-handle was removed, and the outbreak stopped. This was 27 years before Koch's discovery of the germ of cholera, and in fact years before any disease could be definitely ascribed to bacteria.

cholestasis. Stagnation of bile in the liver due to obstruction of the bile passages, a common cause of ◊ *jaundice*.

cholesteatoma. A complication of perforation and chronic infection of the ear-drum: skin from the outer ear grows inwards, is shed in the ordinary way, but cannot escape. It causes damage by pressure and harbours infection, and needs surgical removal.

cholesterol. A fat-like substance in most tissues: blood contains about 0·2 per cent. Chemically, it is a ◊ *steroid*, and bile salts and various hormones are probably derived from it.

Cholesterol is the main component of deposits in the lining of arteries – ◊ *atheroma* – associated with arteriosclerosis and common diseases of middle and old age such as angina and stroke. The amount of cholesterol in the blood is usually (but not always) increased with this condition, but whether the excess causes atheroma is not known. Pending definite proof it is reasonable to reduce the amount of cholesterol by a moderate diet or other means in the hope of allaying arterial disease. Regular doses

of *clofibrate* reduce the amount of cholesterol and other lipids in the blood.

choline. An organic compound of ammonium hydroxide; it is essential to life and is sometimes counted as a vitamin of the B group. But unlike a true vitamin, choline can be synthesized in the body. Deficiency arises only when the diet is so poor that the raw material for choline synthesis is not provided; this is characteristic of *kwashiorkor*, a grave form of malnutrition seen in the tropics. Lack of choline interferes with the disposal of fat and damages the liver.

The compound ◊ *acetyl choline* is released at the ends of nerve fibres to stimulate adjacent nerve or muscle cells.

choline esterase. An enzyme responsible for the formation and decomposition of acetyl choline. Drugs such as eserine inhibit this enzyme and so prevent acetyl choline from being destroyed as soon as it has acted. This reinforces the action of nerves that release acetyl choline, particularly those of the *parasympathetic* system.

chondr(o)-. Prefix = 'of ◊ *cartilage*'.

chorea. 1. *Sydenham's chorea* (chorea minor; St Vitus's dance) is a disorder of children, usually associated with rheumatic fever, characterized by uncontrolled jerky movements, which may involve any part of the body. Unlike a *tic* or habit spasm, which is repetitive, the movement of chorea has no pattern. Mild cases are often dismissed as fidgeting. The cause is not known. The condition clears up spontaneously in two or three months.

2. *Huntington's chorea* (chorea major) is a rare hereditary condition. Although the tendency is inherited as a dominant character, symptoms do not appear until adult life. In addition to the uncontrolled movements of chorea there is progressive mental disorder. Sedative drugs relieve the symptoms to some extent, but no cure is known.

chorioid = ◊ *choroid*.

chorion. The outer layer of the membrane surrounding the foetus.

chorionepithelioma. An extremely rare form of cancer derived from the chorion.

choroid (chorioid). Network of small blood

vessels in the eye, immediately outside the retina.

choroiditis. Inflammation of the choroid, sometimes due to identifiable infection but usually of unknown cause. It may disturb vision, but complications such as detached retina and glaucoma are more serious effects. As a rule, corticosteroid drugs are the most effective treatment.

choroid plexus. Networks of blood vessels in the ventricles of the brain in which cerebrospinal fluid is formed.

chromium. A white metal with many industrial uses. Chromium and its salts can cause various types of skin disease.

chromosome. A particle seen in the nucleus of a cell during cell division (i.e. splitting to form two new cells), but not seen in a resting cell. A chromosome is a collection of a large number of *genes*; each gene determines one element in the hereditary make-up of the body.
   The nucleus of a resting cell contains a jumble of genes. When the cell is about to divide, this material is organized as a set of X- or V-shaped chromosomes; there are 23 pairs in the human set. The members of a pair are similar excepting the pair of sex chromosomes in the male. In the female, the 23rd pair consists of two large X chromosomes; in the male, of one X chromosome and one small Y chromosome. ◊ *genetics.*

chronic. (Disease) of long duration, often of gradual onset (cf. ◊ *acute*).

chrysarobin. Substance extracted from the bark of a Brazilian tree, *Andira araroba* (also grown in Goa); formerly much used in the treatment of psoriasis, but superseded by dithranol.

chrysotherapy. Treatment with salts of gold, now practically confined to rheumatoid arthritis.

chyle. Milky fluid in the lymph vessels of the small intestine: it is an emulsion of tissue fluid and the fat absorbed from food, which is taken up by the lymph vessels (lacteals) and not, like other components of food, by the veins.

chylomicron. Minute droplet of fat suspended in blood.

chyme. Fluid, partly digested contents of the small intestine.

cilia (pl. of *cilium*). **1.** Eyelashes. **2.** Fine hair-like structures, like the pile of velvet, on the surface of some cells, e.g. those of the air-passages. Their constant undulation sweeps mucus and dust particles upwards to be coughed or sneezed away or swallowed.

ciliary muscle. Muscle encircling the lens of the eye for focusing.

cinchona. *Peruvian* (*Jesuit's*) *bark*, the natural source of *quinine*, introduced to Europe from South America in the 17th century as a remedy for malaria, then a common disease throughout Europe (which cinchona cures), and for many other fevers (which it does not affect).

cinchophen. A synthetic drug formerly given for gout.

circle of Willis (**circulus vasculosus**). (Thomas Willis (1621–75), English anatomist and physician.) A circular system of arteries at the base of the brain: blood is carried into the skull by the left and right internal carotid arteries and the basilar artery (formed by the union of the two vertebral arteries) of which communicating branches form a ring. To a limited extent this provides an alternative supply if one artery fails, but the main function of the circle is to balance the pressure of blood delivered to the brain.

circulation. Constant flow of blood and other body fluids. An average man contains about 45 litres of water (70 per cent of body weight). The cells contain 30 litres. Three litres are in the *plasma* of the blood (the suspended cells make the total volume of blood up to 5 litres). The remaining 12 litres fill the spaces between groups of cells. This *tissue fluid* bathes all the cells of the body except those of the liver and spleen, which are directly in contact with the blood. The *cerebrospinal fluid* of the brain and spinal cord is separate from the rest of the tissue fluid. All the substances necessary for life filter into the cells from the tissue fluid, in exchange for waste products. By filtration from the ◊ *capillary* blood vessels the tissue fluid receives fresh supplies and gives up waste. For the system to work, the blood in the capillaries must be continually replaced with fresh blood; otherwise supplies would run out and waste would accumulate. The most urgent need is oxygen. The 5 litres of blood in the body can hold at the most 1 litre of oxygen, which is enough to keep a man alive for 4 minutes at rest, or less than a minute during exercise. Nor can the blood give up all its oxygen to the tissues. Thus the blood must circulate rapidly. At rest, it is pumped at the rate of 5 litres every minute, and this can be increased to every 10 seconds.

The heart is two separate pumps, right and left. The right side pumps blood through the lungs where the oxygen content is restored. This blood returns to the left side of the heart to be sent round the body again. Part of it is diverted to the kidneys for removal of waste products. Another part goes first to the stomach and intestine where it takes up foodstuffs, and from there to the liver where these are processed. All the blood then returns to the right side of the heart to be sent through the lungs again. (◊ *heart*.)

Blood flows from the heart to the periphery in *arteries* which divide into smaller and smaller branches and finally into *capillaries* where the work of the blood is done. The capillaries enter small *veins* which join to form larger and larger vessels on the way back to the heart. The blood is ejected from the heart in spurts; between beats the pressure falls to zero. But the arteries are elastic. They are stretched with each beat, and their recoil maintains the pressure and flow between beats. Instead of falling from 120 mm. of mercury to zero, the pressure in the arteries fluctuates between 120 and 80 mm. It is this smaller difference which is felt as the ◊ *pulse*. The resistance to the flow is greatest in the smallest arteries (*arterioles*), and in them the pressure falls to about 30 mm., while the pulse disappears. The capillaries are even smaller, but they are so numerous that they offer less resistance. The pressure in the veins is very low. Muscular activity keeps the blood moving in the veins, and one-way valves ensure that the flow is in the right direction.

1. REGULATION

The circulation is regulated primarily by the rate at which the heart pumps. The calibre of the vessels is adapted to the needs of the moment, partly by local mechanisms but mainly by the *vasomotor centre*, a group of

nerve cells in the lowest part of the brain, close to the cardiac and respiratory centres. A continuous stream of impulses from the centre, carried in ◊ *sympathetic* nerves along the vessels, keeps the muscle fibres in the vessel walls partially contracted. If the blood pressure rises because of increased flow from the heart, the nervous impulses decrease, the vessels dilate, and the normal pressure is restored. If the pressure begins to fall, the vessels contract. This reflex originates in nerve-endings sensitive to pressure in some of the large arteries. Impulses in these nerves inhibit the centre. Other factors influencing the centre are the same as those which influence the cardiac centre (◊ *heart* (3)). The two centres are co-ordinated to keep the blood pressure within reasonable limits. Emotion affects the state of the blood vessels even more than it does the heart.

The vasomotor centre affects the circulation as a whole, but the varying needs of particular organs are met by local mechanisms. For instance, the carbon dioxide which accumulates in an active muscle causes vessels in that muscle to dilate, so that it receives more blood at the expense of other organs. *Cramp* is a failure of this response. When the activity of the heart is increased, the lowered concentration of oxygen causes the ◊ *coronary arteries* to dilate and admit more blood and oxygen. The cramp of an inadequate blood supply to the heart is *angina pectoris*.

The *kidney* has a unique means of maintaining its blood supply. Defective circulation in the kidney causes an enzyme, *renin*, to be released. This reacts with a substance in the blood to form *angiotensin*, which directly stimulates the arterioles to contract and so raises the blood pressure. High blood pressure is a common complication of kidney diseases.

The small blood vessels in the *skin* are the principal means of regulating the body ◊ *temperature*. If they relax, blood is cooled at the surface of the body, and if they contract heat is retained.

Various disorders involving the circulation are discussed under ◊ *artery; blood pressure; heart failure; oedema; shock; vein.*

2. HISTORY

The circulation of the blood is one of the fundamentals of physiology. Until it was understood the workings of the body made little sense. Many of the most important discoveries in medicine were the result of advances in other sciences: for example, the processes of disease could not be studied until the microscope had been invented. But Harvey's discovery that the blood circulated, announced in 1628, could have been made at any time in the preceding 2,000 years. Harvey had no more idea than Hippocrates of how blood passed from arteries to veins, for he had no microscope. But he deduced that it must somehow do so from facts which the ancient Greeks could have observed.

The valves of the heart and their effect were described in the 4th century B.C. by an adherent of Hippocrates, but the real significance of their permitting flow in only one direction was missed. The arteries of a dead body are empty, all the blood having stagnated in the capillaries and veins. If an artery is opened after death it appears to contain air – as indeed it does after it has been opened. The physicians of antiquity assumed that the arteries were for the transport of air, mysteriously transformed into 'vital spirit'. But for this fallacy Herophilus and Erasistratus, working in Alexandria, would probably have discovered the circulation in the 3rd century B.C. Herophilus distinguished veins from arteries, but thought that the pulse was a property of the arteries themselves. Erasistratus observed that an artery would bleed if it were cut during life, because, he said, the escaping air was replaced with blood which entered by very small vessels between the veins and arteries. He was postulating capillaries, admittedly with the flow in the wrong direction. If this idea had been related to what was known of the heart valves the puzzle would have been solved.

In the 2nd century A.D. Galen went a step further by proving that the arteries carry blood and not air, but he rejected Erasistratus' view that the heart was the terminus of both veins and arteries, and ignored his theory about capillaries. Instead, Galen described the veins and arteries as two separate trees. The veins originated in the liver, where blood was formed from materials brought by the portal vein from the liver. Similarly the arteries originated in the lungs. The arteries were still primarily concerned with the transport of vital spirit. Their blood came from the veins through holes in the wall between the two sides of the heart. In both veins and

arteries blood simply ebbed to and fro.

In 1268 Ibn an-Nafis of Cairo said that there were no holes such as Galen had described, and the blood must reach the left side of the heart from the right by passage through the lungs. In 1552 ◊ *Servetus* said the same thing, and at about that time ◊ *Columbus* proved it. In 1603 ◊ *Fabricius ab Aquapendente* described the valves of the veins, without recognizing their function.

Finally, in 1628 Fabricius's pupil ◊ *Harvey* described the continuous circulation of blood through the body as we should describe it today, and in so doing marked the transition from ancient to modern medical science. It only remained for ◊ *Malpighi*, with the help of a microscope, to demonstrate the actual channels – first suggested 20 centuries earlier by Erasistratus – which complete the circuit.

circumcision. Surgical removal of part of the foreskin (prepuce) of the penis. The medical value of circumcision has been overstated. Infants seldom need the operation, and those who do are often suffering from ill-advised attempts to draw the foreskin back. In fact, an adherent foreskin is normal in infancy, and only later does the foreskin become loose.

There is, however, evidence that cancer of the penis (an uncommon disease in any case) is even rarer in circumcised men. The difference could be due to bacterial growth under the intact foreskin. Wives of circumcised men are rather less liable to cancer of the cervix of the uterus than other women, according to some authorities, but the evidence is open to question.

circumflex (anat.). Describes several structures which wind round other structures (especially bones).

The *circumflex nerve* is a branch of the ◊ *brachial* plexus which winds round the neck of the humerus, where it may be injured by a fracture, with paralysis of the ◊ *deltoid* muscle, and consequent difficulty in raising the arm.

The name of this nerve has recently been changed to *axillary* nerve.

cirrhosis. A disorder of the liver, in which healthy liver tissue has at some time been damaged and replaced by fibrous scar tissue. The changes involve the whole organ. The fibrous tissue hardens the liver. Clumps of new liver cells give the organ a lumpy surface, and their yellowish colour gives the condition its name (Gk *kirrhos* = tawny).

The normal liver has a great facility for regeneration, but in a cirrhotic liver lost tissue is unlikely to be all replaced. The mere loss of functioning tissue would not matter until a great deal was destroyed, because the normal liver has a substantial surplus. A more immediate source of trouble is compression by fibrous tissue of the blood vessels in the liver. A large volume of blood is carried in the *portal vein* from the stomach, intestine, and spleen to the liver, to be chemically processed before returning to the heart by the *inferior vena cava*. When the circulation through the liver is impaired by cirrhosis the blood is dammed and finds other routes to the heart. There are small communications between the normal portal vein and the ordinary veins around the oesophagus and rectum: with severe cirrhosis these are distended and liable to bleed. Similar veins at the umbilicus are distended, and the spleen is congested and enlarged. Jaundice, and poisoning by substances that ought to be neutralized in the liver, are other possible effects. But in most cases, cirrhosis causes no symptoms at all: it is only at an advanced stage that there is a risk of serious bleeding or failure of liver function.

As often as not, no cause can be found. The commonest *known* cause of cirrhosis is heavy drinking over many years. Another known cause is malnutrition, and it seems that the cirrhosis of the chronic alcoholic is in part a special case of malnutrition. Alcoholics seldom eat well; their digestion is impaired by damage to the lining of the stomach; above all, alcohol is used in the body as a source of chemical energy in preference to other fuel and therefore the little proper food that the drinker eats is not used.

Virus hepatitis (infectious jaundice) is under suspicion as a precursor of cirrhosis, but has not been definitely incriminated.

Heart failure with stagnation of blood in the liver, and various chronic disorders of the liver itself, can lead in time to cirrhosis.

Although cirrhosis advanced enough to cause ill health is a serious disorder it is by no means the hopeless condition that it was once thought to be. Alcoholic cirrhosis is sometimes virtually cured by abstention from alcohol. An exactly regulated diet improves most cases. Badly impaired cir-

culation in the liver may be improved by a by-pass operation (◊ *liver* (3)).

cirs(o)-. Prefix = 'varicose'; e.g. *cirsoid aneurysm*, a dilated, tortuous artery.

citric acid. A weak organic acid readily extracted from lemons and other fruit: in the human body it is an intermediate product in the combustion of foodstuffs. The *citric acid cycle* (Krebs cycle) is a series of chemical reactions in which carbon dioxide and water are formed with release of the energy; it is common to carbohydrate, fat and protein combustion, since citric acid is formed from any of them.

claudication. Limping – usually *intermittent claudication*, a cramp-like pain in the legs during mild exercise, due to inadequate supply of blood to the muscles from defective arteries. It is a similar disorder in the legs to angina in the heart, and the usual reason for it is ◊ *atheroma*. Drugs to dilate the arteries are of limited value, because the diseased arteries may not respond to them. The most effective treatment is daily exercise to encourage the growth of new blood vessels. In some cases the artery can be repaired surgically.

clavicle. The collar-bone, a bar joined at its inner end to the breast-bone (*sternum*) and at its outer end to the shoulder-blade (*scapula*). The two joints are bound by very tough ligaments, stronger than the bone itself, so that an injury is much more likely to break the bone than dislocate either of its joints.

The clavicle is more often broken than any other bone: almost any kind of fall involving the upper limb can cause a fracture of the clavicle because it is no more than a light strut and cannot withstand a heavy load. The patient almost announces the diagnosis by supporting the elbow of the injured side with his good hand. Since the whole length of the clavicle lies just below the skin, the fracture is usually obvious.

A bandage to brace the shoulders back reduces (sets) the fracture, and the clavicle heals quickly. Another method, said to give the best cosmetic result, is to keep the patient flat on his back with a pad between the shoulder-blades, so that the weight of the shoulders pulls the fragments into place; this method is described in the

Edwin Smith Papyrus of the 17th century B.C.

In the rare event of a dislocation of the joint at the outer end of the clavicle, the damage may need surgical repair.

climacteric. Change of life; in women it is the same as the ◊ *menopause*, but the male climacteric is a nebulous concept, for although male fertility gradually declines over the years the change is quantitative rather than qualitative.

clinical. Of the sick-bed or its occupant – e.g. *clinical diagnosis* is recognition of disease at the bed-side from the patient's symptoms and signs, as opposed to diagnosis by laboratory tests, X-ray examination etc.

clitoris. A small protrusion at the front of the vulva, sensitive to sexual excitement: its development in the female corresponds with that of the penis in the male.

clofibrate. A drug used to lower the concentration of cholesterol and other lipids in the blood in order to lessen the risk of ◊ *atheroma* and in particular of coronary artery disease.

clomiphene. A synthetic drug able to stimulate the ovary in the manner of the gonadotrophic hormone of the pituitary gland, used for treating certain types of female infertility (◊ *fertility*).

clostridium. A genus of bacteria, including those of *tetanus* and *gas gangrene.* They thrive in the absence of air. Most are by nature soil-dwellers and infect man only by mischance.

clot ◊ *blood* (4).

club-foot (talipes). Deformity of the foot, generally a result of faulty development before birth, but the term may also include the results of any interference with natural growth such as infection of bone or injury to nerves. Taken early, some types do well with simple treatment such as manipulation and splinting. Others need surgical reconstruction of the joints of the foot. Even early treatment may not obviate the need for special footwear, but at least it improves performance.

coagulation. Clotting; ◊ *blood* (4).

cobalt. A metal involved in human chemistry as a component of cyanocobalamine (vitamin B_{12}). A radioactive ◊ *isotope* of cobalt is used in the treatment of some types of cancer.

cocaine. An alkaloid extracted from the South American coca plant, formerly much used as a local anaesthetic. It also has effects like those of adrenaline: the constriction of arteries helps the surgeon by discouraging bleeding, but the stimulation of the heart can be dangerous. It is a notorious drug of addiction, causing temporary elation and hallucinations; habitual use causes grave deterioration of personality and sometimes frank insanity.

coccidioides. A microscopical fungus: an uncommon cause of serious infection of the lungs.

coccus. A spherical or roughly spherical ◊ *bacterium.* Several types can cause disease, including *streptococci* (growing in chains), and *staphylococci* (growing in clumps); these two are the usual causes of pus-formation. *Diplococci* grow in pairs. They include *gonococci* (causing gonorrhoea) and *meningococci* (causing epidemic meningitis).

coccyx. The lower end of the backbone; a small triangular bone projecting beyond the sacrum. It consists of four tiny vertebrae fused together, and is all that remains of a human tail. It is liable to be broken by a direct blow between the buttocks. The fracture is painful but seldom serious.

cochlea. Spiral cavity, like a snail-shell, containing the hearing apparatus (organ of Corti) of the inner ◊ *ear* (3).

codeine. Alkaloid drug from opium, closely related to morphine but less powerful and probably less habit-forming. It is used to relieve pain, generally in small doses mixed with other drugs such as aspirin, to suppress unnecessary cough, and sometimes to suppress diarrhoea.

coeliac artery. A branch of the aorta, carrying blood to the stomach, liver, pancreas, and spleen.

coeliac disease. A disorder of early childhood: the child fails to assimilate certain components of the diet, notably fats, and develops chronic diarrhoea and malnutrition. The cause is unknown, but many of the patients do not tolerate *gluten*, a protein in oats and wheat, and improve when it is omitted from the diet. Complete recovery is the rule, but may take several years. ◊ *sprue*

coeliac plexus (solar plexus). Network of nerves behind the stomach, derived from the sympathetic and vagus nerves, supplying branches to regulate the stomach, intestine and other abdominal organs.

co-enzyme ◊ *enzyme* (4).

coitus interruptus. ◊ *contraception*.

colchicum. The root of *Colchicum autumnale*, the autumn crocus, provides an alkaloid, colchicine, which is an effective remedy for attacks of gout.

cold. 1. Acute inflammation of the mucous membranes of the nose and throat due to a virus infection, or a similar condition due to allergy. ◊ *common cold*.
2. The effects of cold environment on the body are *local* and *general*.
Local effects. The usual response is contraction of small arteries in the skin: this decreases the flow of blood at the surface of the body and prevents loss of heat. It is one of the principal mechanisms for regulating body ◊ *temperature*. The arteries of the fingers, toes, and ears tend to contract less than other superficial arteries, so that frostbite is less common than it would otherwise be. Unlike the small arteries, the minute capillary vessels are dilated by cold, and blood stagnates in the affected skin, which becomes blue as oxygen is consumed. But with extreme cold the tissues cease to use oxygen and the blood in them remains red. ◊ *Raynaud's disease* is an exaggerated response to cold, the arteries contracting so much that the affected parts (usually the hands) are severely deprived of blood. ◊ *Chilblains* are more like an allergic reaction to cold. ◊ *Trench foot* (immersion foot) is the normal response to cold sustained for longer than even healthy tissues can tolerate. ◊ *Frostbite* is damage to skin and other tissues by ice crystals formed in them.
Cold prevents nerves from conducting impulses and so blocks sensation. It has a

limited use as a local anaesthetic; for instance, a spray of ethyl chloride evaporates so rapidly on the skin that the nerve-endings are chilled to numbness and a small abscess can be opened without pain.
The more destructive effect of extreme cold is also put to good use. Carbon dioxide snow is sometimes used to destroy warts and moles. Pin-point application of cold (cryosurgery) is now replacing heat (cautery) in several branches of surgery; it has much the same effect as a localized burn with less risk of harm to surrounding tissue. A cold 'burn' can be used to stick the retina – the sensory membrane of the eye – in place if it becomes detached.
General effects. Acting through the hypothalamus in the floor of the brain, cold causes increased secretion of thyroid hormone and adrenaline, which in turn increases the rate at which heat is produced by combustion of fat and carbohydrate. Shivering is a means of dissipating the energy of muscle contraction as heat instead of as work. The local effect of cold on blood vessels is reinforced by reflex action starting in the hypothalamus and causing contraction of small arteries near the surface of the body generally. After prolonged exposure to cold the mechanisms for maintaining body temperature are overcome and the body cools rapidly. The victim falls asleep; all his bodily functions are slowed, and he is apt to die when his temperature has fallen below 20°C. (68°F.).
Babies and old people have difficulty in keeping warm, and conditions that would be merely uncomfortable to others are dangerous to them. Heat is produced in the mass of the body and lost from the surface. The amount that can be produced varies with weight, and the amount lost with area. A baby weighing 10 kg. has a surface area of about half a square metre. A man weighing eight times as much has about four times the area. Exposure to cold is therefore much less risky for the man, until he grows old and his ability to generate heat begins to fail. Old people living alone in cold houses can die of exposure.
Apart from its direct effect, cold seems to aggravate various chronic illnesses; how it does so is not known.
Controlled cooling of the body is successfully used in surgery of the heart to slow body chemistry and so reduce the need for oxygen. At a temperature of 25°C. (77°F.) the circulation can be stopped for

ten minutes without harming the brain. Cooling may prove useful in treating illness such as shock, where the circulation is temporarily jeopardized.

cold abscess. An abscess, usually tuberculous, developing so slowly that the signs of inflammation are scarcely noticed.

cold sore = ◊ *herpes* simplex.

colic. Intermittent pain, often severe, arising from internal organs. It is due to powerful contraction of involuntary muscle, which stretches the sensory nerve endings. (Organs liable to colic are usually insensitive to other stimuli: e.g. burning or cutting the intestine is painless.) Colic is a symptom either of inflammation, which both stimulates contraction and sensitizes nerve-endings, or of obstruction, when the muscle pushes against resistance. Typical examples are inflammation of the intestine with food poisoning, and obstruction of a bile duct by a gall stone.

coliform. A group of bacteria, not strictly classified, including the normal inhabitant of the large intestine *Escherichia coli*, and several species causing disease of the intestine.

colitis. Inflammation of the *colon* (large intestine, lower bowel). The common causes are bacterial food poisoning and the various types of dysentery.

Ulcerative colitis is a severe, chronic inflammation of the colon of which the cause is still unknown. Bacterial infection plays a part, but the bacteria invade mucous membranes already damaged by some other process. At present the most likely explanation is an allergic reaction in which some component of the mucous membrane is rejected as though it were an extraneous substance (◊ *autoimmunity*). Emotional disturbance is often cited as a secondary cause and sometimes as a primary cause. It is true that emotion affects the intestine – the association of fear and diarrhoea is almost proverbial – but equally the uncontrollable diarrhoea and incapacity of severe colitis must be a potent cause of emotional upset. Probably emotion plays a similar part to infection in aggravating the primary defect.

Ulcerative colitis is dangerous because the continued diarrhoea leads to various chemical disturbances, dehydration, and ultimately severe emaciation. Loss of blood in the stools causes anaemia. Some patients recover completely from an attack and have no further trouble, but most need prolonged treatment.

Antibiotics, or the sulphonamide sulphasalazine, to control infection, and some form of psychotherapy both have a place in the treatment, in order to combat secondary aggravating factors. The dietitian may have some difficulty in choosing a diet to combat the malnutrition without contributing to the symptoms.

Corticosteroids generally bring some improvement and sometimes put a stop to all symptoms, though they cannot be expected to cure the underlying disease. In many cases the only effective treatment is to remove the whole of the affected part of the intestine. Since the rectum is nearly always involved, this means providing an artificial opening to the small intestine above the site of inflammation (ileostomy) through the front of the abdomen. This is very drastic treatment, but the results justify it. Patients in whom every detail of the skeleton could be made out are returned to a normal life, with the ileostomy no more than a minor nuisance. It is far from being an ideal form of treatment, but until much more is known about ulcerative colitis it is likely to be the best that can be offered in severe cases.

collagen. A protein: the principal component of connective tissue. Its molecules are assembled like three-strand ropes. Many of the processes of ageing are apparently due to derangement of this structure.

The *collagen diseases* (connective tissue diseases) have as their common factor a disorganization of collagen strands. This is a group of widely differing disorders, for collagen is found in most parts of the body. Several skin diseases and types of rheumatism are included. In all collagen diseases there is inflammation without infection. Corticosteroid drugs usually suppress the symptoms, but do not affect the underlying process, of which the nature is largely unknown. At least some of the collagen diseases can be partly explained by ◊ *autoimmunity*.

collateral. Alternative route for blood-flow, provided by secondary blood vessels when a primary vessel is obstructed.

Colles, Abraham (1773-1843). Professor of anatomy and surgery, Dublin. Colles wrote an important treatise on surgical anatomy, which includes a description of the fascia of the abdomen and perineum still named after him (1811). He was a bold and skilful surgeon, best remembered for his paper 'On the Fracture of the Carpal Extremity of the Radius' (1814).

Colles' fracture. Colles described a fracture 1½ inches above the wrist, but the much commoner injury now named after him is nearer to the joint. After a fall on the palm of the hand the lower end of the radius is broken off and displaced backwards, carrying the hand with it (the wrist joint is

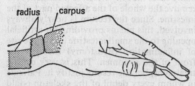

Colles' fracture of the radius.

intact). Since the radius and ulna are joined at the wrist by a strong band of fibrocartilage, there is always a concomitant injury at the ulnar side of the wrist: the fibrocartilage or a ligament is torn, or the tip of the ulna is broken off. In a severe case there may be other fractures or dislocation, and the median nerve may be compressed against the shaft of the radius. These fractures usually do well after manipulation and a few weeks in plaster, but with a bad one the wrist sometimes remains stiff.

coloboma. Congenital absence of a sector of one of the tissues of the eye, usually the iris, giving the pupil the shape of a key-hole. It is much more noticeable to the patient than to anyone else.

colocynth. A sort of wild pumpkin from which a powerful purgative has been extracted since ancient Egyptian times.

colon. The large intestine (lower bowel), excluding the caecum and the rectum; ◇ *intestine* (1).

colostomy. Surgical operation to take on the natural function of the rectum: a loop

of the colon is brought through the muscle and skin of the abdomen, and an artificial anus is made; a flexible bag is worn against it. A temporary colostomy is needed during convalescence after various operations on the intestine. If the rectum has to be removed because of cancer, the colostomy remains. Although the idea is very distasteful, in practice colostomies generally work well. With a well-fitted appliance they give no offence or discomfort, and many patients have them completely under conscious control.

colour blindness. Inability to distinguish between certain colours. Normal eyes see colours as various mixtures of three primary colours, each served by a particular kind of nerve-ending. In much the same way, colour photography records the whole spectrum as various mixtures of three primary dyes.

Several anomalies are possible in this system, but only one is at all common: absence of specific nerve-endings for recognizing red. People with this defect cannot distinguish red from the next primary colour, green. Red-green colour blindness (Daltonism) is a sex-linked character (◇ *genetics*), i.e. one that women may transmit to their sons without themselves being affected. Women can have red-green colour blindness only if they have an affected father and a mother who 'carries' the defect. The rarer forms affect both sexes equally often.

The disability from colour blindness is so slight that many affected men are not aware of their condition until they are examined for a job on the railway or at sea where coloured lights have to be distinguished.

colp(o)-. Prefix = 'of the *vagina*'.

Columbus (Realdo Colombo) (*c.* 1516-1559). Professor of anatomy and surgery at Padua 1544-59; pupil and successor of Vesalius. His text-book, *De re anatomica*, repairs some of his great teacher's omissions. He was the first man to describe the lens towards the front of the eye and not at the centre. He showed that the arteries expand when the heart contracts - all earlier anatomists, unaware of the circulation of the blood, had supposed that both contracted simultaneously. He recognized the function of the valve at the root of the pulmonary artery in preventing reflux of blood into the heart, and demonstrated that blood flows from the heart through the lungs. These discoveries were a step towards the description of the whole circulation by Harvey, who studied at Padua 50 years later.

coma. Unconsciousness from which the subject cannot be roused (as he can from natural sleep); the activity of the brain as a whole is depressed, and reflexes such as coughing that are unaffected by sleep are suppressed. A principal danger of coma is that saliva or vomit may be inhaled and prevent breathing because there is no cough to remove it. When the cause of the coma is increasing (e.g. continued bleeding in the brain; continued absorption of poison) the coma may deepen until the brain ceases to act at all and the subject dies. Even when the cause is stationary or receding a person in coma needs constant supervision to ensure that breathing continues.

The many causes of coma all involve some kind of insult to the brain. They include direct *injury*, *pressure* (bleeding, abscess, tumour), *infection* (meningitis, encephalitis), *poisoning* (alcohol, drugs; also poisons formed within the body as in uncontrolled diabetes or failure of liver or kidneys), *lack of oxygen* (suffocation, obstruction of blood vessels, failure of circulation as in shock), *lack of sugar* (overdose of insulin). An important cause of transient coma, epilepsy, is unexplained.

comedo. Blackhead (◊ *acne*).

commensal. Creature living in or on another species without harm to either, e.g. the normal bacteria of the skin and intestine.

common cold. A virus infection of the mucous membranes of the nose and throat. The familiar symptoms – tickling throat, sneezing, running eyes and nose, cough, headache – set in about a day after exposure and rarely last as long as a week. Inflamed mucous membranes are susceptible to added infection by bacteria, which delays recovery and may lead to bronchitis and other complications; but considering the prevalence of colds, complications are not very common. Immunity is short-lived and is confined to the particular strain of virus that caused the attack – and at least 30 different viruses can cause colds. There is no known way of preventing colds, nor of shortening the attack. Treatment does, however, make a cold less disagreeable and may reduce the risk of complications. The most important part is to keep warm and stay indoors, and popular household remedies such as aspirin and hot whisky are as effective as more sophisticated preparations.

The idea of 'catching cold' is found in many languages, and the belief that one literally does so is likely to die hard. In fact, wet feet, sitting in draughts and the rest do not cause colds; only infection with one of the viruses can do that. But *feeling* cold is often the first symptom of the infection, and is easily blamed for the later symptoms. Secondly, in cold weather people are crowded together in the few warm places such as cinemas and underground trains, where they infect each other. Thirdly, some people react to cold air as others react to pollen; they sneeze and their eyes water. The same kind of thing troubles people with chronic bronchitis, and cold damp air aggravates their wheezing and coughing. But if the common cold were really due to cold and dampness it is hard to believe that sports such as ski-ing and yachting would keep their well-earned reputation for promoting health. Mountaineers and sailors face many hazards, but this is not among them.

compressed-air sickness (caisson disease; dysbarism). A hazard of diving: adverse effects of pressure changes, including 'the bends', ◊ *barotrauma*, and nitrogen narcosis.

Water pressure at 1 atmosphere for each 10 metres of depth forces gas, mainly nitrogen, to dissolve in the body fluids. These may froth when the pressure falls during ascent. The bubbles, foreign bodies in the tissues, cause the bends. Symptoms range from itching, cramp-like pain and vertigo to paralysis, suffocation and coma. By surfacing in timed stages according to established rules the diver lets the gas seep safely away through his lungs. These rules are for experts in perfect physical condition: others need much wider safety margins. Time is as critical as depth: it takes as long to surface from a protracted shallow dive as from a brief deep one.

Barotrauma (physical injury) ranges from nose-bleeds to grave lung injuries. Ears are very vulnerable, and nobody with ear or sinus infection should dive.

Any highly concentrated gas (again mainly nitrogen) can affect the brain as a narcotic like alcohol, dangerously impairing a diver's judgement. In this and some other respects helium to dilute the oxygen is safer than nitrogen. Undiluted oxygen is toxic under high pressure.

The bends are treated by recompression to dissolve the bubbles and decompression over many hours. Symptoms may be delayed and also deceptive. *Any* symptom within 24 hours of a dive needs expert care at once; otherwise a chance of preventing permanent damage may be lost. The doctor must be told that the patient has been diving.

Dysbarism adds to the risk of diving by impairing balance (ear injury) and co-ordination. Nobody should dive alone, and any beginner needs professional super-vision.

concussion. Shaking of the brain, as by a blow to the head or a jolt to the neck, with temporary disturbance of consciousness. In every case, concussion probably puts some of the millions of nerve cells in the brain permanently out of action, and re-peated concussion, such as professional boxers may suffer (a knock-out is concus-sion), causes serious deterioration. Events immediately before concussion are usually not remembered (retrograde amnesia). Anyone who has just recovered from con-cussion still needs observation, because symptoms of more serious damage may be delayed for several hours.

condyle. Rounded end of a bone, e.g. a knuckle.

congenital. Present from birth: not neces-sarily *hereditary*; for example, a child may suffer an injury before birth, which is then congenital though not hereditary.

congestion. Surplus of blood in a part of the body, either from increased supply (e.g. inflammation) or inefficient removal (e.g. heart failure).

conjunctiva. Delicate membrane covering the inside of the eyelids and the front of the eye.

conjunctivitis (pink-eye). Inflammation of the conjunctiva, due to infection with bacteria or viruses. The contagious 'swim-ming-bath conjunctivitis', like the tropical conjunctivitis ◊ *trachoma*, is due to a virus-like parasite that (unlike true viruses) responds to treatment with antibiotics. ◊ *ophthalmia*.

connective tissue. The packaging material of the body, separating, protecting and sup-porting the various organs. Like all tissues, the connective tissues live by the cells they contain, but the importance of connective tissues lies in the inert ground-substance that surrounds the cells. The least special-ized of these tissues is *areolar tissue*. Its soft ground-substance contains a loose tangle of slender fibres. Layers of areolar tissue between organs keep them more or less in place while allowing considerable freedom of movement, e.g. between muscles and skin. *Adipose tissue*, the main store of fat, is like areolar tissue with droplets of fat in its cells. In *fibrous tissue* the fibres of collagen are systematically arranged in bundles or sheets. This is the stuff of ligaments and tendons.

In *bone*, the ground-substance is hardened by a deposit of calcium salts; in *cartilage* it is more rubbery.

Some anatomists include *blood* and *lymph*, where the ground-substance is fluid, among the connective tissues.

connective tissue diseases ◊ *collagen.*

constipation. Constipation is the most over-rated of all symptoms. Because faeces are unpleasant and seemingly poisonous, people have always believed that getting rid of them as fast as possible must prom-ote health. This belief has been convenient for doctors because purgative medicines are easy to find; some that are still in use were known to the physicians of ancient Egypt.

In fact, getting rid of poisons is mainly the job of the kidneys. Faeces are poisonous in the sense that they contain bacteria that can cause trouble if they contaminate parts of the body other than the intestine. But in the intestine these bacteria are harmless, and in any case they cannot be eliminated by purges. They *can* be eliminated with large doses of antibiotics, and the consequences may be serious.

Though most people open their bowels once a day there is no need for everyone to do so. 'Average' is not necessarily the same as 'normal' or 'essential'. In countries with a poor but bulky diet, the national average may be two or three motions a day, but plenty of people stay healthy on two or three motions a week. With the richer, less bulky diets of wealthy societies some people open their bowels much less often without being in any real sense constipated.

On the other hand, a daily motion is no proof that one is not constipated, because the rectum may not completely empty itself.

Normal bowel function has two components. Waste matter in the whole of the large intestine finds its way to the rectum without undue delay; and the rectum is completely emptied at more or less regular intervals. Failure of either is constipation. The effects of constipation are mechanical. Discomfort, lassitude and the rest are reflex symptoms of distension of the rectum. They could equally well be caused by air in the rectum, and have nothing to do with poisoning. If faeces stagnate and harden, their passage may injure the anus and cause cracked skin (fissure), blood blister (external piles), or distended veins (true, internal piles). Motions then become painful, and the constipation becomes worse. It is in these cases more than any others that purgatives are needed. Much constipation is due either to faulty diet – the 'easily digested' foods of Western civilization are all too easily digested and leave no residue – or to mental and physical sluggishness. The easiest remedies are vegetables and exercise. The psychological factor is important but hard to define; worry about constipation may be the main element. The regular use of purgatives irritates the intestine, which in time becomes accustomed to its daily dose and will not perform without drugs; thus imaginary constipation becomes real.

Though constipation is not an important illness in itself, it may be a symptom of something more serious. Constipation does not cause cancer, but cancer of the large intestine causes the bowels to be opened less (or more) often than has been usual for the particular patient. Prompt investigation of this symptom is often life-saving, for these cancers are generally curable in the early stages when symptoms are first noticed.

consumption. Any disease causing serious loss of weight; in particular tuberculosis of the lungs.

contact lens. Glass or plastic shell, ground on the inner surface to fit the front of the eye closely, and on the outer surface to serve as a spectacle lens.

Contact lenses are more expensive and more troublesome than spectacles. For many people, improved appearance is enough to outweigh these disadvantages. There is also less risk of breakage – the eyes are well protected by the structure of the skull and by defensive reflexes. When the front of the eye is misshapen a contact lens is the only kind that will give good vision.

At present, two kinds of plastic lens have superseded glass lenses. Soft plastic is more easily fitted to the eye than hard, but is more expensive and more difficult to look after.

contagion. Transmission of infectious disease by direct contact (as opposed to airborne or water-borne infection etc.).

contraception. Birth control; preventing sexual intercourse from leading to pregnancy. Some methods are designed to prevent the male sperm from fertilizing the female ovum, and others to prevent the already fertilized ovum from developing.

Three methods in common use require no artificial aids. The first, withdrawal, or *coitus interruptus*, is simply withdrawing the penis from the vagina before orgasm. Some people may find this form of anticlimax tolerable, but it is certainly not reliable. Even with careful timing, a few sperms escape before orgasm, and a single sperm is enough.

The second is the safe-period or rhythm method, which depends on the fact that both ova and sperms are short-lived, so that conception is possible only within a few days of ovulation. If intercourse is avoided for five or six days about half-way between menstrual periods, pregnancy is unlikely. For this method to be reliable, one has to know when ovulation is going to take place, which is a fortnight *before the next* period, rather than after the last. Some women are so regular that they can predict quite accurately, but others are not, and for them a temperature chart kept throughout the month is the only guide. The virtues of this technique are theological rather than physiological.

The third is not really a method; it is to apply the fact that when an ovum has been fertilized, i.e. a pregnancy has begun, no further ovum is released until some time after the end of pregnancy, and sometimes not until breast-feeding is over. Once pregnant, a woman cannot conceive again and carry twins of different ages. It has been suggested that the relative infertility of a nursing mother is one reason why breast-feeding is continued for as long as two years in some parts of the world, as a simple means of birth control.

Physical barriers between the sperm and ovum include the sheath or condom worn by the man, and several types of occlusive pessary which close off the opening of the uterus high in the vagina. Condoms are easy to get and to use and are fairly reliable, but either partner may find them aesthetically objectionable. A pessary, e.g. a diaphragm or a Dutch cap, is better in this respect, but professional help is needed in the original fitting and the woman has to learn how to insert and remove the device.

The intrauterine device (IUD) is a little spring, placed in the cavity of the uterus and left there. It does not prevent the ovum from being fertilized, but with an IUD in place a fertilized ovum cannot establish itself and grow: the uterus rejects it. Complications are unusual, and the method has been used in some large-scale birth-control campaigns designed to check over-population.

Various chemical preparations for insertion into the vagina just before intercourse are supposed to kill sperms. They are more effective tnan attempts to kill the sperms afterwards, but on their own they are far from reliable. They may help as an adjunct to a condom or a pessary.

Oral contraceptives – 'the pill' – are hormone preparations that prevent the ovaries from releasing ova in the same way as natural hormones prevent this during pregnancy. They are the most reliable of all contraceptives provided that the woman strictly follows the prescribed schedule. This is usually one pill daily for three weeks, followed by a week's rest during which there is a period of bleeding like a menstrual period. There are certain drawbacks to the method. Some women feel sick, and some put on weight. Thrombosis (the formation of a blood-clot in a vein) is a rare but serious complication. In short, the complications of taking the pill can also be complications of pregnancy: they arise from the same alteration in the balance of hormones. Hence the dictum that it is safer to take the pill than not to. The method is safer now than it was when it was introduced in the early 1960s, because the required dose is less than was at first thought. Most preparations are a mixture of an oestrogen and a progestogen (◊ sex hormones). Instead, the components can be taken during alternating periods, which is said to be more natural, or a progestogen can be taken alone, which causes fewer complications but occasionally allows an unintentional pregnancy.

Lastly, in either sex there is the possibility of ◊ sterilization by a simple operation.

contracture. Shrinkage of connective tissue or scar. All scars tend to contract. With extensive scars, e.g. from burns, this may restrict movement, and in extreme cases plastic surgery may be needed to restore function. If a limb is immobilized by paralysis or plaster, fibrous tissue around joints may contract and restrict movement unless regular physiotherapy is given.

Dupuytren's contracture of fibrous tissue in the hand is described under its own heading. Volkmann's contracture is scarring and shrinkage of muscles from deficient blood supply when a plaster cast is too tight.

contrecoup. Injury to one side of the brain from a blow on the opposite side of the skull.

contusion. ◊ bruise; injury to deeper tissues through intact skin.

convulsion. Involuntary unco-ordinated contractions of muscles; fit; seizure. (◊ epilepsy.) A convulsion is a symptom of irritation of nerve cells. One of the commonest causes is fever in childhood.

Cooley's anaemia. (T. B. Cooley (1871–1945), American physician.) ◊ haemoglobin; genetics.

Cooper, Sir Astley Paston (1768–1841). A distinguished London surgeon and anatomist, and above all the inspiration of a great school of medicine. He taught at St Thomas's Hospital, of which Guy's, founded in 1725, was a sort of annexe. After a disagreement with St Thomas's, Cooper became the leader of a new school at Guy's, and Guy's Hospital separated from St Thomas's. (At that time the two hospitals were both near London Bridge.)

Cooper taught that clinical observation – the recording of symptoms – must be related to postmortem study of the actual changes in the affected organs. In other words, practical medicine needs a scientific basis of anatomy and pathology. This doctrine was brilliantly applied by his young colleagues Bright, Addison, and Hodgkin, under whom Guy's was the leading school in England if not in the world.

cord ◊ *spermatic cord; spinal cord; umbilical cord; vocal cord.*

corium (dermis; cutis vera). Inner layer of the skin, containing fibrous tissue, blood vessels, nerves, sweat glands; covered by the outer skin or epidermis.

corn. A cone of horny dead tissue in the outer layer of the skin formed in response to localized pressure from an ill-fitting shoe, and causing pain by irritating nerve-endings in the corium.

cornea. Circular window at the front of the eye, through which the iris and pupil may be seen. The cornea has no blood vessels, and its nerves transmit only the sensation of pain. A very lively reflex shuts the eyes at the least stimulation of these nerves.

Next to blood transfusion, grafting of a cornea from somebody else is the most successful of all operations in which tissues are transferred from one person to another; it is perhaps because the cornea receives no blood that a foreign one is not rejected. It is for this purpose that eyes are bequeathed to hospitals.

coronary arteries. Two branches of the aorta supplying blood to the heart muscle, which consumes a large amount of oxygen and needs a good supply of blood. The heart can make little use of the blood passing through its cavity, which has a waterproof lining. The arteries encircle the heart and distribute twigs throughout its muscle.

The flow through the coronary arteries is adapted to the needs of the moment by a mechanism independent of the control of arteries in general: if the heart works harder more oxygen is used and more carbon dioxide is formed. The coronary arteries respond to carbon dioxide by dilating to let in more blood and so more oxygen. If a point is reached where the heart is still short of blood and the arteries can dilate no further a severe pain develops; this is ◊ *angina.* Various drugs can be used to dilate the coronary arteries. Their value is limited, because if there is angina the arteries are probably as widely open as they can be. The whole trouble is that they are abnormal

and cannot be fully dilated by any means.

It is possible to inject an opaque fluid into the coronary arteries by way of a tube introduced through an artery of the arm or leg, and then study the arteries with X-rays. This allows blockages to be located with a view to surgical treatment.

coronary thrombosis. Obstruction of a coronary artery or one of its branches by blood clot, depriving part of the heart muscle of blood and causing its death.

Purists object to the term because it describes only the state of the artery. What matters is the suffocation (infarction) of the heart muscle (myocardium), and the term *myocardial infarction* is preferred. Death from infarction is possible without thrombosis (there may be only severe narrowing of the artery), and coronary thrombosis can occur harmlessly, without infarction.

Like most other vessels, the coronary arteries intercommunicate, and blockage of one should not be a disaster. But for thrombosis to occur the artery must be affected with ◊ *atheroma.* The chances are that neighbouring arteries are similarly affected and cannot take over the circulation in the area.

The prime symptom is pain of the kind described under ◊ *angina.* It differs from other angina in that it does not pass off with rest, and the patient commonly shows signs of ◊ *shock.* Some people almost literally drop dead; the heart simply stops beating. Although this is a common disaster it is by no means the usual outcome (as widely supposed). The great majority survive.

For some days after a coronary thrombosis there is some danger that the heart may stop or at least that its rhythm may be disturbed, or the heart may work inadequately with symptoms of heart failure. Any of these conditions can be fatal, but they are all more or less remediable if the right help is at hand. There is also a risk of a second attack which may well prove too much; or the scar at the site of the thrombosis may give way before it is firmly established. These dangers persist for two or three weeks. The patients who survive so long (still a clear majority) are likely to be fully recovered about six weeks after the attack.

The diagnosis is often obvious from the symptoms. It may be confirmed by the electrocardiogram and by chemical changes in the blood.

The most important part of treatment is complete rest so that the heart has as little work as possible while it heals. Emotional rest is as important as physical, and opiates are needed for some days. Anticoagulant drugs, to discourage clotting, may ward off a second attack. Oxygen inhalations are often given in the early stages. Sudden stoppage of the heart or grave disorders of its rhythm can sometimes be corrected by electrical stimulation. Many cardiologists believe that every case should be treated in a hospital unit with all these facilities to hand. But this disease is far too common for the number of hospital beds even in the best equipped countries.

In many countries, coronary thrombosis is the commonest cause of death in men. It is also common in women, but on average they are some years older when they have an attack. In Britain, it kills more men than all forms of cancer together. No positive means of prevention has yet beeen found, but at least one can avoid some of the factors associated with proneness to the disease. These are considered under ◊ *atheroma*, which is the predisposing defect in the arteries; they include smoking, lack of exercise, and overeating. But atheroma is not the whole story, because it was almost as common at the turn of the century as it is now, while coronary thrombosis has increased enormously. The new factor appears to be stress. Coronary thrombosis was once rare in Ghana, but recent studies there show that Ghanaians in 'Western' jobs are quite as liable to get it as Europeans.

The typical patient is usually described as the hard-worked, energetic, driving manager. This is not quite true; the over-anxious, not so successful deputy runs a greater risk, and the most vulnerable of all are the misfits, real or supposed.

corpus luteum (yellow body). A small, yellowish structure formed in the ovary at the site of a released ovum. It forms several hormones, including *progesterone* which stimulates the lining of the uterus to grow in readiness for pregnancy. If the ovum becomes fertilized, the corpus luteum persists; if not, the corpus luteum withers and the lining of the uterus is shed, i.e. menstruation occurs.

corpuscle. A small body; a small well-defined structure within an organ or tissue; a blood cell.

cortex. Distinct outer layer (shell) of an organ, e.g. *cerebral cortex*, the layer of nerve cells (grey matter) on the surface of the brain.

corticosteroid. Any of several hormones formed in the cortex of the adrenal glands, with the ◊ *steroid* chemical structure and effects on body chemistry that are essential to life; or a synthetic derivative with similar effects to the natural hormones.

The actions of these hormones are considered under ◊ *adrenal* (cortex), and the effect of deprivation under ◊ *Addison's disease*.

Until the present century the adrenal cortex was not known to have any function. In 1910 it was shown that animals could not survive without it, and in 1934 E. C. Kendall isolated a hormone from it. (Kendall had isolated thyroid hormone in 1914.) For some time, the only known use of the hormone was for treating Addison's disease. In 1949, Kendall, T. Reichstein, and P. H. Hench described much wider uses; in the following year they shared a Nobel Prize. They had shown that corticosteroids would suppress the symptoms of inflammation and allergy. These two reactions (they are variants of the same fundamental process) occur in a very wide range of diseases – a current handbook lists over a hundred conditions in which corticosteroids may be used to suppress one or the other.

For a short time the new preparations were widely acclaimed as the greatest of wonder-drugs, despite warnings from the discoverers that the practical uses would be limited.

There are grave objections to these drugs, and the disadvantages often outweigh the possible advantages. Inflammation has unpleasant and sometimes dangerous effects, but it is fundamentally a defensive reaction. To suppress it indiscriminately is like abolishing the fire brigade to stop it from breaking windows and doors. Again, allergy is a misapplication of the process by which immunity to infection develops; if allergy is suppressed with corticosteroids, so is immunity. Many of the symptoms of infection arise from these defensive reactions. They can be promptly relieved by corticosteroids, but the infection itself is then unopposed and likely to kill the patient.

In the second place corticosteroids,

affecting as they do many of the chemical processes of the body, have numerous undesirable effects if they are given over long periods. Healing, which depends on inflammation, is impaired, and wounds, gastric ulcers and the like become very troublesome. Bone and fibrous connective tissue are weakened, the patient puts on weight (much of it retained water), his blood pressure rises. As one would expect, the symptoms of prolonged treatment with large doses of corticosteroids are like those of over-activity of the adrenal glands (Cushing's syndrome).

In the third place, giving corticosteroids in time suppresses the natural activity of the adrenal cortex. If the treatment is suddenly stopped the patient is left with no adrenal hormones and develops symptoms of Addison's disease.

If the adrenal cortex is healthy the effects of corticosteroid treatment can be produced indirectly by giving ACTH, the pituitary hormone that stimulates the adrenal cortex. The patient is then treated with his own corticosteroids. The same complications can arise, with the one difference that it is the pituitary that is suppressed: when treatment is stopped the patient does not form enough of his own ACTH to keep his adrenals working.

In spite of this disheartening catalogue, corticosteroids are extremely valuable drugs. Short courses of treatment are practically free from risk, but with long courses the dose has to be exactly regulated, and at the end the drug has to be withdrawn gradually enough for the patient's own adrenals to have time to recover.

Apart from their obvious value in diseases of the adrenal glands, corticosteroids may be life-saving in conditions of violent stress such as shock after extensive injuries or burns (interference with healing is relatively unimportant because the drug is used only to tide the patient over a short period of acute danger). Similarly they can be used in the comparatively rare cases where allergic reactions are violent enough to threaten life (◊ allergy). Their widest use is in controlling the many kinds of inflammation that are not due to infection, including several rheumatic disorders and a whole range of skin diseases. Many of the diseases that respond to this treatment are probably examples of ◊ autoimmunity, where inflammation arises from a kind of allergy to some natural component of the body itself. A few of these conditions can be lethal unless corticosteroids are given. The drawbacks of the treatment are then of minor importance. Far more often the disease is more a nuisance than a danger, and the benefits of treatment have to be weighed against the drawbacks. The decision whether or not to use corticosteroids is among the most difficult in current medical practice. A patient with rheumatoid arthritis who has once experienced the immediate improvement that corticosteroids can bring may take a deal of persuading that on balance her particular case is better treated without them.

There are fewer problems when corticosteroids can be applied directly to a trouble-spot, e.g. by injection into an inflamed joint, or as an ointment on a localized skin disease. In such cases there is not much danger of disturbing the chemical balance of the body as a whole.

A new use for corticosteroids is to suppress the reaction to 'foreign' tissue that causes organs grafted from other people to be rejected.

corticotropin (corticotrophin). Pituitary hormone, stimulating the adrenal cortex; ACTH.

cortisol; cortisone. Two of the ◊ corticosteroid hormones.

Corvisart, Jean-Nicolas (1755–1821). Napoleon's personal physician; author of an important treatise on diseases of the heart (1806). His most influential work was a French translation of Auenbrugger's book on percussion of the chest as a method of diagnosis. More than anyone else it was Corvisart who shook off the scholastic shackles that impeded progress in the Paris school of medicine; under his influence Paris was to lead the rest of the world in scientific medicine. His best known pupil was Laënnec, the inventor of the stethoscope.

corynebacterium. A genus of bacteria, including the diphtheria bacillus.

coryza. Running nose; common cold.

Cos. Aegean island, birthplace of Hippocrates (c. 460 B.C.) and seat of the most influential medical school of antiquity.

costal. Of the ribs.

couching. The simplest operation for ◊ *cataract*: instead of being removed as in the modern operation, the diseased lens of the eye is simply displaced so that it no longer impedes the passage of light.

cough. Explosive release of air from the lungs: the pressure is raised by attempting to breathe out while the vocal cords are closed; then the cords are suddenly relaxed. It can of course be done deliberately, but essentially it is a reflex action provoked by irritation of the larger air-passages. Mucus or an inhaled foreign body is expelled in the same way as a shot from an air-gun – and at a comparable muzzle-velocity. This is a useful function, but coughing is also provoked by inflammation of the mucous membrane of the trachea or bronchi even when there is nothing to expel, and by pressure from outside the bronchi (e.g. by enlarged lymph nodes with whooping cough).

cough medicines. A useless cough is suppressed by drugs such as codeine that diminish the response to irritation, or in some cases by damping sensation at the back of the throat. A *linctus* is a syrupy preparation with, as a rule, both effects.

An *expectorant* mixture stimulates the glands in the mucous membrane of the bronchi to dilute and loosen the sticky material that accumulates with bronchitis, and so makes coughing easier and more useful. Most of the drugs used are *emetics* given in doses too small to cause vomiting.

counter-irritation. Relief of minor symptoms by applying heat or mild irritants to the skin. Liniments are used to ease pain and stiffness in joints and muscles and (with less reason) to soothe hacking coughs; hot-water bottles are laid on aching stomachs; poultices and fomentations are supposed to draw out deep-seated inflammation. African herbalists treat most illness by making cuts in the skin and rubbing in irritant powders, and the acupuncture and moxibustion of traditional Chinese medicine appear to be refinements of the same method.

All these forms of treatment stimulate nerves in the skin, and by reflex action this dilates blood vessels and increases the flow of blood in the affected skin. Why reddening the skin – the only demonstrable effect – should help is not clear. Hippocrates pointed out that one kind of discomfort relieved another (by drawing attention from it?). A poultice on a boil is a special case because it increases the circulation at the site of the trouble. The most potent effect of any form of counter-irritation may well be that the patient sees something positive being done.

cowpox (vaccinia). A virus infection of cattle transmitted to man, resembling smallpox but much milder. An attack confers immunity to smallpox; this is the principle of vaccination.

cramp. Painful spasm (sustained contraction) of muscles. The known causes include shortage of salt from excessive sweating as in miner's or stoker's cramp or heat-stroke, for which the remedy or preventive is to take more salt. Deficient blood supply is another cause: if the arteries of the legs are narrowed they do not admit enough blood for the demands of exercise, and a characteristic pain in the calves develops with walking and passes off with rest. This type of cramp is *intermittent claudication*. *Angina pectoris* is a similar event in the heart muscle. Swimmer's cramp has been ascribed to spasm of the limb arteries together with diversion of blood to a full stomach.

Occupational (e.g. writer's) cramp is thought to be a kind of neurosis, because it is brought on not by using a particular group of muscles but by applying them to a particular job.

There is no satisfactory explanation of the familiar kind of cramp that comes on at any time, even during sleep, and behaves as though the muscle were squeezing and stimulating its own nerve to set up a vicious circle. This cramp is relieved by stretching the affected muscle – e.g. if it is in the calf by pushing the heel down and the toes up. The variety of the recommended drugs only shows how little the disorder is understood.

cranial nerve. Nerve arising directly from the brain and passing through one of the holes in the skull (cf. ◊ *spinal nerve*, arising from the spinal cord). Twelve pairs of cranial nerves are described, but they are not an orderly series like the spinal nerves. Their names and functions are as follows:

I. *Olfactory*; sense of smell.
II. *Optic*; vision.

III. *Oculomotor*⎫
IV. *Trochlear* ⎬ eye movements.
V. *Abducent*   ⎭

VI. *Trigeminal*; ordinary sensation from the face and scalp, movements of the jaw.

VII. *Facial*; movements of the face.

VIII. *Auditory* (acoustic); in two parts: *cochlear* (hearing) and *vestibular* (balance).

IX. *Glossopharyngeal*; sensation from the back of the mouth.

X. *Vagus*; digestive organs, heart, air-passages.

XI. *Accessory*; sternomastoid and trapezius muscles.

XII. *Hypoglossal*; movements of the tongue.

cranium = ◊ *skull*.

creatine. A nitrogenous compound in muscle. Chemical energy is stored by the formation of creatine phosphate and released for muscle contraction by the decomposition to creatine.

crepitus. A crackling sound heard with a stethoscope over inflamed lungs; also the grating sound and sensation over the broken ends of a bone.

cretin; cretinism. Cretinism is congenital deficiency of thyroid hormone, retarding mental and physical growth; a cretin is a person so affected. ◊ *thyroid gland* (2).

cricoid cartilage. The uppermost ring of cartilage around the ◊ *trachea*; it is the principal support of the ◊ *larynx*.

crisis. Time of decision; turning-point or sudden exacerbation during an illness; change for the better.

Crohn's disease. Regional ◊ *enteritis*.

cromoglycate. Sodium cromoglycate is used for treating some allergic diseases, in particular asthma and hay fever. It prevents the release in affected tissues of the toxic substances that cause symptoms. The treatment is continuous. Its purpose is to prevent attacks, not to cure them.

croup. Strained, noisy breathing and harsh cough, as a rule in children. The causes include retarded growth of the larynx (which corrects itself in time), allergy, virus

infection, and bacterial infection such as diphtheria (membranous croup).

cryptococcosis = ◊ *torulosis*.

cryptorchism. Retarded descent of the testicles from the abdomen to the scrotum. ◊ *testis*.

CSF = ◊ *cerebrospinal fluid*.

cubital; cubitus. (Of the) forearm, elbow, or ulna.

Culex. A kind of mosquito found in most parts of the world; it is generally harmless but in parts of West Africa may transmit the threadworm that causes tropical elephantiasis.

culture. Artificial breeding of bacteria for identification, preparation of vaccines etc. ◊ *microbe*.

curare. Ancient South American arrow-poison extracted from various plants (species of *Strychnos* and *Chondodendron*). It causes rapid paralysis of muscles throughout the body.

Curare was used in hunting. An animal wounded with an ordinary arrow had only to go a short distance to be lost in the dense forest. A slight wound from a curare-tipped arrow was enough to prevent it from escaping, so that it could be dispatched with a hunting knife. When the wound had been cut away the flesh was safe to eat. An incidental advantage to the hunter was that the animal died silently, without frightening the rest away.

The arrow-poisons described by early pioneers (including Raleigh) were battle-poisons, unrelated to curare. The first true accounts were by 18th-century explorers. In 1813, an English naturalist Charles Waterton made the important discovery that a poisoned animal could be kept alive by artificial respiration until the effects of the curare had worn off; for curare kills only by paralysing the muscles of breathing. A veterinary colleague, Sewell, suggested that curare might be used to relax the dangerous muscle spasms of tetanus. More than a century later this method was successfully adopted.

In 1850 Claude Bernard published the first of his papers on the action of curare, proving that its action was to prevent impulses from crossing from nerve-endings to muscle fibres. Bernard recognized the potential value of curare in medicine, but insisted that it could not be used until it could be purified and studied in more detail than was then possible. His point was proved by others who tried to use it and found it unreliable.

A pure alkaloid, *d*-tubocurarine, was isolated in 1935. Since 1942 this and other related drugs have been used during surgical operations. Breathing is regulated artificially, and curare provides complete muscular relaxation – a most important aid to the surgeon – while the dose of anaesthetic is kept to a safe minimum. This technique has removed one of the principal risks of major surgery – that a large enough dose of a conventional anaesthetic to relax the muscles may be dangerously large.

Cushing, Harvey (1869–1939). American neurologist, a pioneer of brain surgery. He was both a distinguished scientist and one of the most skilful of surgical technicians – a rare combination but essential to his chosen specialty.

Cushing's syndrome. A disorder of body chemistry, with retention of salt and water, obesity confined to the face and trunk, high blood pressure, weakening of bone and connective tissue, and sometimes diabetes and other symptoms. It is due to excessive production of steroid hormones by the cortex of the adrenal glands or to prolonged treatment with such hormones (♢ *adrenal*; *corticosteroid*).

cutaneous. Of the skin.

cuticle. The outer layer of the skin; epidermis.

cutis (cutis vera) = ♢ *corium*.

cyanide. Cyanides are the quickest acting of all poisons. Inhaled fumes of hydrogen cyanide (prussic acid) kill almost instantaneously; swallowed cyanides in a very few minutes. A victim who survives as long as half an hour is likely to recover.

These poisons inactivate enzymes responsible for the transfer of oxygen from the blood to the actual chemical processes on which life depends. The result is a sort of chemical paralysis of the whole body. It is like suffocation, but instead of the victim's being deprived of oxygen he is unable to use the oxygen that he has.

Among the antidotes used, nitrites and methylene blue permit the haemoglobin of the blood to form a relatively inert compound with cyanide; sodium thiosulphate (photographer's hypo) forms a thiocyanate and ferrous sulphate a ferrocyanide. In all cases, the object is to prevent the cyanide from combining with the iron of the respiratory enzymes.

cyanocobalamine. Vitamin B_{12}.

cyanosis. Bluish complexion from lack of oxygen in the blood circulating through the skin, due either to inadequate intake in the lungs, e.g. pneumonia, or to stagnation of blood in the circulation, e.g. heart failure. Local disorders such as chilblains cause localized cyanosis.

cycloplegia. Paralysis of the pupil of the eye.

cyclopropane. An anaesthetic gas.

cyst. 1. Bladder (mostly in compound words, e.g. cystitis).

2. Abnormal swelling, containing fluid. Cysts are of several kinds. Some are tumours with cells that form mucus or other fluids with no way of escape; some are composed of normal fluid-forming (glandular) cells that have become displaced in the course of early development; some are ordinary glands, e.g. grease glands in the skin, of which the outlets have become blocked. Cysts appear most often in the skin and in the ovaries, where they may grow very large unless removed.

cysticercus. Larval form of tapeworm: the adult worm lives in the intestine, but cysticerci may be widely scattered in the body.

cystic fibrosis. An uncommon hereditary defect of numerous glands, including the mucous glands of the bronchi, the sweat glands, and the digestive glands. It is a recessive character – both parents carry the abnormal gene without showing signs of the disease, and there is a 1:4 chance that a child of the marriage will inherit the gene from both parents and develop cystic fibrosis. In the past, affected children have not survived, but with modern treatment they have every chance of doing so, and of meeting fellow-sufferers at treatment centres. If two of them marry, all their children must be affected.

The symptoms include severe digestive disorders, difficulty with breathing and lung infections (because of blockage by thick mucus), and a tendency to heat-stroke (because the sweat glands pour out too much salt).

Digestion is maintained by an exactly calculated diet with supplementary enzymes. The lungs are kept clear by drugs and physiotherapy to loosen and drain mucus, by prompt treatment of infection with antibiotics, and by providing a fine mist with a nebulizer for the patient to breathe at night – this keeps the mucus in his lungs so wet that he can cough it up.

cystine. An amino-acid; one of the components of protein. It occasionally accumulates in the urine and forms stones in the bladder.

cystitis. Inflammation of the urinary bladder, usually from bacterial infection, but sometimes from mechanical irritation from crystalline deposits in the urine.

Urine is normally free from bacteria. The conditions in which it may become infected are discussed under ◊ *pyelitis* (inflammation at the outlets of the kidneys, commonly associated with cystitis), and the treatment is similar. The symptoms of cystitis – frequent and painful passage of urine – arise from over-sensitivity of the bladder and its outlet.

cystoscope. Optical instrument for examining the inside of the urinary bladder. It is simply a lighted tube with a system of lenses, slender enough to be passed up the urethra into the bladder. A local anaesthetic is usually instilled before the instrument is passed.

cytochrome. Group of compounds related to the haemoglobin of blood, found in all tissues and concerned with the transfer of oxygen from the blood to the cells.

cytology. Study of cells. ◊ *histology.*

cytotoxic agents. Drugs that suppress cell reproduction or ◊ *mitosis,* i.e. they stop the growth of tissues and the normal replacement of degenerated cells. A drug with this property must, in large enough doses, be a general poison. The drugs are useful because rapidly growing cells such as those of cancer are much more susceptible than normal cells, so that a small dose may inhibit a cancer without damaging healthy tissues. In practice, though, an effective dose is likely to be unpleasant, and these drugs are given only with great caution. Not all cancers respond equally well to cytotoxic treatment. Among those that do best are Hodgkin's disease and some types of leukaemia.

Apart from the treatment of cancer, these drugs are sometimes used to suppress the rapidly growing white blood cells that are concerned with ◊ *immunity,* for example to prevent a recently transplanted kidney from being rejected as 'foreign' matter, or to relieve severe symptoms of ◊ *autoimmunity.*

Many widely different substances are in one way or another cytotoxic. They include derivatives of nitrogen mustard, alkaloids derived from the periwinkle, and antibiotics such as actinomycin.

D

Daltonism. Colour blindness, especially the red-green type, from which the chemist John Dalton (1766–1844) suffered.

D. and C. = ◊ *Dilatation* and curettage.

dampness. A damp surface loses heat by evaporation at a rate of about 600 calories per litre of water on a cold day. The primary fault of a damp house is that it is cold. But damp walls suggest other defects such as poor ventilation and rotten woodwork; in extreme cases the house may be structurally unsafe. The moist air and unpleasant smell add to the occupier's discomfort. If the walls are permanently damp, nothing else in the house is ever quite dry, and this includes clothing. Damp clothes are cold not only because of evaporation but because the warmth of clothes is due to insulation: the air enmeshed in cloth does not conduct heat, and therefore the body does not lose heat through it. But if the enmeshed air is damp it becomes a better conductor of heat, i.e. a worse insulator, and the body does lose heat through it.

The direct ill effects of dampness on health can be ascribed to the difficulty of keeping warm.

In very hot surroundings, dampness has the opposite effect. If the air is very moist it will take up no more water vapour; sweat will not evaporate from the skin and one cannot keep cool.

dandruff. A harmless scaly condition of the scalp. The surface of the skin is made of dead cells, which are continuously shed and replaced with new cells from the deeper layer. From most of the body, the fine scales are shed without being noticed, but on the scalp they tend to collect as dandruff. With greasy skins dandruff is more noticeable than with dry skins. Dandruff is associated with acne because both are favoured by greasy skin.

dapsone. A sulphone drug, at present the standard treatment for leprosy.

Darwin, Charles Robert (1809–82). British naturalist. Together with A. R. Wallace he first suggested (1858) that evolution had come about by natural selection, i.e. that the individuals best adapted to their environment stood the best chance of survival and so the best chance of breeding to establish their type. His work aroused great controversy, mainly because it appeared to attack religious beliefs. In fact Darwin did not deny the Creation ; he only pushed it further back in time, and suggested a way in which the earliest creatures might have developed into different and more complicated types. Also, people resented the idea that they were descended from monkeys. This is not quite what Darwin said. According to his theory, men and apes have a common ancestor less highly developed than either.

The direct importance of Darwin's work to medicine is the light it sheds on anatomy and embryology. Its indirect and much greater importance is that Darwin was the first biologist to discuss life in scientific terms, without any preconceived notion that things are so because it is right that they should be so. In other words, he was the first to shake off the fetters of teleology and make a purely objective study of life.

DDT (dichloro-diphenyl-trichloroethane). A contact insecticide discovered in Switzerland during the Second World War. It was much more effective than earlier insecticides, and became a major weapon against insect-borne disease, especially in the tropics. The few insects that survive unfortunately tend to produce offspring that resist DDT – a highly condensed example of evolution by survival of the fittest.

dead space. Air passages (nose, pharynx, trachea, bronchi) through which inspired air passes on its way to the working areas of the lungs. The air in this space takes no part in respiration, and a breath must be deep enough to remove it in order to be effective. Breathing through a tube, e.g. under water, increases the space, and if the tube is long enough effective breathing is impossible and the subject suffocates.

deafness. Hearing depends on a chain of events, and can be impaired or lost through disorders of any link in the chain (◊ *ear*).

The *external* or visible ear carries vibration in the air to the ear-drum. The *middle* ear transmits vibrations of the drum through a series of tiny bones to the *inner* ear, where vibrations are translated into nerve impulses. The *auditory nerve* transmits these impulses to the brain, where they are analysed and recognized as sounds.

The skin of the external ear secretes wax from modified sweat glands. Blockage by accumulated wax is perhaps the commonest cause of deafness; it is cured by washing out the wax – which may first have to be softened with oil.

The middle ear may be damaged by infection (*otitis media*), and before the discovery of antibiotics the operations sometimes needed to cure infection were almost as likely to cause deafness as the infection itself. The risk had to be accepted because untreated infection could spread to the brain.

Inflammation of the Eustachian tubes is a frequent complication of hay fever and common cold. It disturbs the middle ear and may cause some loss of hearing for a while. Poor hearing in childhood is often due to blockage of the Eustachian tubes by large adenoids.

Otosclerosis is a formation of unwanted bone in the middle ear. Hearing may begin to fail in early adult life. The cause is not known. Many of these cases respond well to surgical reconstruction.

The inner ear and auditory nerve can be damaged by physical injury, infection etc. The efficiency of the nerve deteriorates throughout adult life. Numerous poisons and drugs can affect the nerve.

Deafness from birth can be caused by virus diseases (notoriously German measles) in early pregnancy and by various difficulties during labour. A child that cannot hear does not learn to speak; deaf-mutes are mute only because they are deaf. By dint of extraordinary skill and patience, specialist teachers are nevertheless able to get many of these children to speak intelligibly.

The external ear, the ear-drum, and the opening of the Eustachian tube at the back of the nose can be inspected. The rest of the apparatus can be studied only indirectly and by inference.

The distance at which the patient hears a watch or a whisper with one ear closed is a very rough though useful guide. Tuning forks have special uses. If the base of the fork is applied to the skull sound is conducted by the bone as well as in the usual way by air. Defective air-conduction can be distinguished from defective bone-conduction and sometimes from nerve-deafness. This information is often important in the choice of a hearing-aid, since hearing-aids are of two types – those inserted into the ear to amplify air-conducted sound, and those placed behind the ear for bone-conduction.

A *pure-tone audiometer* emits a note of any chosen pitch (frequency) and volume (intensity). From the volume needed for the patient to hear notes of various frequencies a chart of his hearing can be made. Throughout adult life the ears become less sensitive to high-pitched notes: for instance, few adults can hear the cry of bats, though most children can. Deafness in old age is often only loss of the upper range. Such people suffer as much as anyone else from loud noises, and they can hear that they are being spoken to, so nobody believes that they are deaf. But they cannot distinguish consonants – which are high-pitched sounds – and cannot therefore understand what is said. With occupational deafness in very noisy jobs it is the frequencies that have assailed the ear that are ultimately lost.

Like blindness, deafness is not often total. What matters is whether the remaining sensation is useful.

decidua. Lining of the uterus, shed during a menstrual period or after the birth of a child.

decompensation. A defect of the heart (e.g. an inefficient valve) is said to be *compensated* when the beat is strengthened enough to maintain a normal circulation, and *decompensated* when the circulation is impaired, i.e. when there is a degree of ◊ *heart failure*.

decompression. 1. The very gradual return to atmospheric pressure of people such as deep-sea divers who work under high pressure, to avoid ◊ *compressed-air sickness*.
2. Relief of raised pressure inside an organ by an operation to release excessive fluid; especially release of cerebrospinal fluid or blood through a burr-hole in the skull, e.g. after head injury.

decubitus. 1. Lying in bed; position when lying. **2.** Ulcer formed by pressure of lying in one position; ◊ *bed-sore*.

defibrillation. Restoration of rhythmical heart beat by electrical stimulation in case of fibrillation (a completely irregular beat: ◊ *arrhythmia*).

degeneration. Alteration of body cells towards less specialized cell-types as a result of defective blood supply, infection etc. As a result of degeneration muscle or liver cells tend to lose their special functions and resemble the cells of fatty or connective tissue.

déjà vu. The false impression of having previously seen things that one is seeing for the first time; wrongly said to be a symptom of epilepsy and other disorders. In fact, most people experience it from time to time.

Delhi boil = ◊ *oriental sore.*

delirium. Disturbance of the brain by injury, fever, poisoning etc., with confusion, often hallucinations, excitement and other symptoms of disorganized and exaggerated mental activity.

Delirium tremens is a kind of delirium affecting heavy drinkers, especially after injuries or during sudden illness. It is not, as was once thought, an effect of sudden withdrawal of alcohol.

delivery. Childbirth ◊ *labour.* It is the mother who is delivered of the child, and not, as some medical jargon would have it, the child that is delivered (like a parcel at the door).

deltoid. Triangular muscle covering the shoulder. The base of the triangle is the broad attachment to the clavicle and scapula; the fibres converge on the narrow apex half-way down the outer side of the humerus. The muscle abducts the shoulder, i.e. raises the arm sideways.

delusion. An unshakeable belief which a normal person of the same intelligence and background would recognize as obviously wrong and unreasonable. The extreme delusions of grave mental disorder, especially schizophrenia, are easily discerned, but there is no clear line between mild delusion and simple error. In fact it is almost impossible to define delusions without calling one's political and religious opponents insane.

Most delusions are harmless except as pointers to mental illness. Some are danger-

ous: a man who thinks he is the Emperor of Atlantis may also think he has the right to cut off people's heads; or (a much commoner danger) one who thinks he is persecuted may take violent steps to defend himself.

dementia. Originally, mental disorder involving loss of intelligence, as opposed to *amentia*, where intelligence is retarded from birth. Thus *dementia praecox*, premature dementia, now known as schizophrenia. Dementia is now generally taken to mean mental deterioration as a result of physical changes in the brain, e.g. from infection. chronic poisoning, injury, arterial disease. The distinction between these 'organic' disorders and mental disorders without organic change in the brain or evident physical cause may be artificial: it may be simply that in the latter case the changes and causes have not been identified.

Senile dementia arises from the degeneration of brain cells in old age; ◊ *senility*. *Presenile dementia*, fortunately uncommon, is a group of disorders where brain cells start to degenerate for no known reason in middle age.

Dementia paralytica or general paralysis of the insane is an effect of advanced ◊ *syphilis*.

denaturation. Altering the structure and properties of a protein by changing its environment, e.g. 'setting' egg-white by warming.

dengue. A virus infection occurring throughout the tropics, transmitted by the mosquito *Aëdes aegypti*. Symptoms arise about a week after infection; they include fever, skin rash, nausea, headache, and severe pain in joints ('breakbone fever'). The symptoms often subside about the third day but return after a short interval. After the second, usually milder episode the patient recovers completely, though he may need several weeks to get back his strength.

No treatment shortens the illness, but drugs such as aspirin, codeine, and tranquillizers may ease the symptoms. A vaccine is available, but better still the disease can be eradicated by mosquito control.

dentine (dentin). The main substance of a tooth; ivory. ◊ *teeth* (1).

dentistry. There are pre-Roman specimens of artificial teeth, held in place by wires or metal bands attached to the remaining sound teeth. An Egyptian papyrus of about the 16th century B.C. describes filling cavities and splinting loose teeth with gold wire. Greek surgeons carried these skills to the Roman Empire.

Along with the rest of medical science, good dentistry was lost in the Middle Ages. The Renaissance surgeons who revived it include Paré in France and Fabricius ab Aquapendente in Italy. Fabricius seems to have been the first to drill and cleanse cavities before filling them.

Pierre Fauchard (1678–1761) was the first specialist in dentistry and the author of the first treatise on the subject (*Chirurgien dentiste*, 1728). He made complete removable sets of false teeth, fitted artificial crowns, and improved Fabricius's method of treating decay, incidentally refuting the current belief that decay was due to worms.

But apart from the few surgeons who happened to be interested in it, dentistry remained in the hands of men with little if any special training. A few jewellers made false teeth; for the rest, dentists were itinerant tooth-pullers. Dentistry as a profession was hardly known until the middle of the 19th century. Then in 1844 Wells gave the first dental anaesthetic. In 1848 (Sir) John Tomes published a most influential work: *Dental Physiology and Surgery*. In the 1850s professional examinations were introduced in many countries – first in America, which in modern times has consistently led the way in the various branches of dentistry.

Recent developments include vastly improved apparatus, the growth of orthodontics (the correction of deformities of the teeth), of preventive dentistry, and of co-operation between dental and general surgeons in the treatment of injuries and diseases of the mouth and jaws.

In some countries there are two professional grades – licensed dentists and graduate dental surgeons, with various auxiliary grades. The profession was unified in Britain with the formation in 1921 of the Dental Board, associated with the General Medical Council. In 1956 the Board was replaced by an independent General Dental Council.

deodorant. (Means of) removing smells. Unpleasant smells are often due to the action of bacteria: thus fetid breath is generally caused either by bacterial decomposition of food left between the teeth or by bacterial infection of the gums, and strong body smells are due mainly to bacterial decomposition of sweat, rather than to an excess of sweat. Hence careful cleaning of the teeth and dental attention generally deal with the former, and soap (which deals well with most skin bacteria) with the latter. Body deodorants act partly by decreasing the secretion of sweat and partly as disinfectants, i.e. by killing bacteria.

depilatory. (Means of) removing hair. Various chemicals, e.g. barium sulphide, cause hair to fall. They need to be prepared and used with care to avoid injuring the skin. X-rays are also effective; this method was formerly much used in the treatment of resistant cases of ringworm of the scalp, but with newer remedies, particularly griseofulvin, depilation is now seldom needed.

depression. In general: a disorder of mood; protracted and disproportionate melancholy. In a more technical sense: the same exaggerated misery accompanied by impairment of all mental processes and of physical functions such as appetite, sleep, sex, and work.

In some circumstances, melancholy is a normal response. After bereavement, for instance, its absence might imply mental illness. Some people are gloomy by nature but cannot reasonably be called abnormal, and everyone at times feels dejected for no good reason. What distinguishes depression as an illness from a normal fluctuation of mood is that it is deeper and lasts longer than one would expect of the particular person affected. A close friend or relative may notice the early symptoms more easily than a specialist who has not known the patient before. The point is worth making because the sooner the patient is treated the better. Effective treatment not only prevents needless suffering; it can be life-saving, because untreated depression can end in suicide.

To outward appearances there are two kinds of depression. The first looks like a reaction to external events that would upset anyone to some extent, and counts as an illness only because the patient's reaction is greater, in degree and duration, than the circumstances warrant. This can be called *reactive* depression. The second kind, where there seems to be no good reason for misery, can be said to have arisen within the patient himself, and this kind, often associated with the other symptoms of the second definition above, can be called *endogenous* depression. The distinction is useful if only for the sake of discussion, even if reactive and endogenous depression are not so much two distinct illnesses as two factors contributing to the same symptom.

The actions of various drugs support the idea that at least some depression may be endogenous, arising from a disturbance within the patient's own nervous system. Reserpine, a kind of tranquillizer used mainly for the control of high blood pressure, acts by suppressing the action of certain substances that transmit nervous impulses in the brain. It has the drawback that in some patients it causes severe depression. On the other hand, drugs that enhance the activity of these transmitters (MAO inhibitors, see below) relieve depression. Thus, depression might be merely a symptom of deficiency in some part of the brain of one of these transmitters, probably *serotonin*. Unfortunately for this theory, the deficiency might be only a result of depression and not a cause; the question is still open. Exactly the same problem arises with other mental illnesses: does alcohol make people neurotic, or do people drink because they are neurotic? ◊ *schizophrenia*.

A clinical or symptomatic classification is as elusive as one based on causes. Some depression is only a kind of personality at the dark end of a spectrum that leads by way of 'average' personalities to the overwhelmingly merry and ebullient. As with the spectrum of political opinion, the two extremes can be very close to each other. The mood of people with *cyclothymic* personalities alternates between gloom and elation. This looks like a small-scale model, still within normal limits, of the serious disorder known as manic-depressive psychosis, but the relation of one to the other is not clear (◊ *schizoid personality*, in relation to schizophrenia).

Depression may take the form of a *neurosis*, i.e. the patient has understandable reasons for being miserable, and himself understands the nature of his illness: it is the degree and duration of his misery that are abnormal. This is the type that has been called *reactive depression*. Many psychiatrists no longer accept such a diagnosis, feeling that there is more to these cases than a simple neurosis. On the other hand, depression is sometimes a symptom of an anxiety state, which is certainly a neurosis.

Severe depression may be a component of ◊ *manic-depressive psychosis*. Though many people with this psychosis have episodes of mania as well as of depression, some suffer only depressive attacks, and in the early stages at least these may appear to be neurotic or 'reactive', as described above. But the patient is not completely rational, and is liable to have other symptoms of endogenous depression, such as insomnia and loss of weight. Depression of the same type starting in middle age, *involutional melancholia*, is described by different psychiatrists as a disorder on its own or as a variant of manic-depressive psychosis.

The risk of suicide cannot be judged by the apparent depth of depression. The safest course is to regard all depressives as potential suicides. Next to preventing suicide, the object of treatment is to reestablish the patient in society and in his own esteem. He cannot be talked out of his depression: he may not even be interested in the possibility of a cure because he does not consider himself worth saving. But the drugs now available not only relieve the symptoms but get the patient into a frame of mind where he can discuss his illness and listen to advice. Antidepressant drugs brighten the patient's mood, but paradoxically the treatment of a severe case may have to begin with a tranquillizer. Loss of sleep and of weight form vicious circles with depression. They can be difficult to treat at home; the patient needs to be watched because of the suicide risk, and some of the more powerful drugs need close supervision. Therefore severe depression is usually treated in hospital. Some very ill patients lack the initiative and energy to kill themselves, but they may make an attempt to do so as they begin to recover under treatment.

There are two main groups of antidepressant drugs. The first, the monoamine (MAO) inhibitors, was discovered in the early 1950s when the drug *isoniazid*, given for tuberculosis, was found to raise the patients' spirits, sometimes alarmingly. Chemically related drugs were then successfully used to relieve depression. These drugs inactivate M A O, an enzyme that serves to destroy some of the substances (noradrenaline; serotonin) that are released at nerve junctions in the brain to transmit impulses. If these transmitters were not destroyed as soon as their work was done they would accumulate and set up uncontrolled activity in the nervous system. The net effect of M A O inhibitors is to increase the available noradrenaline and serotonin. But M A O has the secondary function of inactivating other potentially dangerous substances. The standard doses of various drugs become highly poisonous to a patient taking M A O inhibitors. And *tyramine*, found in cheese, yeast extract and some other foods (it is probably the ingredient of cheese that can disturb sleep) also becomes poisonous with M A O inhibitors. Since a depressed patient may not care much about being poisoned, these drugs need the closest supervision.

The second group, comprising the tricyclic antidepressants, does not interfere with M A O, but may enhance the action of noradrenaline in some other way. Drugs of the two groups are therefore not used together. Some patients who do not respond to one group may respond well to the other.

Apart from a possible deficiency of serotonin, depression is also associated with an excess of sodium in certain brain cells. Lithium salts displace sodium, and have been used for treating manic-depressive psychosis. They appear to be more effective with the manic than the depressive component.

Some of the most rapid and dramatic recoveries from severe depression are achieved by ◊ *electroconvulsive therapy*, which is the application of small electric shocks to the brain. Nobody knows how the method works, but it is a most valuable stand-by, especially with patients who are so ill that their treatment is an emergency.

It can be argued that even the most up-to-date treatment does not actually cure depression. Neither does a splint mend a broken leg, but it allows a man to walk while the bone heals itself. Certain people are by nature liable to depression, and, having recovered from one attack, they may have another later on. Other people have brittle bones that a slight injury may break: their fractures can be treated and healed, and if they have another accident

nobody pretends that the treatment of the first was a failure.

dermatitis. Literally: inflammation of the skin. But most skin disease involves at least some inflammation, and the term dermatitis is not usually applied to inflammation due to infection. It still covers an assortment of disorders, mostly related in some way to *allergy*. The same can be said of the word *eczema*. There are still differences of opinion, but as a rule the two terms are used indiscriminately for the same ill-defined group of disorders.

Atopic dermatitis is a chronic, patchy, mild inflammation of the surface of the skin. The main symptom is usually itch, often out of all proportion to the apparent severity of the rash. In an average case it is a mild affliction for most of the time but liable to flare up on occasion. The condition behaves like a type of asthma where the patient is a little short-winded at all times and has an occasional attack of real difficulty in breathing, precipitated by a particular allergy, or by emotional stress, or for no apparent reason. There is more than just allergy to such cases of asthma, and more than just allergy to atopic dermatitis. The condition is often associated with other, more definite forms of allergy such as hay fever. Emotional disturbances are common, but they may be as much an effect of the dermatitis as a cause. Of all symptoms, itch is the most dependent on emotional state. In this condition, much of the skin trouble is due to scratching rather than to the original disorder.

The course of atopic dermatitis is unpredictable, but in general the long-term outlook is good. Even if the patient is always predisposed ('a sensitive skin'), he is likely to improve gradually and go for long periods without symptoms, or, with reasonable luck, remain permanently free.

Babies sometimes have this disease or something very like it (*infantile eczema*). They usually grow out of it, but they may be exposed to a dangerous complication: if they are vaccinated, there is sometimes a violent, even fatal flare-up. These babies must not only not be vaccinated; they have to be protected from contact with people who have just been vaccinated.

Contact dermatitis must be the commonest of skin diseases (except acne, which is hardly a disease at all). It is also the commonest occupational disease. The appear-

ance of the affected skin is not characteristic of this disease and no other; it might
be any sort of inflammation, with reddening, raised spots, perhaps some puffiness.
As with atopic dermatitis one cannot be
sure how much of the damage is due to the
actual disease and how much to scratching.
Because the primary cause is contact with
an irritant, exposed skin (hands, forearms,
face) is most often affected, but since the
irritant may be in clothing, soap etc. no
part of the body is exempt. The affected
area is often the best clue to the kind of
irritant.

According to the original concept of
allergy, the causative agent (allergen) must
be a protein. Contact dermatitis is generally due to much simpler chemical substances, which probably act by altering the
structure of one of the body's own proteins
so that it becomes a 'foreign' protein.
Whereas atopic dermatitis is an immediate
reaction to an allergen, contact dermatitis
is a delayed and cumulative response.
Atopic dermatitis is part of a more general
allergic response, which happens to show
itself in the skin but might just as well take
the form of, say, asthma. Contact dermatitis is strictly confined to the skin, and although the rash may spread to some extent
it is always worst at the actual point of contact.

There is no limit to the number of substances that can cause contact dermatitis.
Textiles (and substances used in their preparation), plants (primula, ragweed), cosmetics, drugs, woods, lubricants, synthetic
resins, solvents, even metals (nickel,
chromium) have been implicated.

Actinic (solar) dermatitis is a variant of
the same disorder: too much sunlight will
give anyone dermatitis, but some people
get it after slight exposure because their
skin has been sensitized by a drug, cosmetic
etc. which has just failed to produce a
dermatitis in its own right.

With all these conditions the first and
most difficult problem is to identify the
exact cause. This may prove impossible,
especially with atopic dermatitis, where
other factors than simple allergy are involved; but patience and ingenuity will
generally provide the answer with contact
dermatitis. Cure is then a matter of avoiding contact with the culprit. It may be as
simple as change of bath-soap or as complex as a change of occupation.

Seborrhoeic dermatitis is a common

affliction of people with greasy skins. In its
usual mild form it consists of small scaly
spots on the scalp with excessive formation
of dandruff. Occasionally it spreads to the
face and the back of the shoulders – a similar distribution to acne, which it may
accompany. The cause is completely unknown, but most cases respond well to
simple lotions or ointments for removing
scales and grease.

Stagnation of blood in the skin, generally
due to varicose veins, leads to *stasis dermatitis* (varicose eczema), with thinning and
pigmentation of the skin, which is very
vulnerable to slight injury or irritation.

dermatology. Study of the skin.

dermatophyte. Any of a group of microscopical fungi infecting the skin and causing ringworm and other troubles.

dermatosis. Any affliction of the skin (an
even vaguer term than dermatitis).

dermis = ◊ *corium.*

dermoid. A kind of cyst formed by the
growth of a displaced fragment of skin,
isolated from the surface either by an accident of prenatal development or, rarely, by
injury.

Descartes, René (1596–1650). Although his
direct contribution to medical knowledge
was small, Descartes has an important place
in medical history, because more than anyone since Aristotle he taught scientists to
think clearly. Pure science (on which biology
and medicine should be based) is today
mainly concerned with reducing to a minimum the 'facts' from which natural laws are
derived, and of course with ensuring that
they are true facts. This attitude to nature
springs from Descartes's doctrine that
nothing is so obvious that it can be accepted
without question. Most errors in science
have arisen – and still arise – from neglecting this simple rule, from taking things at
their face value. There are good examples
in Descartes's own writings. In considerable detail he deduced the workings of the
human body, but he argued from wrong
data and therefore came to wrong conclusions. Although he had read and praised
Harvey's clear proof that the heart muscle
pumped blood round the body, Descartes
stated as a self-evident fact that the heart

heated and distilled the blood. From this he argued with inexorable logic that the heat expanded the blood, forcing it into the arteries; that the most refined fraction of the distillate rose highest, to the brain, whence this 'subtle fluid' was carried by the nerves (which must therefore be hollow) to the muscles. 'And how could digestion take place in the stomach, unless the heart sent heat there by the arteries, with some of the more fluid parts of the blood, which help to dissolve the food that is put there?' The purpose of breathing was to cool and condense the blood, making it fit to return to the heart and feed the fire there. The account is grotesquely wrong at every point. It was almost bound to be, for the role of logic is to interpret facts, not to replace them. John Hunter stands far below Descartes intellectually, but he was a much better biologist: he worked on the principle 'Why think? Why not try the experiment?'.

On the other hand, Descartes guessed the nature of reflex action long before anyone else, though he thought it occurred only in animals, which had no soul. He has been much criticized for giving the soul an exact anatomical position – in the pineal body, a small gland in the middle of the brain. But his definition of the soul ('that part of the body of which the nature is simply to think') could as well be applied to the mind, of which the brain is surely the centre if anything so elusive can have a centre. An understanding of sensation and psychology is much facilitated by Descartes's doctrine that qualities such as sounds, colours, or textures are events in our brains rather than inherent properties of the world around us.

Much of the development of modern physiology has taken place in France, and this may be largely due to the influence of Descartes on French thought.

desensitization. A method of treating ◊ *allergy*: first, the substance(s) to which the patient reacts (the *allergen*) has to be identified by showing that it causes allergic inflammation in the skin; the allergen is then injected in gradually increasing doses until the patient is immune to its effects.

In psychiatry; a method of treating certain neuroses. The source of his anxiety having been identified, the patient is exposed in reality or imagination to situations that are increasingly alarming to him, and learns to relax at each stage.

desquamation. Shedding of the outer layer of the skin (a continuous, normal process); peeling after sunburn, scarlet fever etc.

detergent. Cleansing agent, especially one that acts by lowering surface tension – this enables water to penetrate better and remove grease by forming an emulsion. Some detergents are used as ◊ *antiseptics* for the skin. Their action depends on an opposite electrochemical effect to that of soap, so that the two cancel each other and should not be used together.

devil's grip = ◊ *Bornholm disease.*

dextran. Carbohydrate, chemically like starch and cellulose, of which a solution can be injected into a vein to restore the volume of the blood in severe ◊ *shock*, e.g. after extensive burns, where fluid has leaked from the bloodstream into the damaged tissues. A solution of sodium chloride can be used in the same way, but quickly leaks away. Dextran molecules are too large to escape from the blood vessels, so they retain the necessary water by ◊ *osmosis.*

dextrocardia. An unusual arrangement of the heart with the apex on the right, the mirror-image of the common arrangement; sometimes all the other organs are also transposed – liver on the left, spleen on the right etc. – and the condition is then called *situs inversus.* It has no medical significance.

dextrose. Grape-sugar; glucose.

diabetes. Abnormal excess of urine. The two kinds of disease described below have only this symptom in common.

diabetes insipidus. An uncommon disorder, in which a large volume of urine is formed regardless of the state of the body's store of water. In healthy people the flow of urine from the kidneys is regulated to keep the dilution of the blood constant. Diabetes insipidus is a breakdown of this mechanism, usually from failure of the pituitary gland to secrete antidiuretic hormone (ADH). The primary defect may be in the pituitary itself, or in the hypothalamus, the part of the floor of the brain that governs secretion of the hormone in response to changes in the dilution of the blood. The defect is remedied by giving A D H by injection or in snuff or nasal drops. (An extremely rare form of diabetes insipidus is due to congenital inability of the kidneys to conserve water.)

In extreme cases, the daily amount of urine, and therefore the amount of water to be made good by drinking, has amounted to more than half the patient's body weight.

diabetes mellitus. Diabetes mellitus, or simply *diabetes*, is the result of a deficiency of ◊ *insulin*, a hormone secreted by the pancreas to regulate the use of sugar (glucose). The deficiency can be caused in more than one way, so that diabetes is a group of diseases with similar symptoms, not a single disease.

Deficiency of insulin may be *absolute*, when the pancreas does not form a normal amount. Or it may be *relative*, when the patient does not use insulin properly and needs more than even a normal pancreas can secrete. A man whose pancreas has been removed forms no insulin at all. He needs injections of 20 or 30 units of insulin daily to stay healthy. Many diabetics form much more insulin than this for themselves, yet need a larger daily injection than people with none – because they have antagonists to insulin in their tissues and most of the insulin is wasted, or because their body cells (particularly those of the liver) do not respond normally to insulin. The exact nature of the antagonism to insulin is not known. Several hormones (pituitary, adrenal, thyroid, and *glucagon* from the pancreas itself) oppose the action of insulin, and a few cases of diabetes can be blamed on an excess of one of them – e.g. diabetes as a symptom of Cushing's syndrome, which is an excess of adrenal hormones. In most cases, *antibodies* which combine with insulin and neutralize it may be the cause; or it may be that the liver takes up insulin and 'imprisons' it, which has the same effect.

1. EFFECTS OF DIABETES

The symptoms of insulin deficiency range between none at all and those of a debilitating and, unless treated, fatal illness.

Glucose should be released from the liver into the blood and taken up by cells throughout the body to be oxidized (burnt) to carbon dioxide and water. This oxidation is the body's main source of energy. In some way insulin enables glucose to pass through the outer membrane of a cell. If there is no insulin, glucose is not taken up but accumulates in the blood.

The effects are far-reaching. The most obvious and least important are: excess of glucose in the blood (which is quite harmless), overflow of glucose into the urine, and increased volume of urine to carry the glucose. Increased volume of urine causes severe thirst, which may be the first symptom of diabetes.

The secondary effects on body chemistry are more significant. Because glucose cannot be burnt, fat is burnt instead, and the patient loses weight. But the combustion of fat can be completed, i.e. brought to the end-products carbon dioxide and water, only in the presence of reagents formed during the combustion of glucose. Since glucose is not being burnt, fat combustion stops half-way. The intermediate products – *ketone bodies* – collect in sufficient amount to become poisonous. They cause severe *acidosis* and ultimately *coma*, in which the patient is likely to die unless he is given insulin. As well as fat, protein is consumed as fuel, so that muscle and other tissues are weakened.

A third group of symptoms is due to degeneration of small blood vessels. Those of the eyes and kidneys seem the most susceptible; uncontrolled diabetes can lead to defective vision or even blindness, and to a form of Bright's disease of the kidneys. The nerves of the limbs are sometimes affected by diabetic neuritis (neuropathy), with tingling, numbness and other troubles; this may be due to interference with their blood supply.

Diabetics are also prone to disease of large arteries (*atheroma*) with its complications such as angina. This may be due to disturbed fat chemistry.

Another common complication is bacterial infection. A crop of boils is occasionally the first indication of diabetes.

2. TYPES OF DIABETES AND TREATMENT

The depressing account given above applies only to a severe form of the disease, usually starting in childhood or early adult life. This *juvenile diabetes* is considerably more serious than the effect of removing the pancreas. The patient seems to have not merely no insulin activity but some positive activity in the opposite direction. Apart from a tendency to run in families (it is no more than a tendency) no causes of juvenile

131

diabetes are known. Until the discovery of insulin these patients were bound to die young. With the correct daily doses of insulin and a controlled diet, they lead a perfectly normal life.

Since insulin is rapidly digested in the stomach it has to be given by injection. The effect of plain insulin wears off in about 8 hours, but long-acting compounds enable many patients to manage with a single daily injection. The dose has to be found by trial and error; it may be anything from a few units to several hundred in a particular case, and it varies according to the diet. Theoretically the patient could eat as he pleased and work out the right dose of insulin for the day's food, but in practice he takes a more or less fixed diet so that the dose need not be changed. Even then his requirements vary slightly, e.g. after unusual exertion or illness, and the urine has to be tested regularly to ensure that it is kept free from sugar and ketone bodies. Some diabetics ensure against overdosage by taking only enough insulin to leave a trace of sugar in the urine.

Diabetes that starts in middle age is generally a much milder disease. The patient is commonly over-weight when the first symptoms appear. His trouble is a limited supply of effective insulin. By eating less he may well keep his diet within the bounds of what his own insulin can manage. Of those who do need a supplement, many can be kept fit with one of the insulin-substitutes taken by mouth, avoiding the inconvenience of daily injections. These drugs either increase the patient's production of insulin or reinforce the effect of insulin. They cannot replace insulin in people who have none.

3. HISTORY

The term diabetes was first recorded by Aretaeus in the 2nd century A.D., and the sugary taste of the urine by Thomas Willis in the 17th. Claude Bernard's research on sugar in the body in the mid-19th century was the start of a proper understanding of diabetes, and in 1889 von Mering and Minkowski proved the association of diabetes with a deficiency of the pancreas. But severe diabetes remained an incurable disease until 1921, when Banting and Best isolated fairly pure insulin. Insulin was crystallized in 1926, and its formula was established in 1959 (◊ insulin).

It is often pointed out that insulin is no cure, because the patient needs daily injections for the rest of his life. This is a very pessimistic view. To be sure, a dose of insulin is no more a permanent cure of diabetes than a drink of water is a permanent cure of thirst; but while the effect lasts the cure is complete and the patient is in all respects healthy.

More than any other class of patient, diabetics have to be their own physicians, and their doctors have become advisers and teachers rather than custodians of esoteric knowledge.

diagnosis. The identification or recognition of diseases. The methods are precisely those of detectives in novels (and no doubt of real detectives too). Apart from a few cases where the culprit practically gives itself up (e.g. a text-book history of migraine; an unmistakable rash of chickenpox) it is a process of elimination from a group of suspects, starting with the premise that anyone might have any conceivable disease.

The first piece of evidence is the patient's own statement of his troubles – the case-history. Here the physician's skill lies in getting the facts without putting ideas into the patient's head, and in judging the patient's reliability as a witness. His problem is not with blatant liars (about age, habits, or disabilities), who are easily recognized, but with honest people who hide symptoms to avoid making a fuss or hearing bad news, or invent symptoms to rationalize their anxieties. The patient's account of previous illness and family history often gives important clues.

Physical examination is a well rehearsed routine. To record a medical history and make a complete examination would take at least an hour, but even a short history narrows the field of inquiry and indicates which parts of the examination need special care. Although physical examination occasionally reveals something quite unexpected, its main value is in confirming or refuting suspicions aroused by the history.

Finally, special investigations may be needed, such as chemical tests, microscopical study of blood cells or other tissues, and X-ray examination. A few such investigations are done routinely and count as part of an ordinary examination: simple chemical tests of the urine, for example. The current emphasis on early recognition of diseases that cause few symptoms until they reach a dangerous stage is bringing various 'special' investigations into routine practice. But as a rule patients are subjected to X-rays, blood tests and the rest only when the possible diagnoses have been reduced to two or three suspects, or when a provisional diagnosis needs elaboration – e.g., *pneumonia*, but which antibiotic drug will deal with it best?

The level of diagnosis varies greatly. Until fairly modern times diagnosis was almost always *symptomatic*. A diagnosis of gout (*podagra*) put into a word what the patient had described – the sensation that his foot was caught in a trap. It did rather more, because by naming the disease the physician was putting it in the same class as other cases he had seen or heard of, and on the basis of past experience he could predict and prescribe. Today, obvious examples of symptomatic diagnosis would be *asthenia* or *debility* (weakness), *constipation*, *dyspepsia* (indigestion), *hypertension* (high blood pressure). None of these diagnoses says anything about the real nature of the trouble. Less obvious examples include *asthma*, *epilepsy*, *neurosis*, and *rheumatism*. Any of them can be qualified in at least some cases to give a more complete answer. Thus nobody would settle for 'constipation' without asking why, or 'rheumatism' without trying to say which of the several types. But when known causes of a disease have been ruled out the symptomatic diagnosis has to be qualified by an adjective ('essential', 'idiopathic', 'primary'), meaning only that the trouble seems to have started of its own accord. 'Epilepsy' means that the patient has fits; 'idiopathic epilepsy' means that nobody knows why.

The next step is an *anatomical* diagnosis to define the exact site of the trouble. This is obvious enough when a patient breaks his leg; but injuries apart, anatomical diagnosis was hardly possible until medicine began to be founded on a thorough knowledge of anatomy in the 16th century, and it was unusual until pathology – the processes of disease – came under serious study in the 18th and 19th centuries. The change makes the difference between the superb *symptomatic* accounts of Sydenham (17th century), and descriptions by Addison and Bright (early 19th) of the precise location of diseases. From the symptomatic diagnosis *dropsy*, Bright distinguished cases where the primary trouble was heart disease from those where it was in the kidneys, the one responding to treatment with digitalis and the other not. Bright's colleague Addison, investigating cases of progressive and fatal debility, defined two diseases: one of the blood (pernicious anaemia) and one of the adrenal glands (Addison's disease).

When the site of a disease has been defined, something can usually be discovered about its nature (*pathological diagnosis*) and cause (*aetiological diagnosis*). Only then can the treatment be wholly rational. Addison could only describe pernicious anaemia as '"idiopathic", to distinguish it from cases in which there existed more or less evidence of some of the usual causes or concomitants of the anaemic state'. But he had shown his successors where to look, and in the present century pernicious anaemia and Addison's disease have both been brought under control, the one with liver extract (later vitamin B_{12}) and the other with adrenal hormones. Each was due to deficiency of an essential factor. The diagnosis was still not complete, for the deficiency was unexplained. It so chances that both are now ascribed (at least by some investigators) to allergic reactions to parts of the body's own tissues (◊ *autoimmunity*). If this should be proved, the next question will be: why the reaction? Probably no diagnosis will ever be complete. The problem is simply pushed further back; and that is really all that any science achieves.

The level of a diagnosis depends not only on how much is known of the disease, but also on what is necessary or practicable in the particular case. Complete investigation of every illness is out of the question – half the population would be admitted to hospital and the other half would be attending to them, and most of the patients would either die or recover before their diagnoses were complete. In practice a diagnosis is taken far enough to show what has to be done for the patient; only in selected cases does it need elaboration. A fundamental difference between general practice and the narrower specialties is that the general practitioner has to make some sort of diagnosis, however superficial, in every kind of case, and from this rapid diagnosis decide whether detailed investigation is really needed; whereas the specialist meets cases that have already been selected, and is always expected to make a complete diagnosis.

For instance, a patient may be sent to hospital with the vague diagnosis 'acute abdomen', meaning that he has one of half a dozen conditions, any of which needs urgent surgical attention. To carry the diagnosis further before getting him to hospital would only waste precious time. Or an undiagnosed fever may have to be treated as typhoid until further notice, because to prove the diagnosis takes time in which the condition could become dangerous.

Sometimes new forms of treatment demand new methods of diagnosis. Until recently, 'stroke' was an acceptable diagnosis. The kind of stroke did not matter because in any case there was nothing to be done about it. Now that some kinds can be prevented by surgery and others by drugs, it is often necessary to decide which blood vessel is involved and in what way.

In the past, diagnosis has been static and qualitative: it has tried to answer the question: what is the abnormal condition? The present trend is towards dynamic and quantitative diagnosis: how far has the trouble advanced, and what progress is it likely to make? This is dictated by recent developments in the treatment of disease. When people with symptoms from high blood pressure could only be given advice and sedatives, a diagnosis of 'hypertension' was enough. Now that there are highly potent drugs for controlling blood pressure, with undesirable as well as desirable effects, each case has to be accurately assessed: the degree of hypertension, its rate of progress, and the risks of withholding treatment have to be accurately balanced against the properties of the various drugs.

It is too soon to say much about diagnosis by computer, which is still in the experimental stages. Most people find the idea repugnant because it seems inhuman, but they may be missing the point. A diagnosis is made by sifting evidence and deciding which of the suspects is the likeliest culprit in the light of one's past experience of similar cases and of other people's published reports. As in crime detection, the first and most important step is to *suspect* the right answer; proving it is generally a matter of routine. The usual reason for completely missing a diagnosis is not suspecting it. No doctor is likely to overlook malaria in the tropics, because there it is the prime suspect in every case of fever and the parasites can be seen in the blood if they are sought. But outside the tropics a patient who develops malaria may wait for days before the possibility enters anyone's mind, though when once the question is raised it can be answered almost at once. With rare diseases, or unusual manifestations of common ones, the diagnosis may lie outside the physician's experience or reading. and it might take weeks to find the answer in a library. These are the errors that a properly programmed computer would avoid. It would automatically 'suspect' everything that had been fed to it, and it would assess the chances that a given set of symptoms were due to a particular disease, or that a given case would respond to a particular form of treatment – according, of course, to the information it had been given previously. Nobody has seriously suggested that computers could assume all the responsibilities of physicians, but there is no doubt that they can become most valuable tools as a sort of instant reference library.

dialysis. Selective diffusion through a membrane serving as a molecular filter: small molecules, e.g. salts, pass through, while large ones, e.g. proteins, do not. The principle is described in more detail under ◊ *osmosis*. It is applied in the artificial kidney: a membrane divides a stream of the patient's blood, taken from an artery and returned to a vein, from a prepared solution of salts, glucose etc. in the same concentrations as those of healthy blood. Since these substances are balanced across the membrane there is no effective traffic in them. The protein molecules and corpuscles of the blood are too large to pass through. But waste products such as urea flow from the zone of high concentration (the blood) to the low concentration of the prepared solution and are washed away. The apparatus is designed to take over the work of incompetent kidneys, but it may also be life-saving in some types of poisoning, e.g. overdoses of sleeping pills.

diamorphine. Diacetyl morphine; ◊ *heroin*.

diaphragm. Sheet of muscle separating the thorax from the abdomen. Its fibres arise from the lumbar vertebrae, the lower ribs, and the lower end of the sternum. They converge on a flat sheet of dense fibrous tissue, the central tendon. The whole structure forms a sort of dome.

When the muscle contracts, the central

tendon is pulled down, the thorax is enlarged, and air is drawn into the lungs to fill the extra space. This is the most important mechanical factor in ◊ *respiration*. Since the thorax is enlarged at the expense of the abdomen, the muscles of the abdominal wall simultaneously relax. If they do not relax, the diaphragm raises the pressure in the abdomen, e.g. during defaecation.

The origin of the diaphragm is in the neck, from which it has descended in the course of evolution, and in the development of the individual embryo. Any organ that migrates keeps its original nerve. The *phrenic* nerve on each side is formed from spinal nerves in the neck, above the origin of the nerves of the arm. It runs downwards among the neck muscles, into the thorax beside the heart, and through the diaphragm to branch out on its under surface.

Because the phrenic nerve takes this remarkable course one may survive disruption of the spinal cord at any but the highest level. Though the whole body from the shoulders down is paralysed the diaphragm continues to work. A broken neck is fatal only if the spinal cord is torn in the upper part of the neck. On the other hand poliomyelitis may sometimes affect cells in the upper cervical region while sparing the cord lower down; then the patient needs an iron lung although his trunk and limbs are unaffected.

The phrenic nerve is easily accessible in the neck. A small operation to paralyse it prevents one side of the diaphragm from moving and so rests the lung. This used to be a common operation to give tuberculous lungs a chance to heal, but with effective drug treatment of tuberculosis it is now seldom necessary.

Diaphragmatic ◊ *hernia* is a protrusion of part of the stomach through the opening for the oesophagus.

diarrhoea. Frequent passage of watery motions. The contents of the small intestine are always liquid. The main function of the large intestine is to absorb most of the water, leaving a soft but not watery residue of faeces to be passed. If the passage through the large intestine is unduly delayed too much water is absorbed and the faeces become dry and hard and difficult to pass; that is constipation. But if the passage is too rapid, or if there is an excess of water, the faeces are still liquid when they reach the

rectum and defaecation is urgent and frequent.

Most diarrhoea is due to inflammation of the intestine, with excessive production of watery mucus and over-activity of the intestinal muscles both contributing to the symptoms. Inflammation can be caused by viruses (many outbreaks of gastro-enteritis, especially in children), bacteria (bacterial food poisoning, bacillary dysentery), or larger parasites (amoebic dysentery, worm infestation); by irritant drugs and poisons; or by allergic reactions (food allergy, and possibly ulcerative colitis).

A saline purge (e.g. Epsom salt) works by ◊ *osmosis*, retaining water in the large intestine. Inability to digest sugars or other foodstuffs causes diarrhoea in the same way (◊ *carbohydrate intolerance*). In other types of malabsorption – e.g. sprue, deficiency of the pancreas – fat is not digested and causes a sort of diarrhoea.

The functioning of the intestine is much influenced by the nervous system and endocrine glands (thyroid, adrenal), and disturbances of these may cause diarrhoea. Sustained fear or anxiety can lead to overactivity of the intestine.

'Irritable colon' is a common complaint, especially of people who worry about their bowels and take laxatives. In essence it is a failure to keep a regular bowel habit, tackled by laxatives instead of a mixed diet, daily exercise, setting a regular time for opening the bowels, and ignoring an occasional failure. The rectum is irritated by hard faeces and forms too much mucus, which the constipated sufferer regards as diarrhoea.

Most of the common types of diarrhoea clear up in a day or two. The old treatment of a dose of salts or castor oil was rational because it helped to remove irritants, and by emptying the large intestine left the patient constipated for a while. It is seldom used now that most bacterial infection responds to sulphonamides or antibiotics.

Sustained diarrhoea demands attention because unless the cause is correctly treated the patient rapidly develops dehydration (especially if he vomits as well), and acidosis from loss of alkali (bicarbonate).

When the cause of diarrhoea has been established the symptom itself can be relieved with drugs such as codeine or absorbents such as kaolin.

A changed bowel habit always needs investigation (◊ *constipation*).

diastole. Phase of relaxation of the heart muscle during which the cavities of the heart are filled with blood (to be pumped out during the alternate phase, *systole*).

diathermy. Production of heat in a tissue by means of a high-frequency electric current, used for the relief of symptoms due to inflammation or stiff and painful muscles and joints.

diathesis. Hereditary or constitutional tendency to a particular type of disease. With many diseases that run in families, e.g. tuberculosis, angina, some types of cancer, it is the diathesis that is inherited, not the disease, and it may be possible to avoid factors that precipitate the actual disorder.

dicophane = ◊ *D DT*.

diet. Food is needed as fuel (◊ *energy*) and as raw material for growth and maintenance of the body. Even in adult life most tissues are continuously broken down and replaced, and although some of the material can be resynthesized and used again much of it is lost.

The three principal foods are *protein*, *fat*, and *carbohydrate*. All three can be used as fuel. Protein and carbohydrate supply the same amount of energy – about 4 Calories per gramme. Fat provides 9·3 Calories per gramme. But whereas fat and carbohydrate can be freely consumed, a good deal of the protein in the diet must be conserved as building material. In general, the chemical arrangement of foodstuffs differs from that of the body's own components. Digestion breaks down the food into simple compounds that are then rearranged as specifically human materials.

In addition to the three basic components, essential substances that cannot be synthesized in the body have to be supplied ready-made (◊ *vitamin*). The diet must also provide all the chemical elements ('minerals') found in living matter – some in minute amounts (e.g. copper, fluorine) and some in sizeable quantities (e.g. iron, calcium). Many of these minerals are poisonous in excess.

Undigested ballast (roughage) such as vegetable fibre improves the mechanical efficiency of the intestine.

1. BALANCED DIET

The diet must provide enough fuel. At complete rest, an average man needs 1,700 Calories daily. A sedentary worker needs some 2,500 Calories, and heavy manual labour may call for twice as much. The principal ingredients of a proper adult diet are:

(*a*) *Protein*. The minimum may be below 35 grammes daily. This amount of protein is found in a quart of milk, or 5 eggs, or ¼ lb. of meat, fish, or cheese, or 1 lb. of bread, or 2 lb. of cooked peas, beans, or spinach, or 5 lb. of cooked potatoes. But the bare minimum suffices only if there is enough other food to save protein from being consumed as fuel, and if the quality of the protein is right, i.e. if the amino-acids of which protein is composed are in the correct proportions. In practice these conditions are seldom met, and a reasonable diet contains twice the theoretical minimum of protein. Many proteins lack one or more amino-acids of the nine or ten that cannot be synthesized in the body (*essential amino-acids*), and in this respect animal foods are better than vegetable. A vegetarian diet must be well varied so that one food makes up the deficiencies of another. Because protein is used for building new tissue, children (weight for weight) need more than adults; and at any age lost protein has to be replaced after prolonged illness, or loss of blood.

(*b*) *Carbohydrate*. Carbohydrates (starch, sugar) can theoretically provide all the body's fuel, and with few exceptions (e.g. Eskimos, who live mainly on fat and protein) a starchy staple is the main item of food, with the more expensive proteins and fats as relish. Since all digestible carbohydrates are converted to glucose in the body, the particular form of starch or sugar in the diet ought not to matter, but there is evidence that refined sugar hastens arterial disease (◊ *atheroma*).

(*c*) *Fat*. A diet without fat is insipid and difficult to cook. Fat provides more than twice as much energy as other foods and reduces the bulk that has to be eaten. People who live almost entirely on carbohydrate have to consume very large quantities. But fats (the term includes oils) cannot provide all the energy, because the combustion of fat stops half-way unless there is also a supply of carbohydrate. Fuel in the body is ultimately oxidized to carbon dioxide and water. But this does not happen in one stage, as it would in a fire. It involves a long chain of chemical reactions. Some of the intermediate products of fat become poisonous if they are allowed to accumulate, as in ◊ *diabetes mellitus*. In the presence of the products of carbohydrate breakdown, they are promptly converted to harmless substances; but in the absence of these products they persist. With severe diabetes, when carbohydrates cannot be broken down, this kind of acidosis from fat becomes dangerous.

Certain components of fat (*essential fatty acids*) which cannot be synthesized are needed in the same way as essential aminoacids. Vegetable oils are a better source than animal fat. Lack of essential fatty acids is another factor in arterial disease, which is much less serious in people whose dietary fat is mainly vegetable.

The fat-soluble vitamins (A, D, K) are found mainly in fats and oils, and a fat-free diet is likely to be deficient in them.

(*d*) *Vitamins*. A mixed diet generally contains enough of all the vitamins, but the unvaried diet of poor communities in many parts of the world often lacks one or more of them (◊ *vitamin*).

(*e*) *Minerals*. Any sort of diet provides most of the minerals needed, but a few of these essential ingredients are sometimes lacking. Anyone can become short of ◊ *salt* if he sweats much, unless salt is added to his food (some miners put salt in their beer). Most diets contain only enough ◊ *iron* to meet normal demands, and not enough to make up losses from bleeding. Milk and vegetables contain plenty of ◊ *calcium*. Deficiency of calcium is more often due to lack of vitamin D (needed for assimilation of calcium) than to shortage of calcium in the diet. Small amounts of ◊ *iodine* and ◊ *fluorine* are needed, and in many parts of the world food and drinking water do not supply enough.

The principle, discussed under ◊ *vitamin*, that a surplus contributes nothing useful applies to all ingredients of the diet. A varied Western diet, including animal and vegetable foods, is unlikely to lack anything important.

Old people living alone who could afford to eat well may develop malnutrition from neglecting their diet.

2. MALNUTRITION

Millions of people in underdeveloped countries suffer from an inadequate diet. The commonest deficiency is of good protein, because the supply is limited and expensive. Clear-cut diseases are associated with lack of each of the vitamins. But a poor diet is generally poor in several respects, and malnutrition usually involves several ingredients of an adequate diet. The commonest state is not so much positive illness as failure to be really healthy, with vague symptoms such as apathy and weak resistance to infection. Malnutrition is especially serious in children, millions of whom die of what should be relatively mild infections of the intestine or lungs. ◊ *kwashiorkor* is a vicious form of malnutrition of children in many tropical countries.

In most of Europe, North America and other industrialized areas, malnutrition is more often due to illness than lack of food. Failure to assimilate food from the intestine (◊ *malabsorption*) is a symptom of various disorders. Chronic infection makes added demands, while impairing appetite and digestion. Protein and vitamins need special attention during pregnancy and lactation. Young women occasionally develop severe malnutrition from *anorexia nervosa*, an emotional disorder with complete absence of appetite.

3. SPECIAL DIETS

There is little to recommend the traditional insipid slops of 'invalid cookery', seemingly based on a belief that enjoyable food must be harmful. Modern cookery books properly advise attractive food for the sick, a better prescription than discouraging an already depressed appetite. But bulky or flatulent foods are uncomfortable bedfellows, and during almost any illness the sight of an over-loaded tray can be nauseating. The only valid principle seems to be that sick people can best manage small, varied, and agreeable meals; quantity can be made up by eating more often than usual. This may call for much patience and ingenuity.

All kinds of unusual diets are said to promote fitness. They succeed because they encourage people in the habit of eating too much to eat less.

Indiscriminate slimming can be harmful unless the reduced diet is planned to include essentials. ◊ *obesity*.

Several diseases need very special attention to diet. With some (e.g. coeliac disease, gout) certain foods are not tolerated. Some people are allergic to particular foods such as shellfish or eggs and must avoid them unless they can be desensitized by a course of injections. With diabetes the diet is planned to meet the various chemical disturbances affecting fat and carbohydrate. With all digestive disorders the diet is dictated by what the patient can manage. Special diets for kidney disease minimize the waste products to be excreted in the urine.

A major problem in dietetics is to fulfil the medical requirements of a diet while keeping a proper balance of essential ingredients. A second problem is to make the diet palatable: for instance heart disease may call for severe restriction of salt (and also of the size of meals), and salt-free food is extremely uninteresting. It is neither easy nor wise to plan special diets without the help of a dietitian.

differential diagnosis. Distinguishing between conditions with similar symptoms.

differentiation. The process in the development of living cells by which a cell acquires the special characteristics and functions of a particular tissue or organ. The cells of cancers are often poorly differentiated, like those of an early embryo; generally speaking, the less differentiated its cells, the more dangerous the cancer. Julius Cohnheim suggested (1877) that cancers grew from remnants of undeveloped embryonic tissue. This is probably true of a kind of infantile tumour (teratoma), but most cancer probably grows from adult tissue that regresses to a more primitive type.

diffusion. Movement of molecules in a fluid from a zone of high concentration to one of low concentration, tending to produce an even concentration throughout, like a drop of ink in a glass of water.

digestion. Chemical rearrangement of food, essentially a breaking down of large molecules into small ones that can be absorbed through the lining of the intestine, carried in the blood to the liver, and reassembled as needed.

Carbohydrates in the diet are sugars or starches. The common unit is a *monosaccharide* with the formula $C_6H_{12}O_6$ arranged as glucose, fructose, or galactose. Ordinary sugar (sucrose) is a *disaccharide* formed by the fusion of one molecule each of glucose and fructose. Milk sugar (lactose) is a disaccharide from glucose and galactose, and maltose is formed from two molecules of glucose. Starches have large molecules which are chains of glucose molecules.

An enzyme in the saliva, *ptyalin*, begins the digestion of starch by splitting off glucose molecules from the chain two at a time – i.e. as maltose. This is unimportant. Acid in the stomach splits sucrose into glucose and fructose. In the small intestine, the enzyme *amylase* from the pancreas completes the conversion of starch to maltose. For each disaccharide, the lining of the small intestine contains an enzyme to convert it to monosaccharides. These, and only these, are actively assimilated into the blood. In the liver, fructose and galactose are converted to glucose, which is therefore the final form of all dietary carbohydrate.

Fats are compounds of glycerol with fatty acids. The enzyme *lipase* from the pancreas splits fat into these components. The process, once thought to be complete, is now known to be only partial. Much of the dietary fat is assimilated unchanged. But first it must be made into a very fine emulsion, and this requires firstly that *some* of the fat should be split, and secondly that bile salts from the liver should be present. Both pancreas and liver must therefore be working properly for fat to be absorbed. Most of it is taken up not by the blood-stream but by the lymphatic vessels of the small intestine (lacteals) and delivered straight to the general circulation without passing through the liver, to be stored or consumed all over the body.

Protein is broken down to its component amino-acids partly in the stomach by hydrochloric acid and the enzyme *pepsin*, and partly in the small intestine by enzymes from the pancreas (trypsin) and lining of the intestine (erepsin).

Vitamins are assimilated unchanged – they have to be, for by definition they cannot be synthesized in the body. Vitamin B_{12} is not absorbed unless it is accompanied by 'intrinsic factor', formed by the normal stomach. If fat absorption is defective the fat-soluble vitamins A, D, and K may not be absorbed. In particular, vitamin K deficiency follows obstruction of the bile (obstructive jaundice).

◊ *stomach; intestine; diet.*

digitalis. Foxglove and related plants: source of the most valuable drugs for the treatment of heart failure. It was known to medieval herbalists as an emetic and purgative. Only when ◊ *Withering* investigated it properly in the late 18th century were these actions recognized as danger-signs of overdosage. After that it was regarded as primarily a diuretic – a drug for promoting the flow of urine – because in cases of dropsy the urine increased and fluid retained in the body vanished. The direct action of digitalis on the kidneys is now known to be of secondary importance. It is the action on the heart that really matters. Fluid retention (dropsy) is a result of inefficient work by the heart (⟐ *heart failure*). Digitalis increases the efficiency of the failing heart and so relieves the pressure and congestion in the veins that cause fluid to accumulate, at the same time improving the circulation of blood through the kidneys and so enhancing their output of urine. The useful actions of digitalis are firstly that it slows the heart beat, so that each beat is given time to be effective, and secondly that it strengthens the contraction of overtaxed heart muscle (though not of a healthy heart). Few drugs need more careful supervision than digitalis, because it is eliminated so slowly that doses accumulate. Overdosage makes the heart rate dangerously slow and may completely derange its rhythm.

digitoxin; digoxin. Pure substances extracted from *digitalis*, used in preference to the older preparations of digitalis leaves because the dose can be more accurately controlled.

dilatation. Widening or stretching, e.g. the reflex widening of blood vessels to increase flow, or of the pupils to admit more light to the eyes; or mechanical stretching to relieve abnormal narrowing (stricture) of a tubular organ such as the urethra. *Dilatation and curettage* is a common gynaecological procedure: under anaesthesia the muscle of the cervix uteri (normally a closed valve separating the uterus from the vagina) is gently stretched until it relaxes enough to admit a small instrument with which the lining of the uterus is peeled off. This lining is in any case only temporary: it is shed at each period and re-formed. The operation is especially valuable for diagnosis of gynaecological disorders, since microscopical examination of the lining membrane is an accurate guide to the function of the uterus and ovaries.

dimercaprol. ⟐ *BAL*, an antidote to certain metallic poisons.

Dioscorides (1st century A.D.). Greek physician in Rome. His *Materia medica* was the greatest compendium of drugs of antiquity. It remained the standard text until pharmacopoeias began to be compiled about A.D. 1600. And these early pharmacopoeias were little more than commentaries on Dioscorides with a few additions from Arabian and Indian sources.

diphtheria. An acute infection, nearly always of the throat but occasionally of other mucous membranes, by the diphtheria bacillus (*Corynebacterium diphtheriae*; Klebs-Löffler bacillus). In the tropics this bacterium has been known to infect the skin.

The disease is contracted either from a patient or from a carrier who harbours the bacteria without ill effects, by air-borne infection from coughs and sneezes. A few cases have been traced to infected milk. Within a week, and sometimes after only two or three days, the patient develops fever and sore throat. The typical sign is a soft crust (membrane; pseudomembrane) that forms over the affected mucous membrane. The inflamed tissues are swollen and painful, and the lymph nodes at the sides of the neck are commonly involved, but the infection spreads no further. These bacteria stay close to their point of entry; they never invade the blood-stream. Their special vice is that they form *toxins* – chemical by-products taken passively into the blood that are intensely poisonous to nerve cells, heart muscle and other tissues.

The first danger of diphtheria is mechanical: if the membrane is around the entrance to the trachea it may obstruct the airway. An artificial opening (tracheotomy) has then to be made below the obstruction.

The second and more insidious danger is poisoning by toxins. The commonest effects are defective function of heart muscle or of the kidneys, and localized paralysis resembling poliomyelitis. In untreated cases any of these can be fatal, but the toxin can be neutralized with a specific *antitoxin*. When antitoxin is given in time to forestall the effects of diphtheria toxin, the actual infection in the throat generally clears up without serious ill effects.

In many countries diphtheria has been reduced from a major cause of death among children to a very rare disease by routine immunization of children. During an attack of diphtheria the body forms its own antitoxin, but not quickly enough to avert serious risk. But by treating toxin with formaldehyde it is rendered harmless yet still able to evoke antitoxin formation. A child that has been given treated toxin (*toxoid*) is then immune to diphtheria in the sense that he produces antitoxin immediately if he is later infected.

The *Schick test* is a minute injection of toxin into the skin. If the subject is immune, the dose is promptly neutralized and nothing happens; if not, the skin is reddened. The test is used to decide who needs to be immunized during an outbreak.

diphyllobothrium. Giant tapeworm of Scandinavia, Japan and parts of North America. ◊ *worms*.

diplegia. Paralysis of both arms or both legs.

diplopia. Double vision; failure to superimpose the images recorded from the two eyes, nearly always due to imbalance of the eye muscles, which should automatically keep both eyes fixed on the same object. A childhood squint does not cause diplopia because when the child is learning to interpret vision he ignores messages from one or other eye; in time the suppressed eye becomes 'lazy' and its image is no longer consciously perceived even if the squint is corrected.

disaccharide. A sugar of which the molecules are made up of two simple sugars, e.g. *sucrose* or cane sugar, composed of glucose and fructose (◊ *carbohydrate*).

disc. The intervertebral discs are tough fibrous pads joining the individual bones of the backbone (vertebrae), making the whole structure flexible yet strong. ◊ *vertebra* (1).

disinfectant. Substance used for destroying harmful microbes. The term is generally applied to chemicals used for treating things such as apparatus, sickroom furniture or drains, in contrast with ◊ *antiseptics*, used on people: the only difference is that disinfectants need not be harmless to human tissue and are cheaper.

dislocation. Displacement of the moving parts of a joint, with the result that the joint is either immobilized or completely unstable.

The muscles and ligaments that hold a joint together are generally more resilient than the bone to which they are attached, and an injury is more likely to break a bone than to dislocate the joint. In most joints, dislocation is uncommon except as a complication of fracture of one of the bones forming the joint. The two main exceptions are the shoulder and the lower jaw. In the shoulder, instability is the price of extreme mobility. There is very little support below the joint, and the upper end of the humerus is easily twisted out of its shallow socket when the arm is extended above the head, e.g. in self-defence when one is thrown forwards and liable to land on one's head. It is a proverbial hazard of horse-riding. The lower jaw sometimes slips forward in its sockets at the base of the skull during a deep yawn. Injuries of the jaw push it in the opposite direction and are more likely to break the bone.

Sometimes the hip is dislocated from birth, and early treatment is required to prevent permanent disability; ◊ *hip*. Dislocation of the fully developed hip is an uncommon and severe injury. Only great violence will displace this very stable joint.

The small joints of the fingers are occasionally dislocated.

Other dislocations are nearly always accompanied by fractures. They include the two best known of all fractures. Colles' fracture is essentially a fracture of the radius just above the wrist, but there is also displacement of the inner (little-finger) side of the joint. Pott's fracture is a dislocation of the ankle, a joint that cannot be dislocated without breaking one of its supporting bones.

Within a few hours of the injury it is seldom difficult to replace a dislocated bone, even, on occasion, without anaesthetics. But if treatment is delayed the surroundings swell, tissues stick together, and the condition is as hard to correct as any fracture. Mere replacement is not all, for no joint can be dislocated without tearing ligaments, and these need time – sometimes several weeks – to heal. The joint may be weakened and liable to repeated dislocation. Various operations have been evolved for strengthening or replacing weak ligaments.

disseminated sclerosis = ◊ *multiple sclerosis*.

distal. Peripheral; further from the centre of the body or from the trunk (as opposed to *proximal*).

diuresis. Flow of urine; artificially increased flow of urine.

diuretic. Any drug used to promote a flow of urine. The kidneys filter a huge quantity of water from the blood. Most of it is reabsorbed and returned to the blood along with salt and other essentials; unwanted waste products remain in the small amount of water that is passed as urine. An excess of salt acts as a diuretic by ◊ *osmosis*, and in diabetics the excess of sugar has the same effect. Most diuretic drugs impede the reabsorption of salt in the kidneys. The increased output of salt carries with it a corresponding amount of water.

Diuretics are successfully used for treating heart failure, high blood pressure and many other conditions where fluid and salt are retained in the body.

diverticulitis; diverticulosis. *Diverticulosis* is the presence of small bulges or pockets at weak points in the large intestine. X-ray examination reveals such diverticula in many middle-aged people and most old people. The condition is harmless.

Diverticulitis is inflammation of a diverticulum, with symptoms like those of appendicitis but in the wrong place, usually on the left side of the abdomen. Surgical treatment is seldom necessary; antibiotics generally control the infection.

If the inflammation persists and chronic diverticulitis develops, the symptoms may be very like those of cancer of the large intestine: changed bowel habit (sometimes diarrhoea, more often constipation), vague abdominal pain, occasionally bleeding from the rectum, and, rarely, complete obstruction. The condition has to be distinguished from cancer by X-ray investigation and direct inspection of the lower part of the intestine with a lighted tube (sigmoidoscopy). Most cases of chronic diverticulitis respond to medical treatment with an easily absorbed diet, leaving little undigested residue to occupy the large intestine, drugs to relieve spasm and pain, and mild laxatives. Surgical treatment – removal of the affected segment of intestine – is reserved for severe or complicated cases.

diving. Some medical aspects are considered under ◊ *compressed-air sickness*.

DNA. Deoxyribonucleic acid. ◊ *genetics* (1).

doctor. Literally = teacher; since the 13th century, one who has attained a teacher's degree at a university. The first doctorates were conferred at Bologna. Other universities soon followed suit, and throughout Europe 'doctor' soon became synonymous with 'doctor of medicine', perhaps because he had to be distinguished from practitioners with no degree, whereas other learned professions had no untrained competitors. In most of Europe this is only colloquial usage and there is in addition a correct term for a practitioner of medicine (*médecin, Arzt, médico,* etc.). Britain is one of the countries where a doctorate is not automatically awarded on qualification; most 'doctors' have either a bachelor's degree from a university or a diploma from one of the other recognized institutions, and for them 'doctor' is a courtesy title. A doctorate in medicine can be had only some years after qualification, in recognition of research or specialized studies. Yet there is no convenient title other than *doctor* for all the people officially known as registered medical practitioners. The word should be *physician* – it is still so in America – but unfortunately this title is reserved in Britain for specialists in internal medicine (who are known in America as *internists*). The reason seems to be that three professions evolved that were not fused until the 19th century; *physicians* (the real doctors), *surgeons* (barbers), and *apothecaries* (druggists). As each attained professional status, the surgeons, having been denied recognition in the past, refused to accept the title when it was theirs and with nicely inverted snobbery clung to the title *Mr* as a mark of distinction. The apothecaries, who for centuries had been the real family doctors, had no title at all. Their own name had gone to the pharmacists; and they held licentiates and not degrees. But the courtesy title *Dr* has legal sanction. All examining bodies in Britain have to maintain standards set by the General Medical Council, and the Law recognizes only the Council's registration, not the degree or diploma by which it was obtained. To call oneself a doctor is taken to mean that one claims to be qualified and registered.

Domagk, Gerhard (1895–1964). German pathologist. From 1928 he studied hundreds of chemicals to find one which would kill invading bacteria without harming the patient. The only success of the kind had been Ehrlich's use of arsenic against syphilis. But the germ of syphilis was delicate, and the margin between poisoning the germ and poisoning the patient was narrow. Domagk was tackling a much hardier microbe, the streptococcus. Anything capable of destroying a streptococcus must, it seemed, also destroy the patient. The solution was to interfere with a chemical process vital to the bacterium but not used by the patient's cells. This was the effect of Domagk's *prontosil*, the first ◊ *sulphonamide*. Domagk's new method of testing drugs in live mice was the key. With the conventional test-tube methods prontosil would have been inactive. Sulphonamides would not have been discovered, and neither would the ◊ *antibiotics*, because everyone would still have assumed that bacteria could not be attacked in a living patient – as Fleming, the discoverer of penicillin, pointed out.

Domagk later discovered that tuberculosis, which the sulphonamides do not affect, could be treated with ◊ *isoniazid*. He received a Nobel Prize in 1939.

dominant. Character that need be inherited only from one parent, whereas a *recessive* character does not appear unless it is inherited from both parents. ◊ *genetics* (2).

dopa. Dihydroxyphenylalanine, an intermediate in the natural synthesis of adrenaline, and incidentally of the pigment melanin. In the nervous system, dopa is converted first to dopamine and then to noradrenaline and adrenaline.

A derivative of dopa, methyl-dopa, is a useful remedy for high blood pressure, which is caused partly by constriction of small arteries by noradrenaline. Methyl-dopa partly replaces the usual dopa in the synthetic process, and is converted to methyl-noradrenaline. This comparatively inert substance dilutes the active noradrenaline and so reduces the constriction of arteries.

In parkinsonism (shaking palsy) there is a deficit of dopamine in the affected part of the brain. Giving dopamine or adrenaline has little effect on the disease, perhaps because they are dispersed and destroyed without reaching the target. But a form of dopa, L-dopa, does reach the brain, where it is converted to dopamine, and in about 75 per cent of cases it relieves the symptoms. That it does not work in 25 per cent suggests two different types of disease. L-dopa has been in use since 1968, and at present appears to be one of the most effective ways of treating parkinsonism.

dorsal. Relating to the back.

dorsiflexion. Bending backwards; of the ankle – raising the front of the foot (plantar flexion is pointing the foot).

dose. The official dose of a drug, set out in the pharmacopoeia, is a range within which a suitable dose for most adults will be found. The correct dose in a particular case is the least that will produce the desired effect. Theoretically the dose of a drug should be related to the patient's own body weight, but in practice such accuracy is often unnecessary. And with many drugs the size of patients varies less than individual response, which has to be gauged by trial and error, starting with a small dose. If the patient is abnormally susceptible, a dose large enough to be useful may be toxic, and another drug has to be tried.

double-blind. A technique for assessing the effects of a drug. The response of patients to the drug is compared with the response of other patients (or the same ones on another occasion) to either another drug or an inert preparation made up to look like the drug. Neither the patients nor the physician know which preparation is which, because the knowledge can falsify the experiment. ◊ *research*.

Down's syndrome ◊ *mongol*.

dracunculus. A kind of parasitic worm; the ◊ *Guinea worm*.

drainage. A common surgical procedure: provision, e.g. with a rubber tube, of a way of escape for pus or other fluid from an abscess, operation wound etc.

dream ◊ *sleep*.

dressing. Covering applied to a wound to protect it from further injury or infection and give it a fair chance to heal itself. Paré's dictum (16th century) still holds: 'I dressed him. God cured him.'

A gauze dressing helps to stop bleeding by providing a framework for blood-clot, with the disadvantage that it is difficult to remove the dressing without disturbing the clot. Where dry gauze would be especially liable to stick (e.g. burns) dressings impregnated with soft paraffin are useful.

The first requirement of any dressing is that it should be sterile – free from bacteria. Hospital dressings are sterilized in bulk. For domestic use, sterilized dressings with an adhesive backing are convenient. In an emergency, an inner surface of a laundered handkerchief is reasonably safe, because a hot iron destroys bacteria.

dropsy. Excess of water in the tissues; ▷ *oedema*.

drowning. Suffocation by water. In the ordinary sense, drowning is due to inhaling water, but a rather similar condition can arise if water from the body's own fluids accumulates in the lungs as a result of disease. An unconscious patient with a full stomach (e.g. after heavy drinking) risks inhaling fluid regurgitated from the stomach.

Drowning by sea-water has the special danger that a concentration of salt in the lungs attracts water from the blood, so that a comparatively small amount of inhaled sea-water can lead to the accumulation of a larger amount of fluid.

Often the amount of water inhaled is too little to kill the victim simply by displacing air from the lungs, and sometimes people drown without inhaling any water at all. This is because a reflex, designed to prevent foreign matter from blocking the air-passages, holds the larynx closed against the water, and the victim chokes. But these muscles of the throat relax soon after consciousness is lost, and the victim recovers if he is given a chance to breathe.

Artificial respiration, mouth-to-mouth for choice, is the principal means of saving the victim's life. But neither this nor any other treatment is of the least use unless the air-passage is free of mechanical obstruction. The mouth and throat have to be cleared of weeds etc., and the patient's jaw has to be held forward to draw his tongue away from the back of his throat (this manoeuvre is the most important first-aid for unconsciousness from any cause).

drug. In non-technical language, *drug* has come to suggest a narcotic or habit-forming substance. In the technical sense, a drug is any substance taken medicinally to help recovery from sickness or relieve symptoms, or to modify any natural process in the body.

Vitamins are on the border between drugs and foods: given to improve a defective diet they are presumably foods, but in other circumstances they may count as drugs. Other substances given to make up a deficiency include *iron* for some types of anaemia, and *hormones* for disorders of glands. These relatively few drugs used to make up deficiencies of substances essential to health are perhaps the only ones that can be said to improve function directly and without risk of ill effects, because they do no more than restore the normal chemical balance. If there is no deficiency, such drugs can do no possible good, and an excess may be harmful. An overdose of iron is poisonous, and the action of most hormones is dangerously exaggerated by overdosage.

Other drugs – the great majority – act by disturbing the function of a particular tissue or organ or by interfering with a particular chemical process. The immediate effect is nearly always negative, though the result as far as the body as a whole is concerned may be positive and beneficial. It is rather like crime prevention: imprisonment is no boon to criminals, but it helps the rest of the community.

Many drugs are chemically similar to active components of living tissues. The similarity can work in at least three ways, which can be illustrated by drugs related to adrenaline, a substance concerned in the natural function of many organs. First, *isoprenaline* is an effective alternative to adrenaline; the two have similar chemical actions on the cells of the body. Second, *amphetamine* has little direct action on the cells, but the enzyme that serves to destroy adrenaline when it has served its purpose will as readily take up amphetamine, leaving any adrenaline in the tissues to continue its work; thus the net effect of isoprenaline or amphetamine is to reinforce adrenaline, though the methods are quite different. Third, *methyl-dopa* is probably taken up by other enzymes needed for the synthesis of adrenaline, which then waste their effort in synthesizing an inert compound; the net effect of this drug is to suppress the action of adrenaline.

Many widely different kinds of drug depend for their action on their ability to impersonate a natural reagent in the body. It is often impossible to say in advance whether a new product of research will reinforce or suppress the action of the substances that it resembles.

An important class of drugs is directed not at the human body but at its parasites. An ideal drug of this kind would kill bacteria etc. without any effect on human tissue. The trouble is that all life, whether human or bacterial, depends on very similar chemical processes. These drugs depend on relative rather than absolute differences – on disturbing processes that are vital to the parasite but of minor importance to man. Some of the older anti-parasitic drugs, e.g. arsenic compounds for syphilis, are poisonous to all living matter, but the parasite is rather more susceptible than the patient.

All substances – even water and oxygen – are poisonous in the sense that a gross excess is harmful. With few exceptions, all drugs are poisonous when the useful dose is exceeded, because even a 'safe' dose has unwanted effects in addition to the desired effect, and if more than the necessary dose is taken the unwanted effects mount up without any benefit to compensate for them.

The ill effects of a drug may be simply too much of what the drug is intended to do. Digitalis is given to slow a racing heart to an efficient rate. Too much digitalis slows the heart to a dangerous rate. Secondly, a drug given for its action on one organ usually affects other organs, and these secondary actions are as a rule undesirable. They have, however, led to some useful discoveries. Sulphonamides, given to control bacterial infection, have a secondary action on the amount of sugar in the blood, and another on the flow of urine. Research into these actions has produced drugs derived from sulphonamides with, respectively, a useful effect on diabetes and a powerful diuretic action, greatly increasing the amount of urine produced. In general, however, the secondary actions or side-effects of a drug are tiresome and sometimes dangerous. Thirdly, drugs can provoke allergy in the same way as other substances introduced into the body. And finally, an extremely undesirable property of many drugs is that they may be habit-forming ($\diamond$ addiction).

The flood of new and highly active drugs since the Second World War has improved the treatment of countless diseases but has also brought new problems. Early in the 16th century, Paracelsus warned against the possible danger of giving combinations of drugs that might conflict with each other, and the danger is now very real – prescribers have to be constantly on their guard against incompatible mixtures. One drug may be a kind of antidote to another. At the best this prevents the other drug from having the desired effect, and at worst it can be dangerous. For instance, anticoagulant drugs are used to prevent blood clots from forming with arterial disease. Barbiturates inhibit anticoagulants and so increase the required dose. If the patient stops taking the barbiturate, he finds that he is then getting an overdose of the anticoagulant. A greater risk is potentiation of one drug by another, where the combined effect is greater than the sum of the two when the drugs are taken alone. This can be valuable, as with co-trimoxazole, a mixture of small doses of two antibacterial drugs which is far more active than a large dose of either ingredient alone. But other mixtures, such as pethidine with certain antidepressants, can be lethal.

Another problem that has always existed but is much more serious with modern drugs is the difference between patients in their response to some drugs. Some people have a hereditary deficiency of an enzyme needed for inactivating a particular drug, and are unduly sensitive to the drug. This applies to several drugs used in psychiatry, which therefore have to be given very cautiously at first. Similarly a patient may develop an allergy to a drug. Such individual differences are in themselves a justification for having several drugs with similar actions on the market.

The term *bioavailability* has been coined to describe a matter of particular concern to pharmacists. It can safely be taken for granted that manufacturing and dispensing pharmacists will supply the prescribed dose of a drug, within the strict limits of accuracy and purity laid down by the Pharmacopoeia. Unfortunately it does not always follow that the correct dose will find its way into the circulation. The size of the particles of a drug affect the ease with which they are absorbed from the stomach, and it can even happen that a supposedly inert substance used to bind the particles into a tablet may react with them. Thus there are sometimes real differences between 'identical' drugs prepared by rival manufacturers.

The introduction of new drugs is discussed under ◊ *research*. ◊◊ *homoeopathy*; *naturopathy*; *placebo*.

duct. A tube for carrying the fluid secreted by a gland.

ductless gland. Gland of which the secretion (a hormone) passes straight into the circulation; i.e. an ◊ *endocrine* gland, as opposed to *exocrine* gland, which has a duct to carry its secretion to a particular region, e.g. saliva to the mouth.

ductus arteriosus. A blood vessel joining the pulmonary artery to the aorta, enabling blood to by-pass the lungs until birth; at birth the vessel should close almost at once to establish a proper circulation through the lungs as soon as they begin to work. Failure to close (patent ductus arteriosus) is a common type of congenital heart disease, and the easiest to correct – by tying a ligature round the vessel. ◊ *heart* (1).

dumbness. In childhood the commonest cause is deafness, which stops the child from learning to speak. Any mental disturbance that impedes learning may affect speech. In later life, a stroke may disturb either the mechanics or the mental process of speech.

Dumdum fever = ◊ *kala-azar*.

duodenal ulcer ◊ *peptic ulcer*.

duodenum. The first part of the ◊ *intestine*, between the stomach and the jejunum. The name ('twelve') refers to the length, twelve finger-breadths.

Dupuytren, Guillaume (1777–1835). French military surgeon. His name is given to a fracture of the radius a hand's breadth above the wrist with dislocation of the lower end of the ulna, a very unstable combination of injuries often needing operation; and to the contracture described below.

Dupuytren's contracture. Thickening of the fibrous lining of the palm (the *palmar aponeurosis*) which makes it impossible to straighten the fingers. Earlier surgeons had mentioned the condition, but Dupuytren gave the first full account of it in 1831. It is commonest in elderly men; it may be associated with other disorders of fibrous tissue or rheumatism. Many causes have been suggested, including pressure on the palms and alcoholism, but none has yet been proved. It is probably a symptom of a systemic disorder rather than a purely local condition. It can be relieved by removing the aponeurosis, but the present trend is towards less drastic measures.

dura mater. Parchment-like covering of the brain and spinal cord; the outer layer of the ◊ *meninges*.

dwarf. On average, children grow to a height half-way between their parents and the average of the population, but there is wide variation, and even tall parents may have a small but perfectly normal child. A true dwarf is abnormally small because of some defect. The most familiar type – the circus midget – has ◊ *achondroplasia*: the growth of his long bones is defective, but he is normal in all other respects. A much rarer type is due to disorders of the ◊ *pituitary* gland with lack of growth hormone. In addition, almost any chronic disease of childhood may interfere with normal growth.

dys-. Prefix = 'bad'; in many medical terms the implied sense is *difficult* or *deformed*. The hundreds of *dys-* compounds not separately defined below include *dysarthria* (impaired speech), *-chezia* (constipation), *-kinesia* (inco-ordination), *-lexia* (word-blindness), *-pepsia* (indigestion), *-plasia* (defective development), *-tocia* (difficult labour), *-trophy* (defective nutrition of an organ).

dyscrasia. In classical medicine: faulty balance of the four humours, supposed to be the fundamental cause of illness. Later: a constitutional disorder.

dysentery. The original meaning is diarrhoea with blood and mucus, together with pain and *tenesmus* (unproductive straining). In this sense of the word, dysentery is a collection of symptoms indicating severe irritation of the large intestine, of which the possible causes might range from food poisoning to cancer.

In current usage, dysentery means infection of the large intestine either by a protozoon, *Entamoeba histolytica* (amoebic dysentery) or by bacteria of the genus *Shigella* (bacillary dysentery). These infections do not necessarily produce all the symptoms of the first definition.

The large protozoon *Balantidium* is a rare cause of dysentery. The intestinal forms of ◊ *bilharzia* are common in many warm countries; this infection may be called chronic dysentery. Malaria is often blamed for dysentery, but what appears to be malarial dysentery is more likely to be bacillary dysentery added to an attack of malaria.

1. AMOEBIC DYSENTERY

Entamoeba histolytica resembles the amoeba of the school biology class. It is just sufficiently evolved to count as an animal; a creature consisting of a single cell about 25 microns (1/1000 in.) in diameter, which is little more than a living blob of jelly with a nucleus. It feeds by engulfing particles of human tissue, red blood cells for choice, and it can broach and enter the lining membrane of the intestine. It reproduces by splitting into two halves, each of which grows into a mature amoeba. This easy life is possible only while the parasite is inside a human body. During an attack of amoebic dysentery large numbers of amoebae are ejected in the stools and most of them must die. But as the attack settles and the stools become less fluid, amoebae which have not already invaded the mucous membrane may be unable to do so. These take on a new form. They become *cysts*, like the spores of some bacteria and other simple plants. A cyst is a round, inert body, usually with several (2–4) nuclei. It makes no demands on its environment, for it neither feeds nor reproduces. In this form the parasite can live for weeks without human company.

The disease is contracted by swallowing food (e.g. raw vegetables) or water contaminated with these cysts. This is most likely to happen in places where human excrement is used as manure, but unless ideal standards of hygiene are maintained amoebic dysentery can occur anywhere. It is common in the tropics and subtropics, and fairly rare elsewhere.

The natural history varies greatly from case to case. Most of the people who are infected – in some areas over 50 per cent of the population – have no symptoms at all. They come to light only when cysts are found by microscopic examination of the stools, which in the tropics is as much a routine test as measuring the blood pressure. The cysts which they pass can be carried by flies, or, when they have dried, as dust in the wind. When someone else has swallowed them the cysts emerge from their 'hibernation' and become active amoebae again.

Comparatively few people suffer a full-blown attack of dysentery. Usually the symptoms are much vaguer: aches, which may suggest appendicitis; feeling off-colour; occasional diarrhoea; even constipation. The patient may go on like this for years, never really ill but never quite well; or he may have attacks of real dysentery from time to time. This, then, is one of several diseases which can keep people who live in the tropics constantly below par (◊ *tropical diseases*).

The most important complication is infection of the liver by amoebae which enter the veins of the intestine and are carried to the liver in the portal vein. Amoebic abscesses may be formed, causing fever, and pain over the liver. Spread of infection from the liver to more distant organs (e.g. lung) is possible but rare.

Prevention is the best remedy for this disease. Proper sanitary facilities and habits and care in the handling of food prevent the transmission of the amoebae, but against the social and economic background of many tropical countries amoebic dysentery is unlikely to be eradicated for a long time.

Various drugs can be used for treating the infection. Two or more, acting against the amoebae in different ways, are commonly given. One of the oldest and most effective is *emetine*, derived from ipecacuanha. But the required dose may be more than the patient can tolerate, for emetine is safe only in small doses. Other drugs can be used instead of or in addition to emetine.

Intestinal bacteria which are normally harmless can set up severe infection in a mucous membrane already damaged by amoebae, and many of the symptoms of amoebic dysentery are due to secondary infection of this kind. It is often impossible to eradicate the amoebae until the secondary infection has been cured. This can be done with sulphonamides, but certain antibiotics, notably the tetracyclines, are effective not only against these bacteria but against the amoebae themselves. Certain drugs used against malaria can also be used here. Of these, chloroquine is especially successful with amoebic disease of the liver.

Many other drugs are being used. As a general rule, if half a dozen remedies are used for one disease, none is wholly satisfactory. This is no exception.

2. BACILLARY DYSENTERY

The intestinal bacilli are a large family of microbes adapted to a parasitic life in the large intestine. Some are quite harmless as long as they remain in the intestine; in their countless millions they form a large part of its normal contents. The colon bacillus, which everyone harbours from early infancy, is dangerous only if it strays, e.g. to the kidneys. But two groups cause disease in the intestine itself. These are *Salmonella*, of which different species are responsible for typhoid fever and much bacterial food poisoning, and *Shigella*, the germs of bacillary dysentery. An important distinction is that infection with *Salmonella* may be widespread, whereas *Shigella* infections are confined to the intestine.

The severity of bacillary dysentery varies with the species of *Shigella*. The worst type, Shiga dysentery, is common in the Far East. This can be a fulminating disease almost as violent as cholera, with profuse diarrhoea, bleeding, and dehydration. Flexner dysentery is rather less severe. It is common in all warm countries, and there are occasional outbreaks in Britain, most often in institutions. The usual dysentery of temperate climates is the Sonne type, which is much milder than the others. In a typical case the only symptom is diarrhoea lasting at the most a few days.

An attack may last only a day or two with a Sonne infection or some weeks with the severer types, but even without treatment a healthy adult nearly always recovers, though he may be very ill for a while. Dysentery in small children is a different matter, for their reserves of water and salts are quickly depleted. In tropical countries dysentery is a leading cause of death among children whose resistance is lowered by malnutrition, malaria and other afflictions.

In Britain, dysentery is important mainly as a cause of outbreaks of diarrhoea in schools. It is a nuisance rather than a danger. Affected children contaminate either their own fingers or, by way of the lavatory seat, the fingers of other children. Lavatory seats have been unjustly blamed for transmitting many ailments, but they are undoubtedly the vehicle of much intestinal infection. The best safeguard is to wash the hands after using the lavatory. Education in this matter is useful only if the educators remember to provide soap and water.

The sulphonamide drugs have greatly improved the treatment of bacillary dysentery, and many of the newer antibiotics are also effective; but loss of water and salts is more serious than the actual infection. If the patient can drink freely there is no great problem, but small children and any patients who are vomiting may need to have fluids injected into a vein or under the skin.

dysmenorrhoea. Pain with menstrual periods, mainly in the lower abdomen or the small of the back. Secondary (symptomatic) dysmenorrhoea in women who have previously had normal periods can arise from a whole range of gynaecological disorders, and is treated by identifying and dealing with the cause. Much the commoner disorder is *primary dysmenorrhoea*, affecting girls from their first period or soon after. Neither the cause nor even the source of the pain is known, although this must be the commonest ailment (except perhaps acne) of adolescent girls and young women. Pain at the start of a period is vaguely ascribed to reduction of blood-flow by spasm of the uterus (a sort of anginal pain) and pain that comes on later to congestion, and it is true that the early type of dysmenorrhoea is sometimes relieved by drugs that relax spasm, and the later type by lying down, which may help to prevent blood from gravitating to the pelvis. Many cases respond to treatment with hormones, especially those that prevent ovulation (the contraceptive pill). This strongly suggests defective balance of the sex hormones as an underlying cause.

Severe primary dysmenorrhoea can be incapacitating at the height of the attack, but it does not lead to any worse trouble, and its tendency is to get gradually better. Few cases persist after the birth of the first child, and some improve after marriage but before pregnancy. This could be an argument in favour of a hormonal cause or, as some people believe, of an emotional cause. In fact it could be either or both, because the production of hormones and the emotional state are inextricably tangled. Considering that emotional disturbance can completely stop the menstrual periods it would not be surprising if it contributed to painful periods. Although the pain certainly has a physical basis, the amount of distress it causes may well depend on emotional factors. Anything to do with sex is emotionally charged, and if dysmenorrhoea is commoner and more severe in our society than in others, our social taboos and religious teaching may well be to blame.

dyspareunia. Painful coitus. The condition may be secondary, i.e. a symptom of some other disorder, such as inflammation or a structural defect. In men this is the only kind of dyspareunia, the likeliest cause being inflammation of the foreskin. In women there are many causes of secondary dysparcunia, such as an unusually well-developed hymen, inflammation of the vagina or urinary bladder, and shrinkage of the lining of the vagina after the menopause. All these conditions are amenable to treatment, and when the cause of the difficulty has been dealt with, the symptom itself can be expected to disappear.

Primary dyspareunia is due to involuntary contraction of the muscles around the vagina, sometimes making coitus not just difficult but physically impossible. It is a defensive reflex, perhaps the aftermath of painful experience, perhaps due to conscious or unconscious aversion to sex. The ignorance and clumsiness of a young husband is a common cause. Patience and tact are needed to allay the patient's fears – with, of course, adequate medical investigation to exclude physical causes.

dysphagia. Difficulty in swallowing, a symptom of blockage or muscle spasm in the throat or gullet.

dyspnoea. Difficulty in breathing; undue shortness of breath; sometimes defined as awareness of the effort of breathing. Its essential character is that the effort is inappropriate. Nobody is more short of breath than a runner at the end of a race, but that does not count as dyspnoea because the effort is appropriate, it quickly passes, and it causes no real distress. Dyspnoea arises if the circulation through the lungs is sluggish, so that the lungs are not given a chance of oxygenating the blood at the required rate (as with heart failure); if the flow of air in and out of the lungs is impeded (asthma, bronchitis); if the blood cannot carry enough oxygen (anaemia); if the supply of oxygen is limited (high altitudes).

E

ear.

1. OUTER (EXTERNAL) EAR

The *auricle* or *pinna* – the visible part of the ear – has a core of elastic cartilage, which does not extend down to the lobe (lobule). Several vestigial muscles are attached to the auricle; they represent muscles which other animals use to amplify and locate sounds. The canal (*external auditory meatus*) is directed inwards and forwards. It is about 3 cm. long, and ends at the ear-drum. Since the canal is not quite straight the auricle has to be pulled back and up before the drum can be examined. The canal is widest where it meets the drum; thus the objects which children push into their ears can be difficult to remove. The sweat glands of the canal are modified to secrete a kind of wax.

Much nonsense has been talked about the shape of the auricles, which does not often indicate anything of importance. But protruding ears can be a source of real misery to a child, and the appearance can be greatly improved by plastic surgery.

The three common afflictions of the canal are small boils, which can be extremely painful; accumulation of wax causing temporary deafness; and foreign bodies such as beads. All are easy enough to manage given the right tools; but the ear-drum is delicate, and unskilled probing in the canal can do irreparable harm.

2. MIDDLE EAR

The middle ear is a cavity in the temporal bone, a part of the skull. Its outer wall is the tympanic membrane, the fibrous drumhead of the ear-drum. The cavity is bridged by three tiny bones which transmit the vibration of the membrane to the inner ear. At the back of the cavity is a small hole leading to the *mastoid antrum*, a hollow in the bone immediately behind the ear. In front is the opening of the *Eustachian tube*, leading to the back of the nose, by which the middle ear communicates with the outer air. This communication ensures that the air pressure is the same inside and outside the drum.

Inflammation in the nose causes the mucous membrane of the tube to swell. If the tube is completely blocked hearing is impaired and the ear aches. More seriously, in-fection can spread up the tube to the middle ear. Pus cannot escape by the congested tube, and the pressure rises and causes a violent earache (◊ *otitis media*). The infection may spread still further back and involve the ◊ *mastoid* antrum. Untreated, these are very dangerous conditions. They respond very well to antibiotics, but earache – especially in a child – is still a real emergency.

◊ *Otosclerosis* is a familial disorder in which an abnormal deposition of bone in the middle ear interferes with the movement of the small bones – it is treated surgically.

3. INNER EAR

(i) *Hearing.* The inner ear is a small but very elaborate structure deeply embedded in the temporal bone. It includes two distinct organs, one for hearing and the other for balance. The first is the *cochlea*, a snail-shaped container for the *organ of Corti*, in which vibration (sound) produces nervous impulses for transmission to the brain. The receiving cells are arranged on a flat membrane which divides the cochlea into two spiral compartments. The fibres of this membrane gradually increase in length towards the apex of the spiral, which suggested to Helmholtz that they acted as resonators like the undamped strings of a piano – if the dampers of a piano are raised with the pedal the appropriate strings will take up their note from another instrument or a voice. This theory was accepted for about a century, but has lately been rejected.

The slightest movement of the organ of Corti initiates an electrical current. The greater the movement, the higher the voltage, up to about 5 mV. This is quite unlike a nervous impulse, which is single or repeated discharge of fixed amplitude.

High notes, i.e. rapid vibrations, die out near the beginning of the spiral. The lowest notes are carried the length of the organ of Corti to the apex of the spiral. A note of any given pitch always dies out at the same level, opposite the same cells. The sum of the electrical currents produced is an electrical replica of the vibrations of the original sound: the organ of Corti behaves exactly as a microphone or a pick-up. But this electri-

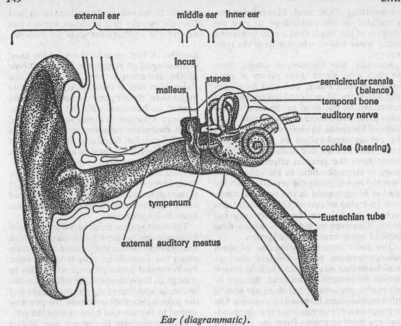

external ear   middle ear   inner ear

incus

stapes

malleus

semicircular canals (balance)

temporal bone

auditory nerve

cochlea (hearing)

tympanum

Eustachian tube

external auditory meatus

Ear (diagrammatic).

cal record cannot be relayed directly to the brain, if only because a nerve fibre can transmit only a few hundred impulses per second whereas a high note would need several thousand. What the brain apparently identifies is the distance that a particular sound travels along the organ of Corti. Each level in the organ has a corresponding pathway (nerve fibre) to the brain, so different pathways from the ear transmit different frequencies. Louder sounds produce more impulses per second. Low notes stimulate not only the cells to which they are carried, far round the spiral, but also the cells on the way. Higher notes, which do not travel so far in the cochlea, stimulate fewer cells. The brain evidently gets much more information than it needs, and there must be some still unidentified means of suppressing unwanted impulses.

The range of a young ear is about 10 octaves, say from $\frac{1}{2}$ octave lower than a piano to $2\frac{1}{2}$ octaves higher. It is most sensitive to the upper 3 octaves of the piano, and it can also best distinguish pitch in this range. (The fundamental tone of a 64-foot

organ pipe is too low to be heard; it is the harmonics that are audible.)

Throughout adult life even a healthy ear becomes gradually less sensitive. and it is the highest notes – which stimulate the fewest cells – that are most affected. The fundamental tone of a woman's speaking voice is around middle C; of a man's, an octave lower. Both are below the most sensitive range of the ear and well below the range that is normally lost with age. But the quality or *timbre* of a sound depends not on the fundamental but on higher pitched accompanying sounds. Without these it is impossible to distinguish between vowels. And consonants, on which intelligible speech so much depends, are very high-pitched. Thus, if the higher frequencies are lost, speech may be heard but not understood.

(ii) *Balance.* The part of the inner ear concerned with balance, the *vestibular apparatus,* is in two parts. The sensitive cells of the *otolith organ* have fine hairs with chalky particles suspended from them. They record the gravitational pull on the hairs, which varies in different groups of hairs with different positions of the head. This information is collated in the cerebellum to give the position of the head: thus a man swimming under water knows whether he is the right way up.

Secondly, the *semicircular canals*, three on each side, lie in three planes at right angles to each other, and also have cells with fine hairs. They record not position but movement of the fluid in the canals. This takes place when there is acceleration in the plane of the canal. In view of the position of the canals acceleration in any direction must affect at least one pair. Rotary movements have the greatest effect. When the rotation stops the fluid in the canals continues to move, giving the sensation that the head is being turned in the opposite direction. In trying to correct this apparent disturbance of balance the subject may fall down. This type of giddiness, with a false sense of movement, is called *vertigo*.

The most important function of these balance organs is to regulate the eye muscles so that an object can be held in view despite movement of the head. Balance itself is also important, but there are several other mechanisms involved (◊ *posture*). The impression with vertigo that the surroundings are moving comes from the disturbed reflexes between ear and eye. The ear signals, wrongly, that the head is turning, and the eyes flicker in an attempt to keep the passing scene in focus. The flickering movement is called *nystagmus*.

4. AUDITORY NERVE

Hearing and balance are conveyed in the acoustic and vestibular divisions of the auditory (8th cranial) nerve. The nerve runs across the floor of the skull into the brain-stem just below the pons. Here the impulses are relayed to consciousness and to various reflex pathways.

Disorders of this nerve cause symptoms such as vertigo, hissing or ringing in the ear (*tinnitus*), and deafness, which are also common symptoms of trouble in the ear itself. The diagnosis of these symptoms is briefly discussed under ◊ *deafness*.

The auditory nerve is easily damaged by pressure with head injuries, meningitis, or bleeding, abscess, or tumour of the brain. It can be affected by various drugs, including *aspirin, quinine,* and *streptomycin*. Certain viruses have a special affinity for the auditory nerve: nerve-deafness is a rare complication of *measles* (which can also give

trouble by way of the Eustachian tube); and *German measles* in a pregnant woman can destroy the auditory nerves of the embryo.

earache. A bad earache is one of the most distressing of all symptoms. The membrane of the ear-drum is very sensitive. If the Eustachian tube is blocked, e.g. with a cold in the nose, the air pressure inside the drum cannot be balanced with the atmospheric pressure. Changes of atmospheric pressure, as in mountain railways or aircraft, may then be painful. Similarly, the pressure of wax or a foreign body such as a bead in the ear can cause earache, especially after ill-advised attempts to remove the obstruction. Even a very small boil in the canal of the ear is enough to cause severe pain, from spread of the inflammation to the drum rather than from direct pressure.

The most violent earache is due to inflammation inside the drum (*otitis media*), which nearly always arises from spread of infection along the Eustachian tube from the nose. Pus is formed under pressure which may be enough to burst through the inflamed membrane, in which case the ear discharges and the pain is relieved; otherwise the pus may spread to the *mastoid* bone behind the ear.

Pain apparently in the ear may in fact arise in a diseased tooth or still further afield.

All the conditions likely to cause earache respond well to early treatment, but little can be done for an earache until the cause has been determined. Since one of the conditions – acute otitis media – is extremely dangerous a painful ear needs to be examined as soon as possible.

Eaton agent. A parasite, probably a very small bacterium rather than a virus, causing a common type of pneumonia formerly known as *primary atypical pneumonia*. Unlike true virus infections this disease responds to treatment with some antibiotics. Even without treatment it is much less dangerous than other types of pneumonia.

ecchymosis. Bruise; bleeding into the skin either from injury or from spontaneous leaking of blood as in the rashes of some fevers and in disorders of blood-clotting.

ECG = ◊ *electrocardiogram.*

ECHO. A group of viruses (Enteric Cytopathic Human Orphan). ◊ *virus* (1).

echo-encephalogram. Pattern of echoes from within the skull, obtained by transmitting high-frequency (ultrasonic) impulses across the skull, and recording their reflections from structures in their path. The same device, a piezo-electric crystal, generates the ultra-sound and picks up the echoes, which are conveyed to a cathode-ray tube like a radar screen. The method is especially useful for showing displacement of the brain, e.g. by bleeding from a fracture of the skull.

eclampsia. Convulsions occurring at the end of pregnancy as a result of toxaemia. ◊ *toxaemia of pregnancy.*

ECT = ◊ *electroconvulsive therapy.*

ectoderm. Layer of cells in an ◊ *embryo* from which the skin and nervous system develop.

ectopic. In an abnormal anatomical situation. *Ectopic pregnancy* occurs when a fertilized ovum, instead of passing down the Fallopian tube and implanting itself in the lining of the uterus, settles in the tube or elsewhere. Such a pregnancy seldom lasts more than 2 or 3 months, though cases have been reported in which an infant has survived in the cavity of the abdomen for long enough to be born live – of course by Caesarean section. In most cases the embryo dies early and is absorbed. Occasionally the Fallopian tube bursts and bleeds, and an immediate operation is needed to repair the damage.

eczema. There is no clear distinction between eczema and ◊ *dermatitis.* The commoner types are discussed under that heading.

EEG = ◊ *electroencephalogram.*

effort syndrome (Da Costa's syndrome, 'disordered action of the heart'). A form of anxiety neurosis, with symptoms suggestive (at least to the patient) of heart disease: pain over the heart, palpitation, breathlessness, fatigue. The pain is due to tension of the pectoral muscles, and the other symptoms are familiar accompaniments of anxiety. The heart is normal, and the symptoms vanish with the source of anxiety, if it can be eradicated. This was a common complaint during the First World War, but is now a rarity.

effusion. Leakage of fluid into a body cavity (chest; abdomen) due to inflammation or congestion.

ego. According to ◊ *Freud,* that part of the self or personality that keeps in touch with the material world; the conscious mind. It holds the balance between instinct (the *id*) and conscience (the *superego*).

Ehrlich, Paul (1854–1915). German scientist. One of the pioneers of bacteriology, he also distinguished himself in several other branches of medical science. Ehrlich's discoveries included:
  1. A method of staining and identifying the bacilli of tuberculosis;
  2. A method of assaying the potency of diphtheria antitoxin, essential to correct dosage;
  3. A rational theory of how the antitoxin worked, and arising from this study a theory to explain the whole process of ◊ *immunity* to infection as a chemical combination of antigens and antibodies, for which he received a Nobel Prize in 1908;
  4. The drug salvarsan (606), later modified to the safer compound neosalvarsan, the first drugs to be prepared for treating the cause of a disease – in this case, syphilis.
All subsequent work on immunity and allergy springs directly from Ehrlich's research, and his salvarsan is the prototype of scores of drugs now used against infection.

Einthoven, Willem (1860–1927). Dutch physiologist, of Leyden, awarded a Nobel Prize in 1924 for his invention of the electrocardiogram.

ejaculatio praecox. Premature ejaculation, a minor but sometimes distressing disorder of coitus, where the male climax arrives too soon. ◊ *sex.*

elastic tissue. Ordinary connective tissue with the addition of many fibres of the protein *elastin*; it is like draper's elastic in which cotton weave is laced with rubber threads. This tissue is found in some ligaments and in the walls of arteries.

elbow. Two joints are combined at the elbow: a hinge between the humerus and ulna, and a ball-and-socket between the humerus and radius. A notch in the shaft of the ulna turns on a fixed roller (*trochlea*) in the centre of the lower end of the humerus, and a shallow socket at the top of the radius moves round a fixed ball (*capitulum*) at the outer side of the trochlea. The joint is set at an angle about 10° off centre, so that the hand swings clear of the hip when the arm is at the side (*carrying angle*). The ulnar joint can only be bent or straightened. The radius perforce moves with the ulna, since the two bones are joined at both ends, but its ball-and-socket also allows it to be twisted at the elbow in pronation of the forearm. This movement is described under ◊ *radius*. In essence the elbow is a hinge between the ulna and the humerus; the radius is only incidental. Indeed, the head of the radius can be surgically removed without serious disability. At the ◊ *wrist* it is the other way round: the hand articulates with the radius, and the ulna is unimportant. Stress is transferred in the forearm from one bone to the other.

Fractures and dislocations of the elbow are common. They may come together. The notch in the ulna is deep, and if it is wrenched free of the humerus one or other bone is likely to be damaged. Usually the ulna, carrying the radius with it, is forced backwards. The vessels and nerves in front of the joint are then stretched against the lower end of the humerus and may be injured. A fracture of the lower end of the humerus with backward displacement of the lower fragment has the same effect. Thus the complications may be more serious than the original injury. If the upper end of the ulna is fractured and the radius remains intact, the deformity of the ulna pushes the radius out of place; this injury may be harder to treat than fracture of both bones. The greatest problem with injuries of the elbow is that this joint is more liable than any other to remain stiff after treatment. The correct anatomical position of the bones can usually be restored, either by manipulation or by operation, but the functional result is often disappointing.

electrocardiogram (ECG). A record of the electrical changes in the heart muscle. The currents are very small and can be detected only with a highly sensitive galvanometer. Such an instrument was invented in 1903 by Einthoven, who was awarded a Nobel Prize in 1924.

Currents were originally recorded across three pairs of electrodes: both wrists; each

wrist in turn with left ankle. The tracings from these three standard leads give a good impression of the heart as a whole. The most important refinement of Einthoven's work is the use of additional electrodes placed on the chest wall; these may pick up small defects which would be obscured with the standard leads, and also localize them.

The ECG reveals disturbances of rhythm (◊ *arrhythmia*), damage to the heart muscle, especially with ◊ *coronary artery* disease, imbalance between the two sides of the heart where one side is overloaded, and various kinds of poisoning which affect the heart muscle (e.g. ◊ *digitalis*, ◊ *potassium*).

electroconvulsive therapy (ECT). Treatment of mental illness by applying a small electric shock to the scalp. This causes a brief loss of consciousness and, with the original method of applying the treatment, a convulsion like an epileptic seizure. The convulsion had nothing to do with the efficacy of the treatment, and though the patient remembered nothing of it, there was a risk that it might cause him to injure himself while unconscious. Furthermore, the very idea of ECT alarms most patients. The present method is to give a light anaesthetic and a muscle relaxant, which suppress the convulsion but preserve the useful effect of the treatment. Nobody knows how ECT works, but it remains one of the best ways of treating severe depression, and it is sometimes effective with other types of mental illness.

electroencephalogram (EEG). A record of electrical events in the brain. Nerve cells generate small electric currents that can be picked up from the surface of the scalp and shown on a cathode-ray tube. By using several leads from different parts of the scalp the electrical patterns from different regions of the brain can be studied.

The interpretation of the EEG is still empirical. Certain patterns are regularly found with normal brains, and other patterns suggest some interference with normal function. So far, the greatest value of the EEG has been in confirming the diagnosis of epilepsy and distinguishing between certain types of epilepsy. In some other disorders of the brain it may help to locate the trouble.

electromyogram (EMG). A record of nerve

impulses to muscles and the response of the
muscle, for the diagnosis of faults of nerve
conduction and muscle contraction.

elephantiasis. Gross thickening of the skin
and underlying connective tissue due to
chronic obstruction of the lymphatic vessels, usually by thread-worms (◊ *filaria*).

embolism. Blockage of an artery by an
embolus (fragment of blood-clot, air bubble
etc.) carried in the blood-stream. The effect
of embolism depends on the size of the obstructed vessel, the presence or absence of
alternative routes for the circulation of
blood beyond the stoppage, and most of all
on the importance of the tissue, if any, deprived of blood. Embolism of a small artery
in an area with a good network of arteries
has no ill effects. Embolism of an artery of
the brain is one of the causes of *stroke*.

Embolism is commonly due to a fragment
of clotted blood from a vein, carried through
the heart to a lung. The usual effect is a kind
of pneumonia in the affected zone; but a
blockage of a main artery may be rapidly
fatal. Some lives have been saved by surgical
removal of large fragments of blood-clot
from arteries in the lungs.

The usual type of embolism, by blood-
clot, arises as a complication of disease in
the wall of an artery (◊ *atheroma*) or a vein
(◊ *phlebitis*) which allows blood to clot in
the vessel.

embolus. Clot, bubble etc. blocking an artery, causing ◊ *embolism*.

embryo. In human biology: an unborn offspring from the time of fertilization until
the time, some two months later, when it is
sufficiently developed to be unmistakably
human. (For the rest of pregnancy it is
known as a foetus.) During the first month a
human embryo much resembles that of any
other vertebrate; during the second month,
that of any other mammal.

An embryo starts as a fertilized *ovum*, a
single cell 0·1 mm. in diameter, just large
enough to be seen with the naked eye. This
small object is much larger than other cells
of the human body. By the time it has travelled down the Fallopian tube and implanted
itself in the lining of the uterus it is about a
week old. Until then it has no means of
growing larger, but its one large cell divides
into two smaller cells, then the two into four
and so on until a colony of 100 or more cells
has been formed, the whole mass (*blasto-*

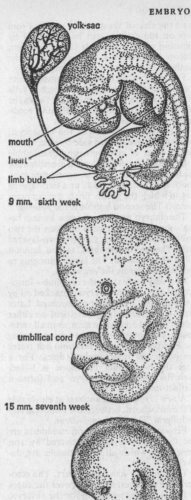

9 mm. sixth week

15 mm. seventh week

30 mm. end of eighth week

cyst) the size of the original ovum. From now on the embryo can be nourished by diffusion of raw materials (water, oxygen, glucose, amino-acids, salts etc.) from the mother's blood, and it grows very quickly.

The embryo gets its nourishment from the mother through the outer layer of cells of the blastocyst. Later, this layer forms the *placenta* and one of the enveloping membranes of the foetus, the *chorion*.

In the *inner cell mass* of the blastocyst, two bubbles are formed side by side, with a double layer of cells between. One bubble will form the inner enveloping membrane of the foetus, the *amnion*. (The two membranes, chorion and amnion, make up a two-layered bag in which the foetus floats during pregnancy.) The second bubble is the *yolk-sac*.

The embryo proper – the new human being – grows from the cells between the two bubbles. At first this is simply a two-layered disc. The layer belonging to the amnion forms the *ectoderm*. The layer belonging to the yolk-sac forms the *endoderm*.

At a very early stage the mid-line – longitudinal axis – of the embryo is marked off by a straight rod of cells, the *notochord*. Later growth is practically symmetrical on either side of the notochord. In man, as in all vertebrates, the notochord mostly disappears as the backbone grows (◊ *skeleton*) but traces persist in the intervertebral discs. For a time the developing backbone is longer than the rest of the embryo and forms a distinct tail.

A new layer of cells appears at either side of the notochord, between the ectoderm and endoderm. This is the *mesoderm*.

Ectoderm, mesoderm, and endoderm are the three germ-layers, discovered by von Baer, from which all other tissues are derived.

The disc now has three layers. The ectoderm grows fastest and spills over the edges to form an outer wrapping for the embryo. The endoderm curls to form an inner tube. The mesoderm remains between the two. Along the future back of the embryo a deep groove appears in the ectoderm, which then grows over to convert the groove into the *neural tube*. The front end of the neural tube is later folded and expanded to form the brain; the rest keeps its original shape as the spinal cord. Thus the ectoderm provides both skin and nervous system.

The endoderm lines the whole digestive tract. Offshoots form the digestive glands (liver, pancreas etc.) and also lungs.

Muscles, bones, connective tissue and blood vessels are all derived from mesoderm. The heart is formed in mesoderm at the head of the embryo next to the developing brain; it is displaced towards its final position as the mouth grows between heart and brain.

In the first few weeks, nerves grow outwards from the developing brain and spinal cord. As the various parts of the body take up new positions they keep their original nerves. In adult anatomy, the source of a nerve indicates the origin of the part it supplies. For example, the diaphragm – a muscle separating the heart from the abdomen – gets its nerves from the spinal cord high in the neck, because this muscle is first formed just below the original position of the heart.

By the end of the second month all of the main structures of the body are more or less in place. The proportions are strange: the head is relatively huge and the legs are small, while some organs are still rudimentary. There is little bone, but the whole skeleton is already formed in cartilage. The backbone no longer extends beyond the buttocks as a tail. The embryo is now about 4 cm. ($1\frac{1}{2}$ ins.) long. Its further development is considered under ◊ *foetus*.

embryology. Natural history of animals (generally vertebrates) from conception until birth; in particular the study of the development of the various tissues and organs.

In general biology, embryology helps to explain the course of evolution and the relations between different species of animal; for although the old dictum that the development of the individual recapitulates the evolution of the species has been much overworked, it is still true that the embryos of very different species are very similar, and that in its early stages an embryo almost certainly imitates the embryos (not the adults) of its remote ancestors.

Medical students learn embryology to bring order to the seeming chaos of adult anatomy, and to understand how congenital defects arise.

Embryology, like several other sciences, began with Aristotle in the 4th century B.C. His biological studies included an investigation of the developing chick – a most convenient subject, for one has only to set a clutch of eggs and remove and open one each day. He left a good account of development from the third day of incubation, when the embryo becomes visible to the naked eye. He found that the organs are formed in succession, not all at the same time. He regarded reproduction as a purely female function; the male only set the process in motion.

No further progress was made until the 17th century, when embryology was revived by the great anatomists of Padua, such as Fabricius and Harvey. A fellow-student of Fabricius, Volcher Coiter, wrote the first treatise on embryology since Aristotle. But since none of these men had a microscope they could not add much to Aristotle's account.

The development of the chick as seen through the microscope was described in 1673 by Malpighi. This work was a great step forward, but introduced a serious fallacy that was to last until the 19th century. Malpighi's earliest embryos had already been incubated for several hours; long enough for him to see the rudiments of organs that Harvey and others had missed. He concluded that all the organs were present in miniature from the start. Aristotle's view that the organs were formed in succession was fully restored 150 years later by Saint-Hilaire in France and von Baer in Germany. Von Baer, perhaps the greatest of embryologists, identified the egg or ovum of a mammal in 1827, and showed the development of all tissues and organs from the primary germ layers, ectoderm, endoderm, and mesoderm. He formulated the *biogenetic law*, foreseen by Aristotle and Harvey, that all embryos are alike.

A detailed account of embryology would be out of place here. There are short notes under ◊ *embryo* (early stages) and *foetus* (later stages).

emerods (archaic) = ◊ *haemorrhoids*.

emetic. Drug given to cause vomiting. In former centuries, emetics were very widely used as an alternative or addition to purging, blood-letting, sweating – anything that would allow noxious matters to escape. They still have a limited use in treating recent poisoning.

Emetics are of two kinds. Some act by irritating the stomach; they include the household standby – common salt – ammonium carbonate, and ipecacuanha. Small doses of the last two, not enough to cause vomiting, cause reflex stimulation of mucous glands in the lungs and are used in cough mixtures to loosen sputum. A second type of emetic stimulates a reflex centre in the brain. Morphine sometimes does this, which is why a few people cannot tolerate it. A related drug, *apomorphine*, regularly acts as a powerful emetic. It has successfully been used to create an aversion to alcohol in alcoholics who have not responded to more humane methods.

emetine. An emetic drug extracted from ipecacuanha, given by injection in the treatment of amoebic dysentery and its complications.

EMG = ◊ *electromyogram.*

emotion. The great obstacle to rational discussion of the emotions is that sooner or later one's own emotions enter the fray at the expense of reason. People have always paid lip-service to ideas like 'worried sick' or 'broken-hearted', and they have always accepted in principle that emotion and physical health or sickness are related. But as soon as it comes down to cases a barrier descends. The barrier may be of disbelief ('he's putting it on'), exasperation ('he should pull himself together') or even sympathy ('poor fellow'). Any of these may happen to be the right answer in a given case, but the choice depends not on the merits of the case but on the mood of the speaker.

Much misunderstanding comes from supposing that emotions are (or should be) the same for everyone, or that normal and abnormal physical responses to emotion can be defined: 'if I can suffer frustration without getting a duodenal ulcer, so can he.' But both his frustration and his physical reaction may be quite different from mine.

Civilization demands self-control, and self-control is learning not to act as emotion dictates. Even this is more than anyone can manage at all times, and reflex physical responses to emotion can hardly be controlled at all. A man can more or less learn not to punch someone on the nose whenever he is angry, but he cannot stop his pulse from racing, or a host of internal adjustments of which he is not even aware. It is these adjustments – disturbances of equilibrium – that can in time lead to physical illness, and self-control does not improve them. (If anything, it may make them worse. Properly controlled emotion is more likely to upset digestion, blood pressure and the rest than savagery.) This is the fallacy behind 'pull yourself together'. If, for example, a man is ill because he is constantly afraid, 'pulling himself together' may stop him from running away, that is from *behaving* fearfully. But it does not always stop him from being afraid, and it is the internal and uncontrollable effects of fear that make him ill. Only if not running away teaches him that there was nothing to be afraid of can pulling himself together cure him; but as long as his fear lasts, self-control cannot help him. (It may, of course, make him a more useful citizen, but that is a social and not a medical cure; he is still not healthy.)

The emotional background to particular kinds of illness is discussed under ◊ *psychosomatic disease*; ◊◊ *anxiety*.

Empedocles (5th century B.C.). Greek philosopher whose theory that all matter was compounded of four humours (earth, air, fire, water) remained the basis of theoretical medicine for some 22 centuries.

emphysema. *Pulmonary emphysema* is an ill-defined condition of the lungs. There is over-inflation of the air-spaces with loss of the thin dividing walls between spaces where exchange of oxygen and carbon dioxide should take place. Probably three factors contribute to the damage: the physical stress of constant coughing, excessive inspiration in an attempt to overcome narrowing of the bronchi, and destruction of lung tissue by bacteria. All three are present in *chronic bronchitis*, and emphysema is most often seen at an advanced stage of this disease, though it may complicate other long-standing disease of the lungs. Since lost lung tissue cannot be replaced the only effective way of dealing with emphysema is to treat the preceding disease before it reaches this stage.

Surgical emphysema is air introduced into connective tissue by injury or operation. The air is gradually absorbed: the condition is of no importance.

empyema. A kind of abscess: with most abscesses the infection excavates a cavity in the tissues, but with an empyema the pus occupies a natural cavity in the body. The term is most often applied to a collection of pus in the pleural space, between a lung and the outer wall of the chest. Before the discovery of antibiotics, empyema was a frequent and dangerous complication of pneumonia. In the influenza pandemic of 1918 and 1919 many people died after the sequence of influenza, pneumonia, and empyema.

Empyema has to be treated surgically. The pus is first drawn off with a hollow needle and syringe. Later, when as a result of inflammation the lung is firmly stuck to the chest wall around the abscess an opening can be made for the pus to drain away completely. A London physician in 1919 found that his patients with empyema died much more often than those of his assistant. This, it turned out, was because he was the better diagnostician and able to recognize an empyema at an earlier stage. It was then the practice to operate as soon as the diagnosis was made, and with early diagnosis the operation was being done too soon, and the lung collapsed like a pricked balloon. The assistant diagnosed his cases only at a later stage, when the adhesion to the chest wall kept the lung inflated.

enamel. The coating of the crown of a tooth; it is mainly a complex of phosphate and fluoride of calcium, like the mineral component of bone but with a much denser crystalline structure. ◊ *teeth*.

encephalitis. Inflammation of the brain; the infectious agent is nearly always a virus. (Bacterial infection is usually confined to the coverings of the brain: ◊ *meningitis*.)

Perhaps the only virus that invariably settles in the brain is that of *rabies*, a fatal but fortunately rare disease occasionally transmitted from animals to man. In many parts of the world (Russia, N. America, Japan) local forms of virus encephalitis are carried by insects. These are mostly diseases of animals, only accidentally affecting man. They are seldom dangerous.

Even *poliomyelitis*, the best known form of encephalitis, is not primarily an infection of the brain. In the great majority of cases it is a harmless infection of the intestine, and involvement of the brain is a dangerous but unusual event. Most other viruses can cause encephalitis, but only very rarely. The severity of the disease varies widely: anything is possible from a transient headache to paralysis or death, but, apart from poliomyelitis, lasting ill effects are unusual when the infection has passed.

The encephalitis that follows some of the common infectious fevers has not yet been explained. It appears to be not an actual infection of the brain, but an allergic reaction to the virus. But these cases are so rare that it is difficult to study them.

Encephalitis lethargica was a widespread epidemic in the closing years of the First World War and some time after. It was also known as 'sleepy sickness' (nothing to do with African sleeping sickness). Many of its victims were left with a severe disturbance of muscular co-ordination (post-encephalitic parkinsonism). At the time there was no known way to isolate a virus, and after about 1923 the disease vanished; but everything about the epidemic suggests a virus infection. Historically, it is an interesting example of a serious disease that has appeared from nowhere and mysteriously departed, like some of the plagues of antiquity.

encephalopathy. Any disease of the brain, especially with physical changes from causes other than inflammation, e.g. lead poisoning.

endarteritis. Inflammation of the lining of an artery.

end-artery. A terminal branch of an artery that does not communicate with other branches. The importance of end-arteries is that if one is blocked, the tissue it supplies is completely deprived of fresh blood and dies.

endemic. (Disease) always present in a given region or population (whereas an *epidemic* arrives, spreads, and disappears).

endocarditis. Inflammation of the lining of the heart, especially that of the heart valves. This tissue is unaffected by most diseases, but it becomes involved in rheumatic fever (rheumatic endocarditis), ◊ *mitral stenosis*. Heart valves deformed by congenital defects or rheumatic fever are sometimes infected with streptococci or other bacteria (bacterial endocarditis). This is dangerous, because fragments of the infected tissue are carried in the blood and can cause blockage of arteries (embolism) anywhere in the body. Rheumatic endocarditis does not always need treatment, but seriously damaged valves can often be repaired surgically. Bacterial endocarditis, formerly incurable, responds to antibiotic drugs.

endocrine (a Greek form of Claude Bernard's term 'internal secretion' (1885)). An endocrine or ductless gland is one which releases its product (a *hormone*) directly to the blood-stream to act on other parts of the body. It is distinguished from an *exocrine* gland, of which the secretion (e.g. sweat, digestive juice) flows into a duct to be used locally.

The *pituitary*, *thyroid*, *parathyroid*, and *adrenal* glands are purely endocrine. The *pancreas* is an exocrine gland of digestion, with a duct leading to the duodenum, and also an endocrine gland releasing insulin into the blood. The *ovaries* and *testicles* produce eggs and sperms and are also endocrine glands; their hormones regulate sexual functions throughout the body.

No other organs are generally regarded as endocrine glands, though several might be added to the list. The kidney produces a hormone which affects the blood pressure, and another controlling the formation of red blood cells, and the duodenum produces *secretin* which stimulates the pancreas.

The particular functions of hormones are described with the glands which produce them. Here, it need only be stressed that none of the glands acts independently of the others. There are feed-back mechanisms between the pituitary and most of the other glands. The pituitary can secrete *trophic* hormones to stimulate these glands, and the hormones from the glands suppress the corresponding trophic hormones. If, for example, the thyroid is not secreting enough thyroxine, the pituitary hormone stimulates more secretion. An excess of thyroxine suppresses the pituitary; the thyroid is thus deprived of its stimulus and the balance is restored. In this way the amount of various hormones in the blood is kept at the right level. But the 'right' level depends on circumstances, and the setting of the feed-back mechanism is determined by the nervous system acting on the pituitary. Thus the nervous and chemical functions of the body are closely interrelated.

Several glands may be involved in a single function. Growth, for example, depends on the pituitary acting in its own right (growth hormone) and also on hormones from the thyroid and sex glands under pituitary control. The combustion of sugar involves both parts of the adrenal (two distinct glands), the pancreas, the thyroid, and the pituitary.

1. HISTORY

The workings of the endocrine glands could not be studied until chemistry was well advanced, in the late 19th century, though the glands themselves had long been known. The anatomists of antiquity thought that the pituitary secreted mucus to cool the blood, and that the thyroid lubricated the larynx. Galen recognized that ovaries corresponded with testicles (which is by no means obvious). The adrenals were first described in the 16th century; the little parathyroids only in the 19th.

In the 12th century Roger of Palermo treated goitre with burnt seaweed – a rich source of iodine and an admirable remedy (◊ *thyroid* (2)). Paracelsus (1516) found many cretins where goitre was common. The first account of toxic goitre was by Caleb Parry of Bath, published posthumously in 1825, and followed in 1835 and 1840 by the reports of Graves (Dublin) and Basedow (Berlin). The function of the thyroid was fairly well understood by the end of the 19th century, and in 1915 E. C. Kendall announced his discovery of its hormone, thyroxine.

Thomas Addison described adrenal failure (Addison's disease) in 1849. Exactly a century later Kendall and his colleagues opened a new field of medical treatment by treating rheumatic and other diseases with adrenal hormones.

Thomas Bartolin of Copenhagen (1616–80) found an association of diabetes with pancreatic disease. The pancreatic origin of diabetes was proved by von Mering and Minkowski at Strassburg in 1889, but the hormone, *insulin*, was not isolated until 1921, by Banting and Best at Toronto. One of their collaborators in this work, Collip, isolated the parathyroid hormone in 1925.

Sex hormones were first isolated in about 1930. For this work Butenandt of Berlin and Ruzicka of Zurich shared a Nobel Prize in 1939. The study of these hormones is complicated by the fact that they are formed in the adrenals as well as the sex glands.

The pituitary has set physiologists more problems than any other gland. Defects of the pituitary cause several completely different types of illness: diabetes insipidus, major disorders of growth giving rise to giants or dwarfs, the diseases named after Cushing, Fröhlich, and Simmonds, and probably certain types of goitre and of diabetes mellitus. The pituitary is not a uniform structure but a mosaic producing at least half a dozen unrelated hormones. Fairly pure extracts of several have been made, and ACTH, first isolated by Collip, has been synthesized.

One more name must be mentioned: in 1775 a Paris physician, Théophile de Bordeu, suggested that the bodily changes which follow castration must be due to the loss of some substance formed by the testicle and passed into the blood-stream. He thought that other organs might behave in the same way, each making its special contribution to the general economy. Bordeu's shrewd guess was the beginning of endocrinology.

endoderm. A layer of cells at a very early stage in the development of an ◊ *embryo*, the inner of the three germ-layers. The digestive organs and lungs are derived from it.

endometriosis. The presence of fragments of mucous membrane of the same kind as the lining of the uterus in other situations – either embedded in the muscle of the uterus or in other organs, especially the ovaries. The fragments of membrane pass through the same monthly cycle as the normal uterine membrane: they swell before a period and then bleed, but they have no outlet, and therefore cause severe pain for several days before a period. The symptoms disappear during pregnancy and after the menopause. In effect, this is a severe form of dysmenorrhoea.

In mild cases, analgesic drugs (aspirin etc.) may suffice. Sometimes, but not often, the offending tissue can be found and removed surgically. All symptoms are relieved by bringing on the menopause by irradiation or removal of the ovaries, so that the uterus and the abnormal tissue cease to be stimulated by ovarian hormones. But the hormone pills used for contraception may work as well without sterilizing the patient. Since she may well need hormonal replacement if her ovaries are removed, hormones instead of operation are a good bargain.

endometrium. The lining of the uterus.

endoscopy. Internal examination by direct vision through a lighted tube, generally with a system of lenses – e.g. gastroscopy (stomach); cystoscopy (bladder).

endotoxin. A poison (toxin) forming part of a bacterium and damaging only tissues in the infected area. (An *exotoxin* is released into the circulation and affects distant organs.)

enema. Medication injected into the rectum (1) to relieve severe constipation or wash out the colon before an operation, (2) to instil water and nutrients, for which it is not a very satisfactory method, (3) to get an effective concentration of a drug to the large intestine, e.g. corticosteroids for the treatment of ulcerative colitis.

energy. Apart from the obvious demands of voluntary movement, the body needs a constant supply of energy to maintain breathing, heart beat, temperature, and chemical activities.

Energy exists in various forms – mechanical, electrical, chemical etc. – and one form can be converted to another. Energy may be stored in a system. For instance, energy is rapidly fed into a clock by winding and gradually released as the spring unwinds. When a battery is charged, electrical energy is converted to chemical energy and stored, to be converted back to electrical energy when the battery is used.

All chemical processes involve energy. Some store energy; others release it. When a chemical process is reversed, energy flows in the opposite direction: when hydrogen burns it combines with oxygen to form water, and energy is released. But if energy is fed into water as an electric current, the water is split into hydrogen and oxygen.

Animals get energy by slowly burning foods; this releases stored chemical energy. Protein, fat, and carbohydrate can all be burnt. The final products are always carbon dioxide and water. Plants carry out the same process in reverse. They combine carbon dioxide with water and provide the ultimate source of all food (herbivores eat plants; carnivores eat herbivores), and of the energy that animals need. But the formation of the foods is the opposite to burning, and instead of releasing energy

plants take up energy from sunlight. Thus the sun is the ultimate source of all energy in the body.

Foods undergo chemical change during and after digestion. Those that are to be stored as fuel are converted either to ◊ *glycogen* (animal starch) and stored in the liver and muscles, or to fat, which is stored all over the body but mainly under the skin where it also serves as an insulator. Glycogen is simply a chain of glucose molecules, and before use it is converted to glucose. Fat is similarly converted to fatty acids and glycerol.

Outside the body one gets energy from fuel by setting fire to it, i.e. causing it to combine with oxygen and release energy in the process. In the body, the same end-point is reached in a series of steps. The same amount of energy is released, but gradually; and instead of all being dissipated as heat, some of it is transferred as chemical energy to intermediate products.

These intermediates are then available for any chemical process, such as muscular contraction or secretion by glands, that requires energy. The most important intermediate is ATP (adenosine triphosphate), one of the fundamental components of living matter. It readily transfers one of its three phosphate groups to other compounds, together with a parcel of immediately available energy for use in chemical reactions such as the synthesis of new substances. The lost ATP is re-formed when fresh energy is supplied by the oxidation of various substances derived from glucose or fat. These oxidations need numerous reagents, of which some can be synthesized in the body and others must be supplied in the diet as vitamins of the B group. (Chemical reactions in the body are discussed further under ◊ *enzyme*.)

The amount of energy used in the body can be calculated from the amount of oxygen consumed, which is easy to measure in a laboratory. The result is expressed as units of heat (Calories) for convenience, but since any form of energy can theoretically be converted to an equivalent amount of any other form, any other unit would do as well. An average man at rest uses some 1,700 Calories per day for his vital functions, and this is equivalent to about 80 watts, or 1/10 h.p. This resting amount is the *basal* rate. The additional energy needed for mechanical work depends on occupation. A sedentary worker may need an additional 1,000 Calories or less, but a manual labourer needs much more.

The *efficiency* of a machine is the ratio between the energy provided by the fuel and the amount of work done. With a good petrol engine the figure may be as high as 25 per cent; with a steam engine it is much lower. With a human body at rest, mechanical efficiency is zero because the energy used to remain alive does no external work. During exercise the efficiency of the body as a whole rises to about 20 per cent, and a muscle considered on its own achieves 25 per cent. As with any other engine, the remaining energy is mostly dissipated as heat. Some of the heat is of course needed to maintain body temperature, except in a very hot environment.

Directly or indirectly, most of the hormones affect the output and use of energy. Adrenaline releases glucose from the glycogen stores into the blood-stream. Insulin enables the glucose to enter the cells where it is to be consumed. Thyroid hormone acts on the *mitochondria*, the compartments within the cell where the transfer of chemical energy by ATP takes place; it causes more energy to be converted to heat.

All kinds of food can be converted to glucose, and there are no grounds for supposing that special foods increase the amount of energy that the body can exert.

Entamoeba. A genus of protozoon (amoeba) *Entamoeba coli* is a harmless inhabitant of the large intestine. A related species, *E. histolytica*, causes amoebic ◊ *dysentery*.

enteric fever. A group of infectious diseases including typhoid and paratyphoid fevers; or simply typhoid fever.

enteritis. Inflammation of the intestine, a symptom of many diseases, including infection with bacteria or viruses and allergic reactions. The commonest types – the digestive upsets of summer holidays, and a distressing illness of babies – include inflammation of the stomach and count as ◊ *gastro-enteritis*.

Regional enteritis (Crohn's disease) is a disease of unknown cause, with inflammation confined to one segment of intestine, often the last part of the small intestine. It can cause vague pain, or diarrhoea, or symptoms suggesting appendicitis or even

obstruction. Treatment includes adequate relaxation, drugs of the belladonna type to relieve spasm, and a well planned diet. Corticosteroids sometimes give complete relief. The affected intestine may have to be removed surgically.

enuresis = ◊ *bed-wetting*.

enzyme. An enzyme (or ferment) is a substance produced by living cells which promotes chemical change. Since each enzyme is responsible for only one type of change the number of different enzymes in the body is large, perhaps several thousand. The properties of a living organism largely depend on the chemical reactions it can perform and so on the enzymes it can produce. Differences between species or between members of the same species are generally speaking differences between their enzymes. Heredity transmits the ability to form particular enzymes (◊ *genetics*). An enzyme is a highly specific *catalyst*. The following section simply expands this statement.

1. CATALYSIS

A chemical reaction is a rearrangement of atoms to form new compounds. Thus a metal, zinc, and an acid, hydrochloric acid, react to form a white salt, zinc chloride, and an inflammable gas, hydrogen:

$$Zn + 2HCl \rightarrow ZnCl_2 + H_2.$$

The atoms are unchanged, but they are rearranged by transferring chlorine (Cl) from the acid to the metal. The change is fairly rapid, but it is not instantaneous; the mixture does not explode.

A spark causes hydrogen and oxygen to react, forming water:

$$2H_2 + O_2 \rightarrow 2H_2O.$$

This is a very fast reaction, and the mixture does explode.

Similarly hydrogen and nitrogen combine, to form ammonia:

$$3H_2 + N_2 \rightarrow 2NH_3.$$

But this reaction is so slow as to be useless. The gases can, however, be attracted to the surface of specially prepared iron. Held to the iron, the atoms of hydrogen and nitrogen react quickly. Ammonia is formed and released, leaving the iron free to take up a fresh batch of hydrogen and nitrogen. This is the Haber process for manufacturing ammonia. A small quantity of iron changes a very slow reaction into a reasonably fast one, and the iron undergoes no chemical change. This is *catalysis*; iron is a catalyst to the reaction.

The equation shown above implies that all the hydrogen and nitrogen combine to form ammonia. This is untrue, for the reaction can take the opposite direction, when ammonia breaks down to hydrogen and nitrogen:

$$2NH_3 \rightarrow 3H_2 + N_2.$$

This latter reaction is favoured by high temperature or low pressure. But at any temperature and pressure the two reactions take place simultaneously. While there is little ammonia in the mixture, the first reaction predominates. If there is much ammonia to be broken down the second predominates. At a critical concentration the two reactions balance, and although the three constituents are constantly reacting ammonia is re-formed as fast as it breaks down:

$$3H_2 + N_2 \rightleftharpoons 2NH_3.$$

The catalyst works equally well in both directions. Therefore it cannot affect the point of balance. It accelerates both the formation and the destruction of ammonia to the same extent. All it can do is to hasten both reactions so that a balance is attained more quickly.

One more example from inorganic chemistry shows how a catalyst may act by forming an *intermediate compound*. Sulphuric acid (H_2SO_4) is readily formed from sulphur trioxide (SO_3) and water. The equation is a simple addition:

$$SO_3 + H_2O \rightarrow H_2SO_4.$$

Sulphur *di*oxide (SO_2) is easy to get, but it is very reluctant to take on a third oxygen atom to form SO_3. On the other hand nitric oxide (NO) easily takes on oxygen to form a dioxide (NO_2). This compound reacts, again easily, with sulphur dioxide:

$$NO_2 + SO_2 \rightarrow NO + SO_3.$$

Thus the difficult conversion of SO_2 to SO_3 is done in two easy stages by means of a catalyst, NO. The catalyst acts as vehicle for conveying oxygen. The intermediate compound, NO_2, promptly reverts to NO in the second stage, so that at the end the catalyst is intact. The equation may be written:

$$2SO_2 + O_2 \xrightarrow{NO} 2SO_3.$$

In the body, a substance which would normally react very slowly if at all forms with its enzyme an intermediate compound which can react quickly.

2. NATURE OF ENZYMES

Like any other catalyst, an enzyme acts in very small quantities; it is unchanged at the end of the reaction on which it works; it affects only the speed and not the nature of the reaction; it facilitates the converse reaction to the same extent.

Carbon dioxide (CO_2) combines with water to form carbonic acid (i.e. to make soda-water). It is a slow process. A sparklet siphon needs a good shake before any appreciable amount of carbonic acid is formed after the CO_2 has been released. In the living body CO_2 is a by-product of many vital reactions, and it must be removed by the blood and taken to the lungs to be exhaled. The blood cannot convey it as a gas; the CO_2 must form soluble carbonic acid and bicarbonates, and it must do so quickly as the blood flows past. The enzyme carbonic anhydrase in the red blood cells increases the speed of this reaction 18,000 times: an hour's work is done in a fifth of a second.

The converse reaction (carbonic acid to CO_2) is equally possible. But the continual production of CO_2 in the tissues keeps the balance tilted in favour of forming carbonic acid. In the lungs, on the other hand, CO_2 is continually removed by breathing, which favours the breakdown of carbonic acid to release more CO_2. And the same enzyme accelerates this breakdown to the same extent as it did the formation.

Enzymes are highly selective. A given enzyme will catalyse one kind of reaction and no other. But since it works by forming an intermediate compound with the substance to be transformed it may well form similar compounds with other closely related substances. The importance of this is explained in section 3 below.

Since living chemistry is largely a matter of compounding substances in one place and decomposing them in another (as carbonic acid in the example given) most enzymes have the double function of promoting both forward and backward reactions.

All known enzymes are proteins, and all proteins are very sensitive to changes of acidity and changes of temperature. Only a few, such as pepsin in the stomach, can act in an acid medium. All are destroyed by heat. They work best a little above normal body temperature (37°C.). But at, say, a temperature of 50°C. the enzymes are put out of action, and with them the whole body chemistry. Thus the principle that chemical reactions are accelerated by warmth is true of living reactions only within narrow limits.

3. ENZYME POISONS

Some chemicals attach themselves almost indiscriminately to others, including catalysts. If this happens the catalyst is unable to work, because the part of its molecule which should be forming an intermediate compound (section 1, above) is already occupied by the invading chemical. Chemicals of this type include cyanides, and many compounds of arsenic and mercury. These are, of course, among the deadliest of mineral poisons. Cyanides have a remarkable affinity for iron. The enzyme *cytochrome oxidase*, by means of which oxygen is used in the body cells, contains iron, and if this iron is occupied by a cyanide the enzyme ceases to act. Death is almost immediate.

The poison gas lewisite and other arsenic compounds behave in the same way as cyanides, though with less immediately vital enzymes. The antidote, British antilewisite (BAL), has the same structure as the vulnerable portion of the enzymes. Arsenic attaches itself to BAL, leaving the enzyme free to do its work.

Other poisons act because they closely resemble the compound on which an enzyme usually acts. Many bacteria need a supply of para-amino-benzoic acid in order to grow. But the bacterial enzymes will accept instead a similar but useless compound, para-amino-benzene sulphonamide (sulphanilamide). This compound therefore prevents the bacteria from growing, and is a valuable drug. Many drugs act against human enzymes in this manner. Their effect may be to suppress some activity, or it may be to stimulate by preventing an enzyme from destroying an active natural substance too rapidly.

4. PRECURSORS AND CO-ENZYMES

Some enzymes are not wanted in the cells which produce them. Powerful enzymes for digesting proteins are formed in the pancreas, but the pancreas is not intended to digest itself. These enzymes are inactive until they join other enzymes formed in the intestine, where they can act on food; the intestine is protected from them by a film of mucus. Similarly the enzymes which clot blood are in the blood all the time. Circulating blood does not clot because the enzymes are inactive until they are joined by substances only released when there is an injury to be repaired. Such enzymes are like bombs which do not receive their war-heads until they are ready for action. They are not strictly enzymes but only precursors.

A co-enzyme is a substance needed to activate an enzyme and usually serving as a bridge between two enzymes: it may be the end-product of one reaction and the starting point of the next. Nearly all of the ◊ *vitamins* help to form co-enzymes.

5. ENZYME DEFICIENCIES

In general, hereditary characters reflect the ability to form particular enzymes. Differences between healthy individuals could probably be traced to slight differences in unimportant enzymes, and inherited illness to greater differences or defects. In some disorders a missing enzyme has been identified. A small amount of the amino-acid *phenylalanine* in the diet is necessary to health, but if large amounts are allowed to accumulate they are harmful. Any excess of phenylalanine is normally converted to its hydroxide, *tyrosine*, by means of an enzyme. Children born without this enzyme become mentally defective. The condition is known as *phenylketonuria*. If phenylalanine is almost excluded from the diet these children can develop normally. At the next stage, tyrosine is partly converted to the pigment *melanin. Albinos* lack an enzyme needed for this conversion. Other enzymes convert tyrosine to thyroid hormone (◊ *thyroid gland*); if one of these is missing the child will be a *cretin.* Many other disorders, most of them rare, have been traced to particular enzymes, and it becomes increasingly clear that some common diseases are of the same type, though why some of them remain dormant until adult life has not been explained.

Enzyme poisons have already been mentioned. One can guess that many common symptoms of disease are due to suppression of enzymes. Vitamin deficiencies deprive enzymes of essential co-enzymes. Viruses, which cause more illness than any other agent, live at the expense of their host's enzymes. Some bacteria may do the same, and many bacteria produce harmful enzymes of their own. Cancer is a disorder of cell growth and therefore, presumably, of enzymes. But this sort of argument can be extended until it becomes sterile: all illness disturbs normal function; function is orderly chemical change, and chemical change depends on enzymes. So illness is a matter of disturbed enzymes – this is a truism, and it hints at knowledge of cause and effect which nobody yet has. One thing, however, is certain: that the next major advance in medicine is more likely to come from the study of enzymes than from any other field of research.

eosin. A red acidic dye, much used in staining biological specimens for microscopic examination, usually with a contrasting blue alkaline dye; different components of the specimen take up one or other colour.

eosinophil. A kind of white blood cell, containing granules readily stained with eosin. The number of circulating eosinophils increases during illness due to allergy.

ephedrine. A drug originally extracted from a plant *Ephedra* or *ma huang*, used in China for many centuries but not adopted by Western medicine until about 1930.

The chemical structure and behaviour of ephedrine resemble those of ⟡ *adrenaline*, but adrenaline is inactive when taken by mouth whereas ephedrine is active. Disorders such as asthma which respond to adrenaline can be treated with ephedrine without the need for injections.

The enzyme ⟡ *monoamine oxidase* decomposes adrenaline and also ephedrine; it may be that ephedrine acts not directly but by drawing the fire of this enzyme and so enhancing the effect of adrenaline on the bronchi and elsewhere.

epicanthus. Vertical fold of skin at the inner corner of the eye, usual in Mongolians but uncommon in other races.

epidemic. (Disease) introduced to a region or population, spreading, and apparently disappearing until the next outbreak. (cf. *endemic*, always present in the region.)

epidermis. The outer layer of the skin.

epigastrium. The upper part of the abdomen, in the angle of the ribs over the stomach.

epiglottis. A flap of cartilage behind the tongue; at rest it is upright and the breath passes behind it between the vocal cords. During swallowing the epiglottis drops back to cover the vocal cords and prevent food from being inhaled.

epilepsy. An ill-defined group of disorders characterized by fits (seizures). A fit is an episode of disorganized and excessive activity in some part of the brain, causing disturbances of sensation, movement, or consciousness according to the area of the brain that is involved. With *petit mal* epilepsy the only symptom is fleeting loss of consciousness. The patient – usually a child – may even be unaware that anything has happened. *Grand mal* is the well known type of fit in which the patient – sometimes warned by preliminary symptoms – falls unconscious, often with a cry. His muscles stiffen and then twitch violently, often causing him to bite his tongue. His bladder may empty. The attack lasts a couple of minutes. Some patients then go into a deep sleep. A few patients, instead of sleeping the attack off, pass into a trance-like state in which they behave unaccountably and in some cases antisocially.

The preliminary symptoms or *aura* indicate the area of the brain where the disturbance begins, before spreading to other parts. The aura may be an uncontrolled movement in some part of the body, or a sensation, or even, in very rare cases, a bizarre pattern of behaviour. There is no aura if the attack starts in a 'silent' area of the brain – one that is not concerned with perception or action – and in many cases the disturbance spreads so rapidly that the patient is unconscious before he has time to notice anything. In *focal* (Jacksonian) epilepsy the aura is the most prominent part of the attack: it generally starts with localized twitching that rapidly spreads to more and more muscles, and may or may not culminate in a *grand mal* attack.

No other disease arouses as much superstition as epilepsy, for none is quite so suggestive of 'possession'. Hippocrates' treatise *On the Sacred Disease*, probably written about 400 B.C., tried to debunk the superstition indicated by the title and present epilepsy as a disease like any other, a result of natural causes. Yet even now many people are uneasy in the presence of epileptics, and not only in primitive societies.

In discussing the nature of epilepsy, the

first point to be made is that anyone can have an epileptic fit. A head injury, an electric shock, various drugs, asphyxia, or a severe bout of fever can all cause fits. These fits are not merely *like* epilepsy; they *are* epilepsy, as defined in the first two sentences of this article. The only difference between an epileptic and anyone else is that he is unduly liable to this kind of disturbance.

In *symptomatic epilepsy* the fits are set off by a detectable physical agent such as a blood-clot or displaced fragment of bone after an injury, a tumour, pressure of oedema (excess of fluid, e.g. with very high blood pressure), or infection. Children often have fits (convulsions) at the beginning of a fever such as measles; their brain cells are more sensitive than adult cells to a rising body temperature. The location of the cause can often be inferred from the type of fit, since the origin of a particular movement or sensation is a known area of the brain. If the cause can be dealt with, symptomatic epilepsy is of course curable.

Idiopathic epilepsy – apparently spontaneous, without detectable cause – is the commoner type, and what most people mean by epilepsy. Either the brain cells are unduly susceptible to minor irritation, or there is an unrecognized agent setting off fits. In support of the former idea, idiopathic epilepsy generally starts in childhood and the children often gradually improve, just as children soon stop having convulsions in response to fever. But even if this should be so it cannot be the whole story, and many neurologists believe that *all* epilepsy is symptomatic, though the centre of the disturbance may be no more than a minute scar, too small ever to be traced.

Epilepsy, then, is no more a disease in its own right than high blood pressure or fever. It is a reaction that can be evoked in many ways. It is called symptomatic when a cause can be found, and idiopathic when the cause is unknown.

Since most epilepsy is 'idiopathic' only the symptom can be treated, not the cause. But most epileptics can be kept free from attacks, and many remain well after all treatment has been given up; the young epileptic has the best chance of complete recovery.

The unsuitability of certain jobs has been exaggerated. Employers and workmates are naturally anxious about the risk, but in fact there are very few jobs that are wholly unsuited to epileptics. Driving heads the

list, and nobody who is known to have fits can get a licence. In some countries, people who are kept free from fits with drugs are allowed to drive. An unreasonable objection is that if the person needs drugs he must still have the disease and should therefore not drive. A reasonable objection is that the drugs used for controlling the fits slow a driver's reactions. Many authorities, medical and legal, hold that the patient should not drive until he no longer needs drugs.

Many drugs are used to suppress the symptoms of this condition. Bromides are obsolete, but after more than half a century phenobarbitone is still the main standby. The chief objection to it is that it is a powerful sedative and causes drowsiness. Newer drugs for *grand mal* include phenytoin and primidone. Patients differ, and the best drug or mixture has to be found by trial and error. The right dose is the least that will keep the patient free from attacks. In time – it may be several years – the dose can often be reduced and finally given up. If fits start again the dose has to be increased again. Such disappointments are inevitable because the only way to find out whether it is safe to reduce the dose is to try. Patients who have gone two years with neither drugs nor fits are generally regarded as cured.

Petit mal is treated with a different type of drug, e.g. ethosuximide. It is essentially a disorder of childhood, and complete recovery is the rule, especially if there has been no associated *grand mal*.

Hereditary factors play only a minor role in epilepsy, and the disease is not a reason for not having children. On the other hand an intending marriage partner has to know what is involved; marriages have been dissolved on the grounds of unrevealed epilepsy.

Epilepsy is commonly thought to be associated with mental defect. Probably one reason for this belief is that injury to the brain in infancy can cause both epilepsy and mental defect. But most epileptics are normal people in all other respects.

epinephrine. Official name in USA for ◊ *adrenaline*.

epiphysis. Accessory part of a bone, developed in infancy as a separate bone and later joining the main structure. Until a year or two either side of puberty, epiphyses (mainly the ends of the limb bones) are joined to the shafts of bones by cartilage. The age at which a particular cartilaginous bridge is converted to bone is more or less constant; this sometimes gives the age of a skeleton at the time of death.

episiotomy. Surgical division of the perineum to enlarge the outlet of the birth-passage in cases of difficult birth.

epistaxis. Bleeding from the nose. ⬦ *nose* (1).

epithelium. Coating or lining tissue; skin or mucous membrane.

Erasistratus (3rd century B.C.). Physician of Antioch and Alexandria, regarded as the founder of scientific physiology. He and his contemporary Herophilus established a school in Alexandria that was not surpassed until the rise of the Italian universities after the Middle Ages. Erasistratus showed that all organs received nerves, arteries, and veins. He made experiments to show the motor and sensory functions of nerves and their dependence on the brain. He recognized that the heart valves permitted flow in only one direction, but could not infer the circulation of blood because (like everyone until Galen in the 2nd century A.D.) he thought that arteries contained air and not blood. He attributed much disease to congestion of blood vessels.

erection. Engorgement of penis or other sex organs with blood: it is a reflex action depending on parasympathetic nerves. Muscles around the veins contract and prevent blood from leaving, and the erection is maintained by the pressure of blood in the arteries.

erector spinae. Complex system of muscles supporting the backbone, forming a rounded ridge at either side of the mid-line where the spinous processes of the *vertebrae* separate the two halves of the system. The component muscles, some joining adjacent vertebrae, others spanning several, are attached to the backs of the vertebrae and to the base of the skull, the ribs, and the pelvis.

These muscles are arranged to twist the backbone and to bend it sideways or backwards. They cannot actively bend it forwards because they are all behind the vertical axis; this movement is done in the neck by the ⬦ *sternomastoid* and in the lower part of the back by the abdominal muscles. But in practice gravity is the principal flexor of the backbone, and erector spinae has the important task of regulating and resisting the force of gravity to maintain the erect posture.

erepsin. Intestinal enzymes for digesting protein.

ergot. The fungus *Claviceps purpurea*, a parasite of rye. It contains numerous alkaloids, which account for its poisonous properties and its medicinal uses.

Ergot interferes with the stimulant action of adrenaline on the muscle of arteries and on some other tissues, but itself directly stimulates involuntary muscle. The net effect of these contrary actions is unpredictable, and therefore crude extracts are no longer used. Some of the pure alkaloids have a more limited and manageable action. *Ergometrine* acts mainly on the muscle of the uterus. Injected immediately after childbirth, it causes the uterus to contract firmly and so stops bleeding. *Ergotamine* acts on blood vessels in the head and sometimes prevents migraine.

Outbreaks of ergot poisoning have been due to bread made from contaminated rye. Many victims have died. Others have lost fingers and toes from gangrene due to sustained constriction of the arteries, and still others have had convulsions and mental derangement.

The alkaloids of ergot are compounds of lysergic acid and thus related to the hallucinogen LSD.

erysipelas. A severe, contagious infection of the skin with streptococci, causing diffuse, spreading inflammation, high fever, and sometimes grave complications such as pneumonia and nephritis. Until the discovery of sulphonamides, erysipelas was a dangerous and fairly common disease; but now it is seldom seen and rapidly cured.

erythema. Reddening (inflammation) of the skin. *Erythema nodosum*, with red lumps in the skin, is an uncommon complication of various types of infection; it probably represents an allergic reaction.

erythrocyte = red blood cell (⬦ *blood*). *Erythrocyte sedimentation rate* (ESR) is a clinical laboratory test: the rate at which the red cells settle in a column of blood in a glass tube is measured. Rapid sedimentation suggests that the disease under investigation is still active.

erythromycin. An antibiotic with similar activity to penicillin, used especially against bacteria which have become resistant to penicillin.

Escherichia. A genus of bacteria, mostly harmless; including *E. coli*, a normal inhabitant of the large intestine that causes trouble if it strays to other parts of the body such as the kidneys.

ESR ◊ *erythrocyte*.

ethanol. Ethyl ◊ *alcohol*; spirits of wine.

ether. A group of chemical compounds derived from alcohols; usually *diethyl ether*, $C_2H_5.O.C_2H_5$, a volatile anaesthetic. Ether was one of the first general anaesthetics to be used. It was difficult to administer because it made the patients choke, and it was soon replaced by chloroform. But chloroform was more insidiously dangerous and ether came back. It was easy enough to handle if the early stages of anaesthesia were done with another agent – chloroform or nitrous oxide, and it was safe. In recent years, less irritant anaesthetics have tended to displace ether, to avoid post-operative vomiting and coughing.

ethical. A term used to describe medicines, not necessarily those of which the sale is controlled by law, that are advertised only to the medical and allied professions. Reputable companies back the advertisement of their ethical products with information about the underlying research, references to published reports, and warnings of known risks. Products advertised to the general public are described as 'over-the-counter'. By maintaining this distinction the manufacturers have undoubtedly saved a good deal of disappointment, embarrassment and confusion between doctors and patients. ◊ *research*.

ethics. Many people, including some doctors, are baffled by the intricacies of medical ethics.

Doctors everywhere are supposed to accept a code of conduct more or less based on the ◊ *Hippocratic Oath*. In many countries they have to take an oath when they qualify, though not in Britain, where a partly unwritten code should be taken for granted.

The Hippocratic Oath was not only an undertaking to act in the best interests of the patient; it was also an initiation to a guild. Some of its provisions lay down the doctor's behaviour towards his patient, and others, his behaviour towards his colleagues. This division has remained, and it is with the rules about ethical procedure between two doctors that the general public mostly quarrels, feeling that the profession is concerned mainly with its own interests.

Misbehaviour by a doctor may be a criminal offence, or malpractice, or negligence, or a breach of ethics, or a combination of the four. Before the laws in England were relaxed, abortion was, with a few exceptions, a crime. If it was carried out regardless of the patient's best interests, purely for the sake of a large fee, it was also unethical, and if it was decidedly the wrong treatment for the particular case (e.g. a young married woman wanting a child but afraid of pregnancy and needing only reassurance) then it was malpractice as well. Professional abortionists, sometimes erring in all these ways, went to prison for breaking the law, and lost their right to practise for their unethical behaviour ('infamous conduct'). But there were also doctors who performed abortions for a reasonable fee or sometimes without charge because, despite the law, they thought the operation medically justified. Some of these went to prison too. The operations were illegal, but were they unethical? Adultery with a patient, on the other hand, is not a crime in law, but it is highly unethical and can cost the doctor his right to practise.

Incompetence is unethical in that a doctor has a moral duty to know his own job. It is most likely to be penalized when a patient is awarded damages because of wrong or inadequate treatment. On the whole, the Courts are reasonable in their demands on doctors. They do not expect a country practitioner to have the special skills of a brain surgeon, nor a brain surgeon to be an expert on antenatal care. Each is expected to provide the skill normally expected from someone working in his chosen branch of medicine.

Negligence means falling below this standard. In most cases, including some incurring very heavy damages, negligence arises from a lapse of attention, such as failing to check a dose or taking a telephone message too lightly.

Among the skills required of any doctor is a knowledge of his own limitations. A country doctor doing his best in an emergency is not blamed if *his* best is not as good as the best of a specialist in that particular operation. But a town doctor would be negligent if he attempted the same operation knowing that a specialist was within easy reach. This is the modern equivalent of the Hippocratic clause that forbids inexperienced doctors to operate. It extends far beyond surgery. Medicine is now so specialized that nobody can be expert in all its branches, and every doctor meets a variety of cases that need a second opinion.

Malpractice can mean the same as negligence, but it is often used in a much wider sense to include deliberate wrong treatment, such as unjustified surgery, and unethical behaviour such as breach of confidence.

This matter of confidence or professional secrecy raises problems. In principle, anything that a doctor learns about his patients is to be kept secret. It may be in the patient's best interests for the doctor to discuss the case with the wife or husband, but he is not supposed to do so without the patient's permission. More than one doctor has paid heavy damages for an unguarded word to a patient's spouse. Many parents feel that they have an absolute right to know what their children have told the doctor. But what if an adolescent consults a doctor precisely because he trusts him not to talk to his parents? Sometimes it is clearly ethical for the doctor to discuss a patient with the family, e.g. with mental disorders where the patient cannot reasonably be asked for permission, or with a gravely ill patient. A doctor called as a witness does not have the same privileges as a lawyer: he cannot withhold information on the grounds that it is confidential. This can put ethics in direct conflict with the law. To make it still worse the enforced breach of confidence may be actionable unless the doctor first insists that he is giving evidence under protest.

As regards the behaviour of doctors towards each other, the first cause of misunderstanding is that etiquette is often confused with ethics. To advise a patient (except in an emergency) knowing that he is under the care of a colleague is usually more a breach of etiquette than of ethics. Blatant advertising, on the other hand, is unethical. Another breach of ethics that, like advertising, can cost a doctor his licence, is 'covering', which means using a medical qualification to shield an unqualified practitioner, e.g. by signing certificates or prescriptions on his behalf. Some unqualified practitioners may be very good at their job, but professional standards have been established to protect the public, and it is not surprising that doctors should be penalized for undermining them.

A set of written and unwritten rules discourages doctors from stealing patients from one another, and these are the ones that most annoy the public. Some of them surely started as measures to protect the guild rather than its clients, but as they now stand they do serve – perhaps clumsily – to protect the patient. It is at best undesirable, and at worst really dangerous, for two doctors, unknown to each other, to be treating the same patient. Alternative forms of treatment, both justifiable, may be dangerously incompatible. And, for all the advances of scientific medicine, confidence is still an important factor in most cures. A patient who plays one doctor off against another presumably distrusts both, and neither is likely to do him much good. People often ask doctors whom they meet on holiday or over a dinner table for advice about their health, often with the implication that their own doctors are wrong. When they get a non-committal answer, they complain about stuffy medical etiquette. To give a detailed opinion in these circumstances would be a breach of etiquette; it would make difficulties for the other doctor. But it would also be, as often as not, a breach of ethics because any such opinion would be based on insufficient information and therefore negligent. If a patients loses confidence in his doctor, it is much better for him to change doctors completely than seek casual advice.

A word is needed here about the relation of specialists and hospital doctors to general practitioners. In Britain the specialist is traditionally a *consultant* whose primary function is to advise general practitioners rather than patients. In principle it is the practitioner, the family doctor, who calls him in, rather as a solicitor takes counsel's opinion on his client's behalf. In practice, the consultant usually advises the patient directly, if only to save time, but he does so on behalf of the family doctor, to whom he returns the patient when he has given the advice or treatment that he was asked to give. In many other countries the patient is transferred rather than referred to a specialist. Events there may take the same course as in Britain, but without the feeling that the patient's own doctor is still his doctor even if for the time being he is in the background. The British system gives the family doctor a most valuable function – that of a kind of referee who in an age of over-specialization can still see the wood for the trees.

Historically, this is why a specialist will often refuse to see a patient without a letter from his doctor. Pressure of work is perhaps a stronger reason in hospitals, but it is not the original one, which is basically a rational division of labour.

The system is open to abuse by doctors who refer patients without sufficient thought, and by consultants who do not send adequate reports to the doctor, but that does not condemn the system. Nor does the form of abuse known as dichotomy, where an unscrupulous doctor refers a patient to an expensive specialist and then shares the fee, an offence for which both can be immediately struck off the Register.

Professional standards are maintained in several ways. The most important is undoubtedly the long and closely supervised training, during which approved behaviour is instilled like a series of conditioned reflexes. By the time that they are ready to qualify, most medical students find that pretty women who are also patients no longer disturb them, and that to discuss patients in public would be gross blasphemy: this can happen even if in all other ways they are still lecherous and garrulous.

The General Medical Council, a statutory body, keeps the Medical Register, which is the official list of people licensed to practise as doctors. Its disciplinary committee deals with breaches of ethics (infamous conduct). It is perhaps unfortunate that there is no intermediate penalty between warning an offender and depriving him of his livelihood by striking his name off the Register. Formerly, doctors had no right of appeal against decisions of the GMC and no right to legal representation before it, but this has now changed. A doctor who has been struck off can apply for readmission to the Register. He can be struck off for any serious breach of ethics. An alcoholic doctor may be let off with a warning, subject to his undergoing treatment, and a drug addict may be allowed to practise but forbidden to prescribe certain drugs.

A doctor convicted of any serious crime can also be struck off when his conduct has been reported to the GMC. Negligence can bring him to the Civil Courts with a claim for heavy damages. Doctors employed by the National Health Service can be fined by their local committees for not looking after their patients, and also for over-prescribing, i.e. for prescribing needlessly expensive remedies against public funds.

Contrary to what many people think, the British Medical Association has no powers to discipline its members other than that of persuasion. But it has an ethical committee to advise doctors on questions of professional ethics. Most doctors subscribe, as professional insurance, to one of the organizations that offer legal advice and indemnity against the costs of legal actions. These organizations also keep a close watch on professional standards.

All the professions allied to medicine, such as dentistry, nursing, and pharmacy, are subject to similar codes and disciplinary bodies.

ethmoid. A small bone of the skull, forming the roof of the nose. Its name (= sieve-like) refers to the large number of holes for the olfactory nerves, carrying the sense of smell, which led the anatomists of antiquity to suppose that mucus was formed inside the skull in the pituitary gland and flowed down to the nose.

ethyl chloride. An anaesthetic agent similar to chloroform but with a more rapid action. It is very volatile, and when sprayed on the skin it evaporates so quickly that the skin is cooled to the point of insensibility. Thus it can also be used as a local anaesthetic.

eu-. Prefix = 'good', 'easy' (the converse of dys-; e.g. eupepsia, healthy digestion, as opposed to dyspepsia, indigestion).

euphoria. Abnormal elation.

Eustachian tube. Narrow passage between the cavity of the ear-drum and the back of the nose. Its opening in the side of the naso-pharynx is above the soft palate (◊ *pharynx*). Eustachius described the tube in 1562 in the first detailed account of the ear, but Alc-maeon of Croton had mentioned it 2,000 years before.

Eustachius (Bartolomeo Eustachio) (?1520–1574). Anatomist in Rome; physician to the Pope. One of the few great anatomists of the time who did not work at Padua (◊ *Vesalius*). He was a more accurate but less imaginative worker than his contemporary Vesalius: he recorded details which Vesalius missed, but he did not see the body as a dynamic, inte-grated system. His accounts of particular organs – ear, larynx, kidney, nervous system – are admirable, but few were published in his lifetime. By the time they appeared (1714) they were no longer needed; the suc-cessors of Vesalius at Padua had already stolen Eustachius's thunder.

evolution. The derivation of different species from common ancestors; a process of grad-ual change from generation to generation.

Although no general theory of evolution was formulated until the 19th century (◊ *Lamarck; Darwin*), scientists had toyed with the idea since the time of ◊ *Aristotle*. Darwin not only produced convincing evi-dence that species were not ready-made but had evolved from simpler forms of life; he also indicated that change was established by 'natural selection'. If in any way an individual is better adapted to its environ-ment than its fellows, and can transmit the advantage to its offspring, then in time the descendants of the new type outnumber and ultimately supersede the older type. The process is summed up in Herbert Spencer's phrase 'survival of the fittest'. Darwin could not offer any explanation of how changes had taken place, because nothing was known of genetics. It is now clear (◊ *genetics*) that change occurs by mutation, which as a rule is harmful but occasionally confers an advantage that can be transmit-ted to the offspring.

The theory of evolution is important to medical science in several ways. Firstly, it brings order to biology, of which rational medicine is a branch. Many of the puzzles and seeming illogicalities of anatomy make sense in the light of the past history of the race, and the growth of an embryo from a single cell to a fully developed infant is like an epitome of the evolution, over millions of generations, of the human race from the first living cells. Physiology deals with the working of the body and its component organs, and everything in physiology can be seen as a means of adaptation to the environ-ment. The 'fittest' that survive are those that are best adapted.

As regards hereditary ailments, most of which take the form of enhanced liability to a disease, effective treatment tends to neu-tralize the effect of natural selection and so, in a sense, weaken the population. But this is a very slow process, and if the diseases can be cured it does not matter. And in ad-vanced human society mere physical fitness – the ability to hunt and fight – is no longer a measure of adaptation to the environment. What distinguishes man from other animals is his ability to use his brain to adapt the environment to suit him. In his struggle for survival, ingenuity is a much more import-ant factor than strong teeth.

A disquieting form of evolution takes place at the other end of the natural scale among the microbes that cause infectious diseases. Successful treatment of infection can encourage the rapid evolution of modi-fied microbes that resist the treatment (◊ *antibiotic*). This has occurred mainly among bacteria, but malaria is showing a similar tendency.

exanthem(a). 1. Skin rash as a symptom of an infectious fever (chickenpox, measles, typhus etc.). **2.** The disease itself.

excretion. Elimination of by-products of digestion and body chemistry, also of excess requisites such as salt. The principal organs of excretion are the *kidneys* (water, nitrogen compounds, salts, acids), the *lungs* (carbon dioxide, water), the *skin* (water, salt), and the *liver* (bile pigments and salts, extraneous poisons). Technically speaking, the undi-gested food waste in the faeces is not ex-creted, because the body has never assimi-lated it; it is merely in transit.

exercise. Although few people would deny that exercise promotes health there is not much evidence to show that it does so; nor is it quite clear what the evidence ought to show, because nobody can define 'health' and 'fitness' or say whether they mean dif-ferent things. Since most people feel fitter with regular exercise than without it there is not much need for scientific proof that they are materially better off for a daily walk. It is by no means clear that *being* fit is any different from *feeling* fit.

Exercise strengthens muscles, and disuse causes them to waste. This is only one example of the general principle that tissues with no work tend to shrink, presumably because a decreased supply of blood keeps them under-nourished.

Training is more complex. Increased bulk and strength of muscle is only one part of it. Improved skill is of course another, but in unknown ways exercise also increases mechanical efficiency – the amount of work from consuming a given amount of fuel.

But health cannot be measured as muscular strength, and exercise must have more subtle effects. For example, among people with high blood pressure the mortality is highest in those who take least exercise (but it is influenced by many other factors such as overeating and smoking, and causes are hard to distinguish from effects or from mere coincidences). A muscle at rest needs very little blood. Even the heart can carry on with a very poor circulation in its coronary arteries when there is no exertion. During exercise, the amount of blood flowing through a muscle increases at least ten-fold. This is achieved partly by widening the vessels, partly by raising the pressure, and partly by opening up new channels. If these auxiliary channels are in regular use, they are always available for emergencies. But if muscles, especially the heart, have not worked hard for years, then when their arteries begin to degenerate there is nothing in reserve.

Although the main purpose of exercise would be to forestall damage to the heart as the arteries age, it may well help even when some damage is already done, and at some centres patients with angina are treated with carefully graded exercises.

The effect of exercise on the state of mind is quite as important as its effects on the muscles and circulation. In fact, mental and physical effects are not really distinct, because exercise promotes mental relaxation and thus helps to overcome stresses that contribute to physical illness.

exocrine. An exocrine gland is one with a duct to carry its secretion to its site of action, e.g. saliva to the mouth or enzymes from the pancreas to the duodenum (cf. *endocrine*, having no duct and secreting into the bloodstream).

exophthalmic goitre = toxic goitre with protruding eyes as a symptom. ◊ *thyroid gland* (2).

exophthalmos. Protruding eyes. There are many possible causes, e.g. injuries and diseases of the orbit, but the only common one is exophthalmic goitre.

exostosis. Superfluous mass of bone. ◊ *osteoma.*

exotoxin. Poison released by bacteria into the circulation and causing damage away from the site of infection. For instance, tetanus bacilli do not stray from the wound where they have a foothold, but their exotoxins injure the central nervous system.

expectorant. Medicine to loosen mucus in the lungs and facilitate coughing. ◊ *cough medicines.*

extension. 1. The movement of straightening a joint (opposed to flexion). **2.** Treatment of a broken bone by a steady pull on the limb. The purpose is to overcome the tendency of the patient's muscles to contract automatically and cause overriding of the broken ends of bone. ◊ *fracture.*

exteroception. Sensation or perception of things other than one's own body – the 'five senses', as opposed to *proprioception*, which informs about the position of joints, balance etc.

extrasystole. A common irregularity of the heart beat ('dropped beat'). ◊ *arrhythmia.*

extravasation. Leakage of fluid from a vessel into the surrounding tissues, as a result of injury. Internal bleeding is the obvious example, but the term may apply to urine, bile or other fluids.

exudation. Seepage of watery fluid from the blood through intact vessels, e.g. as a result of inflammation.

eye.

1. STRUCTURE

The eye is a sphere with a slight bulge in front and a stalk behind, a little to the inner side of the mid-line. It has a firm shell, the *sclera*, with a transparent bulge in front (*cornea*). The stalk at the back carries the *optic nerve*, transmitting visual impulses to the brain.

The sclera is lined first with a layer of pigment and fine blood vessels (*choroid*) and second with a mesh of nerve fibres and their light-sensitive endings (*retina*).

Behind the cornea is a pigmented diaphragm supported by muscle (*iris*), and behind the iris, again supported by muscle, is the *lens*. The *pupil* is a hole in the middle of the iris.

The space between the cornea and the lens is filled with watery fluid (*aqueous humour*), and the rest of the eye is filled with a clear jelly (*vitreous humour*).

Light passes freely through cornea, aqueous humour, pupil, lens, and vitreous humour to the sensitive retina. The pigmented choroid behind the retina prevents reflection of light.

The *orbit* is a socket in the skull considerably larger than the eye. The dead space is filled with loose fat, leaving the eye free to move. Six small muscles attach the sclera to the orbit.

A thin membrane, the *conjunctiva*, lines the eyelids and covers the front of the eye. The conjunctiva is constantly lubricated and washed with tears. The tears are secreted by the *lacrimal gland* under cover of the outer part of the upper lid, and drain into the nose through a small opening at the inner corner of the eye.

2. FUNCTION

The optical system of the eye, that is, the arrangement for focusing a sharp image on the retina, is simple. The 'lens' is only a minor component of the effective lens, for most of the work is done by the curved cornea, which on its own (with its backing of water) is a powerful fixed-focus lens. The named lens behind it is flexible; its curvature is adjusted by its surrounding muscle. It is supplementary to the cornea, and the means of varying the focus.

The iris contracts or relaxes to adapt the size of the pupil to the amount of light. It incidentally constricts the pupil when the eye is focused for near vision.

The sensitive nerve-endings in the retina are of two kinds: *cones*, which function in good light and register colour, and *rods*, which need very much less light but are colour-blind. As in colour photography, all colours are recorded as different mixtures of three primary colours, perceived by three kinds of cone. Again as in colour photography, vision depends on chemical reactions promoted by light; the rods and cones are sensitive to the products of the reactions.

The cones are most sensitive to yellow, which therefore seems brighter than other colours of the same intensity. The rods are sensitive only to blue and green: hence the apparent brightness of grass by moonlight.

Rhodopsin (visual purple) is the light-sensitive chemical of the rods. It is inactivated by bright light, and thus the rods are switched off when the light is good enough for the less sensitive cones (otherwise the glare would be intolerable). Adaptation to night-vision depends on the slow re-synthesis of rhodopsin. The process requires vitamin A, and night-blindness is an early symptom of vitamin A deficiency.

Impulses from the retina are carried back to the brain in the optic nerve. A cross-over system between the two optic nerves carries impulses from the left halves of both eyes (representing objects to the observer's right) to the left side of the back of the brain, and from the right halves to the right side. The brain takes several years to learn to interpret the slightly different images from the two eyes.

There are several relay stations in the nerve-path from the eyes to the back of the brain, concerned with reflex activity such as focusing and adjusting the pupils, and also remoter functions such as maintaining the posture and balance of the body. As an organ of balance the eyes are secondary to reflexes governed by sensation from the muscles and joints of the limbs.

3. DISORDERS

Optical defects (astigmatism, myopia etc.) are considered under ◊ *vision*. Most of the conditions mentioned in the following notes are described further under their own headings.

Working from front to back: the *conjunctiva* is protected from injury by the eyelids and the very rapid blink reflex, and from infection by the flow of tears. Infection, leading to *conjunctivitis*, is nevertheless very common. Even very slight injuries are troublesome if they involve the *cornea*. Small foreign bodies in the eye - and unskilled attempts to remove them - may cause ulcers on the cornea. These small wounds heal only slowly because the cornea has no blood supply, and if they are at all

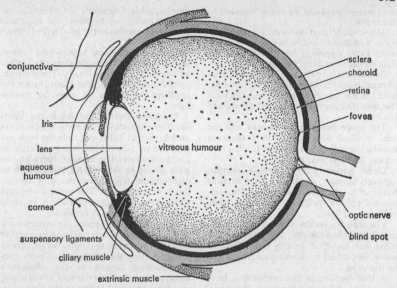

conjunctiva

sclera
choroid
retina

fovea

iris

lens

vitreous humour

aqueous humour

cornea

optic nerve

blind spot

suspensory ligaments

ciliary muscle

extrinsic muscle

Eye (diagrammatic).

deep they may leave opaque scars that interfere with vision. An eye can be blinded by severe scarring of the cornea. This is the type of blindness that can be cured by grafting a cornea from someone who has bequeathed his eyes to a hospital.

The *aqueous humour* is secreted from the tissues behind the iris and kept at a pressure (between 10 and 24 mm. of mercury) by compensatory leakage in the angle between the outer rim of the iris and the back of the cornea. The flow is through the pupil from behind. Disturbances of this mechanism may cause the pressure to rise: this is *glaucoma.*

The *iris*, its supporting tissue, and the *choroid* form a single layer, the uveal tract. Inflammation from various causes (and often from no known cause) may involve the whole tract (*uveitis*) or one part of it (*iritis, choroiditis*). If possible, the cause is treated, but in most cases treatment is directed to preventing complications such as glaucoma or damage to the retina, while the inflammation settles in its own time. Corticosteroid drugs have become the standard treatment for most of these cases. Drugs such as atropine are used to keep the

iris dilated and prevent it from sticking to the lens.

The one common disorder of the *lens* is *cataract* or opacity, which can be due to congenital defect, injury, or ageing. Because the lens is only an accessory (see previous section) it can be removed and spectacles will give satisfactory vision.

The *retina* cannot function unless it is evenly applied to the back of the eye. *Detachment* of the retina may follow injury or may occur spontaneously; it occasionally complicates other conditions such as *choroiditis.* Vision is lost in the affected area. Detachment is treated by making minute injuries to stick the retina in place, by heat, cold, or other means. Inflammation – *retinitis* – may complicate inflammation elsewhere in the eye; other cases are ascribed to various more general ailments including diseases of blood vessels, chronic alcoholism, and nutritional deficiencies. Much the commonest retinal disorders are due to diabetes and high blood pressure. In all these cases it is the underlying disease that is treated.

The *optic nerve* arises in an area to the inner side of the mid-point of the retina;

there are no rods or cones in this area (optic disc) and it is therefore a blind spot. (Since the image on the retina is reversed, the blind spot corresponds with a small area in the field of vision to the *outer* side of centre.) The nerve is liable to damage by increased pressure within the eye (glaucoma) or inside the skull, by the same conditions as cause retinitis, and by *multiple sclerosis*, a disease of various parts of the nervous system.

Squint is a failure to balance the muscles controlling movement of the eyes. Since the eyes do not point in the same direction the images do not correspond. With the common squints of childhood, the brain resolves the conflict between disparate images by ignoring one. If the squint is neglected, the habit of ignoring impulses from one eye becomes fixed and the eye – although perfectly healthy – is in effect blind. It is for this reason, and not for the sake of appearance, that childhood squints need to be treated early. The much less common squints that come on in adult life, after the brain has

learned to resolve the two images, cause double vision.

eyelid. An eyelid is a crescent of rubbery cartilage, covered with skin and lined with conjunctiva. The muscles are mainly under conscious control, but the muscle raising the upper lid also responds to involuntary stimulation from sympathetic nerves.

Small glands in the lid margins may become blocked and form painless cysts, easily removed, or they can be infected by bacteria in the same way as skin glands elsewhere – a *stye* (hordeolum) is a boil on an eyelid.

eye-strain. Working in a poor light is inefficient and tiring but unlikely to do physical harm to the eyes. Much of the fatigue and discomfort can be ascribed to bringing the work too close in an attempt to compensate for bad lighting. Uncorrected optical defects – not wearing glasses when they are needed – have much the same effect.

F

Fabricius ab Aquapendente (Girolamo Fabrizio d'Acquapendente) (*c*. 1537–1619). Professor of anatomy and surgery at Padua (1565–1604); pupil of Fallopius. He continued the detailed study of anatomy that had begun with Vesalius, and picked up ◊ *embryology* more or less where Aristotle had left it. In a detailed account of the formed human foetus he described the two short-circuits in the foetal heart (◊ *heart* (1)).

He also described the valves which allow blood in the veins to flow only towards the heart, but did not recognize their function. He accepted Galen's theory that blood flowed in the other direction, and thought the valves ensured that the small branches should be fed, by checking the flow. The mistake did not matter, for Fabricius inspired his pupil Harvey to find the correct answer.

Fabricius Hildanus (Wilhelm Fabry (Faber)) (1560–1634). German anatomist and surgeon; a founder of the medical renaissance in Germany, often compared with Paré in France. He introduced the new anatomical learning from Italy and added important studies of congenital abnormalities. His classification of ◊ burns (3 degrees) still stands, as do his principles of amputation for gangrene.

facial. Of the face.
Facial artery. A branch of the external *carotid* artery. Its pulse can be felt at the side of the jaw.
Facial nerve. The 7th cranial nerve: it sends branches to all the muscles of facial expression. The sensory nerve of the face is the *trigeminal* (5th cranial). Paralysis of the facial nerve is common ; ◊ *Bell's palsy.*

facies. The face; or the appearance of the face as a clue to diagnosis. The *Hippocratic facies* of grave illness is described in the *Prognostics*; ◊ *Hippocrates.*

faeces. Rejected waste from the intestine, consisting of the undigested remains of the food (largely cellulose), bacteria, and a variable quantity of water and mucus. The colour is due to bile pigment (a breakdown product of blood pigment), and the odour mainly to nitrogen compounds produced by bacterial action. Examination of the faeces is important for the diagnosis of diseases of the intestine. Blood is not necessarily due to piles: traces detectable only by chemical tests may be highly significant, for any blood in the faeces is abnormal. It may be the earliest sign of cancer, at a curable stage. There are of course many other possible causes, but they have to be positively identified before cancer can be excluded.

Chemical examination may indicate faulty digestion if substances that should have been assimilated are found. Infection of the intestine is identified by studying the bacteria of the faeces, and worms and other parasites, or their eggs, are recognized by microscopy.

failure. The word is much used in a relative sense, when it may alarm the uninitiated who take it in an absolute sense. Failure of an organ (heart, lungs, a gland) seldom means that it has ceased to work. It means that the organ does not fully meet the demands made on it, and if performance cannot be improved it may still be possible to relieve failure by reducing the demands. (◊ e.g. *heart failure.*)

faint (syncope). Sudden unconsciousness from lowered blood pressure in the arteries of the brain. A faint is a reflex effect. Overactivity of the vagus (parasympathetic) nerves, from emotional or other causes, slows the heart and at the same time relaxes blood vessels in the abdomen, to which much of the blood promptly gravitates. As soon as the subject's head comes down to the level of his heart, as it must if he falls or lies down, the flow of blood to his brain is restored.

Faintness from standing to attention is due to pooling of blood in the legs. It can be relieved by twitching the muscles. Faintness on suddenly standing is due to delay in the reflex adjustment of the blood vessels to the new position.

Fallopian tubes. A pair of tubes open at one end to the cavity of the abdomen and at the other to the upper part of the uterus. The abdominal end, which looks not unlike a sea anemone, is next to the ovary. It collects the ovum that is shed each month and conveys it to the uterus. Sperms swim up the tubes from the uterus, and fertilization takes place in the Fallopian tube; the fertilized ovum begins to develop into an embryo before it reaches the uterus.

Occasionally an embryo remains in the tube instead of migrating to the uterus (◊ *ectopic* pregnancy).

Inflammation of a Fallopian tube (*salpingitis*) is due to bacterial infection. An abscess may form and need surgical treatment. In some cases the inflammation causes scarring and obstruction of the tube; if both tubes are so affected the woman is sterile. The tubes can be closed surgically in order to sterilize a woman.

Fallopius (Gabriele Fallopio) (1523–62). One of the great school of anatomists at Padua, a pupil of Vesalius. He added numerous details to his teacher's work, including the first good description of the tubes named after him.

Fanconi syndrome. (Professor G. Fanconi, contemporary Swiss paediatrician.) A congenital disorder of the kidneys, as a result of which various essential nutrients pass into the urine along with waste products, causing malnutrition and especially weakness of the bones. A very carefully balanced diet helps, but affected children cannot always be kept free from symptoms.

farmer's lung. An allergic reaction to fungal spores in mouldy hay, with symptoms of bronchitis: fever, cough, wheezing, and, after repeated attacks, loss of weight. The disease has only recently been identified, and no means of preventing it has yet been found.

fascia. Fibrous tissue wrapped round muscles and other organs; the packing material of the body. A bewildering array of different layers can be described, but the arrangement seems simple if one imagines that the organs grow into a pool of connective tissue and compress it into thin sheets between them. The fibrous covering of bones (*periosteum*) merges with the fascial sheaths of the neighbouring muscles.

The fascia covering the body just under the skin is said to be in two layers, deep and superficial; but the superficial 'fascia' is simply a layer of fat divided into compartments by fibrous strands. The deep fascia is rudimentary over the chest and abdomen to allow for expansion, but elsewhere it is tough and unyielding. A layer of fascia is an effective barrier against the spread of infection through the tissues, but pus very readily tracks along a fascial plane. Thus although in itself fascia is the least interesting of tissues it is important to the surgeon.

fat. Strictly, fats and oils are *triglycerides* – compounds of *fatty acids* neutralized by *glycerol* (glycerine). The usual fatty acids of dietary fat are oleic, palmitic, and stearic acids. In the body they can be converted to, or synthesized from, acetic acid. Glycerol and acetic acid are both consumed by the same process as sugar to provide energy, and the end-products are water and carbon dioxide.

There is no difference between a fat and an oil except consistency. At body temperature, human fat is liquid – in fact it is an oil. Animal fats solidify at room temperature; their vegetable equivalents remain oily. (Mineral oils are an entirely different class of substance.)

Several unrelated compounds, the *lipoids* (lipids) are often classed as fats. Like fats, they are insoluble in water but soluble in alcohol etc., and their disposal in the body is closely linked to that of fat. Much the most important of them is *cholesterol*.

Small amounts of fats and lipoids are incorporated in the structure of the body-cells and are not available as fuel. The rest is stored in *adipose tissue* in various parts of the body, mainly under the skin. It serves as an insulator and shock-absorber, and can at any time be mobilized as fuel and consumed.

Fats and lipoids can be synthesized in the body from carbohydrates and so should not be essential to the diet. They are convenient food, because a small amount provides much energy: weight for weight, twice as much as protein or carbohydrate, and fat is eaten more or less pure, without the large amount of water that goes into the cooking of starchy food. A diet with little fat has to be very bulky to provide enough energy. But beyond convenience, some fat seems to be needed for good health. The reason is unknown. It is true that a diet short of fat often lacks the fat-soluble vitamins A and D, but that is not the whole story.

The quality of fat also affects health. If some 'essential' fatty acids are lacking, excessive amounts of cholesterol accumu-

late and damage arteries (◊ *atheroma*). These essential acids are found in vegetable oils but much less in animal fats.
◊ *obesity*.

fatigue. The body-systems likely to suffer fatigue are the muscles and the nervous system.

Under experimental conditions a muscle can be tired by rapidly repeated stimulation, when the by-products of muscle chemistry accumulate faster than they can be carried away in the veins. To what extent, if any, this accounts for the fatigue of ordinary exercise is not known, but swelling from seepage of fluid is probably a more important factor. But during sustained exercise, tired muscles often recover to some extent. This, and the whole phenomenon of second wind, is still unexplained.

Again under experimental conditions, reflexes become sluggish after prolonged repetition. This is a sort of fatigue, but it cannot be equated with ordinary tiredness.

No amount of artificial stimulation impairs the efficiency of nerves, under laboratory conditions.

Mental fatigue is often associated, and perhaps identical, with boredom; and even fatigue that seems purely physical comes on much sooner with dull tasks than with interesting ones. Drugs such as amphetamine that give temporary respite from fatigue may do so simply by elevating mood.

The healthy tiredness at the end of a busy day cannot be properly explained. It has to be largely mental, because typically it does not come on until a satisfying task is completed. And in every sport it is the loser who feels exhausted. But to say that this kind of fatigue is mental is to state the obvious: it is a feeling and like any other feeling can only be defined as a state of mind. The origin of the feeling is still a mystery.

Extreme tiredness stops all activity, and sleep becomes imperative. Until more is known of sleep and the reasons for it, tiredness has to be defined as need of sleep, and sleep as that which relieves tiredness.

fatty degeneration. A disorder of nutrition in various tissues, notably liver and heart muscle. If these tissues are deprived of certain foods, or of oxygen (e.g. because of anaemia or poor circulation), their cells are unable to dispose of fats. As a result fat accumulates in the affected tissue and impairs its function. Hence an excess of useless

fat in the liver is sometimes a result of starvation.

Poisons such as alcohol interfere with the consumption of fat throughout the body so that fat is deposited in the liver and elsewhere.

fauces. The back of the throat; the region between the mouth and the pharynx, containing the tonsils.

favism. Poisoning by a kind of bean, *Vicia fava*, found in Italy. It affects only certain people and is apparently a severe allergy, with diarrhoea and anaemia from destruction of red blood cells. Blood transfusion is sometimes needed.

febrile. Affected with, or related to, ◊ *fever*.

feed-back. A term borrowed from electronics: numerous systems in the body are kept constant by using a product of the system to regulate its own output. For example, the adrenal glands are stimulated to produce cortisol by a hormone, ACTH, from the pituitary. But an excess of cortisol suppresses the release of ACTH and so inhibits the production of more cortisol until the level returns to normal.

felon. A common type of septic finger, with the infection confined to the pad (pulp) of the finger-tip.

femoral. Of the femur (thigh-bone), or of the thigh as a whole.
Femoral artery. Main artery of the lower limb, the continuation of the *external iliac* artery. It enters the front of the thigh halfway along the fold of the groin, where its pulse can be felt. The femoral artery runs between muscles to the back of the knee, where it continues as the *popliteal* artery. A large branch, the *profunda femoris*, is the main artery of the thigh itself; the femoral is more concerned with the parts below the knee.
Femoral nerve. Nerve of the extensor muscles (*quadriceps*) at the front of the thigh. It is formed from the lumbar spinal nerves, and enters the thigh at the outer side of the artery.
Femoral vein. The vein corresponds closely with the artery.

femur. The thigh-bone; a massive column of bone, with a slight forward curve, and a

girder-like ridge behind. At the hips the two
femora are separated by the width of the
pelvis. At the knees the femora come together. Hence the bones are set at an angle
in the form of a V. The upper end of the
femur is turned inwards and forwards; the
neck is set at an angle of about 130° with the
shaft. The angulation is more pronounced in
women than in men, to compensate for the
broader V of the shafts made by a woman's
relatively wide pelvis and short thighs. The
head of the femur is almost a perfect sphere
to fit the hemispherical socket (*acetabulum*)
of the hip-bone. The lower end of the femur
is widened to form two projections, the
condyles, on which the ◊ *tibia* slides when
the knee is flexed.

The femur is very strong, but it may be
subjected to great strains, and fractures are
common. Loss of blood may be severe with
no external wound, for there is room in and
among the muscles for profuse bleeding.
Very rarely the nerves behind the knee are
involved in a fracture of the lower end of the
femur, but usually the problem with a
broken thigh is the fracture itself. The
muscles pulling the broken ends are so
powerful that displacement, overlapping,
and shortening can be difficult to overcome.
If the bone is correctly set, a plaster cast
cannot be trusted to keep it in place because
there is so much room for play in the yielding mass of muscle. With few exceptions,
these fractures need either a continuous pull,
maintained by a system of weights and
pulleys while the bone heals, or internal
fixation by splints screwed to the bone or
inside the medullary cavity.

The neck of the femur is especially vulnerable in elderly people, who can sustain a
fracture here from an apparently trivial
fall. The head of the bone can usually be
held in place with a fluted nail driven into
the neck from the outside. But with this
treatment the patient has to remain in bed
while new bone forms round the nail, and
with old people prolonged bed-rest brings a
risk of pneumonia and other complications.
This risk can be overcome by removing the
head of the femur and fitting a metal
replacement. The patient is able to stand
within a day or two of the operation.
    ◊ *hip; knee; fracture.*

fenestration. A surgical operation for the
relief of deafness due to advanced ◊ *otosclerosis*: an artificial window is made
between the middle ear and the organ of

hearing of the inner ear. Fenestration is now
largely superseded by less drastic and more
reliable operations.

Fernel, Jean (1497–1558). Professor of
medicine in Paris; author of a treatise on
medical practice that was a standard work
of reference for two centuries. He divided
his work into three parts: physiology,
pathology, and treatment, in the manner of
a modern text-book. Pathology – the nature
of disease – was his special study. He
summarized current views and added many
observations of his own, including one of
the few descriptions of appendicitis before
the 19th century. He made no startling
discoveries but he was the first to classify
medical knowledge in a way that made
scientific progress possible; in other words
he formulated the problems that his successors were to solve.

ferric; ferrous. Iron compounds are ferric or
ferrous, according to the electro-chemical
state of the iron. Both sorts have been used
for treating iron-deficiency anaemia, but
ferrous salts are preferable because they are
better assimilated. Ferrous sulphate is cheap
and effective, but a few people do not
tolerate it well, and other salts, e.g. ferrous
gluconate, have to be used instead.

fertility. Though most married couples
produce children without undue difficulty,
some manage only after years of disappointment and some not at all. Medicine
cannot always help, but every case is worth
investigating.

In the first place it is the couple that
needs attention and not one or other
member. Some husbands resent any
suggestion that they should be examined,
as though it were an insult to their man-
hood. In fact, infertility has little to do with
impotence, of which they think they are
accused, and among civilized people
neither diagnosis need be taken as an
insult.

Even in these enlightened times a few
infertile couples need no more than simple
instruction about sex. And apart from mere
technique, the timing of coitus is important.
A woman is most likely to conceive a
fortnight before a period, when ovulation
occurs.

If it is hard to see what the emotional
climate can have to do with fertility, the
fact remains that the successful treatment

of a neurosis may incidentally cure infertility. Sometimes adopting a child seems to have the same effect. All kinds of physical ill health also reduce fertility.

Examination of the seminal fluid may show that the number or the motility of the sperms is abnormally low. Measures to improve the man's general health, and perhaps a brief term of abstinence followed by coitus timed to coincide with ovulation may help, and artificial insemination from the husband (AIH) is sometimes advised.

Various gynaecological disorders that impair fertility can be treated surgically. But sometimes the ovaries fail to release an ovum each month because of a deficiency in the pituitary gland. This gland below the brain should secrete a hormone to stimulate the ovaries. If this mechanism fails the patient can be given injections of the hormone or the synthetic substitute *clomiphene*, with a warning that the treatment sometimes leads to twins, triplets or more.

In a few cases where both partners are normal there seems to be some chemical antagonism between sperms and uterine secretion. In these cases, as in those where the sperms are defective, the question of artificial insemination from a donor other than the husband (AID) may arise. This is technically simple, but it presents grave ethical and legal problems.

There remains a large group of couples in whom no treatable cause of infertility can be found. For them, adoption is often a complete remedy.

fertilization. The union of male and female germ cells (sperm and ovum). In the ordinary way, cells multiply by splitting (binary fission). When the cell splits the complete set of 23 pairs of chromosomes is duplicated. But when the immediate precursors of the germ cells split, one member of each chromosome-pair goes to a finished germ cell. A sperm or ovum therefore has 23 single chromosomes. ◊ *genetics*.

Each month an ovum leaves an ovary and is picked up by the Fallopian tube to be fertilized if sperms swim up the tube from the uterus, and one of them fuses with the ovum. The fertilized ovum then has 23 pairs of chromosomes, one member of each pair from either parent. Later events are described under ◊ *embryo*.

fetishism. A form of anomalous sexual behaviour, where the patient is sexually excited by an object such as an article of clothing, his fetish, in preference to more conventional sources of excitement. ◊*sex*.

fever. Raised body temperature (= *pyrexia*), or any disease of which pyrexia is a leading symptom.

Fever is usually associated with infection, but is also a symptom of other kinds of illness.

The normal body temperature is maintained by a centre in the brain, which meets any threatened alteration with appropriate reflexes: reduced flow of blood through the skin and shivering to conserve heat, or increased flow (flushing) and sweating to lose heat. The critical temperature to which the centre is adjusted varies slightly during the day, and in women also during the month. The body temperature may rise by several degrees after a hot bath or strenuous exercise because the reflexes for cooling cannot keep pace, but the centre is unaffected and the temperature is quickly brought back to normal. But with fever the setting of the centre is altered, apparently by the chemical action of substances formed either by the destruction of bacteria or by damage to the body's own tissues.

When fever comes on rapidly it is often accompanied by a *rigor*, an attack of violent shivering, and in children by a convulsion like an epileptic seizure. If the fever subsides rapidly (i.e. by *crisis*) the patient sweats profusely. A typical attack of malaria is a series of short periods of fever alternating with periods of normal temperature, with a rigor at the beginning of each outburst and sweating at the end.

Fever increases the pulse rate and most other processes in the body. The accelerated chemical turnover may contribute to natural defence against infection, but the value of fever is uncertain.

◊ *temperature*.

fibrillation. Rapid unco-ordinated twitching of muscle fibres.

Auricular (atrial) fibrillation occurs in the muscle of the atria, the receiving chambers of the heart, which should set the pace for the more important ventricles. At irregular intervals an impulse gets through to the ventricles and sets off a heart beat. *Ventricular* fibrillation is much rarer and more dangerous, because it stops the heart from doing any effective work.

Auricular fibrillation, a symptom of various heart diseases, can be treated with drugs. Digitalis reduces the number of impulses that get through and allows the ventricles to beat more efficiently, though still irregularly. Quinidine can sometimes be used to restore regular rhythm by stopping the fibrillation, but if the trouble is of long standing clots may have formed in the atria and a normal beat could dislodge them into the circulation and cause them to block an artery. Ventricular fibrillation can be corrected with an electric pulse if there is one to hand; otherwise cardiac massage may restore a normal beat.

fibrin. An insoluble protein, the basis of blood-clot; ◊ *blood* (4).

fibrocystic disease = ◊ *cystic fibrosis.*

fibroelastosis. Proliferation of elastic connective tissue in the lining of the heart, leading to serious heart disease in infancy. The cause is unknown, and no cure has yet been found.

fibroid (fibromyoma). A tumour of the uterus, forming a round fibrous lump, or more often several distinct lumps. Fibroids can cause excessive menstrual bleeding, sometimes discomfort, and sometimes fairly severe pain. They are not a danger to life and are in no way associated with cancer. Untreated fibroids can grow so large as to become a serious physical burden. Some fibroids can be shelled out, leaving the uterus intact and still capable of child bearing, but more often the uterus has to be removed entire. The only after-effect of the operation is that the woman cannot have children, but in many of these cases the fibroids themselves would have made pregnancy unlikely, and most patients are near the end of or past the age of child-bearing.

fibroplasia ◊ *retrolental fibroplasia.*

fibrositis. A vague but convenient term for ill-defined pain in and around muscles – 'muscular rheumatism'. The pain comes and goes for no apparent reason. Most sufferers are without symptoms for long periods; this enhances the reputation of whatever remedy was last tried. In many but not all cases the pain is confined to one group of muscles. Movement may be restricted, but by pain rather than real stiffness.

Apart from the minority of cases where 'fibrositis' is a symptom of some recognized disease, this complaint is an unsolved puzzle. Some authorities deny that it exists, i.e. that the pain has anything to do with inflammation of connective tissue (fibrositis) or of muscle (myositis). Explanations include localized muscle spasm, squeezing a nerve and causing further spasm; weak spots in the fibrous coating of muscles, allowing tissue to be pinched as it bulges through; and minor disorders of the backbone, interfering with nerves as they emerge between vertebrae and causing referred pain in the muscles to which the nerves are destined. This last certainly accounts for many cases.

Faulty posture (which could affect either the backbone or the muscles where the pain seems to be) is an important factor in bringing on attacks. Sitting in an awkward position, or sitting *tensely* in any position can start the pain. Tension, in turn, has many causes, including all kinds of anxiety. In treating this disorder, relaxed and mechanically efficient posture generally does more good than aspirin and massage. The remedy may be as simple as using a different chair for typing, or wearing glasses to avoid having to sit hunched over a book.
◊ *backbone.*

fibula. A slender bone at the outer side of the leg. Its upper end does not quite reach the knee, but its lower end takes part in the ankle, where it forms the outer side of a square socket. The fibula takes no weight, but it is an important anchorage for muscles.

Both ends of the bone lie under the skin. The lower end is the *lateral malleolus*, the knob at the outer side of the ankle. The *lateral popliteal nerve* passes from behind the knee round the upper end of the fibula to reach the peroneal and extensor muscles.

The fibula is easily broken. It seldom remains intact with a fractured tibia, and the two bones may break at quite different levels. A bad 'sprain' of the ankle is often in fact a fracture of the lower end of the fibula, but since bones heal better than ligaments a fracture may be preferable to a sprain. The fibula is fractured in Pott's fracture-dislocation (◊ *Pott, Percivall*).

Rarely, a fracture of the upper end involves the lateral popliteal nerve, which is also liable to compression by a tight bandage.

filaria. A very slender parasitic worm of the tropics. Several kinds affect man. *Wucheria bancrofti* is fairly common in Africa. It is transmitted by a mosquito, and grows in the lymphatic vessels, where it sets up inflammation. The infection also causes occasional attacks of fever. After years of repeated infection the skin and connective tissue of the legs or the genitals may become grossly thickened, a condition known as *elephantiasis*.

Onchocerca, a Central American and African filaria, has a predilection for the eyes and can cause blindness ('river blindness'). Some other species confine themselves to the skin.

Most filariae are killed by the drug diethylcarbamazine.

fissure. A split in skin or mucous membrane; it is really a very narrow ulcer. *Anal fissure*, at the junction of skin and mucous membrane of the anus, probably results from straining because of constipation. It is painful and therefore encourages further constipation. It is one of the comparatively few really good reasons for taking laxatives. An anal fissure may require a small surgical operation.

fistula. A penetrating wound or ulcer, creating an abnormal passage between two body surfaces (body surfaces include the skin and the linings of hollow organs). For instance a stab-wound of the belly may create a fistula between the intestine and the skin, or a surgeon may make an artificial temporary fistula between the bladder and the skin to relieve obstruction in the bladder. Such fistulae usually close themselves if they are kept free from bacterial infection, and if they are not acting as safety valves to an obstructed passage. A spontaneous fistula is nearly always due to infection of a minor injury. An example is *fistula-in-ano*, between the rectum and the skin. This kind of fistula starts with infection of a small blemish in the mucous membrane of the rectum or anus. It does not heal on its own because of constant reinfection by faeces; but it can be cured by a surgical operation to open the track and convert it into a shallow groove: despite contamination, open wounds of the anus heal well.

fit ◊ *epilepsy*.

flagellate. A minute, single-celled animal (protozoon) able to swim with one or more whip-like structures (flagella). Several kinds are parasites of man. Some cause serious disease, e.g. *trypanosomes* (sleeping sickness). Others cause only local irritation, e.g. *trichomonas* in the vagina, and *giardia* in the intestine.

flat foot ◊ *foot* (2).

flatulence. Gas in the stomach and intestine causes a good deal of discomfort. Most of it is swallowed, but some is produced in the lower part of the intestine by fermentation, especially in constipated people. Air is swallowed by gulping food or drink and by unsuccessful attempts to belch, and some nervous people do it at any time. Recognizing that these habits exist is the most important step towards breaking them.

flexion. The movement of bending a joint (opposed to *extension*).

flexure. Line along which skin folds when a joint is flexed.

fluorine. A chemical element with similar properties to chlorine, found in many minerals and in the human body as an ingredient of bones and teeth. Although the amount in these tissues is small – about 1 part in 10,000 – it is essential to their stability.

During the 19th century there were numerous suggestions that fluorine might protect the teeth against caries (decay), but a report from Naples in 1901 that fluorine actually *caused* disfigurement of the teeth discouraged further inquiry for a time. In 1939 a study carried out in four towns in Illinois showed that too little fluorine in the drinking water was associated with frequent caries, but that too much caused unsightly mottling of the teeth. With about one part per million of fluorine in the water, there was enough to keep down the incidence of caries but not enough to cause mottling. These findings were confirmed in other surveys, and in 1946 fluorine was added to the water supply of Grand Rapids, Mich. At once there were complaints of ill-effects

from the 'adulterated' water, but it tran-
spired that the fluoridation had had to be
delayed, and the ill-effects arose before any
fluorine was added. After a quarter of a
century of fluoridation in towns all over the
world there is still no evidence that it is
harmful, and countless children have
escaped dental fillings and extractions. But
some people still oppose fluoridation – in
Antigo, Wisconsin, so strongly that it was
stopped in 1960. All school children were
examined at once and the prevalence of
caries was recorded. By 1966, the prevalence
among Second Grade children had more
than trebled, and the opponents of fluorine
were overruled. It is, however, true that
fluorine is more important to children
whose teeth are still developing. Fluoridation of the water supply means that everyone gets the same treatment, including
adults who may not need it, and some of
them object. Direct application of fluorides
to the teeth in a mouthwash or toothpaste
does not seem to help, but some Russian
and American experiments on painting the
teeth with stannous fluoride have shown
good results.

Fluorine in any form does not abolish
dental caries, but in places where the water
contains enough fluorine, either natural or
added, there is less than half as much
caries as in places where the water lacks
fluorine.

fly. The common house-fly contaminates
food by carrying bacteria from animal or
human excrement on its feet. The danger is
slight where there is efficient water-borne
sanitation but very real under more
primitive conditions. Apart from intestinal
infection such as bacillary dysentery, flies
may be involved in the spread of wound
infection, conjunctivitis (pink-eye), and
poliomyelitis. Even in countries with a high
standard of hygiene it is worth while to keep
flies away from food. In the tropics, houses
are usually sprayed with insecticides to
prevent mosquitoes from spreading malaria; this also keeps down flies, which in
tropical countries can be a serious menace.

A few tropical and subtropical fevers are
transmitted by the bites of flies. They
include sandfly fever and African sleeping
sickness. In these cases the flies are actually
infected by sucking blood from someone
with the disease, unlike house-flies which
merely have dirty feet.

foetus. Unborn infant that has developed
from an ◊ *embryo* to a stage where it is
recognizably human, i.e. from about the
eighth week of pregnancy.

At this time the foetus is about 4 cm. long,
measured from crown to rump. Nearly half
of it is head, and the limbs are very small.
The skeleton is of cartilage – gristle – but the
first flecks of bone are just appearing. Its
heart is pumping blood through its body
and out to the placenta to receive the
ingredients of growth filtered from the
mother's blood. The lungs are still rudimentary. Neither they nor the intestine
serves any purpose until birth. The liver
grows quickly: as the main centre of chemical synthesis and storage it has much to do.
For a time the liver is so large relative to the
abdomen that part of the intestine is
pushed through the umbilical cord.

The various organs grow at different
rates and the proportions of the foetus
gradually change to those of a new-born
baby. At 16 weeks, the foetus is about 10
cm. long, crown to rump, and weighs about
100 g. (4 ins. and 3½ oz.). At 24 weeks it has
grown to 20 cm. and 650 g., and it is
approaching the stage at which it would
stand a chance of survival if it should be
born early. At 28 weeks from the start of the
mother's last period – about 26 weeks after
conception – it is considered viable under
English law, though in practice it would
still be dangerously premature and would
survive only with expert nursing. A foetus
of this age has very little fat, and therefore
great difficulty in keeping warm, and very
little stored fuel. Its reflexes for breathing
and other vital functions are not yet wholly
reliable.

During the remaining ten weeks of
pregnancy the foetus – now definitely a
baby – grows about 50 per cent longer and
increases its weight five-fold.

The next stage in development is described under ◊ *birth.*

folic acid. A vitamin of the B group, present
in all green plants; ◊ *vitamin B.*

folie à deux. Symptoms of mental disorder,
usually paranoid, affecting two closely
associated people at the same time. The
patients are most often sisters. Although
both seem equally deranged the primary
disorder is always with the dominant one;
the 'junior partner' adopts her delusions

and as a rule recovers as soon as they are separated.

follow-up. Periodic examination of a patient after the completion of a course of treatment. Naturally, it is in the patient's interests that a surgeon who has operated on him, or a physician who has treated him for a serious illness, should see him from time to time to ensure that his recovery is maintained or suggest further treatment if necessary. But follow-up examinations are also an important part of clinical research. It is not enough to know that an operation or a new drug gives temporary relief; the long-term results may be equally important, and the possibility of delayed complications has to be considered. Often an extensive follow-up study is needed before a new treatment can be assessed in relation to older methods.

food. ◊ *diet*.

food poisoning.

1. Chemical contamination (lead, arsenic etc.) is rare. Poisoning from lead water pipes has been reported, and accidents can happen during the processing of food. Unwashed fruit from recently sprayed trees may carry poisonous pesticides.

2. Many plants are by nature poisonous (fungi, berries), and some need preparation to make them safe, e.g. a kind of cassava that is the staple diet in parts of S. America and Africa is very poisonous until it has been soaked. ◊◊ *favism; mushroom*.

3. Susceptible people may suffer allergic reactions to particular foods that are wholesome to everyone else; ◊ *allergy*.

4. 'Ptomaine' poisoning is a myth. Ptomaines are substances formed in the decomposition of meat and other organic matter. They are indeed poisonous, but they are also very evil-smelling, and any food so putrid as to contain a dangerous quantity of ptomaines would be quite uneatable. The decomposition that forms ptomaines is due to bacteria, and what used to be called ptomaine poisoning was in fact bacterial infection of the intestine.

5. Most food poisoning is caused by bacteria. One type is an acute infection of the intestine, with inflammation of the mucous membrane, pain, diarrhoea, and sometimes vomiting. The bacteria are species of *Salmonella*. A carrier of these bacteria who handles food can cause large outbreaks. Some outbreaks spread to man from animals; duck-eggs are a notorious source. An attack is unpleasant but not often dangerous. In addition to general measures (◊ *diarrhoea*), sulphonamides or antibiotics may be needed to combat the infection. A second type of bacterial food poisoning is due not to infection of the patient's intestine but to irritant toxins formed by bacteria growing in the food before it is eaten. Cooking kills bacteria and prevents infection, but may not destroy these toxins. This type of poisoning is usually due to staphylococci, but several other kinds of bacteria can produce toxins in the same way. Only one illness of this type – ◊ *botulism* – is really dangerous, and fortunately it is also very rare.

foot. In principle, the anatomy of the foot is almost identical with that of the hand. Only the proportions differ.

The 7 *tarsal* bones correspond with the carpal bones of the hand. Only one takes

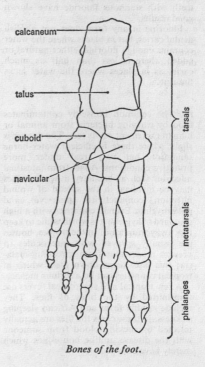

Bones of the foot.

part in the ankle joint, the *talus*. The *calcaneum*, on which the talus rests, is the largest bone in the foot. It protrudes backwards to form the heel and to provide a lever for the Achilles tendon. These two bones are the base on which the rest of the foot turns, e.g. in walking on uneven ground. Turning the sole inwards is *inversion*; turning it outwards is *eversion*. The rounded front of the talus fits the hollow of the *navicular* bone, making a shallow ball-and-socket joint. In front of the navicular are 3 small *cuneiform* bones side by side, each supporting a metatarsal. In front of the calcaneum is the *cuboid* bone, which supports the 4th and 5th metatarsals. The toes articulate with the rounded heads of the metatarsals. As in the hand, the 1st (big) toe has two phalanges, and the others each have three.

The weight of the body is taken by the calcaneum and the heads of the metatarsals. The other bones are raised from the ground as an arch. Since the first 3 toes are supported by the talus, which is above the calcaneum, the arch rises higher on the inner than the outer side. These are the *longitudinal* arches. With the feet together the metatarsals of each side form half of a *transverse* arch. The shape of the bones does little or nothing to maintain the arches, but the very strong ligaments of the sole are an important factor. Most of all, the arches depend on the support of the muscles, of which the strongest are those of the big toe. If these muscles are flabby the ligaments stretch and the arches are flattened.

As in the hand, the most important muscles arise higher in the limb: the *extensors* beside the shin, and the *flexors* deep in the calf. A third group, the *peronei*, joins the fibula to the outer side of the foot. In addition there is a complex system of small muscles in the foot, arranged as those of the hand but to less purpose. They are presumably inherited from ancestors which used their feet for grasping. The really significant movements of the foot are inversion and eversion, and the powerful flexion of the big toe which gives the final thrust to the forward stride.

1. INJURIES

Fractures of the *toes* are nearly always due to direct violence, e.g. by a heavy object falling on the foot, which also crushes the soft tissues of the toe. Such fractures are less important than the damage to the toe as a whole. They are troublesome only if it is the big toe that is broken; any other toe can be lost without disability. *March fracture* is a spontaneous fracture of a metatarsal, usually the 2nd. Most spontaneous fractures (i.e. fractures without obvious causes) happen in unhealthy bones, but this one can affect a perfectly normal foot during unaccustomed exertion. Since a metatarsal is firmly splinted by its neighbours the fracture heals quickly and well.

In contrast, fractures of the tarsal bones are always serious, both in themselves and because the violence needed to produce them is likely to cause other injuries. Hippocrates in the 5th century B.C. singled out fractured calcaneum as one of the most difficult fractures to treat, and the same can be said today. Manipulation is seldom easy, and some form of surgical operation is often needed to replace the fragments. Even with perfect alignment, tarsal fractures can be troublesome, because one or other of the many joints between the bones is often involved, and a broken joint surface does not readily recover its smoothness. Thus the patient may be left with a stiff and painful foot. An operation (*arthrodesis*) to seal off the affected joint, converting the components to a single bone, restricts movement but leaves the foot painless and stable. Paradoxically, arthrodesis may render the foot *more* supple, by relieving the pain that had made any movement intolerable.

2. DEFORMITIES

Various congenital defects are known as ◊ *club-foot* or talipes. Of the acquired deformities – due mainly to unsuitable footwear – the commonest is *hallux valgus* or bunion. The big toe is inclined towards its neighbour. Once this happens the tendons, which should pull straight along the line of the toe and its metatarsal, pull somewhat across this line and increase the deformity. Thus the head of the metatarsal protrudes, and the overlying skin becomes calloused in response to the unaccustomed pressure. If splinting and a change of shoes fail, the deformity can be corrected by a small operation.

Flat foot is incompetence of the arches. Anyone who stands still for long enough will find that his soles begin to ache, because the muscles tire and allow too much of the load to fall on the ligaments. If the muscles are weak or the person is unduly heavy, the ligaments become stretched and cannot recover. A greater load is then thrown on the already overloaded muscles. Treatment is largely a matter of educating the muscles, and it is obviously most likely to succeed if it is started before the condition has become serious. On the other hand, the importance of flat feet can be exaggerated. Some good athletes appear to have very flat feet, which give them no trouble, perhaps because their muscles are sound enough to prevent symptoms. When flat feet ache, either the muscles need to be stronger or the weight which they support needs to be less.

foramen (anat.). Hole or passage through a bone or other structure, e.g. *intervertebral foramen* (between neural arches for spinal nerves leaving the backbone); *foramen magnum* (at the base of the skull for passage of the brain-stem to the spinal canal); *obturator foramen* (between the pubis and the ischium, two of the bony elements of the pelvis); *foramen ovale* (between the left and right atria of the heart before birth).

forearm. The forearm extends from ◊ *elbow* to ◊ *wrist*. The skeleton is two parallel bones, the ◊ *radius* on the side of the thumb, and ◊ *ulna*. The muscles are in two groups, both extending from the front of the humerus (i.e. above the elbow) to the wrist and hand. The flexors spring from the inner side of the humerus and the front of the forearm bones; the extensors from the outer side and the back. The rather unexpected attachment of the extensors in front of the humerus leads them straight to the back of the hand when the limb is in the natural working position, with the elbows bent and the palms facing each other.

The three main nerves are ◊ *radial*, ◊ *ulnar*, and ◊ *median*. The arteries are ◊ *radial* and ◊ *ulnar*. Veins accompany the arteries, but there are also large veins under the skin. From the veins of the back of the hand the *cephalic* vein follows the line of the radius and the *basilic* vein that of the ulna.

Movements are described under ◊ *radius*, ◊ *elbow*, and ◊ *wrist*. ◊◊ *skeleton*.

foreskin ◊ *circumcision*.

formaldehyde. A pungent gas, soluble in water; it is a powerful disinfectant, used for sterilizing instruments that would not withstand heat. *Formalin* and *formol* are solutions in water.

Concentrated formaldehyde is an irritant. A few people are sensitive to very small amounts and develop skin rashes from contact with fabrics processed with formaldehyde.

forme fruste. An attack of a disease without the usual or expected symptoms – an abortive form of the disease.

Fracastorius (Girolamo Fracastoro) (1478–1553). Physician and all-round scholar of Verona, author of the earliest rational account of infectious disease (◊ *microbe*) and of a poem which includes the first treatise on syphilis, a disease which he named.

fracture. A broken bone. Healthy bone is extremely strong. The construction is generally tubular, and parts liable to special stress are often supported by ridges in the form of buttresses or girders. The thinner bones may be broken by a direct blow, but unless the initial force is very great the thicker bones seldom break without leverage. If a bone does break it usually snaps completely; only young bones break partly (green-stick fracture). The break is often transverse if it is close to the actual injury, e.g. Colles' fracture just above the wrist from a fall on the palm. But the line may be oblique or spiral with a less direct injury, e.g. a fracture half-way up the shin from a fall with the foot caught in an obstruction.

Many terms have been applied to different types of fracture. A *compound* fracture is one in direct communication with an open wound, as opposed to a simple or closed fracture. The distinction matters because a compound fracture is likely to be contaminated with bacteria, and infection of bone is dangerous. Until Lister's discovery of antiseptic surgery, compound fractures were usually fatal, and as recently as the First World War amputation was often the only way to save the patient's life. The antibiotic drugs have practically removed the danger.

A *complicated* fracture is one where the broken ends of bone injure other organs (nerves, arteries etc.). A *comminuted* fracture is splintered. A *spontaneous* or *pathological* fracture is due to an injury that would not be enough to break a normal bone but breaks one that is abnormally weak.

The commonest sites of fracture are the

clavicle (collar-bone), the radius at the wrist (Colles' fracture) and the ankle (Pott's fracture). In old people whose bones are weakened by osteoporosis (a loss of bone-substance) fractures immediately below the hip are also very common. Other sites of fractures are mentioned under the names of the various bones.

The principles of treatment apply to all fractures, and they have not changed since medical knowledge began to be recorded. First, the fracture is *reduced*, i.e. the broken ends are restored as nearly as possible to their natural position. Second, the reduced fracture is held in position while it heals.

When these two principles are applied, bone heals like any other tissue. The process begins with ◊ *inflammation*. The flow of blood increases, and fluid, protein and white blood cells are extruded from the blood vessels. The blood-clot at the site of the fracture is gradually removed and replaced firstly with the same kind of delicate spongy tissue as precedes the formation of a scar in the skin. Secondly, this tissue is hardened by chalky deposits to form *callus*, a firm, but not rigid, structureless mass. Thirdly, the callus is replaced by fully developed bone. When a fracture can be exactly reduced the final result is indistinguishable from the uninjured bone; in fact bone is the only tissue that is invisibly mended.

In practice not every fracture needs to be perfectly reduced. The pull of muscles makes the broken ends overlap, but if the ends are in the same mass of blood-clot, callus and ultimately bone will fill the gap. In the leg the bone needs to be pulled out to its original length because shortening impairs function. But in the arm a little overlap and shortening may not matter if the line of the bone is preserved. There are a few situations where perfection matters. Colles' fracture is so close to the wrist joint that any displacement interferes with the mechanical efficiency of the joint, and as a general rule fractures near joints need more exact reduction than others. With any fracture, reduction should obviously be as near perfect as is practicable, but too much manipulation can do more damage than leaving a slight deformity. If for any reason a fracture has to be exposed surgically it is seldom necessary to accept less than perfect reduction.

Most fractures stay in position when they have been reduced if they are kept still, e.g. in a plaster-of-paris cast. A few do not. The thigh is so heavily padded with muscle that no external cast prevents the broken ends from overriding with consequent shortening the leg. In some other situations an oblique fracture tends to slip inside a cast. The problem can be overcome by continuous *traction*, usually with a system of weights to balance the pull of the muscles. Alternatively the fracture can be held in place by a splint fixed directly to the bone or passed down the middle of the shaft as a dowel.

Movement prevents a fracture from healing because the callus breaks before it has time to consolidate. If it continues, the broken ends become sealed with hard bone and healing is then impossible. Instead, a mobile joint forms between the fragments.

Natural healing is also prevented if one fragment loses its blood supply as a result of the injury.

Surgical repair of fractures is generally reserved for cases where natural healing is unlikely, or where the fracture cannot be adequately reduced by manipulation, or the reduction cannot be maintained.

The rate of healing depends on the site of the injury (the thigh may take two or three times as long as the collar-bone, and the shin still longer), and on the patient's age and general health. But even extreme old age does not prevent bones from healing; it only delays the process.

Freud, Sigmund (1856–1939). Viennese physician; a pioneer of modern psychiatry and psychology. Freud had already achieved some distinction as a neurologist, i.e. as an expert on the physical properties of the nervous system, before turning his attention to psychology. He founded the analytical school of psychiatry (◊ *psychoanalysis*).

Few men have been more misunderstood than Freud, and few have less deserved to be misunderstood, because he explained his doctrines in several good books addressed to the general public. Much of his work dealt with the conflicts between the conscious mind and the unconscious instincts, suppressed memories and so on; and the effect of these conflicts on behaviour and health.

Freud's influence is very great, even on people who think they disagree with everything he said. Most of his ideas were not exactly new – 'conscience' is an older word than Freud's 'superego'. His great contribution was to crystallize ideas that had always lurked at the back of people's minds without finding expression. *Ego, id, libido* are now household words.

More than anything else it was Freud's insistence on sex as the mainspring of behaviour that turned people against him. His opponents (some of whom had never read a word of his writings) thought he saw a wanton or a rapist in every cradle, that he was blaspheming against the innocence of childhood. In point of fact, Freud was endearingly sentimental about children. 'Sex' is an unfortunate word in Freud's context. It arouses emotion rather than thought if only because it is taken to mean adult sex. Perhaps 'sexuality' would be better, or some word that would imply an instinct of which sex is one expression. And sex may not be the real stumbling block. The resentment may well arise not from Freud's mentioning things that were not mentionable, but from the implication that a thinking man is sometimes at the mercy of his instincts. In the 17th century Spinoza (with whom Freud had much in common) had been reviled for much the same reason, though he thought the driving force behind human behaviour was the respectable motive of self-preservation.

frigidity. Lack or inhibition of sexual feeling, sometimes amounting to aversion. ◊ *sex.*

frontal. Of the forehead. The two *frontal bones*, left and right, are usually, though not invariably, fused during infancy to form a single bone (◊ *skull*).

The *frontal lobes* are the part of the brain covered by the frontal bone, and extending back some little way into the territory of the parietal bones. The part under the parietal bones controls voluntary movement. The rest, the prefrontal area, has less clearly defined functions. It is concerned with learning, judgement, and behaviour, but in adults it can suffer severe injury without great inconvenience to the patient. In the operation of prefrontal ◊ *leukotomy* the nerve fibres from this part of the brain are cut for the relief of certain mental disturbances.

frostbite. Damage to skin and sometimes deeper tissues by freezing. Prolonged exposure to cold even without actual freezing can seriously damage the skin by interfering with the circulation of blood (◊ *trench foot*), but with true frostbite ice crystals are formed and some loss of tissue is inevitable. The effect is very similar to burning.

The safest way to warm frostbitten skin is in water at blood-heat. Anything warmer is very liable to cause burns. Friction is also wrong. It warms living tissues by stimulating the circulation, but since frostbitten tissues have no circulation to stimulate, friction can only add to the damage.

Frostbitten skin needs to be covered with the cleanest possible dressing, because like burnt skin it is vulnerable to infection, having lost all resistance to bacteria.

frozen shoulder. Pain and stiffness of the shoulder, probably due to inflammation of a ◊ *bursa* that normally prevents friction between the joint and the surrounding structures. Recovery often takes several months, but in the meantime the symptoms can be relieved with analgesics and cautious physiotherapy.

fructose. A simple sugar in fruits; cane sugar is a compound of fructose with glucose. Fructose is assimilated as easily as glucose. Its molecule contains the same atoms as glucose ($C_6H_{12}O_6$) but differently arranged. It is converted in the liver to glucose.

fugue. An episode of apparently automatic behaviour which the patient cannot later remember, most often a symptom of hysteria, but sometimes associated with epilepsy.

fumigation. Disinfection by fume or gas, such as sulphur dioxide from burning sulphur, or formaldehyde. It is used for treating rooms where patients have been nursed with diseases such as smallpox.

functional. A term applied to various disorders, sometimes with misleading effect. The body is conventionally studied in terms of its structure (anatomy) and function, i.e. how it works (physiology). The same division has been applied to the study of its ailments. If symptoms are accompanied by detectable changes in an organ, such as injury, inflammation, faulty development or a chemical anomaly the disorder might be called structural, but the correct term is *organic*. But, if the working of an organ is disturbed without apparent physical cause, the disorder is said to be *functional*. If a muscle is tense because an adjacent structure is inflamed, the tension is organic. If it is tense because the patient is anxious, the tension is functional. An unusual sound (murmur) heard over the heart is organic if it arises from a faulty heart-valve, but functional if it is due to the normal eddying of blood through a healthy valve. Epileptic seizures caused by a head injury are organic, but if the momentary disturbances of the normal working of the brain cells have no apparent cause the seizures are functional – until someone points out that they are probably due to a birth injury too slight to be detected. So 'functional' comes to mean little more than 'of unknown origin', and a useful word is corrupted.

fundus. The part of a hollow organ remotest from its opening: e.g. *fundus oculi*, the floor of the eye; *fundus uteri*, the top of the uterus, the furthest part from the *cervix* or neck of the womb (it is shaped like an inverted flask).

fungus. A very simple kind of plant. Fungi lack the green pigment, chlorophyll, that enables other plants to form carbohydrates (sugar, starch, cellulose) from the carbon dioxide of the air. They are more closely related to bacteria than to green plants, but whereas a bacterium grows to form a colony of individual bacteria, most fungi form a network of branched threads – a *mycelium*. The usual method of reproduction is by forming *spores*. A spore is a minute body, no larger than a bacterium, able to start a new mycelium elsewhere. These tiny seeds can be carried great distances in the air. All dust contains them, and any suitable breeding ground such as exposed food is bound to be contaminated in time and grow a *mould* which is simply a kind of mycelium. Some fungi with their mycelium in the soil grow large fruiting bodies, e.g. *mushrooms*, from which spores are scattered. *Yeasts* differ from other fungi in that they form no mycelium; like

bacteria they form colonies of separate microorganisms.

Fungi are medically important in several ways:

1. A few kinds of ◊ *mushroom* are very poisonous, and although accidents are rare those that do happen can be serious.

2. Certain moulds and yeasts cause infection in the same way as bacteria; indeed the distinction between these fungi and bacteria is vague.

The commonest fungal diseases (mycoses) are superficial infections of the skin (◊ *ringworm*) and mucous membranes (◊ *thrush*).

Ordinary 'household' moulds are mostly harmless, but cases have been reported of infection of the lungs and other organs by such law-abiding moulds as *Aspergillus* and *Mucor*. *Actinomyces*, which can be regarded either as an elaborate bacterium or a simple fungus, causes 'lumpy jaw' in cattle and sometimes infects man. Some uncommon but dangerous fungal infections, e.g. with *Blastomyces*, *Histoplasma*, have been seen more often in the Americas than elsewhere. All these internal infections have been rare in the past, but they are on the increase, and this is not simply an apparent increase due to better diagnosis. Much of it is a real increase due to better treatment of bacterial infection. For bacteria in the body compete with fungi, and when bacteria are eliminated with drugs the field is open to fungi that would otherwise be harmless.

Some fungi provoke allergic reactions; for instance, *farmer's lung* is a form of allergy to moulds in contaminated hay.

3. Some important drugs are obtained from fungi. Yeast is a good source of the B vitamins. ◊ *penicillin* and other ◊ *antibiotics* are produced by moulds.

furuncle = ◊ *boil.*

furunculosis. A crop of boils.

fusion. Surgical fixation of a joint, e.g. *spinal fusion*, bridging adjacent vertebrae with a bone-graft to prevent movement of a chronically inflamed joint.

G

galactose. A simple sugar, combined with glucose to form *lactose* or milk sugar. Galactose is converted in the liver to glucose. Infants with a very rare congenital defect (absence of the necessary enzyme) cannot convert galactose: it accumulates in the blood and causes persistent and sometimes fatal vomiting. They remain perfectly well as long as they are given no milk products.

Galen (Galenos) (c. A.D. 130–200). Greek physician and biologist, 'the Prince of Physicians', the most influential man and one of the most prolific writers in medical history. For fifteen centuries after his death, Galen's doctrines carried almost the authority of scripture. A few pioneers of the Renaissance committed the heresy of questioning Galen – Paracelsus condemned him along with all other medical writers except himself, and Vesalius made a list of Galen's anatomical errors, both in the 16th century, but neither managed to reduce his stature. Even Harvey, in the 17th century, accepted Galen's authority in most things, and tried to show that his own great discoveries had all been anticipated by Galen. In our own century doctors have prescribed remedies that have stood the test of time – but could have stood no other test – since the 2nd century.

Galen was brought up in Pergamon, near the Aegean coast of modern Turkey, then a great centre of learning. There, and later in Smyrna and Corinth, he studied philosophy. He took up his real profession in Alexandria, then the leading medical school in the Empire, carrying on the tradition laid down in the 3rd century B.C. by Herophilus and Erasistratus. These two men were the real founders of human anatomy and physiology and so of scientific medicine, and our knowledge of them is due largely to Galen. Indeed, Galen's readiness to acknowledge these predecessors, and above all Hippocrates, does much to redeem his self-satisfaction. At times he tried to debunk these great men – not always wisely, for his own theories were apt to be further from the mark than theirs. Unfortunately for posterity it was Galen's theories that prevailed.

The greatness of Galen lies not in his theories but in his observations. He wrote an exhaustive account of human anatomy. There had been nothing like it before, and there was to be nothing like it again until 1543 when Vesalius published the *Fabrica*. The mistakes in Galen's anatomy are of two kinds. Firstly, his dissections were of animals. He did not go far wrong when he used monkeys, because their anatomy differs from ours only in matters of detail, but sometimes he used other animals. Secondly, if what he saw conflicted with his preconceived ideas he described what he thought he should have seen. Nevertheless, Galen's anatomical errors are nothing beside the wealth of accurately recorded fact.

Galen carried out some important experiments. He showed conclusively that the arteries contain blood and not, as had been supposed, air. He studied the functions of the spinal cord, showing the effects of injury at various levels. 'The experimental path', he said, 'is long and arduous but leads to the truth'. It was a path that he did not take often enough. When he made experiments they were usually good, but his philosophical training was apt to be too much for him and then he fell back on theorizing. And unlike the real philosophers he presented his theories as established facts. He had an elaborate theory to explain the movements of the blood (◊ *circulation* (2)). The body was pervaded by three kinds of vapour or spirit: natural spirit, formed, with the blood, in the liver; vital spirit, formed in the heart; and animal spirit, formed in the brain and distributed by the nerves. These spirits had their origin in the inspired air. We see Galen the observer at his best when he says that the nerves carry something from the brain: he had made experiments to prove it. And we see the theorist at his worst when, having examined the nerves and found them solid, he states that they are tubular because it suits his theory. (Centuries later we find a much greater thinker than Galen, ◊ *Descartes*, doing the same kind of thing.)

As a physician Galen was the most successful of his day. He travelled widely, but spent most of his professional life in Rome, where he looked after Marcus Aurelius and his son Commodus. Galen's clinical methods were more or less those of Hippocrates five centuries before him, but without the compassion and humility of Hippocrates. In his travels Galen built up a great store of drugs, which he listed and recommended quite uncritically.

The tragedy of Galen was that he needed a successor, and there was none. If someone more self-critical had been there to continue Galen's experiments, scientific medicine might have begun in earnest in the 2nd instead of the 16th century. But in all history there is no full-stop more emphatic than the death of Galen. When he died, rational medicine was extinguished for fourteen centuries. The nature of some of his theories contributed to the eclipse. He tried to show that every detail of the human body was perfectly adapted to the body's needs and a part of a preordained plan, in other words an expression of God's will (◊ teleology). It is all very well for a scientist to have this idea in mind, but stated so baldly it stifles all further inquiry. This was the part of Galen's work that the Dark Ages and Middle Ages preserved, together with the interminable catalogue of drugs, in garbled Latin translations of Galen's Greek. His experiments, and his priceless accounts of earlier doctors whose works had been lost, were all forgotten. But they did not altogether vanish. The Nestorian heretics translated them into Syriac, which Moslem scholars put into Arabic. They returned to Western Europe at the end of the Middle Ages, in Latin translations from the Arabic made in Cordoba.

galenical. Unrefined vegetable drug, or crude extract of a plant used medicinally; e.g. opium is a galenical, but morphia is a refined active principle. Now that the active principles of most vegetable drugs can be isolated and purified, galenicals are seldom used, because doses are difficult to standardize.

In many countries, 'galenical' means much the same as 'pharmaceutical' – concerning the preparation of drugs.

gall = ◊ bile.

The gall bladder is a small bag attached to the under-side of the liver, in which bile is stored and concentrated. When food passes from the stomach to the intestine the gall bladder contracts and ejects bile into the duodenum.

The common disorders of the gall bladder are inflammation (cholecystitis) and gall stones, which are insoluble deposits precipitated from the bile. The two are often associated. They cause pain and indigestion, easily confused with stomach disorders; intolerance of fatty food (because fat needs bile for its digestion and stimulates the gall bladder); sometimes jaundice. Occasionally gall stones are found by chance, having caused no symptoms. Troublesome gall stones are removed surgically, together with the gall bladder. Many attempts have been made to dissolve gall stones by medical treatment, to avoid an operation. A course of chenodeoxycholic acid is said to dissolve cholesterol stones, the commonest type, but at present the treatment is expensive and tedious. It is in the gall bladder that stones form, because it is there that the bile is concentrated and cholesterol is precipitated. When the gall bladder is removed, the tendency to form stones is removed. The occasional apparent relapses after operation are probably not relapses, but previously formed stones that have found their way out of the gall bladder into an inaccessible part of one of the bile ducts.

gamete. A sex-cell, either ovum or sperm.

gamma-globulin. The fraction of the proteins of blood that includes the antibodies responsible for immunity to specific infections. Gamma-globulins can be separated from the other proteins in the blood of someone who has previously recovered from an infection, and used to boost the resistance of others who are at special risk from the same disease. For instance, a full dose of gamma-globulin can be given to protect a child during an epidemic of measles. Or a smaller dose can be given to mitigate an attack while allowing the child to develop his own immunity. This method is now being superseded by vaccination against measles.

Unlike the other blood proteins, which are formed in the liver, gamma-globulins are formed in the lymphatic system.

ganglion. 1 (anat.). A collection of nerve cells, a relay station, in the course of a nerve.

2 (surg.). Cyst of a tendon sheath or joint

capsule, producing a tense, round, usually painless swelling. Ganglia are seen almost only on the back of the hand or wrist. They are quite harmless, but if a ganglion is unsightly or large enough to be a nuisance it can be removed. The time-honoured method of squashing a ganglion with a heavy object (the family Bible was preferred) achieved temporary success, but the ganglion usually reappeared.

ganglion-blockers. A class of drugs used to suppress over-activity of certain nerves. Nerve impulses in the sympathetic and parasympathetic systems, regulating the activity of the organs of digestion, circulation of blood etc., have to cross relay stations (ganglia) where the impulse is transmitted from one nerve fibre to the next nerve cell in the chain by the chemical action of acetyl choline. Ganglion-blockers interfere with the action of acetyl choline at these ganglia. They have been used for treating various disorders, especially high blood pressure. Their disadvantage is that they are not selective: they affect organs that were giving no trouble. Some of the newer drugs block particular groups of nerves, and are replacing the ganglion-blockers.

gangrene. Mortification; death and decay of part of the body. The usual cause is loss of the supply of blood through injury or disease of the artery of the region. Not all localized death of tissue is gangrene; the dead tissue may be replaced by a scar, without any decay (which is due to bacterial action). If, for example, part of the heart muscle loses its blood supply through coronary thrombosis, there is no decay because there are no bacteria in the heart. True gangrene involves body surfaces where there are bacteria. ◊ *infarct.*

Blood supply can be lost through injury to an important artery where the alternative channels for the circulation are inadequate; frostbite; obstruction by clotting of blood in a diseased artery (thrombosis); severe spasm of arteries (e.g. ergot poisoning) and so on. By definition, some tissue must be lost. The great danger is that bacteria in dead tissue multiply without opposition; natural defences and drug treatment are equally powerless against them, and gangrenous tissue is a focus from which infection may spread to and kill healthy

neighbouring tissue. It always has to be removed surgically.

Gas gangrene is a complication of severe wounds where tissue is crushed or torn. The bacteria (*clostridia*) breed in damaged tissue and spread to healthy tissue, which they rapidly decompose, with formation of gas. Clostridia form at least half a dozen different lethal toxins, of which the effect is mitigated by giving antitoxic serum. Penicillin destroys the bacteria at the margins of the gangrene, but tissue already affected has to be removed. These bacteria breed only in the absence of oxygen – they are *anaerobic* – and the treatment of gas gangrene has been much improved by maintaining a high concentration of oxygen in the affected area.

gastrectomy. Surgical removal of (part of) the stomach. Partial gastrectomy involves only the lower part of the stomach, subtotal gastrectomy all but the uppermost portion in contact with the diaphragm, and total gastrectomy the whole organ.

Gastroenterostomy is making an artificial passage between the stomach and the intestine, e.g. when the natural passage is blocked or (less often now than formerly) for the treatment of an ulcer. Some form of gastroenterostomy is of course needed after gastrectomy: when part of the stomach has been removed the remainder has to be joined to the intestine.

The operation is used for duodenal and gastric ulcers (◊ *peptic ulcer*) and for cancer of the stomach. With duodenal ulcer the object is to remove the part of the stomach in which excessive acid is being formed; with gastric ulcer it is to remove the ulcer itself if it will not otherwise heal, and with it the part of the stomach in which new ulcers are likely to appear or in which a cancer may develop; with cancer it is to remove the growth together with the surrounding tissue which may be invisibly affected.

The stomach is not essential to life, or even to satisfactory digestion. Protein can be digested in the intestine without the normal preliminary breakdown by acid and enzymes in the stomach. But if the whole stomach has to be removed the intrinsic factor by means of which vitamin B_{12} is absorbed is lost, and the vitamin may have to be injected. The intact stomach is useful as a reservoir from which a large amount of food can be passed to the intestine in small quantities. After gastrectomy the whole meal arrives in the intestine at once, and some of it may pass through too rapidly to be absorbed. This can lead to under-nourishment and in particular to iron deficiency and therefore anaemia. Some patients describe attacks of nausea and faintness after meals, which may be a reflex response to sudden distension of the intestine, or possibly a transient upset of blood chemistry by too rapid absorption of carbohydrate; it is known as the dumping syndrome.

Many patients escape all these complications of gastrectomy and manage a completely ordinary diet. Others suffer some inconvenience, if only for a time, but at the worst they have only to make their meals smaller and more frequent, and perhaps take supplementary vitamins and iron.

gastric ulcer. Ulcer of the stomach; ♦ *peptic ulcer.*

gastrin. A hormone released into the blood by cells in the lower end of the stomach in response to protein foods such as meat. It stimulates the flow of acid from the upper part of the stomach.

gastritis. Inflammation of the lining of the stomach; a rather vague term covering a range of disorders from mild indigestion to a dangerous emergency.

Unlike most parts of the body, the stomach is rarely inflamed from direct invasion by microbes, because its acid secretion is strongly antiseptic. Gastritis may, however, complicate infection centred elsewhere; and in cases of *achlorhydria* (absence of acid) swallowed bacteria may get a foothold.

Some gastritis is due to *allergy*, e.g. to shellfish. But the likeliest cause is simple chemical irritation. The common irritants include alcohol, tobacco smoke, and many drugs.

♦ *gastro-enteritis.*

gastrocnemius. Prominent muscle of the calf.

gastro-enteritis. Inflammation of stomach and intestine; a group of diseases characterized by vomiting, abdominal pains, diarrhoea, and in severe cases prostration. Bacterial food poisoning, poisoning with heavy metals, infections such as typhoid and dysentery, and food allergies can all be included, but unspecified gastro-enteritis is usually a virus infection – 'summer diar-

rhoea', 'gastric flu', and the sometimes dangerous diarrhoea and vomiting of infancy. As with all true virus infections, the cause cannot yet be dealt with: symptoms have to be treated on their own merits while the infection subsides. Infants have limited reserves of water and are quickly dehydrated by diarrhoea and vomiting. Their stores of bicarbonate and salt are easily depleted. In infants, as in severely affected adults, treatment is mainly a matter of replacing these vital substances. If fluids cannot be kept down when given by mouth, they have to be injected. Painful spasm of the intestinal muscle is relieved by drugs that depress parasympathetic nerves, of which the prototype is belladonna. The diet has to be sloppy and bland.

gastro-enterostomy ♦ *gastrectomy.*

gastroscope. A lighted tube passed down the oesophagus for inspecting the lining of the stomach. With the back of the throat anaesthetized this procedure is much less distressing than one would suppose.

general paralysis of the insane (GPI). (*General paralysis*; *dementia paralytica.*) Widespread involvement of the nervous system at a late stage of untreated ♦ *syphilis.*

genetics. The study of heredity.

If there is a single property that distinguishes living matter from any other, it is the ability to synthesize proteins. These very complex substances, produced from the simplest raw materials, are the chemical basis of life. All living processes depend on a class of proteins, the *enzymes*, because every process represents chemical changes promoted by particular enzymes. This is equally true of breathing or growing red hair or suffering from gout.

Some proteins are common to all living creatures, some to a large category such as animals or mammals, and some to a single species. Some are peculiar to races, families, or individuals within a species. The difference between a man and an oak tree or a typhoid bacillus, or between two men, is largely the difference between the proteins that they can make. This is what they inherit from their forebears, and all that they inherit, and it is all that they transmit to their offspring.

The business of genetics is to show how

the pattern is passed on more or less intact from generation to generation, and to explain how it comes to vary in its finer details.

1. Genes and Chromosomes

Every living cell includes a quantity of *nucleic acids*. One type, DNA (deoxyribonucleic acid), is enclosed in the central *nucleus* of the cell. The other, RNA (ribonucleic acid), is more widely distributed.

A molecule of DNA is a chain with four kinds of link. Any combination or sequence of links is possible, each sequence giving a different DNA. Since there is apparently no limit to the possible length of the chain, there could be an infinite number of different kinds of DNA.

To every kind of DNA there is a corresponding RNA. In some way, a molecule of DNA evokes equivalent units of RNA, which pass to the cell-substance.

The RNA then becomes a mould for the synthesis of a protein.

A molecule of protein is also a chain, but with twenty different kinds of link (aminoacids). Each of the amino-acids is attracted to a particular sequence of three links in a molecule of RNA. The properties of a protein depend on the sequence of aminoacids, which is determined by the sequence of links in the RNA chain, or ultimately by the kind of DNA in the nucleus of the cell. Therefore the whole nature of a cell, and of the body, which is composed of cells, depends on the kinds of DNA at its disposal.

DNA has a second unique property: it can make an exact copy of itself. Cells multiply by splitting into halves, and in the process the entire complement of DNA is duplicated. All the millions of cells of a human body arise by division and subdivision of the single cell formed by the fusion of an ovum from the mother and a sperm from the father; and every cell includes a replica of the DNA of the fertilized ovum.

Before a cell divides, its DNA is organized into paired structures called *chromosomes*. Human DNA forms 23 pairs of chromosomes. The two members of a pair are very similar but not identical (except that the sex chromosomes form a dissimilar pair in the male: see below). During division of a cell, each chromosome splits down its length as the DNA duplicates itself.

But when the germ cells (ovum or sperm) are formed, the chromosomes do not split.

Instead, only one member of a pair goes to a germ cell, which then has 23 *single* chromosomes. When the ovum is fertilized, new pairs are formed with one member from either parent.

The body contains thousands of different kinds of protein, each determined by its own unit of DNA. One such unit, governing the synthesis of one protein (usually an enzyme, promoting one chemical process), is a *gene*.

A chromosome is an assembly of hundreds of genes. A gene is a unit of DNA.

2. Dominant and Recessive Characters

The two members of a pair of chromosomes correspond very closely. In all major respects, any two creatures of the same species are alike, and to this extent their genes are identical. Each parent contributes one member of a pair of chromosomes, and in everything that makes the chromosomes merely human the contributions are alike. But in many points of detail, individuals differ, and the genes that determine these points differ. At a particular point on a chromosome there may be a gene that determines the colour of the eyes. One parent may contribute a gene for blue eyes, and the other for brown eyes. If this happens, the child's eyes will not be of an intermediate colour; they will regularly be brown. The 'brown' gene in some way suppresses the 'blue' gene, and brown eyes are said to be *dominant* while blue are *recessive*. Only if both parents contribute a 'blue' gene will the child's eyes remain blue. A recessive character will appear only if it is represented by both chromosomes of a pair, but a dominant character needs only one. There is no difference to be seen between the brown eyes where both parents contribute brown and those where only one does so. (This example is taken only because it is so familiar: in fact eye colour is rather more complicated and may involve more than one pair of genes.)

The colour of the parent's eyes does not always indicate what gene the child will receive. A brown-eyed parent may well have one blue and one brown gene in his pair, and the germ cell that he passes to the child will have one or the other; the chances are even.

If both parents have the same *recessive* character, both must have a pair of identical genes, and their children have no choice but to take after them as regards that character.

If one parent has inherited a *dominant* character from both of his parents, then he must pass it on to all his children. But if the children get the dominant gene from one parent and the recessive gene from the other, they are 'hybrids'. Although they outwardly show the dominant character, *their* children have an even chance of getting the recessive gene from them.

If two 'hybrids' (both of course showing the dominant character) marry, there are four possible combinations for their children: (1) dom./dom., (2) dom./rec., (3) rec./dom., (4) rec./rec.

Of these possibilities – all equally likely – only (4) will show the recessive character.

In human genetics, matters are not always so simple. Many characters depend on the interaction of several genes. For instance, the original discovery of dominant and recessive characters (Gregor Mendel, 1866) was made with garden peas, which grew either very tall (dominant) or very short (recessive). But normal men are not either tall or short; they are of all heights from about 20 per cent above to 20 per cent below the average, because so many genes are involved that there can be no simple 'either–or'. Most human characters are of this kind. Secondly, alternative genes are not always dominant or recessive. One may *tend* to dominate the other, rather than do so completely. And with some characters the hybrid is in a sense intermediate between pure dominant and recessive.

3. Sex Chromosomes and Linkage

A woman has 23 matched pairs of chromosomes in each cell. In a man, the 23rd pair do not match: instead of two large X chromosomes he has one large X and one small Y chromosome. Evidently the Y chromosome carries a gene for maleness, and this acts as a dominant character. When the germ cells are formed in the ovary or testis, each getting only one member of a pair of chromosomes, the mother *must* contribute an X chromosome to the child, but the father has an equal chance of contributing X or Y. The effect of the Y chromosome is that a testis develops in the embryo instead of an ovary; the hormones formed by the testis account for other male characters.

The X chromosome carries many genes that have nothing to do with sex, but the small Y chromosome does not. For example, colour vision depends partly on a gene of the X chromosome. Red-green colour-blindness is a recessive character determined by a variant of this gene. If a man has this abnormal gene on his one X chromosome, he is colour-blind, because he has nowhere to carry the corresponding normal, dominant gene. But if a woman inherits the colour-blind gene its effect is suppressed by the normal gene on her other X chromosome, unless she is unlucky enough to inherit the same gene from both parents.

A man contributes an X chromosome to a daughter and a Y chromosome to a son. Therefore a colour-blind man cannot pass the defect to a son. If his son should be colour-blind the gene must come from the mother, who is a 'carrier', i.e. she has the abnormal gene on one X chromosome, but a normal and dominant gene on the other; her vision is normal. Any daughter of a colour-blind man *must* be a carrier.

Recessive characters determined by genes on the X chromosome are described as *sex-linked*.

4. Genetic Variation

In principle, a molecule of DNA is everlasting: 'The germ cell is immortal' because DNA, while on the one hand setting the pattern for the living individual, on the other hand goes on replicating itself for succeeding generations. The genes that are common to most creatures must have persisted unchanged for hundreds of millions of years. But if genes never changed at all there could be no evolution and no different species. In fact, accidents can happen to DNA, so that its self-made replica is not exact. If one of the thousands of links in a DNA chain is altered there will be a corresponding alteration in the protein directed by that gene. If the DNA of a germ cell is affected, the alteration is perpetuated (supposing that the offspring survive).

As a rule, a change or *mutation* is a disadvantage. It decreases the chance of survival; either it is promptly lethal, in which case it eliminates itself at once, or the affected individuals fall behind in the evolutionary struggle and are gradually eliminated. But from time to time a mutation confers an advantage in the struggle for survival, and the mutants thrive at the expense of their 'normal' fellows. This is the likeliest explanation of evolution.

The people of West Africa show an instructive example of mutation. A defective recessive gene causes a minor chemical change in the blood cells. Anyone who inherits this gene from both parents develops sickle-cell anaemia and is unlikely to survive till puberty. In the course of generations the gene should gradually disappear unless fresh mutations of the same kind occur, because it confers a disadvantage.

But the gene is not wholly recessive. The 'hybrid' carriers, with the sickle-cell gene on only one chromosome of a pair, have slightly affected blood cells. It is not enough to cause a fatal anaemia, but what it does do is enhance their resistance to malaria. The carriers therefore have a better chance of survival than people with completely normal blood cells, and this advantage outweighs the disadvantage of losing some children from anaemia. Thus the abnormal gene has become very common in West Africa. It can be expected to decrease when malaria is eliminated.

5. MEDICAL GENETICS

Many human disorders are due to defective (mutant) genes. They are seldom very common because the ordinary process of evolution tends to eliminate them but a fresh mutation may occur at any time and a hereditary type of disease then appears for the first time in a family. For instance, the best known type of dwarfism, *achondroplasia*, is a dominant character. As such, it should be transmitted only by a parent who is a dwarf, because one cannot carry a dominant gene without showing its effect. But more often than not the parents of an achondroplastic dwarf have normal bones, and the child is affected by mutation in an ovum or a sperm. The mutant gene is a part of the child's make-up; half of his germ cells will carry it and, on average, half of his children will be affected. His unaffected children have escaped the mutant gene – they got the other chromosome of the pair – and cannot transmit the defect to the next generation. But the gene is not part of the make-up of the normal parents of this dwarf; it affected one group of germ cells, not the whole testis or ovary; and there is no reason why their later children should be affected.

In Britain, the commonest disease due to a single pair of *recessive* genes is *cystic fibrosis* which is a serious danger to life.

Both parents must transmit the abnormal gene for the disease to appear, and it must be assumed that both are 'hybrid' carriers of the gene. The gene may have passed harmlessly down their families for many generations: there is no knowing, because actual cases appear only when two carriers happen to marry. Any child of such a marriage has one chance in four of getting the disease, two chances of being a carrier, and one chance of getting normal genes from both parents. Parents of a child with cystic fibrosis have to decide whether to risk having another child, knowing that it will have three chances of being healthy to one of inheriting the disease.

In these two examples the arithmetic is simple. It is often more complex. The odds have been worked out for many genetic disorders, and the geneticist can help prospective parents to decide whether to have children of their own or to adopt. Known risks are often no worse than the unknown risk that all parents must run: the chance than *any* child will be born with a serious genetic defect is about one in fifty. If a known risk is no greater than this it is best ignored – or nobody would dare to have children.

Healthy people with a family history of a genetic disorder may seek advice before marrying. With a dominant condition such as achondroplasia there is no problem: the normal brothers and sisters cannot possibly have the abnormal gene, and their children are as safe as anyone else's.

With a recessive condition such as cystic fibrosis, normal brothers and sisters have two chances in three of carrying the abnormal gene. In the population at large, one person in twenty-five carries it. If two carriers marry, the chance that a child will be affected is one in four. Taking these factors together, the chance that any child of a person whose brother has cystic fibrosis will inherit the disease is $2/3 \times 1/25 \times 1/4$, or $1/150$. And in Britain this is the *commonest* recessive disorder. With all others, the odds are even longer. With recessive disorders, then, healthy relatives do well to ignore the slight risk, except that first cousins, or other couples who both have a family history of the disease, have to reckon with a greater risk.

In some parts of the world, there are harmful recessive genes so common as to present a major hazard to the public health. Sickle-cell anaemia in Africa is one, and a very similar disease, Cooley's anaemia in southern Italy, is another. ⟡ *haemoglobin.* Carriers can be identified and advised not to marry each other, and this measure, together with the eradication of malaria, has already made Cooley's anaemia less common in Italy.

Carriers of a few other recessive disorders can be identified and advised; or at least the risk to their children can be recognized so that treatment is not delayed. Research in this important branch of genetics has still a long way to go. An example of the need is *haemophilia*, transmitted by a sex-linked gene, and therefore practically confined to males. The sister of a haemophiliac has a 50/50 chance of being a carrier. If she is one, then there is a 50/50 chance that any son will be a haemophiliac and any daughter a carrier. But she has no means of telling in advance whether she is a carrier or not; hence many perfectly normal people are discouraged from having children.

Some genetic disorders can be cured, e.g. *pyloric stenosis*, a constriction of the outlet from the stomach causing fatal vomiting. After a simple operation the affected baby is normal, but there must be no delay. If the risk is known in advance, precious hours may be saved in making the diagnosis. *Phenylketonuria* is a rare cause of mental deficiency due to a recessive gene. The patient has no enzyme for disposing of the amino-acid *phenylalanine*, of which small amounts are a necessary ingredient of the diet but large amounts poison the nervous system. If the condition is recognized at birth the child develops normally on a diet with little phenylalanine, and a chemical test shows whether the parents are carriers.

A few diseases are due to faulty allocation of whole chromosomes. Such defects are usually lethal to the embryo, but some can be survived. These include a wrong number of sex chromosomes (⟡ *hermaphrodite*), and mongolism, in which one of the smaller chromosomes appears in triplicate instead of in duplicate (⟡ *mongol*). Such disorders cannot yet be corrected, but now that the site of the trouble is known research workers at least know which way to look.

The examples so far have been of wholly genetic disorders, which follow well-defined rules. A much larger group of diseases is only partly genetic; environment does the rest. Such diseases tend to run in families without observing any known rules

of inheritance, and the effects of heredity and environment cannot always be distinguished. Tuberculosis is caused by a known bacterium. It can affect several members of a family because they catch it from each other. Or men whose fathers died of coronary thrombosis are more liable than average to die of the same thing; but that could be because they often lead similar lives. In both cases, however, the family tendency persists even if the environment is quite different. Both diseases are precipitated by external factors: bacteria, rich living and so on. But a greater than average *tendency* to them is inherited. The same is true of many of the commonest diseases, including cancer. Even with the little that is known, one can go some way to avoiding some of them. People with a family history of heart disease can take special pains to keep fit, and people with a family history of lung cancer to avoid cigarettes. It may be just enough to tip the uncertain odds in their favour.

In time, research is likely to reveal some of the genetic factors in diseases such as cancer, and when that happens the control of the diseases must soon take a long step forwards.

genital. Concerning reproduction; or (more often) the organs of reproduction (*genitalia*).

gentian. Bitter extract of gentian root, used to promote appetite.

genu. Knee. *Genu valgum* = knock-knee; *genu varum* = bow-leg. ⟡ *valgus.*

genus. Category in biological classification, embracing closely related species – e.g. *Felis*, the cats (*Felis leo*, lion; *Felis pardus*, leopard; *Felis catus*, wild-cat).

geriatrics. Medical care of old people.

germ ⟡ *microbe: infection.*

German measles (rubella). A very common virus infection in childhood, with slight fever, swollen lymph nodes, and a characteristic rash. It is a much milder illness than true measles (*rubeola, morbilli*). After an incubation of 2–3 weeks, the attack starts with headache, fretfulness and a rising temperature, followed a day later by a pink rash spreading from the face. Lymph nodes – typically, behind the ears – are enlarged and sore. The symptoms seldom last more than 3 or 4 days. The patient is infectious from the day before symptoms begin until the day after they disappear.

German measles was thought unimportant until in 1941 it was shown that if a woman contracts it early on in pregnancy, the developing infant adopts the virus instead of rejecting it. This may cause stillbirth, or serious defects – deafness, blindness and disorders of the heart, lungs, nervous system and other organs. Some 40 per cent of such babies are likely to be affected, so that German measles in pregnancy is widely held to justify abortion.

15–20 per cent of girls reach puberty without becoming immune from an attack (which should be confirmed by blood test, for a clinical history is not reliable). For these, vaccination is a safeguard, though it could endanger the foetus if given within 2 months of conception. Or the disease might be eradicated by vaccinating all children.

germ cell. Cell by which an organism reproduces itself; sperm or ovum. That the germ cell is (potentially) immortal is one of the fundamental principles of biology.

gestation. Pregnancy, especially duration of pregnancy. Human gestation lasts on average 38 weeks from conception to confinement, but is more easily measured from the beginning of the last menstrual period as 40 weeks. It varies much more than in other animals.

giant. Growth is determined by a hormone of the ◊ *pituitary* gland. The normal limits are very wide, and even small parents sometimes have very large and perfectly normal offspring. True giants, i.e. people who grow *abnormally* large, have an excess of growth hormone from an over-active pituitary gland. This condition (*gigantism*) is rare. If the trouble starts in adult life when the bones cannot grow longer, characteristic deformities appear (◊ *acromegaly*).

giardia. A microscopical parasite of the intestine; it is a ◊ *flagellate*. Infestation (giardiasis) is so common in healthy children that some experts have doubted whether giardia does any harm at all. But in some cases symptoms such as grumbling bellyache clear up when the parasite has been eliminated with a drug such as quinacrine.

gibbus. Hunch-back; forward angulation of the backbone. It was a common deformity when tuberculosis of the backbone (Potts' disease) was a common disease.

gigantism ◊ *giant*.

gills. Respiratory organs in various aquatic animals. Small and primitive creatures breathe through the skin. Larger and more complex animals cannot get enough oxygen in this way and have evolved more efficient systems.

At a fairly early stage of evolution gill-slits appeared as openings from the side of the pharynx. Their original function is to filter off food from water taken through the mouth, but as fish advanced from a diet of microorganisms to larger prey the gills were adapted to taking oxygen dissolved in the surrounding water into the blood. Land-dwelling vertebrates breathe with lungs, but the gills of their aquatic ancestors have persisted in a modified form. Gills can be recognized at some stage in the growth of every vertebrate, including man. In amphibia, e.g. frogs, the gills are actually used for breathing, but when a tadpole becomes a frog the lungs take over and the gills vanish.

In all but the most primitive vertebrates the forward gills are adapted for use as jaws. In land-dwelling vertebrates the remaining gills have been put to various uses. The larynx, the inner ear, and the thyroid and parathyroid glands are derived from them.

(Strictly speaking it is from the branchial arches and pouches, which support the gills proper, that these structures are derived: real human gills do not appear.)

gingiva. The soft tissue of the gums. *Gingivitis* is inflammation from bacterial infection of the gums. The mouth teems with bacteria, and its tissues are highly resistant to infection. Accumulation of food particles and a chalky deposit from the saliva (tartar, calculus) seem to provide a refuge from which bacteria can infiltrate the gums. Neglected gingivitis loosens the teeth; probably more teeth are lost from this cause than from decay.

gland. 1. An organ that forms and releases (secretes) substances that act elsewhere; if the secretion is carried to the surface of the body or the lining of a hollow organ the gland is *exocrine* (e.g. sweat glands, digestive glands); if it is carried in the blood-stream, the gland is *endocrine* (e.g. pituitary, thyroid).

2. A ◊ *lymph* node; these small bodies are collected in the neck, armpits, groins and elsewhere, and are an important factor in resistance to infection. 'Enlarged glands' are swollen lymph nodes, e.g. in the neck responding to infection of the throat or scalp, or in the armpit to a septic finger.

glandular fever (infectious mononucleosis). An infectious disease, or perhaps group of diseases, of which the agent is still unknown but is presumed to be a virus. As its more common name suggests, it is a fever with which the glands (lymph nodes) are particularly involved. The alternative name, *infectious mononucleosis*, refers to character-istic forms of white cell found in the blood. The attack may take various forms: the main symptom may be enlarged lymph nodes without much else, or digestive upset, or sore throat; skin rashes sometimes occur. Serious complications are most unusual, but some cases drag on for several weeks before complete recovery and leave the patient feeling exhausted. Convalescence lasts longer than after most other infections.

glaucoma. Abnormally high pressure within the eye, causing disturbances of vision and ultimately, unless the condition is treated, blindness. Acute (sudden) glaucoma is painful, but the commoner chronic type is insidious and may pass unnoticed until there is permanent damage to the optic nerve.

The part of the eye in front of the lens contains a watery fluid, the aqueous humour. It is divided by the iris into two compartments: the anterior chamber in front of the iris and the posterior chamber behind. The aqueous humour is secreted behind the iris and circulates through the pupil to be absorbed in the narrow gutter between the rim of the iris and the back of the cornea or window of the eye. If for any reason aqueous humour is secreted faster than it can be reabsorbed into the veins, the pressure rises and glaucoma develops.

In the cases where a cause can be found, it is obstruction to the outlet of fluid rather than excessive production. The filtration angle between the iris and the cornea is never very wide, and in some eyes it is so narrow that bunching of the iris, when the pupil is widely dilated, may be enough to block it.

In other cases, the pores in the angle are deficient. Some glaucoma follows inflam-mation of the iris (*iritis*), and rare cases are due to congenital defects of the eye. But the cause of most glaucoma is unknown.

Acute glaucoma is usually recognized from the symptoms, but chronic cases with few if any early symptoms may need careful investigation. A *tonometer* is a simple instrument like a tiny letter-balance that measures the resistance of the eyeball to light pressure and shows at once whether the pressure in the eye is raised.

Pilocarpine and other drugs that constrict the pupil often relieve the congestion in the filtration angle and allow the excess of fluid to drain normally. Acetazolamide, a drug used to encourage the flow of urine, inci-dentally decreases the formation of aqueous humour. But most types of glaucoma need surgical treatment. The simplest operation is a small hole near the rim of the iris, allowing fluid to drain from the posterior chamber directly to the filtration angle. Other operations are sometimes used to open up the angle.

glioma. A tumour of *neuroglia*, the con-nective tissue of the brain. (The actual nerve cells do not form tumours, because they are unable to multiply.) Glioma differs from the cancers of other parts of the body in that it does not spread to other tissues or organs, but it is equally dangerous because of its situation.

globulin. A class of protein found in the blood and elsewhere. The molecules are relatively large (molecular weight *c.* 200,000). The antibodies responsible for immunity to infection and for allergic reactions are globulins.

glomerulus. Tangle of minute blood vessels in the ◊ *kidneys*, from which fluid is filtered to form urine.

gloss(o)-. Prefix = 'of the tongue'.

glossina. Tsetse fly; found only in tropical Africa; infects man with sleeping sickness, and cattle with a similar disease, *nagana*.

glossitis. Inflammation of the surface of the tongue. The tongue is so resistant to infec-tion that glossitis is unusual in otherwise healthy people, but it is a common complica-tion of anaemia and malnutrition.

glottis. Entrance to the main airway from the pharynx, i.e. the gap between the vocal cords. Oedema of the glottis – swelling due to the inflammation of allergy – is a serious emergency (◊ *pharynx* (1)), since the airway is liable to be obstructed.

glucose. A simple sugar; its combustion with oxygen to form water and carbon dioxide is the principal source of energy in the body. Even without oxygen, some energy is got by converting glucose to lactic acid.

Food contains little if any glucose as such, but all starch and sugar in the diet is changed to glucose by digestion. Glucose can also be synthesized in the liver from protein or fat. Hence glucose has no special advantage over ordinary foods. But when a patient has to be fed through a vein, glucose must be used, because the processes of digestion are bypassed and other carbohydrates would not be converted for use.

gluten. A protein of various cereals (wheat, oats, rye). For most people it is a good food. Patients with ◊ *coeliac disease*, a serious disorder of digestion, cannot tolerate gluten; they often recover quickly when this protein is excluded from the diet.

gluteus. *Gluteus maximus* is the principal muscle of the buttock and the most powerful in the body. *Gluteus medius* and *gluteus minimus* are smaller muscles covered by gluteus maximus.

glycogen. A complex carbohydrate, *animal starch*, similar to ordinary vegetable starch. Its large molecules are chains of glucose molecules.

All carbohydrates in the diet are first digested to glucose; later, much of this glucose is recombined to form glycogen, which is stored in the liver and muscles as a reserve of energy to be called on as needed. The glycogen stores are broken down to glucose at the same rate as glucose is burnt to provide energy, so that the concentration of glucose in the blood and tissue fluid remains fairly constant. The process is regulated mainly by the hormones of the pancreas: *insulin* promotes, and *glucagon* inhibits, the deposition of glycogen. Several other hormones act: *adrenaline* and *thyroid* hormone accelerate the breakdown of glycogen, and *corticosteroids* increase its synthesis, via glucose, from protein.

glycoside. A class of substances extracted from certain plants, including the active principles of *digitalis*.

goitre. Enlargement of the thyroid gland; ◊ *thyroid gland* (2).

gold. Dentists have used gold since very early times for splinting or replacing teeth. The soluble compounds of gold, like those of all heavy metals, are indiscriminately poisonous to proteins and therefore to all tissues, and the effect of all such compounds is cumulative because the body has no ready means of excreting them. Chronic poisoning with heavy metals is successfully treated with chelating agents such as BAL. The medicinal uses of gold are very limited. Only a few of its salts are soluble and stable enough to be used, e.g. sodium aurothiomalate. These preparations were strongly recommended for *rheumatoid arthritis* around 1930, fell into disrepute, and have recently been restored to favour for the treatment of certain cases. Their action is not known: perhaps they act as *cytotoxic* agents to depress a kind of allergic reaction that is a factor in this disease.

gonad. Primary sex organ: ovary or testis.

gonadotropin. Hormone formed in the pituitary gland and acting on the gonad. *Chorionic gonadotropin* is supposedly formed by the embryo to suppress its mother's menstrual cycle during pregnancy.

gonococcus. *Neisseria gonorrhoeae*, the bacterium of gonorrhoea.

gonorrhoea. The commonest of the venereal diseases; a bacterial infection due to the gonococcus, which invades the mucous membranes of the urethra and uterus. After a short incubation period (2–10 days; as a rule 3 days) a man develops pain and discharge of pus from the urethra; a woman may have the same, but she may feel no symptoms, in which case she can pass the infection on without being aware of it. Untreated infection can be protracted and lead to obstruction of the flow of urine in the male and sterility in either sex. The later complications include arthritis and infection of the eyes. Although gonorrhoea does not infect an unborn infant in the uterus, the infant's eyes are liable to infection while it is being born; and this can cause blindness.

The sulphonamide drugs were very effective against this disease when they were first used, but from the original few gonococci that resisted the drugs many resistant strains have now evolved. In some large towns where the infection circulates rapidly, sulphonamides now cure only a minority of cases. To a lesser extent the story has been repeated with penicillin. Some of the newer antibiotics are still reliable, but that will not necessarily last.

There is little natural immunity to gonorrhoea; it can be caught again as soon as an attack has been cured. Because a woman with gonorrhoea often has no symptoms she may not seek treatment, and reinfection of the man who has been treated is all too likely.

Contraceptives are a very unreliable defence against gonorrhoea.

⇨ *venereal disease.*

gout. A chemical disease with precipitation of uric acid crystals in the tissues. Most of the symptoms are caused by crystals around joints, often a single joint.

There are numerous sources of the uric acid in the body. It is a breakdown product of nucleic acid, an essential component of all living matter. All foods contain some. The highest concentrations are in animal products such as kidney and liver, and vegetable seeds such as peas. A more important source than the diet is the regular breakdown of the body's own cells; and uric acid is also synthesized from ammonia formed in the body. In a healthy person the concentration in the blood and tissue fluids is kept to about 0·02 per cent by excreting any excess in the urine. The solubility of uric acid is about 0·06 per cent. Above this level, crystals may be precipitated and gout develops. The excess could arise in three ways: too much in the diet, too much synthesized in the body, and too little excreted by the kidneys. Unfortunately, diet is usually the least important, otherwise gout could be controlled simply by cutting out unsuitable food. Over-synthesis, due to an inherited biochemical anomaly, is much more significant. Defective excretion may arise from a similar fault, and also gout is occasionally a complication of kidney disease.

A classic attack of gout begins without warning, often in the middle of the night. A single joint, proverbially at the base of the big toe, is suddenly inflamed and extremely painful. After a day or two the symptoms vanish, but the attack may be repeated at any time, not necessarily in the same joint. Injury predisposes a joint to gout. A bout of heavy drinking can set off an attack by interfering with the excretion of uric acid, but as often as not there is no evident reason for the attack to start.

After many attacks a joint can become permanently deformed, with large deposits of uric acid (*tophi*) in the bones, e.g. of the knuckles. A tophus in the skin of the ear is sometimes seen with long-standing gout.

Many cases of gout take the form of a grumbling arthritis without acute attacks.

Although the main symptoms arise from affected joints, the real danger of gout is damage to the kidneys by uric acid crystals, which can ultimately lead to a condition like advanced Bright's disease. Untreated gout is also associated with degeneration of arteries (⇨ *atheroma*) and its complications. Many people with a persistent excess of uric acid have few if any symptoms, and now that suitable drugs are available it may be that they should be treated in order to protect their kidneys. The question still awaits a clear answer.

The shower of crystals that causes an attack acts as a foreign body in the tissues, and is dealt with by phagocytes (wandering scavenger-cells, like white blood cells) which attempt to engulf the crystals. The resulting damage to the phagocytes causes them to release toxic substances which cause the actual symptoms; the crystals on their own would not be painful.

Colchicum (autumn crocus), the oldest and still one of the best drugs for relieving an attack, seems to act by inhibiting the phagocytes. It has little effect on other types of joint pain. Other analgesics such as phenylbutazone are also effective.

Between attacks, steps can be taken to lower the concentration of uric acid in the body fluids. Numerous drugs enhance the excretion of uric acid by the kidneys. Analgesics such as aspirin do so, but not very efficiently. The usual drugs for this purpose are *probenecid* and *sulphinpyrazole*. In the early stages of this treatment, while deposits of uric acid are being mobilized, acute attacks are very apt to occur, but the final result is usually good.

The penultimate stage in the synthesis of uric acid in the body is a harmless substance, *xanthine*. The drug *allopurinol* is related to xanthine. It diverts the enzyme that oxidizes xanthine to uric acid, so that less uric acid can be formed. In this way the amount of uric acid in the blood can be kept within the limits of its solubility, and gout is then controlled. The only known drawback of this treatment is that it usually has to be continued for life, but most people who have experienced severe attacks of gout accept this price.

People with gout do well not to look for trouble by heavy drinking or overeating, and many of them can afford to lose some weight; also the most unsuitable foods (liver, kidney, meat extract) are easily avoided. But strict dieting is no longer essential with adequate treatment, and many patients controlled by the new drugs find that they can eat more or less to please themselves.

GPI = ◊*general paralysis of the insane.*

graft. Most tissues can be transferred from one part of the body to another if a blood supply is provided; but they can be transferred from one person to another only if steps are taken to prevent rejection of the 'foreign' substance by the recipient's tissues (◊ *transplantation*).

Skin is grafted to a new site much more often than other tissue. A skin-graft is an ideal dressing for injuries such as deep burns where an area of the original skin is lost. It shortens the time of healing, is much stronger than the scar that would gradually form if no graft were done, does not contract like a scar (burn scars can seriously restrict movement), and looks better than a scar.

A split-skin (Thiersch) graft is cut from a suitable donor area thinly enough for the blade to cut across the hair follicles, which are small pits in the surface of the skin. Fresh skin grows from the follicles to cover the donor area, and the graft is nourished by minute blood vessels in the raw recipient area. Full-thickness grafts are used where there is much wear and tear or where a split-skin graft would not look well. The vessels of the recipient area will not usually suffice for these thicker grafts for a time while new vessels grow; therefore the graft is left attached to the donor area by a stalk carrying a few blood vessels. This is separated after a couple of weeks when the graft has had time to establish itself. The donor area is covered with a split-skin graft

unless it is narrow enough for its edges to be stitched together.

Another tissue sometimes grafted is bone. A bone-graft may encourage an indolent fracture to heal by acting as a live scaffolding into which new bone can grow.

granulation tissue. Delicate tissue composed mainly of minute blood vessels and fibres, formed at the site of a wound or bacterial infection as the first stage in healing.

granulocyte. A kind of white blood cell; ◊ *blood* (3).

granuloma. A superfluous mass of granulation tissue formed at the site of a protracted, localized bacterial infection such as tuberculosis. *Granuloma inguinale* is a tropical venereal disease caused by a bacterium, *Donovania.*

gravel. small deposits in the urine of the same nature as the larger 'stones' (◊ *calculus*).

Graves' disease (toxic goitre). (Robert Graves (1797–1853), Dublin physician.) ◊ *thyroid* (2); *Basedow's disease.*

grey matter. Cellular tissue in the nervous system. The brain and spinal cord are composed mainly of nerve cells and their conducting fibres. The actual cells are gathered into well-defined zones which have a pale muddy colour, in contrast with the pure white of the nerve fibres in the remaining zones. The two kinds of tissue are known as grey matter (or substance) and white matter. In the spinal cord the grey matter is gathered into a central column, surrounded by white matter. In the brain, this central grey matter is clumped into *nuclei*, and there is an additional grey zone (cortex) over the surface of the cerebrum and cerebellum.

griseofulvin. An antibiotic from the mould *Penicillium griseofulvum*, chemically unrelated to penicillin. It is effective against certain fungal infections of the skin (ringworm), and is a valuable standby if simpler and older remedies fail.

groin. The junction of the muscles of the belly-wall with those of the thigh; the fold in front of the hip-joint. It is a weak point in the structure of the abdomen because the femoral nerve and blood vessels need a free passage from the pelvis to the thigh, and in the male the duct and vessels of the testis also pass through the muscles. A structure that belongs to the abdomen, such as a loop of intestine, may bulge through the gap provided for one of these vessels; this is the commonest type of ◊ hernia.

group therapy. A form of psychotherapy where a group of patients with similar problems meet to discuss them and the therapist plays an unobtrusive role as chairman. When group therapy works it makes better use of the psychiatrist's limited time than individual psychotherapy, and it is a way round one of the central problems of psychiatry, that the patient so easily becomes as dependent on the psychiatrist as an addict on a drug. In fact, group therapy is sometimes better than individual psychotherapy. People with emotional disturbances are almost bound to feel isolated, and the sense of isolation adds to the anxieties. As one would expect, group therapy works best with neuroses (disorders where the patient's insight is not impaired), but there are also encouraging reports with conditions where conventional psychotherapy often fails, including personality disorders and schizophrenia. Much depends on choosing the right patients for the treatment.

guanethidine. A drug used for treating high blood pressure. It prevents sympathetic nerves from raising the blood pressure by their action on small blood vessels.

Guinea worm (Dracunculus medinensis). A long slender worm, parasitic to man. The larvae enter the body in infected drinking water and migrate from the intestine. The female worm settles under the skin, often near the ankle, and emerges to lay eggs when the patient stands in water. The traditional remedy is to pull her slowly out by winding her round a stick over the course of a week or more. Otherwise, the worm can be killed with phenothiazine.

The disease is confined to West Africa and a few other tropical regions.

gullet = ◊ oesophagus.

gum ◊ gingiva.

gynaecology. Medicine and surgery of the female reproductive system. Obstetrics – the management of pregnancy – is generally counted as a separate specialty, though practised by the same specialists.

gynaecomastia. Enlargement of the male breasts. It can be induced in any man by giving female sex hormones. Since small amounts of these hormones are part of the normal male complement (as normal women have male hormones: the difference is only proportional), the balance is easily upset, and some degree of gynaecomastia is common in adolescence. Except that it may embarrass a young man it does not matter and does not usually last.

A few drugs can cause gynaecomastia.

gypsum. Calcium sulphate; plaster-of-paris.

gyrus. A natural fold on the surface of the brain.

H

habit. A habit is much the same as a conditioned reflex – an action that has become an automatic response to a given stimulus. It may be watering of the mouth at the sight of food or lighting a cigarette in response to boredom or worry. A *habit spasm* or *tic* is an involuntary, purposeless movement, probably representing a movement that once had a purpose. For *drug habit*, ◊ *addiction.*

haematology. Study of blood and its disorders.

haematoma. Swelling from bleeding into the tissues.

haematuria. Blood in the urine, a symptom of injury or disease of the kidneys or bladder. The source has to be identified as soon as possible. Most of the causes, including cancer of the bladder, are curable at an early stage. The cause may be obvious from the other symptoms. In doubtful cases examination of the bladder by cystoscopy usually provides the answer.

haemoglobin. The red pigment of the blood, carried by the red blood cells (◊ *blood* (2)). It is composed of a protein, *globin*, and an iron compound, *haem*. It is the means of transporting oxygen from the lungs to the rest of the body.

Very primitive microscopical animals can get their oxygen by diffusion from the surrounding air or water. But even an insect cannot get enough oxygen in these ways, and all but the simplest creatures have evolved *respiratory pigments* which form loose chemical compounds with oxygen. Human blood carries about sixty times as much oxygen as can be dissolved in it. In the lungs, where breathing provides a constant supply, haemoglobin takes up oxygen. In the rest of the body, where combustion creates a deficit, this oxygen is released. Since the tissues are never wholly depleted of oxygen, haemoglobin never gives up its whole supply. Five litres of blood – the total amount of the body, and also the amount circulating through the lungs in one minute at rest – carry one litre of oxygen, but only a quarter of this is actually used.

During exertion, the rate of circulation is increased, and at the same time a larger proportion of the oxygen is given up, because the carbon dioxide which accumulates in working tissues promotes the release of oxygen from haemoglobin.

The structure of this highly complex substance was established in 1960 by Perutz at Cambridge (Nobel Prize 1962). Globin consists of two alpha chains of 141 amino-acids, and two beta chains of 146 amino-acids. Each chain carries a molecule of the iron compound, haem, which can take up and release one molecule of oxygen. This is normal adult haemoglobin (HbA). Other haemoglobins are known in which the amino-acids of globin are differently arranged from those of HbA. (Haem does not vary.) Before birth, globin is formed from alpha and gamma chains, in which some 30 of the amino-acids differ from those of adult beta chains. This gives foetal haemoglobin (HbF), which is thought to work at a lower concentration of oxygen than HbA. Since the foetus gets its oxygen second-hand via the mother's blood and the placenta, this property of HbF would be an advantage. During the first four years of life HbF is gradually replaced by HbA.

Certain hereditary forms of anaemia are due to faulty synthesis of globin. In the haemoglobin of *sickle-cell anaemia* (HbS) a single amino-acid in the beta chain is out of place. This causes distortion and fragility of the red cells, which are liable to break up more rapidly than they can be formed. If a child inherits the faulty gene from both parents he is unlikely to live long enough to pass the disease on to the next generation. If he has it from only one parent, his red cells carry a certain amount of HbS, but not enough to harm him. If, however, he marries someone of the same type a quarter of their children will have the disease, and a further half will be able to transmit it like their parents. Only one child in four will be quite free of it.

The statistics of evolution and heredity are such that a gene which confers even a marginal disadvantage remains rare. Yet in parts of Africa no less than 40 per cent of the population have the HbS gene, of which a double dose is lethal. This is more than a marginal disadvantage, and after a few generations it should almost obliterate the disease. But malaria is the commonest disease in these regions. The malaria parasite lives off its victim's red blood cells, and in some obscure way the parasite seems to dislike HbS. This protects carriers of the disease, and the lessened chance of dying of malaria outweighs the disadvantage of the HbS gene.

Cooley's anaemia (thalassaemia) is found mainly around the Mediterranean. The haemoglobin is normal except that HbF still exceeds HbA after childhood; the trouble is inability to make enough of it. The effects are similar to those of sickle-cell anaemia: why these cells should be abnormally fragile is not known. A similar relation to malaria has been suggested but the evidence is not as strong as with sickle-cell anaemia.

Carbon monoxide is poisonous because haemoglobin takes it up in preference to oxygen, and does not readily release it. In fact, carbon monoxide usurps the place of oxygen and makes haemoglobin useless. A concentration of more than 0·1 per cent in the air is quite rapidly lethal, and much lower concentrations are dangerous if breathed for a long time.

The *colour* of haemoglobin is bright scarlet when it is saturated with oxygen, as in the arteries. As the oxygen is released the colour becomes more and more blue. The blood in the veins is normally still about 70 per cent saturated with oxygen, and the colour is a rich red-purple. But if blood stagnates because of impaired circulation, heart failure etc., or if the lungs are deprived of oxygen, the blood becomes much bluer and this colour is seen through the skin (◊ *cyanosis*). The compound with carbon monoxide is a vivid cherry red, and people with carbon monoxide poisoning have a bright pink complexion although they are in effect asphyxiated.

haemolysis. Breakdown of red blood cells. Each cell is a parcel of the oxygen-carrying pigment haemoglobin. When the enclosing membrane gives way, haemoglobin is spilled into the plasma. Some very simple animals have their haemoglobin dissolved in the plasma, but not nearly enough can be dissolved for the needs of a warm-blooded animal such as man; hence the red blood cell.

Haemolysis may be due to destruction of red cells by parasites (malaria), or allergic reactions. ◊ *anaemia* (A.2).

haemophilia. An uncommon familial disease, one of the ◊ *bleeding disorders*, due to absence of one the factors needed for normal clotting of the blood. The missing factor (factor VIII) is a protein, which haemophiliacs are unable to synthesize. The symptoms are prolonged bleeding from the least injury, and a tendency to bleed internally without any obvious cause. Firmly applied dressings may stop external bleeding, and several preparations which promote clotting, including the venom of Russell's viper, are useful. Transfusion of healthy blood or plasma, which of course contains factor VIII, is needed to control severe bleeding. Many haemophiliacs die in childhood; only a few achieve a normal life-span.

Haemophilia is inherited as a *sex-linked recessive character* (◊ *genetics*). This means that an affected woman 'carries' the disease without suffering from it, but that affected men are actual haemophiliacs. Children of female carriers have a 50 per cent chance of inheriting the defect – girls as carriers, boys as sufferers. If a male haemophiliac marries, all his daughters will be carriers, and all his sons will be normal. A girl can have true haemophilia only in the extremely unlikely event that her parents are a carrier and a sufferer. But girls can inherit some very rare deficiencies of other clotting factors.

Several royal families have been afflicted with haemophilia.

Haemophilus. A genus of small bacteria. *H. influenzae* is an inhabitant of healthy throats. When resistance is lowered, e.g. by influenza, it can cause pneumonia and occasionally meningitis. Another species, *H. ducreyi*, causes the venereal disease *chancroid*. These infections can be controlled with sulphonamides or antibiotics.

haemoptysis. Blood-spitting; a symptom that calls for prompt investigation because the possible causes include tuberculosis and cancer of the lung. It can also occur with infection in any part of the air-passages and with heart disease (from raised blood pressure in the lungs).

haemorrhage = ◊ *bleeding*.

haemorrhoids (piles). Distended (varicose) veins at the junction of rectum and anal canal, about an inch above the opening of the anus. (The word haemorrhoids is used here in preference to the simpler *piles* only because other disorders in the same region are also commonly called piles. *Haemorrhoids* is from the Greek of Hippocrates. The obsolete *emerods* is a French corruption of the same word.)

As a rule there is no evident cause. Straining because of constipation may contribute but is unlikely to be the sole cause; on the other hand the discomfort of haemorrhoids encourages constipation and so the two disorders aggravate each other. Of the causes that can be defined, compression of veins in the pelvis by a pregnant uterus is the commonest. Cirrhosis of the liver restricts the normal flow of blood from the intestine to the liver and overburdens the alternative routes by the veins of the rectum and oesophagus.

The name haemorrhoids implies the main symptom, bleeding. There is usually some discomfort, but true haemorrhoids are seldom really painful. Even a small daily loss of blood is enough to deplete the body's reserves of iron in time, and anaemia is a common symptom of long-standing haemorrhoids.

Small haemorrhoids often subside with suppositories, to reduce congestion, and mild laxatives. Larger ones can be treated by injection of an irritant fluid that causes a scar to obstruct the distended vein. Because the base of a haemorrhoid is above the limit of the pain-sensitive nerve-endings of the skin, the injection is not painful, though it may cause a disagreeable sensation of distension, like the discomfort of the haemorrhoids themselves. The principle is different from that of injecting varicose veins in the leg. The object is to cause scarring *around* the haemorrhoid, whereas in the leg it is to stick the walls of the vein together from inside.

The definitive treatment of severe haemorrhoids is a surgical operation, much as Hippocrates described 24 centuries ago. The affected veins are isolated and closed off with ligatures.

All haemorrhoids are worth treating because correct treatment relieves much needless distress; but that is not all. The great danger of this condition is that cancer of the rectum at an early, curable stage gives similar symptoms, and unless the diagnosis is proved as soon as possible, a cancer may be neglected until it is no longer curable.

Hahnemann, Samuel (1755–1843). German physician, founder of ◊ *homoeopathy.*

hair. A hair, like a finger-nail, consists mainly of a dense form of the same substance (keratin) as the outer layer of the skin. Dark hair contains a central core of pigment. The follicle from which a hair grows is a small pit in the surface of the skin. In the side of each follicle is a sebaceous (grease) gland.

The growth of hair alternates between an active phase when the hairs lengthen and a resting phase at the end of which hairs are shed and new ones grow from the same follicles. In animals that moult with the seasons the phases are obvious. In man, the phases of individual hairs are not synchronized: while some are active others are resting and still others are moulting.

In the last three months of pregnancy an infant develops a profuse down of very fine hair (*lanugo*). Except in premature babies most of it is shed before birth, to be replaced by rather stronger hairs. The distribution of hair is under the influence of hormones, mainly the sex hormones. Unwanted hair, e.g. on a woman's face, may be no more than inherited tendency; but a serious excess is due to a faulty balance of hormones.

Despite popular belief, cutting hair has no effect on its growth. Shaving is thought to thicken hair only because recently shaved stubble feels rough.

◊ *baldness.*

Hales, Stephen (1677–1761). English parson and scientist; a pioneer of experimental physiology. He showed that some reflexes were mediated by the spinal cord, independently of the brain; and he measured the pressure and rate of flow of the blood in various animals. He also campaigned for better hygiene in ships, hospitals, and prisons.

Haller, Albrecht von (1708–77). Swiss biologist, physician and writer; a pupil of Boerhaave at Leyden, he taught at Göttingen and Berne. Haller was a distinguished botanist; his many contributions to anatomy included a correct explanation of hernia; but most of all he is remembered as a physiologist. His particular concern was the response of living tissue to stimulation – *irritability*.

hallucination. Sensation without physical origin, as 'hearing voices' or 'seeing things', or a waking dream. Hallucinations that the subject insists are real may suggest mental disturbance; they are commonly associated with schizophrenia but can occur with hysteria or mere fatigue, and with physical illness such as alcoholism (delirium tremens) and fever of any kind.

hallucinogen. Drug that causes hallucinations. The hallucinogens include *cannabis* (hemp, marihuana, dagga, bhang), *mescaline*, from a Mexican cactus, *bufotenin*, a toad poison, and *LSD* (lysergic acid diethylamide), a synthetic alkaloid related to ergot. In the past, cannabis has been used as a narcotic, and recently LSD has been used for studying mental disorder, but none of these drugs has any proven medical value. Probably none is a true drug of addiction. Their devotees take them because they enjoy the episodes of temporary insanity. Mescaline and LSD seem to interfere with the natural action of *serotonin* in the brain, and this might suggest that schizophrenia, of which the symptoms resemble those of the drugs, has the same cause.

hallux. The big toe. *Hallux valgus* is a common deformity: tight shoes deflect the big toe across the next toe, and a ◊ *bunion* develops over the protruding joint.

halothane. Anaesthetic related to chloroform. It is a volatile liquid, $CHClBr.CF_3$. Halothane is probably the safest of the known general anaesthetics that are powerful enough for major surgery. Like all chlorine-containing anaesthetics, it is said to damage the liver on occasion, but very few cases have been reported.

hamstring muscles. The group of muscles at the back of the thigh: *semimembranosus*, *semitendinosus*, and *biceps femoris*. The muscles flex the knee and also help *gluteus maximus* to extend the hip.

hand.

1. STRUCTURE

The base of the hand is supported by the 8 carpal bones, roughly arranged in 2 rows. Three of them articulate with the radius to form the wrist-joint: the *scaphoid, lunate,* and *triquetral*. Beyond these lie the *trapezium, trapezoid, capitate,* and *hamate*. The 8th bone, the *pisiform*, lies in front of the main cluster, embedded in a tendon.

The principal muscles of the hand make up the fleshy mass of the forearm. Their tendons pass in front of and behind the wrist, where they are held in position by a system of fibrous bands. Friction is prevented by the slippery synovial sheaths, like the linings of joints, that envelop the tendons.

In addition there are numerous small muscles within the hand. One group forms the ball of the thumb (thenar eminence), and there is a smaller corresponding group for the little finger (hypothenar eminence). Many other slips of muscle arise in the palm and control fine movements of the fingers.

Flexion of the fingers – grasping – is a much stronger and better controlled movement than extension: a musician's problem is not striking the notes but raising his fingers in time to play the next note.

The hand is well supplied with blood by the 2 arteries at the front of the wrist: the ulnar artery leading towards the little finger, and the radial towards the thumb. It is the radial artery that is felt when the pulse is examined. The 2 arteries join in the palm, and if either is obstructed the other can provide a sufficient flow. If the veins accompanied the arteries in the usual way they would be squeezed flat whenever the hand was used for gripping. Blood therefore returns from the hand in large veins on the back of the hand and wrist.

The median nerve supplies the muscles of the thumb and the ulnar nerve the remaining muscles. Sensation is shared between branches of these nerves and the radial nerve.

2. DISORDERS

Injuries of the hand are commoner than any others, for by nature man uses his hands to explore his surroundings: they are his antennae. They are also his first line of defence. In nearly all other animals the head serves these functions.

In proportion to the amount of actual damage, injuries of the hand are much more disabling than any others. Injuries of the thumb are especially serious, because half the value of the hand is lost if the thumb cannot be brought to bear on the fingers. On the other hand the loss of a single finger need not greatly impair function.

Infection may follow very slight injuries. Because the skin is tough and unyielding there is little room for swelling; therefore a small pocket of inflammation can easily cause enough pressure to stop the circulation in, for example, an infected finger-tip. There is also the danger that infection may pass rapidly up the sheath of a tendon from a finger to the palm. An infected finger is thus an emergency. In most cases, anti-

hands: in particular, *rheumatoid arthritis* has a predilection for the bases of the fingers and the wrists.

Other disorders of the hands described elsewhere are *ganglion, Dupuytren's contracture,* and the *carpal tunnel syndrome.*

Hansen's bacillus. The leprosy bacillus, discovered by Gerhard Hansen (1841–1912), a Norwegian physician, in 1868, 14 years before Koch's discovery of the closely related tubercle bacillus.

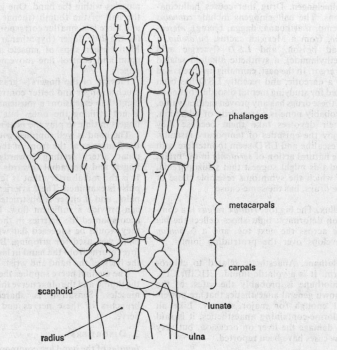

phalanges

metacarpals

carpals

scaphoid

lunate

radius

ulna

Bones of the hand.

biotics will overcome the infection, but if pus begins to form it must be released surgically without delay.

With all kinds of injury or infection of the hand, much care is needed to preserve function, for even a single stiff joint can be a great nuisance. Physiotherapy to keep the joints mobile is often the most important part of the treatment.

Rheumatic diseases commonly affect the

hapten (haptene). A substance, other than a protein, that arouses allergy. The discovery of haptens did not invalidate von Pirquet's theory that allergy was always a reaction to a protein foreign to the tissues: haptens probably act by modifying a protein in the tissues so that it becomes 'foreign'. ◊ *allergy* (1).

harelip ◊ *palate.*

Harvey, William (1578–1657). English physician. He studied at Caius College, Cambridge, and later under the great anatomist Fabricius at Padua; he was physician to St Bartholomew's Hospital, London, and, as Lumleian lecturer at the College of Physicians, the equivalent of a professor of medicine (London had then no university).

In showing that the blood circulated constantly through the body Harvey made the most important discovery in the history of scientific medicine; almost everything else that is known of the workings of the body depends on it. The place of Harvey in medical science is like that of Newton in physics.

His work on the circulation (see *De Motu Cordis*, below) is so great that Harvey's distinction on several other counts is overshadowed and often overlooked. His appointments at St Bartholomew's and the College of Physicians suggest that he was a highly esteemed practising doctor; he was also physician to the royal family and as near as any commoner could get to being a friend of Charles I. If Harvey's colleagues thought little of his prescriptions (Aubrey) that may well be because in an age of gross over-prescribing Harvey tried not to order treatment that could do no good. He was an able surgeon and obstetrician; he was one of the first Englishmen to study the nature of disease by postmortem examination. In his own opinion his most important work was his treatise on embryology (*De Generatione Animalium*, 1651). This book is based on extensive studies of embryos of various species. It offers few facts that were not known to Harvey's teacher Fabricius or indeed to Aristotle, for until the advent of good microscopes embryology could scarcely advance. But Harvey was more careful than any earlier scientist to argue only from the evidence before him, and to avoid pure speculation. By sticking to the facts Harvey was able to draw several conclusions that were confirmed in later centuries. He inferred that every animal begins as an egg, though he was not able to find the egg of a mammal (nor was anyone else for the next 200 years). Since an egg might be too small to be seen, there was no need to suppose that insects and the like arose spontaneously; Harvey was an early opponent of the theory of spontaneous generation, still widely held until Pasteur disproved it.

Harvey correctly stated that the various structures of the body are not all present in miniature from the time of conception, but are formed in sequence. This had been Aristotle's teaching, but Harvey's contemporaries and most of his successors until the 19th century rejected it. Again in the steps of Aristotle, and anticipating von Baer (1792–1876), Harvey noted the close similarity between embryos of widely different species.

1. DE MOTU CORDIS

Harvey's greatest work was published at Frankfurt in 1628. Its full title is *Exercitatio Anatomica de Motu Cordis et Sanguinis in Animalibus* (Anatomical Treatise on the Movement of the Heart and Blood in Animals).

In Harvey's day, Galen's teaching was still generally accepted, and Harvey himself scrupulously followed Aristotle and Galen except when he had clear proof that they were wrong. Galen had said that the purple blood in the veins was formed in the liver and enriched with 'natural spirit' derived from the food. Some of this blood found its way into the arteries by seeping through invisible pores in the dividing wall of the heart; it was enriched with 'vital spirit' from the lungs to become bright scarlet. Veins and arteries carried their respective spirits away from the centre to the rest of the body as the blood in them ebbed and flowed. The heart served only to warm the blood. Its beat and the pulse in the arteries were due to alternating expansion and collapse of the whole apparatus as vital spirit was released and then absorbed.

Since this account was wrong in every particular, and since Galen's opinions were almost a religion for doctors, Harvey's task was comparable with that of the astronomers of his day in proving and persuading others that the earth was not the centre of the universe.

Only a few small cracks had begun to appear in the crust of the old doctrines. Vesalius and the other Paduan anatomists had rightly denied that blood could get through the dividing wall of the heart, but could not explain what it did instead. Ibn-an-Nafis in the 13th century and Servetus and Columbus in the 16th had suggested that blood from the heart might percolate through the lungs and return to the heart. Cesalpino and Leonardo da Vinci both suggested that blood left the heart by the arteries and returned by the veins, and Leonardo recognized the heart as a muscle (but thought its action was to generate heat). None of these men realized that the heart was a pump, or that the blood circulated continuously and rapidly through the body. Even Cesalpino, the only one to use the word 'circulatio', was apparently thinking of occasional seepage rather than a steady flow. And apart from Leonardo none of them supported speculation with evidence. Each has been credited at some time or other with 'discovering' the circulation, but this is like saying that a man who writes science fiction about trips to Mars has invented an interplanetary rocket.

Each step in Harvey's argument was carefully reasoned and then demonstrated by experiment and observation ('first I shall show that this may be so, and then I shall prove that it is so in fact').

He found that the heart is a muscle like any other, and that its beat is due to muscular contraction. The muscle encircles the blood in the heart, and by contracting it squeezes the blood out.

The valves of the heart are so arranged that the blood can be expelled in only one direction: into the arteries but not into the veins. Having entered the arteries, the blood is prevented from returning to the heart.

The valves of the veins allow blood to flow only towards the heart.

From the evidence so far it might be argued that the blood sent out by the arteries is used up in feeding the body, and that the veins bring newly formed blood to the heart for transmission to the arteries. Harvey refuted this theory by pointing to the quantity of blood involved. At the lowest possible estimate the whole mass of blood must pass through the heart in half an hour (we now know that it does so in a minute or less) and this least possible rate of flow greatly exceeded the rate at which new blood could be formed from the food, or at which blood could be used to feed the body. The veins would rapidly be drained, and the arteries would burst 'unless the blood should somehow find its way from the arteries into the veins, and so return to the right side of the heart; I began to think whether there might not be a motion, as it were, in a circle'.

Harvey made countless simple but irrefutable experiments to show that the blood did in fact circulate: that the heart sent a continuous and rapid stream of blood into the arteries and that the same blood returned from all over the body in the veins. In snakes, with their sluggish circulation, he watched the action of the heart in slow motion; in mammals he observed that a part becomes distended with blood if its veins are blocked, and drained of blood if its arteries are blocked and its veins left open. In various dissections he injected water into arteries and recovered it from veins. Anyone can repeat his best-known experiment. The arm is bound above the elbow so that the veins stand out, and their valves are seen as knots or swellings. A vein is compressed with a finger, and the blood is milked upwards to the next valve. The vein between the finger and the valve remains empty until the finger is released; the vein then fills from below. This may be repeated until so much blood has passed along the segment of vein, always in the same direction, that 'you will be convinced of the fact that it circulates'.

2. HARVEY'S INFLUENCE

Harvey had less trouble than most pioneers in persuading his contemporaries that he was right. A few would not listen, but most schools accepted the new doctrine within Harvey's lifetime. But for a long time nobody but Harvey seems to have appreciated the importance of his discovery. He saw that it must affect every part of medicine; yet it hardly began to do so for over a century.

One obstacle was that nobody could explain why blood should circulate until body chemistry, and especially oxygen and its function, began to be understood. Anyone but Harvey would have put forward a theory (masquerading as established fact) 'proving' the need for the circulation, for science was still called 'natural philosophy'. Not even Descartes, the best philosopher since Aristotle, was fully aware of the gulf between philosophical argument and scientific experiment. Harvey is perhaps the first modern scientist in the history of medicine. He concerned himself solely with what he could prove by repeated demonstration. Of reasons for the blood to circulate he said 'I am of opinion that our first duty is to inquire whether the thing be or not, before asking wherefore it is'. No physician had ever spoken in such terms before, and what to us may seem a commonplace remark can have had little meaning for Harvey's contemporaries.

Harvey could find no path to carry blood from the smallest twigs of the arteries to the smallest veins, because he had no microscope and he was looking for vessels much less than 1/1000 inch across. Centuries before, Galen's theory of the blood had required small holes in the dividing wall of the heart. Therefore, said Galen, there are such holes; and everyone believed him, in just the same way as they believed him when he *demonstrated* the presence of blood in the arteries and disproved the old theory that arteries contained air. Until Harvey, doctors did not make any clear distinction between things inferred and things demonstrated by experiment. Anyone else would have said that since blood evidently flowed from arteries to veins there were passages to carry it. Harvey described at length how in one experiment after another he had utterly failed to find any such passages. As later in the century Newton ended his work on optics with a list of problems still to be solved, so Harvey set out more clearly than his critics the questions that he had failed to answer.

Some historians have blamed Harvey for being too conservative, too ready to rely on Aristotle and other ancient authorities. He was a complete teleologist – the ultimate reason for all things was that it was right for them to be so – and his practical medicine was that of Galen. One may as well blame him for being called Harvey and not Darwin or for living in the 17th instead of the 19th century. And in a sense Harvey's conservatism is a very modern trait, arising from the impact of pure science on practical medicine. A pure scientist can afford to reject all previous theories and start afresh, like Descartes. But a scientific physician has to look after sick people who cannot wait for new theories to mature. Today as 300 years ago his best guide is Harvey's doctrine that he must stick to established methods until he can prove that they are wrong.

Hashimoto's disease. Inflammation of the thyroid gland, probably a case of ◊ *auto-immunity*, leading to thyroid deficiency. ◊ *thyroid gland* (2).

hashish = ◊ *hemp.*

hay fever. A common form of ◊ *allergy*; strictly speaking hay fever is a seasonal complaint due to grass pollens, but the term can be stretched to include any allergic reaction involving the lining of the nose.

Tree pollens cause hay fever in the spring, grass pollens in summer; anything to which a person happens to be allergic in the dust of the air can set off an attack at any time. Occasionally stimulation by hot or cold air seems to produce the symptoms of hay fever. Emotion plays some part in most forms of allergy, but is much less important with hay fever than with asthma or allergic skin disease. A few people appear to sneeze with emotion, but generally hay fever is a straightforward response to contact with a particular substance to which the patient is sensitive.

The symptoms are those of an acute inflammation in the nose, often spreading to the throat and the covering membrane of the eye (conjunctiva). Tickling at the back of the nose is followed by sneezing and watering of the eyes and sometimes headache. An attack seldom lasts long, but in some cases where the irritant is perennial a chronic disorder, with the nose always more or less blocked, may develop. Over-enthusiastic use of nose-drops for treating hay fever is one cause of chronic inflammation and catarrh.

The immediate cause of the symptoms is *histamine*, a product of the allergic reaction, and most cases respond well to antihistamine drugs. The particular irritant can often be identified by sensitivity tests. Avoiding it would solve the problem, but that is seldom possible. Desensitization by a rather tedious course of injections works in about 75 per cent of cases. ◊ *cromoglycate.*

head. The head accommodates the brain, several sense organs, and inlets for air and food. In most animals other than man it is also the part of the body that leads the way; but man explores and defends himself with his hands, and in comparison with other mammals his face is rudimentary. With the recession of his nose, his eyes have been able to take a position where they work as a single, stereoscopic unit. He compensates for a rather narrow visual field with a very mobile neck.

The underlying structure is briefly discussed under ◊ *skull.* The soft tissues (nerves, blood vessels, muscles etc.) form a most intricate pattern. All the nerves are derived directly from the brain and not the spinal cord (◊ *cranial nerve*). Blood is delivered by three pairs of arteries: *external carotid* for the face and scalp, *internal carotid* and *vertebral* for the brain. It returns by the *jugular* veins. Apart from the tiny bones for conducting sound in the inner ear, the only mobile joint in the head is the temporo-mandibular joint between the lower jaw and the base of the skull. It is provided with the powerful muscles of *mastication*. In addition, there is a complex array of muscles in the face and scalp. Unlike most voluntary muscles, they are attached to bone only at one end; the other end merges with the skin.

headache. Headache is perhaps the commonest and certainly the least informative of all symptoms. It may accompany almost any general illness, including all kinds of acute infection from a boil on the back to smallpox, poisons such as alcohol, tobacco and many drugs, high blood pressure, decayed teeth, and anxiety. The source of the pain is seldom clear. Even the severe pain of migraine has not been fully explained, beyond saying that it has something to do with blood vessels inside the skull. The brain itself is surprisingly insensitive, but its covering membranes, the *meninges*, perceive pain, and headaches arising from disorders within the skull are often due to irritation of the meninges. The skull itself is the source of the pain of *sinusitis*. The headaches of worry and fatigue – the commonest of all – may arise from tension of the muscles of the neck and scalp.

Persistent headaches, and headaches that do not respond to mild analgesic drugs, need to be investigated; but the mere statement 'I have a headache' gives little more clue to the diagnosis than 'I do not feel well'.

head injury. Hippocrates, who devoted a whole treatise to the subject, observed that while even very grave head injuries were not always hopeless, none was so trivial that it could be ignored.

The special danger is that the skull allows no room for expansion. A small amount of blood is enough to irritate or compress the brain. Although actual damage to the brain cannot be repaired, much can be done to prevent further harm, or to avoid any harm.

A second's unconsciousness is proof of concussion. As a rule there are no after-effects, but repeated concussion such as a boxer may suffer inevitably does permanent damage; and anyone who has been concussed needs to be watched for signs of

further trouble, especially slow bleeding which may need prompt surgical attention.

Suffocation is the commonest cause of death after head injuries. The tongue is slung from the lower jaw. If a man is deeply unconscious his jaw may be so relaxed that the back of his tongue blocks his throat; and because his protective reflexes are suppressed he cannot breathe. Anyone can put two fingers at the angle of the jaw and two more under the point of the jaw, and bring the jaw gently upwards and forwards. The tongue comes with it and the patient can breathe.

It is essential to be sure that the space behind the tongue is not blocked by false teeth or a particle of food. Many lives can be saved if the first person on the scene of an accident gently explores this space with a finger. Any unconscious patient is liable to vomit, and may suffocate from inhaling fluid from the stomach. The danger is largely averted if he is laid on his side with his mouth downwards – provided that the jaw is drawn forwards to keep the tongue clear of the back of the throat.

After severe head injuries some patients develop a kind of ◊ *epilepsy*. Taking all head injuries into account, this is a very rare complication, but after localized damage to certain areas of the brain surface, e.g. by a fragment of the skull, it is not uncommon. The attacks may persist despite surgical treatment of the apparent source of irritation, in which case they are treated in the same way as the usual type of the disease.

Fractures are further discussed under ◊ *skull*.

healing ◊ *inflammation* (1).

heart.

1. DEVELOPMENT

Blood vessels are muscular tubes. In very simple creatures such as worms, ripple-like contraction of the vessels serves to keep the blood flowing around the circuit. There is no clear starting point, and no distinction between arteries and veins. In more complex animals a segment of one vessel, more muscular than the rest, takes over the work of pumping the blood. This is the most primitive type of heart, and the form in which the heart first appears in a human embryo. The direction of flow is from tail to head. Vessels *entering* the tail end of the heart are veins; vessels *leaving* the head end are arteries.

At a later stage, seen in fish, constrictions divide the heart-tube into a series of three or four *chambers*. These are the *sinus venosus* where the veins enter, the *atrium* (or auricle), the *ventricle*, and the *conus arteriosus* where the aorta leaves (in most fish the conus is not distinct from the aorta). The heart becomes folded on itself, so that in a fish viewed from the right side the heart is Z-shaped, the

The left atrium receives the *pulmonary* veins and the right atrium all the others.

The heart is now two separate pumps, the right side serving the lungs and the left side the rest of the body.

This arrangement is useless to the unborn child, which gets oxygen not from its lungs but from its mother's blood by the *placenta*. This oxygenated blood is carried in the umbilical vein to the inferior vena cava and so to the *right* atrium. But oxygenated blood

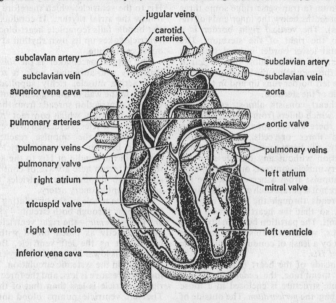

Section of heart, slightly modified to show the four chambers; in fact the right ventricle lies in front of the left.

ventricle lying below the atrium. In man, the heart is later twisted sideways, and when its development is complete the ventricle is to the left of the atrium, not in front of it. In principle, the heart is a mid-line structure, but the preponderance of the ventricle makes it seem left-sided.

Finally a partition (*septum*) grows across the atrium and another across the ventricle, dividing each into left and right chambers.

There is a *valve* at the exit from each of the four chambers to prevent blood from flowing back. A spiral septum divides the primitive aorta into the definitive aorta opening from the left ventricle, and the pulmonary artery from the right ventricle.

is needed in the *left* atrium to be sent round the arteries. Until birth it passes through an opening in the atrial septum, from right to left and so to the aorta. Even so a considerable amount of blood, mainly from the superior vena cava, reaches the pulmonary artery. It is diverted from the lungs by a slipway, the *ductus arteriosus*, joining the pulmonary artery to the aorta.

Before birth, the unexpanded lungs resist the flow of blood; the pressure is thus higher in the right side of the heart than the left, and blood is driven through the two short-circuits from right to left. At birth the first breaths (probably stimulated by cold air) fill the lungs. The pulmonary vessels widen and the pressure in them is relieved. Now – and throughout life – the blood pressure is much greater in the left than the right side of the heart. The flap-like opening in the atrial septum is pushed to and soon becomes sealed off. The ductus arteriosus closes by contraction of its muscular wall and in a few days begins to wither.

2. ADULT HEART

The top of the heart is level with the angle of the sternum (a transverse ridge some three finger-breadths below the inner ends of the clavicles). The vertical right border is a little to the right of the sternum. The horizontal lower border is level with the lower end of the sternum: on the left it reaches the *apex* below the left nipple. From here the left border runs up and in towards the angle of the sternum.

The heart consists almost entirely of muscle, which differs from ordinary muscle in that there are no apparent boundaries between fibres or cells. The essential property of heart muscle is rhythmic contraction without any outside stimulus (ordinary muscle contracts only in response to an impulse from a nerve). Because the fibres are not separate each wave of contraction spreads through the whole mass of muscle, so that the heart contracts as a single unit. The partition between atria and ventricles, which contains no muscle, is bridged by a leash of conducting fibres, the *bundle of His.*

The inside of the heart is lined with a smooth membrane, the *endocardium*, and the whole structure is enclosed in a loose fibrous bag, the *pericardium.* The outside of the heart and the inside of the pericardium are covered with a slippery membrane like the lining of a joint, which prevents friction as the heart beats.

A small and primitive heart gets enough oxygen and other supplies from the blood flowing through it, but the thick walls of a more evolved heart need their own blood vessels. The two ◊ *coronary* arteries arise from the root of the aorta, and their branches are distributed throughout the heart. The returning veins open directly into the chambers of the heart, most into the right atrium.

3. ACTION

The sole function of the heart is to pump blood from the veins into the arteries. The heart is hollow; when its walls contract blood is squeezed out, and the valves ensure that the flow is only in one direction.

The two phases of the action are *diastole* when the heart relaxes and fills, and *systole* when it contracts and empties.

Rhythmic contraction is an inherent property of heart muscle. Left to its own devices the atrium contracts about 140 times a minute, and the ventricle about 30 times. In the intact heart the impulse from the atrium is transmitted by the bundle of His to the ventricle, which therefore has to follow the atrial rhythm. If conduction in the bundle fails (complete heart-block) the ventricle takes up its own rhythm at 30–40 beats per minute.

The natural pacemaker is the *sinu-atrial* (formerly sino-auricular) *node,* a zone of very active muscle, richly supplied with nerves, in the wall of the right atrium. Each wave of contraction spreads from the node through the atria, which contract together while the ventricles are relaxed to receive the blood. When the impulse reaches the junction between atria and ventricles it is carried in the bundle of His to the apex of the heart: from here a wave of contraction spreads up through the ventricles to the aorta and pulmonary artery.

Since the whole of the circulating blood has to pass through both circuits – *pulmonary* and *systemic* – the right ventricle must pump exactly as much blood with each heart beat as the left ventricle. But the resistance is lower in the pulmonary circulation than in the systemic circulation. Therefore the pressure is less, and the force of the right ventricle is less than that of the left. The left ventricle pumps blood into the aorta at a pressure of about 120 mm. of mercury (0·16 atmosphere; 2·4 lb./sq. in.), while the right ventricle pumps at about 25 mm. of mercury.

An essential property of heart muscle is that within reasonable limits it exactly meets the demands made on it; in other words it will expel whatever volume of blood enters. The volume pumped by either ventricle at a beat (*stroke volume*) may be increased from 70 c.c. at rest to 200 c.c. during exertion. But apart from extreme exertion, the volume pumped per minute (cardiac output) depends more on the rate of the heart beat than on the stroke volume. The rate can be increased from about 70 to 200 beats per minute. Thus the extremes of cardiac output are about 5 litres per minute at rest and 40 litres during severe exercise. Increased return of blood (e.g. from active muscles) has two effects on the heart. Firstly, the more the ventricles are filled in diastole the more they contract in systole (*Starling's law of the heart*). Secondly, distension of the atria increases the heart rate (*Bainbridge effect*). ◊ *Heart failure* simply means a breakdown of this mechanism.

Only inherent properties of the heart have so far been considered, but there is also remote control. An isolated atrium beats at about twice the normal resting heart rate. In the intact living body the rate is kept down to about 70 beats per minute by a continuous stream of impulses from the cardiac centre in the brain, carried in the ◊ *vagus* (◊ *parasympathetic*) *nerve* to the sinuatrial node. Most nerve impulses stimulate: these inhibit. This 'vagal tone' is the main factor regulating the heart rate. The heart is accelerated by decreasing the activity in the vagus nerves. But if this were the only factor the maximum rate would be 140 or 150, the fundamental rate of the atrium. In fact, rates over 200 are possible, because the negative effect of withdrawing vagal inhibition is reinforced by the positive effect of the ◊ *sympathetic* nerves, which stimulate the sinu-atrial node.

The reciprocal action of the two sets of nerves is co-ordinated in the *cardiac centre*, a collection of nerve cells in the ◊ *medulla oblongata*, the lowest part of the brain. The centre is close to a similar centre for the control of ◊ *respiration* and responds to similar stimuli, for both centres serve the same needs. Blood carries oxygen, and a greater demand for oxygen is met by increasing the intake (respiration) and simultaneously increasing the circulation of blood. The cardiac centre increases the heart rate in response to diminished blood pressure, lack of oxygen, raised body temperature, and emotions such as fear and anger. The heart itself can respond to an established demand, i.e. an actual increase in the volume of blood returned, but the cardiac centre can anticipate a demand. The angry or frightened man is prepared for action by his increased heart rate by ◊ *sympathetic* nervous activity.

4. CONGENITAL DEFECTS

The development of the heart (section 1 above) can be arrested or go astray at almost any stage. With gross defects the child is stillborn or dies soon after birth, but various malformations are compatible with life. Some do not appear to affect the child's health; others cause degrees of disability up to complete invalidism. For instance, where the right and left sides of the heart are not completely separated the stronger left side may transfer some of its blood to the right. The right ventricle and pulmonary circulation are then constantly overloaded, and unless the hole between left and right chambers is repaired the expected life-span is halved. Another hazard is bacterial ◊ *endocarditis*. Bacteria seldom survive long in circulating blood, but they thrive in a stagnant backwater, such as a ductus arteriosus which has failed to close at birth, or a mis-shapen heart valve.

Often there is more than one defect. If there is a hole between the right and left sides of the heart and also an obstructed pulmonary artery, venous blood which should be sent through the lungs for oxygenation is forced into the left ventricle. The baby appears blue because the blood in his arteries lacks its complement of oxygen.

One septum divides the developing ventricle into left and right chambers; another, growing towards it, divides the emerging artery into aorta and pulmonary artery. If these septa do not meet in the right way the aorta may arise from the right ventricle and the pulmonary artery from the left. Oxygenated blood is then returned to the lungs, and venous blood without oxygen to the rest of the body. A child with this defect is able to survive if there is also a hole between the two sides of the heart which allows oxygenated blood to leak across. Such a hole can be made surgically, and the child may then live long enough to be fit for a larger operation to divert the blood in the atria to the correct channels.

Most of the common congenital defects can now be treated surgically. The operations themselves are still fairly hazardous, but they offer the chance of a completely normal life.

5. HEART DISEASE

As the heart has only one function, to pump all the blood it receives from the veins into the arteries, so in a sense it has only one disease, failure to do so. But ◊ *heart failure* has many causes. The heart has to pump a sufficient *volume* of blood against the *resistance* of the smaller arteries, which requires a certain *force* of contraction. Failure may follow increased volume, increased resistance, or decreased muscular force. Common disorders of the heart may be considered under these three headings.

Increased volume. The total volume of circulating blood seldom varies, but the volume to be pumped from a ventricle with each beat may vary greatly: in a normal heart as much as eight-fold. The volume is abnormally increased with certain *congenital defects* (section 4 above), where blood leaks from one side of the heart to the other and is added to the proper load of the affected ventricle. An incompetent ◊ *valve* allows blood that has already been pumped out of a chamber to leak back, adding itself to the new load arriving from the veins. Incompetence of a valve may be congenital, or a result of inflammatory disease (◊ *rheumatism*, ◊ *syphilis*). It sometimes follows other heart disease, where the heart is enlarged and the valve is stretched. An abnormal load of blood, whatever the cause, means that the heart at rest works as hard as a normal heart during exercise, and has no reserve for the added demands of exertion.

Increased resistance. If the resistance to the flow of blood increases, the pressure must rise for the circulation to be maintained. Again, the heart must work as hard at rest as a healthy person's heart during exercise, at the expense of its reserve strength. If the pressure in the systemic arteries rises (◊ *blood pressure*) the left ventricle is overworked. The pressure in the pulmonary arteries rises, with a similar risk to the right ventricle, in various chronic disorders of the lungs (e.g. ◊ *bronchitis*, ◊ *emphysema*) and also when the left side of the heart is inefficient and allows blood to accumulate in the lungs instead of pumping it to the aorta. Narrowing (*stenosis*) of a ◊ *valve* increases the resistance before the blood ever leaves the heart. Stenosis of a heart valve may be a congenital defect or a complication of rheumatic fever. The fault can often be corrected surgically.

Decreased force. Any debilitating disease may affect the muscular strength of the heart. Various disorders specifically weaken the heart muscle. They include *lack of oxygen*, from deficient blood supply in ◊ *coronary* artery disease, from defective blood in ◊ *anaemia*, and from ◊ *lung* disorders; *malnutrition*, especially ◊ *beriberi*; *poisoning* by bacteria as in ◊ *typhoid*, ◊ *pneumonia*, and other infections, and also by certain drugs; and several types of *degeneration* which are difficult to classify because

their causes are not understood. The weakening of the heart muscle by severe rheumatic fever is in the last category; the obvious effect of rheumatic heart disease is damage to the valves, but there is also a direct effect on the heart muscle. Finally, disturbances of *rhythm* (◊ *arrhythmia*) weaken the action of the heart.

Over-exertion has not been mentioned because it is not a disease, and because an intact heart meets the demands that are made on it. Rickshaw porters, who often die young of heart failure, appear to disprove this. It may be that these men have to exert themselves beyond anything known in other parts of the world, but malnutrition is a likelier explanation.

One condition, ◊ *effort syndrome*, must be dismissed. The heart responds to emotion, and an emotional disturbance may cause symptoms which suggest heart disease. But such hearts are intact; the disorder is elsewhere.

To insist that failure of the heart to meet natural demands is the only real heart disease may be over-simplification, but it seems better than to stigmatize as 'diseased' or 'weak' an organ which is in fact able to meet normal demands. To be sure, a heart aged 60 years has less in reserve than one aged 20, but the demands on it are also less. Football may be too strenuous at 60, but most men of sixty do not wish to play football, if only because their legs are no longer up to it. Football is no longer a normal demand. But even football might be safer than taking no exercise at all for fear of injuring the heart. A daily walk or a spell of gardening *is* a normal demand, and like any other part of the body the heart degenerates if no demands are made on it.

The three types of abnormal demand which may lead to heart disease can all be created artificially. Heart disease is the main cause of death in affluent urban societies, and much of it is man-made. Lack of exercise and overeating have the same effect as increasing the load to be pumped with each beat. Continual worry, with a continual emotional stimulus to the cardiac centre, keeps the circulation at a pitch which would normally be reserved for times of special effort; this corresponds with increasing the resistance. The heart muscle may be weakened by unsuitable eating and drinking or by lack of natural demands on it. Such hearts are no more at fault than motor cars that are constantly overloaded, or run with the choke out, or filled with the wrong fuel. They are potentially normal hearts, prevented from behaving normally.

◊ *atheroma*.

6. EXAMINATION OF THE HEART

The state of the whole patient reflects the state of his heart, and an assessment of the heart therefore amounts to a fairly complete physical examination, with particular attention to the ◊ *pulse* and ◊ *blood pressure*. The sounds heard with a stethoscope are an important guide. When the ventricles are full at the end of diastole the pressure in them rises as they begin to contract. This pressure closes the valves between atria and ventricles. At the end of systole, when the ventricles cease to contract, the pressure in the aorta and pulmonary artery closes the valves at the outlets of the ventricles. Each closure produces a characteristic sound. If the pressure is abnormally high the sound is accentuated. If the two sides of the heart are not synchronized, the second sound is doubled or 'split'. Eddies and crosscurrents, sometimes with defective valves and sometimes in healthy hearts, produce a variety of additional sounds or *murmurs*. The interpretation of heart sounds has become much more accurate in recent years with mechanical recording and comparison of the sounds with more precise tests, but diagnosis from sounds alone is still unreliable in many cases.

Special investigations include X-ray examination of the size and shape of the heart, electrocardiography (◊ *electrocardiogram*), and measurements of the pressure changes and oxygen and carbon dioxide concentrations in the four chambers of the heart by means of fine tubes passed along blood vessels: this last is essential to the exact diagnosis of congenital defects before surgery. The same technique is used to inject solutions that are opaque to X-rays into the heart or the coronary arteries so that their outlines can be shown by X-rays.

heart failure. The word 'failure' is misleading, for it suggests that the heart no longer works and that the patient ought to be dead. This can of course happen, but in the medical sense failure is usually only relative: the heart works, but not as effectively as it should.

As fast as blood arrives from the veins a healthy heart pumps it into the arteries. The heart is in 'failure' when it does not pump the blood quite as fast as it arrives. As a result the veins become congested with blood and the pressure in them rises. The circulation then goes on as before, but with a constant backlog of accumulated blood. The heart no longer empties itself with each beat. Because its muscle is stretched it actually beats harder than a healthy heart (as a stretched spring pulls harder), but without increasing its output. The situation is familiar to anyone who has allowed correspondence to pile up: he may answer letters as fast as they arrive, but he remains a week behind with his work. This inefficient person often works longer hours than his more productive colleagues. He has neither time nor energy for recreation. Since he hardly manages his routine work he cannot take on extra duties at busy times.

The symptoms of heart failure are in two groups : those due to poor output (forward failure) and those due to congestion in the veins (backward failure). Forward failure affects the whole body: all tissues need an adequate supply of fresh blood, and when the supply is reduced nothing in the body functions quite as well as it should.

The left side of the heart receives blood from the lungs and pumps it to the whole body. If this side fails, the burden of backward failure falls on the lungs. If the right side of the heart, which receives blood from the whole body, fails the congestion is spread throughout the body. In health, the blood vessels of the lungs contain only half a pint of blood, whereas those of the rest of the body contain a gallon. A small amount of extra fluid is enough to embarrass the lungs, and thus the laboured breathing of left-sided failure comes on quickly, sometimes without warning. The swollen feet and other symptoms of congestion due to right-sided failure are much more insidious because so much more space is available.

The symptoms of congestion are due not so much to over-filling of the veins as to leakage of water into the tissues, causing *oedema* (dropsy). The various ways in which tissues can become waterlogged are considered under ◊ *oedema*. At least three mechanisms operate in heart failure. The most obvious is the raised pressure in the veins, which raises the pressure in the capillaries and prevents them from absorbing water from the tissues. Secondly, poor circulation deprives the capillaries of their full quota of oxygen and causes them to leak.

Thirdly, poor circulation in the kidneys causes too much salt to be retained in the body; since the concentration of salt is automatically kept constant, any excess of salt is automatically accompanied by an excess of water.

The relation to other disease is very complex, for on the one hand heart failure lowers the efficiency of other organs and on the other hand chronic disease in other organs, especially the lungs and kidneys, can lead to heart failure.

The performance of a failing heart can often be improved by drugs, of which the most important is ◊ *digitalis*. Many causes of heart failure can be treated directly: high blood pressure, disorders of the thyroid gland, anaemia, and various kinds of defective heart valve are treatable and in some cases completely curable. Chronic bronchitis is among the commonest causes of heart failure, at least in Great Britain, and if it cannot be cured much can be done to prevent it from becoming worse. Accumulated fluid can be removed by ◊ *diuretic* drugs, which increase the amount of urine, or simply by restricting salt in the diet (since the excess of water in the body is partly due to an excess of salt). A salt-free diet is insipid, but many patients gladly put up with it when they have once experienced its good effect. The demands made on the heart have to be limited to what it can manage. With severe or sudden failure this may mean complete bed-rest. Here we meet a paradox: severe attacks of difficulty in breathing due to heart failure (cardiac asthma) are most likely to occur when the patient is asleep in bed, probably because during the day any excess of fluid tends to gravitate to the legs, but in bed it is free to overload the lungs. Therefore some patients with heart failure sleep best sitting upright.

Adapting a patient's mode of life to the limits set by an inefficient heart often needs delicate judgement and the closest co-operation between patient and doctor. It must be repeated that failure is a relative term. If the patient's activities are within the set limits, so that the heart can work without a backlog, then he cannot be said to suffer from heart failure. All the other forms of treatment serve to extend the limits. But to restrict activity too much – for instance, to stay in bed when he might be in the garden or to stay at home when his heart would let him be at his office – does no good to a man's heart and does great harm to the man as a whole. There is increasing evidence that carefully graded exercise may be the best treatment of some types of heart disease.

heatstroke. Illness from overheating of the body. Excessive heat can cause at least three different kinds of disturbance. The commonest is lassitude, cramp, and in extreme cases collapse, due to loss of salt from sweating. It is promptly cured by replacing the salt. People about to exert themselves in hot places, such as stokers, avoid it by taking salt in advance.

Fainting is another reaction; in extreme cases it may amount to a state indistinguishable from shock after severe injury, but as a rule the patient recovers promptly as he cools down. A third, sometimes dangerous, reaction to heat is sudden fever if the mechanisms for regulating the body temperature break down. This can happen when the air is not only hot but humid; sweat cannot then evaporate and the body has no natural means of keeping cool.

hebephrenia. A severe mental disorder; adolescent ◊ *schizophrenia*.

hellebore. Several related species of plant (*veratrum*), used from early antiquity as purgatives and emetics. Some lower the blood pressure, and others may assist a failing heart in the same way as digitalis, but their effects are too unpredictable for safety.

hemiplegia. Paralysis of one side of the body (from interference with the opposite side of the brain).

hemp. The plant *Cannabis indica* or *Cannabis sativa*; bhang; dagga; 'pot'; marihuana (the dried tops of the plant – 'grass'); hashish (cannabis resin). It has long been used as a mild narcotic in parts of Asia and Africa where alcohol is forbidden. Its medicinal value is limited because (1) the activity of different samples varies widely, (2) the effect on the individual is unpredictable, (3) it can have disconcerting effects on behaviour, (4) a dose remains in the body for a long time – weeks rather than days – so that the effects are likely to last too long and repeated doses accumulate. To some extent the first of these objections applies to all plant drugs; it is overcome by isolating the active principle and, if possible, synthesizing it. The second and third apply, though not to the same extent, to various accepted drugs and to alcohol. The fourth is, as regards medicinal use, the gravest. The best safeguard with any drug is its natural elimination. It is the tendency to accumulate that makes digitalis an awkward drug to handle, but there has been no alternative to digitalis whereas there are many to hemp.

Next to alcohol and tobacco, hemp has become the most commonly abused drug in Western society during recent years, and there is now considerable pressure on governments to relax the restrictions on its use, since (it is argued) hemp is no worse than alcohol, and if it were legal its *habitués* would avoid the corrupting influence of pedlars anxious to convert them to more dangerous drugs. But the laws are not likely to change while there is still more than a suspicion that hemp can cause lasting mental deterioration. ⟡ *addiction*.

heparin. A substance extracted from liver and other tissues that delays the clotting of blood.

hepatic. Of the ⟡ *liver* (Lat. *hepar*).
Hepatic artery. The liver receives a large supply of blood from the *portal vein*; this is the raw material on which it has to work. But the portal blood has already given up its available oxygen to the intestine, and like any other organ the liver needs oxygenated blood. As the lungs have a private supply from the ⟡ *bronchial* arteries, so the liver has from the hepatic artery, which comes from the aorta via the *coeliac* artery. Its branches in the liver accompany those of the portal vein.
Hepatic coma. Coma from liver failure, due to poisoning by substances (especially ammonia) which a healthy liver destroys.
Hepatic duct. Channel into which bile flows from the liver. Left and right ducts join to form the common hepatic duct; this is joined by the duct of the gall bladder to form the common bile duct, which opens into the duodenum.
Hepatic flexure. Part of the ⟡ *colon*, where it turns to the left under the liver.
Hepatic veins. Blood from the portal vein and hepatic arteries (see above) irrigates the cells of the liver and leaves by a single system of veins, which open straight into the inferior vena cava at the back of the liver.

hepatitis. Inflammation of the liver, mostly ascribed to virus infection. There are two acute forms: epidemic jaundice and serum hepatitis.

Epidemic jaundice is spread from person to person or by contamination of food or water supplies. Serum hepatitis is conveyed by traces of blood or serum on hypodermic needles used, e.g., for immunization or blood transfusion. It has nothing to do with the jaundice that follows transfusion from an incompatible donor. Since it became generally known that ordinary methods of sterilization may not destroy the minute traces of contamination that cause it, this disease has become much less common, except among drug addicts, who catch it from their needles, and whose resistance to the disease is low.

The reason why these diseases were not recognized for what they are until the Second World War is the very long incubation period, which makes it difficult to prove the source of infection. Symptoms of epidemic jaundice do not appear for about a month, and with serum hepatitis the delay can be as long as six months.

Probably most people infected with either virus have few if any symptoms. Susceptible people feel sick for a few days, and often feverish. They then develop *jaundice*, which commonly lasts about a week. After that, they gradually recover, but they often need several weeks to become completely fit. Serious complications are not usual, but some cases of cirrhosis of the liver may have started with hepatitis.

hermaphrodite. A true hermaphrodite is both male and female. This is the natural state of most plants and a few animals, but true hermaphroditism in man is mythical. Nearly all so-called human hermaphrodites are people with the wrong number of sex chromosomes (⟡ *genetics*). They have the primary sex organs (ovaries or testes) of one sex but many secondary characters of the other, or their external appearance is ambiguous.

There have been rare accounts of an ovary and a testis in the same person, presumably from the formation of one embryo from the elements of two. This is as near as one gets to a true human hermaphrodite; but neither organ is fertile.

Adrenogenital syndrome (⟡ *adrenal*) can cause a sort of hermaphroditism in girls, but the ovaries are normal and if the condition is treated the girls develop normally.

Newspaper accounts of sex-change operations refer to plastic surgery done at the request of people with male sex organs to give them the outward appearance of females. These are people whose emotional make-up is female and who wish to equate their physical state with their feelings.

Homosexuality is a matter of emotion and behaviour and bears little relation to physical constitution. ◊ *sex*.

hernia. Protrusion of an organ from one compartment of the body into another, e.g. of a loop of intestine into the top of the thigh, or of an intervertebral disc into the canal for the spinal cord.

Common types of hernia include the following.

Diaphragmatic hernia. The diaphragm is a strong layer of muscle and fibrous tissue separating the cavities of the chest and the belly. Its weakest point is the opening for the oesophagus (gullet) to enter the stomach. Sometimes part of the stomach bulges up through the opening. This kind of hernia is so common as to be almost the rule after middle age, especially in fat people. Generally it gives little if any trouble, but it can cause indigestion and, rarely, symptoms confused with gastric ulcer or even angina. Adjustment of diet to avoid irritating or over-filling the stomach is often enough to relieve the symptoms. Surgery is very seldom needed.

Femoral hernia. A loop of intestine can bulge into the groin alongside the blood vessels to the thigh. The effect is very similar to an inguinal hernia.

Inguinal hernia. This is the commonest form of 'rupture'. The weak point is the small gap in the abdominal muscles where the testis descended to the scrotum. Its vessels pass through the gap, which therefore cannot be sealed off. In older men, coughing or straining may cause a bulge at the gap. In some boys and young men the hernia is into a preformed space: the testis during its descent drags with it a pocket of peritoneum – the lining of the abdominal cavity. This normally withers, but it may persist like the finger of a glove, and a loop of intestine or other abdominal structure easily slips into it.

A femoral or inguinal hernia sometimes causes little trouble, but it can be uncomfortable, and it is always a source of anxiety because without warning it can become *strangulated*: a loop of intestine is pinched at the entrance to the hernia. Its contents are obstructed, and worse still fresh blood no longer reaches it. Prompt operation is needed to save the patient's life. The usual practice is to treat these hernias on sight, without waiting for trouble. A *truss* is simply a pad held firmly against the weak point to stop any organ from entering the hernia. It does not cure, and is seldom really comfortable. Unless there are strong reasons against surgery in a particular case, the best treatment is to repair the defect surgically, either by bringing its margins together or by covering it with a graft of the patient's own fibrous tissue or a synthetic support.

Umbilical hernia. Many babies have a hernia at the navel. These usually close themselves in a year or two without any trouble; but umbilical hernias that develop later need surgical repair.

heroin. Diamorphine; diacetyl morphine; a synthetic derivative of morphine intended to have the pain-killing properties of morphine without causing addiction. It turned out to be even more addicting than morphine, but was nevertheless used because in some cases of severe pain it was more effective.

The use of heroin is prohibited in the United States and some other countries, because of the very serious risk of addiction. In Britain it is still occasionally prescribed for intractable pain, but doctors are not encouraged to use it. Under the latest regulations (1973) only designated specialists can treat heroin addicts.

Herophilus (3rd century B.C.). The first anatomist in history; a native of Chalcedon in Asia Minor, and with Erasistratus one of the founders of the great medical school of Alexandria. He paid particular attention to the nervous system, distinguishing nerves from blood vessels and sensory from motor nerves, and giving a detailed account of the brain. His works have been lost, but were much quoted by Galen in the 2nd century A.D.

herpes. Two quite different virus infections are known as *herpes*. **1.** *Herpes simplex* is a clutch of inflamed blisters ('cold sore') around the mouth or occasionally some other mucous membrane. Most people carry the virus all their lives, without symptoms. A few develop blisters when they have some other infection; exposure to very hot or very cold weather may also cause an eruption. Apart from rare cases of serious infection in infants, this is a harmless disorder.

2. *Herpes zoster* is caused by the same virus as chickenpox. The virus, like that of herpes simplex, lies dormant in the tissues and may flare up many years after the chickenpox. The virus establishes itself around sensory nerve cells about to enter the spinal cord, and causes painful blisters in the area of skin served by the affected nerves. The pain characteristically precedes the blisters. The patient is often unwell and sometimes feverish for some days. A second attack is unusual, but in a few cases pain (neuralgia) persists when the infection has subsided. The symptoms have to be treated on their own merits; there is no known means of shortening or preventing the attack.

Hilton, John ◊ *rest*.

hip. Ball-and-socket joint between the spherical head of the *femur* (thigh-bone) and the cup-like *acetabulum* at the side of the pelvis. The acetabula face outwards and are tilted slightly downwards and backwards, which helps to take the powerful thrust of the thigh in walking.

In contrast with its counterpart the shoulder, the hip is extremely stable. The head of the femur is firmly seated in the deep socket, and the joint is reinforced by stout ligaments, especially in front. The surrounding muscles, those of the buttock and thigh, are the strongest in the body. The price of stability in a joint is limitation of movement, yet the hip is surprisingly mobile in all directions except backwards (extension). When the hip seems to be extended, as in swinging the leg back before taking a kick, it is the whole pelvis that swings on the opposite hip.

Dislocation of a fully developed hip is unusual. It requires great force, such as a collision on the road, and is likely to be only one of several injuries.

Congenital dislocation of the hip is also rather uncommon, but it is important because it can usually be prevented. The primary disorder, present at birth, is no more than a laxity of the ligaments that allows the as yet unformed joint to slip in and out of place. If this state continues, the bones fail to develop and when the child begins to walk

a permanent deformity is established. But if the instability is recognized soon after birth and the hip is splinted in the correct position, the bones develop normally and there is no further trouble. Until about 1960 these dislocations were ascribed to faulty development of the acetabulum, but this was putting the cart before the horse: the acetabulum develops only if the head of the femur lies in it.

The only common *fracture* near the hip is of the neck of the ◊ *femur*, an inch or two from the joint. This occurs mostly in old age.

Children sometimes suffer from a deformity of the head of the femur, ◊ *Perthes' disease*.

The hip is subject to great mechanical strain, and ◊ *osteoarthritis*, ◊ *rheumatoid arthritis* and other rheumatic diseases commonly affect it, causing pain, stiffness, and sometimes great disability. In most cases, treatment is conservative (rest, analgesic drugs, physiotherapy etc.), but there is also a place for surgery for relieving severe pain or restoring function. The oldest method is to immobilize the joint (arthrodesis). By stopping movement it cures the pain, and paradoxically it makes the limb as a whole more mobile by preventing movements of other joints from disturbing the affected hip. Realignment of the femur, which changes the direction of the stresses, has also had some success. A newer method, which was not possible until suitable materials were found, is to replace the whole joint with an artificial ball and socket. In many cases patients who were practically bedridden are enabled to walk normally soon after the operation.

Hippocrates of Cos (around 400 B.C.). By common consent the greatest physician of all time; 'the father of medicine'.

He was probably born in 460 B.C. and lived to a notable age – over 100, some say. He was venerated in his lifetime, and has been held up ever since as the model of what a doctor should be, almost as a religious leader or patron saint. Many legends have grown around him, but that does not justify the belief sometimes expressed that he never existed, that he is an imaginary ideal. Several early writers, including his young contemporary Plato, describe him as a real person. Nor need we insist that Hippocrates wrote none of the many books traditionally ascribed to him. He could not have written them all: some are more recent and some older than Hippocrates, and some of the doctrines are incompatible with others. But half a dozen or more of the finest seem to be the work of one man of Hippocrates' time. Somebody had to write them, and there are no other claimants. They do not reflect the philosophy that Plato has put into Hippocrates' mouth, but this means nothing, for writers of the time often used real people as pegs for their own ideas. Plato's Socrates talks differently from Xenophon's, and perhaps neither is much like the real Socrates. But these are problems for classical scholars. As far as medicine is concerned Hippocrates was a practising physician and surgeon, the leader of a medical school and guild based on the island of Cos, and the author of some of the medical writings of the school. The content of the books, the wealth of original observation, the unerring sense of what is relevant, would set them among the great works of genius. What makes them unique is the spirit in which they are written. They establish for all time how medicine ought to be practised and what doctors should try to be. The superstition and magic of primitive medicine are rejected, and the doctor is no longer a priest or benevolent sorcerer but a humane observer, counsellor and servant of the sick.

The whole collection of seventy or more books known as the *Hippocratic Corpus* represents the teaching of one school and not of Greek medicine in general. Other schools kept the old superstitions alive, much as astrology and the flat-earth theory survive alongside scientific astronomy. In succeeding centuries the Hippocratic ideals were more and more obscured; they all but vanished 600 years later when Galen died, and medicine deteriorated until they were restored in the 16th century.

The book *On Ancient Medicine* says that history is shaped by man's search for food and congenial surroundings, and that medicine is an extension of this search – a means of adapting ourselves to our environment. It therefore concerns everyone.

'Whoever treats of this art should treat of things which are familiar to the common people. For of nothing else will such a one have to inquire or treat, but of the diseases under which the common people have laboured, which diseases and the causes of their origin and departure, their increase and decline, illiterate persons cannot easily

find out for themselves, but still it is easy for them to understand these things when discovered and expounded by others'.

So much for the mystery of health and sickness and for trade secrets in medicine. And this doctrine – that the physician should explain things to his patients – has lain dormant until the present century, and it still has some way to go. To clear up any lingering doubt, Hippocrates continues:

'For it is nothing more than that everyone is put in mind of what has occurred to himself. But whoever does not reach the capacity of the illiterate vulgar and fails to make them listen to him, misses his mark'.

The same idea appears in the first and best known of the *Aphorisms*:

'Life is short, and the Art long; the occasion fleeting; experience fallacious, and judgement difficult. The physician must not only be prepared to do what is right himself, but must also make the patient, the attendants, and externals co-operate'.

Nothing could be further from the aloof oracular physician-priest. Here, the doctor enlists the patient's help, and that of the 'externals' – the forces of Nature.

Death and disease arise from natural causes. *On the Sacred Disease* is a treatise on epilepsy, of all diseases the most likely to be blamed on supernatural causes. The theme of the book is that epilepsy is no more 'sacred' than any other disease; it is a natural event, and epileptic patients are to be studied and cared for like any others.

Diseases have many causes. Any theory that tries to explain disease and death on the basis of one or two causes must be false. Most present-day systems of unorthodox medicine are nonsensical because they ignore this fundamental truth. Hippocrates taught that diseases were disturbances in the balance of the four ◊ *humours* (a view not seriously challenged for more than 20 centuries). The balance might be disturbed by all manner of external factors, especially diet and climate.

From a study of carefully recorded case-histories, Hippocrates identified many predisposing factors. *Airs, Waters and Places* deals with environment. In places with a warm southerly exposure people tend to be fat and sluggish, and they are prone to dysentery but not pneumonia. In places that face north it is the other way round. Foggy regions are the unhealthiest. This book is incidentally one of the earliest on anthropology and psychology. Mountainous country, it says, breeds enterprising and warlike people; in warm low-lying countries the men are small and dark and peaceloving: 'courage and laborious enterprise are not in them'.

'A climate which is always the same induces indolence, but a changeable climate, laborious exertions both of body and mind'.

'It is changes of all kinds which arouse the understanding of mankind, and do not allow them to get into a torpid condition'.

The *Aphorisms* mention various predisposing causes to particular diseases and to illness in general. From a list like Shakespeare's seven ages we learn that babies are prone to sore mouths, vomiting, disturbed sleep, discharging ears. With teething come irritable gums, fevers, convulsions, and diarrhoea. Later come tonsillitis, asthma, worms, goitre. The catalogue takes us through adult life to old age with shortness of breath, urinary troubles, insomnia, and poor sight and hearing.

Strokes are commonest between the ages of 40 and 60.

Fat people are apt to die before slender people.

Consumption is commonest between the ages of 18 and 35.

Hippocrates is much concerned with prognosis – predicting the course of an illness. It may not seem a very useful occupation, but he explains why it is necessary:

'for by foreseeing and foretelling . . . he will be the more readily believed to be acquainted with the circumstances of the sick; so that men will have confidence to entrust themselves to such a physician. And he will manage the cure best who has foreseen what is to happen from the present state of matters'.

The most famous passage in the *Prognostics* describes the appearance of someone likely to die, known as the Hippocratic facies: 'a sharp nose, hollow eyes, collapsed temples; the ears cold, contracted, and their lobes turned out; the skin about the forehead being rough, distended [taut] and parched; the colour of the whole face being green, black, livid, or lead-coloured'. It is finely observed, but Hippocrates does not allow his reader to form an opinion yet, for the patient's grim appearance could be explained in more than one way. Other symptoms have to be considered: lack of sleep, diarrhoea, starvation, any of which might show the same picture. And the patient must be watched for a time for any sign of improvement. The physician does not speak of impending death until he has ruled out the other possibilities. All this is presented as prognosis, but in forming his prognosis the physician has to make a diagnosis – to identify the patient's ailment. No other medical writer before the 18th century approached Hippocrates as a diagnostician. He studied each patient and related what he found to what he had learnt of other patients, and that is the whole science of diagnosis.

Another lesson that was to be slowly forgotten during the next 2,000 years was that medicine, like all science, cannot advance unless it is honest with itself. Prognosis is important here, because the doctor is forced to commit himself openly and expose his mistaken opinions. The test of a theory is to use it to predict an event.

All other medical writers until quite modern times dwelt on their successes. The case-histories of Hippocrates are mostly accounts of patients who died under his care, written for others to learn from his failures.

Treatment is almost disappointingly simple, because it is based on the two principles that Nature will cure most ailments if she is given a chance, and that if a doctor cannot do good he must at least do no harm. Diet and general hygiene take first place. Under-feeding is as bad as over-feeding, especially with children, and the foods that the patient enjoys do him more good than those that he dislikes – on the other hand a change of diet may help.

Drugs are used sparingly, mostly for the relief of pain, flatulence, and constipation (real or supposed). Surgery is reserved for cases where drugs will not help; but when he has to operate the doctor must be bold, quick, and neat. Fractures, dislocations, and wounds are treated by the methods handed down from ancient Egypt and still, in principle, used today. The chapter on the surgical treatment of piles could be slipped into a current textbook without much editing.

From the book *On Regimen* one can put together the elements in the management of a typical case, say of a severe cold or influenza. The patient and his family are exhaustively questioned about the symptoms and circumstances of the illness. The doctor inspects the patient, with special attention to the eyes and mouth, and asks to see the urine and stools. The patient is put to bed, and a hot-water bottle is ordered with strict instructions about protecting the skin from burns. He is given a dose of hellebore as a purgative, and oxymel (honey and vinegar) to soothe his throat. He must drink plenty of *ptisan* (something like barley-water), and is allowed wine within reason as a sedative; for the night he may have a small dose of opium. He is to have light but appetizing meals, and stay where he is while the fever lasts.

If we replace hellebore with a milder purgative, or leave it out altogether, and put the oxymel and opium together in the same bottle of linctus, this could be an account of good practice in the 19th or 20th century. The patient is better cared for than he would have been at any time between the age of Hippocrates and the modern era. In Galen's time he would have been filled with nasty and useless drugs, and later he would have been starved, purged, sweated or bled according to the fashion.

The code of behaviour named after Hippocrates is set out in the next entry, ◊ *Hippocratic Oath.*

It would be silly to pretend that Hippocrates or anyone else achieved single-handed all that is in these immortal writings; they are obviously distilled from centuries of experience. One need not insist that he invented anything at all, for his is not that kind of fame. Other great medical pioneers are remembered for particular and tangible contributions to medical science.

Hippocrates gave medicine a soul.

Hippocratic Oath. The best known of the Hippocratic writings. Its origins may be Egyptian, and the early Indian physicians had a similar oath. The Oath as we know it was presumably taken on admission to the medical school and guild of Cos.

'I swear by Apollo the physician, and by Asklepios, Hygeia, and Panacea[1] and all the gods and goddesses, and call them to witness that I will keep this oath and contract[2] to the best of my ability and judgement: to regard him who teaches me this art as equal to my own parents; to share my living with him, and provide for him in need; to treat his children as my

own brothers, and teach them this art if they wish to learn it, without payment or contract; to give guidance, lectures, and every other kind of instruction to my own sons and those of my teacher, and to students bound by contract and oath to medical law, but to nobody else.

'I will prescribe treatment to the best of my ability and judgement for the good of the sick, and never for a harmful or illicit purpose. I will give no poisonous drug, even if asked to, nor make any such suggestion; and likewise I will give no woman a pessary to cause abortion. I will both live and work in purity and godliness. I will not operate, not even on patients with stone, but will give way to specialists in this work.[3] I will go into the houses that I visit in order to help the sick, and refrain from all deliberate harm or corruption, especially from sexual relations with women or men, free or slave. Anything I see or hear about people, whether in the course of my practice or outside it, that should not be made public, I will keep to myself and treat as an inviolable secret.[4]

'If I abide by this oath, and never break it, let all men honour me for all time on account of my life and work; but if I transgress and break my oath, let me suffer the reverse.'

1. Asklepios (Aesculapius) was a real physician, later deified as a son of Apollo. His daughters Hygeia and Panacea personify health and healing. He is the patron of the guild of Cos.

2. 'Contract' (*syngraphe*) might be 'articles of apprenticeship'. The Oath appears to be both a general code of ethics and an initiation to the guild, the Asklepiades.

3. The prohibition of all operative surgery cannot apply to all physicians, as many critics have have suggested. Medieval physicians chose not to operate, but until the time of Galen, 600 years after Hippocrates, surgery was a part of medicine. The Hippocratic writings include detailed and competent surgical instruction. The suggestion that only the operation for stone was forbidden is not justified. The Oath says literally 'I will not cut, not even sufferers from stone'. This particular operation may have been mentioned because a stone in the bladder was a common and excruciating illness (as it was until the 19th century) that might tempt a student or

young doctor to operate without the necessary surgical training. Instead, he must call in an experienced colleague.

4. For the second time, the doctor is reminded that he is never off duty. He must both live and work in purity, and he may not discuss secrets that he learns outside his practice.

Hirschsprung's disease = ⬦ *megacolon.*

histamine. A degradation product of protein that can be extracted from most tissues; it may well be an artefact produced by damaging the tissue while investigating it. In living tissue it is probably not formed unless the tissue is injured in some way. It then causes ⬦ *inflammation* as a means of repairing the damage done. Many of the symptoms of allergy are due to release of histamine into the affected tissues, and these effects are suppressed by drugs that antagonize histamine (⬦ *antihistamine*).

histology. Study of ⬦ *tissue.* Traditional anatomy is concerned with organs, and histology with the fabric of the organs. Anatomy would see a building as a system of rooms and corridors; histology would see it as brickwork, woodwork, plaster, and paint.

In effect, histology is anatomy with a microscope, although the first man to recognize that all the organs of the body are arrangements of the same few tissues (M. F. X. Bichat, 1771–1802) worked without a microscope, which he despised as a toy.

The study of the individual cells of which tissues are largely composed is *cytology*, but this science need not be distinguished from histology.

An average human cell is about 1/1000 inch (0·02 mm.) across. The standard light microscope has a useful magnification of 1000 diameters, and shows cells as fairly large objects, containing numerous smaller structures. No details smaller than about 1/100 of the cell diameter can be distinguished, because light waves cannot be used to distinguish objects smaller than the waves themselves. Ultraviolet waves are shorter; they are invisible but can be photographed and used to double the effective magnification. The electron microscope gives magnification up to 1/4 million or more. This brings objects as small as the larger molecules into view, so that histology and chemistry now overlap.

Little detail can be seen by looking at the surface of a lump of tissue. One has to examine a thin slice with a light shining through it. Even this shows only a shadowy pattern of pale greys, unless the specimen is first stained. Two or more dyes may be used together; some structures will take up one dye in preference to the other. For routine work a blue alkaline dye, haematoxylin, is used with a pink acidic dye, eosin. The nuclei of the cells attract haematoxylin and are stained blue, while most of the other structures are stained pink. Special stains are used for studying particular chemical components: starch gives a blue compound with iodine; iron can be converted to prussian blue, and so on.

Certain dyes can be applied to living tissue without killing it (*intravital staining*). Unstained living tissue is examined with oblique lighting against a dark background, which greatly increases contrast (as a shaft of sunlight in a dark room reveals dust particles).

Histology has greatly enhanced our understanding of anatomy and physiology, and in the hands of Rudolf Virchow (1821–1902) it became the principal source of information about the underlying processes of disease. In clinical medicine, it is a most valuable method of diagnosis. Only a very minor surgical operation is needed to remove a small piece of suspect tissue, in which a histologist can identify abnormalities. This technique (*biopsy*) is much used for the early detection of cancer.

Hodgkin, Thomas (1798–1866). Physician at Guy's Hospital (⬦ *Cooper*), specializing in pathology – the study of the underlying processes of disease rather than of their outward symptoms. There were great pathologists before Hodgkin (e.g. Morgagni, Bichat, Hunter), but doctors in general did not recognize the practical as opposed to purely scientific value of their work. Hodgkin's appointment as pathologist to Guy's marks the beginning of the present era, in which the pathologist is an essential member of the clinical team, working in the direct interests of individual patients.

Hodgkin's account of what is now known as Hodgkin's disease appeared in 1832.

Hodgkin's disease. An uncommon disorder of the lymph nodes and spleen, and occasionally of other organs. Strictly speaking, it is a disorder of lymphoid tissue, found mainly in the lymph nodes and spleen but also in bone marrow and elsewhere, and concerned with defence against infection. The cells of this tissue proliferate, and the affected nodes become much enlarged. Fever and other symptoms of ill-defined sickness are usual. The patient may die of a chance infection, to which his resistance is lowered (the proliferating lymphoid tissue does not function); or from pressure on vital organs by enlarged lymph nodes; or from exhaustion, for the disease is slowly progressive.

Chronic infection such as wide-spread tuberculosis can produce a very similar picture, but no microbe has been incriminated in Hodgkin's disease. For the present it has to be regarded as an unusual form of cancer. Although rare, it is important firstly in the diagnosis of the many other diseases which can mimic it, and secondly because although in the long run it is still not curable, it is by no means untreatable. Most cases respond to X-ray treatment and to drugs such as nitrogen mustard, also used for leukaemia, which in some ways resembles Hodgkin's disease. Some patients have been kept in fair health for as long as 25 years.

homeostasis. The processes of maintaining constant physical and chemical conditions within the body despite external change. It is the primary function of most organs. ($\diamond$ *milieu intérieur*' under *Bernard, Claude*.)

homoeopathy. A method invented by Samuel Hahnemann at the end of the 18th century, based on the principle that like cures like. Hahnemann observed (inaccurately) that an overdose of quinine causes symptoms like those of malaria. But a moderate dose of quinine cures malaria. Therefore, he argued, small doses of a drug cure symptoms like those that larger doses would cause. The smaller the dose, the greater this paradoxical effect. Homoeopathic drugs are diluted by *trituration* with milk sugar. A 1:10 mixture is finely ground. Of the resulting powder, a fresh 1:10 mixture with sugar is made, and at each subsequent step the drug is diluted a further 10 times. At the 30th dilution or 'potency' there is one part of drug to 10^{30} parts of milk sugar. With the supposedly most potent remedies it is only by an outside chance that the patient will get a single molecule of the drug.

Homoeopathy is not concerned with the processes and causes of disease, but with its symptoms. Perhaps its greatest merit is that it compels the doctor to study all the personal idiosyncrasies of the patient – to regard him as a unique individual and not as just another 'case' of some kind.

Although the theory of homoeopathy does not stand scientific inquiry, Hahnemann was no charlatan. He was a sincere and able physician, disgusted by the excessive, sometimes brutal treatment meted out by his orthodox colleagues.

homosexuality. Sexual desire for members of one's own sex. But it would be absurd to call everyone who has such feelings, even if they lead to homosexual acts, a homosexual. In adolescents a homosexual phase is so common that it must be considered part of normal development. And the heterosexual (towards the opposite sex) feelings of adults are very often at least faintly tinged with homosexual feelings. There are all grades, including some people who seem equally attracted to either sex. American and British surveys suggest that about 4 per cent of men in those societies remain predominantly homosexual through adult life. The condition seems to be less common in women.

There have been many attempts to find a constitutional basis for homosexuality, but so far there is little evidence that physical make-up plays more than a small part. The popular image of a typical homosexual as a parody of the opposite sex applies only to a minority, and these are not in any physical sense intermediate: they affect mannerisms copied from the other sex.

Nor is there general agreement about the psychological background. It has probably been a mistake to look for a single cause when homosexuality may well arise in more than one way. The condition is itself an anomaly of behaviour or personality, and it is very often associated with other anomalies. Thus homosexuals as a class (not necessarily as individuals) include more people who are too easily swayed by their own feelings, insecure, or discontented than one would find among heterosexuals. All these tendencies may well have been exaggerated by centuries of systematic persecution. Incidentally they are not far removed from a kind of artistic temperament, and all the arts owe a great deal to homosexuals. In a way, homosexuality is like promiscuity with the opposite sex, also common among artists, in that it reflects an immature, adolescent pattern of behaviour. And if maturity means the ability to settle down and form a stable marriage, then a touch of immaturity is perhaps the price of being able to achieve anything out of the ordinary. Creative men are seldom ideal husbands. As Francis Bacon, a noted homosexual, put it, 'wife and children . . . are impediments to great enterprise, either of virtue or mischief.' It does not, of course, follow that enterprising men have to be bachelors, less still homosexuals, but it is true that such men are in many ways more childish than their fellows. If we could analyse personalities like finger-prints, we should probably find that a completely mature, rounded, 'normal' personality was so rare as to be almost abnormal, and we should still not know why some people fail to develop a stable heterosexual relationship. The advances of a homosexual adult to a child are often said to cause the child to become homosexual, but there is little evidence to support this view. Indeed, one might expect this to put a child off homosexuality. A much likelier theory is that the wrong kind of parental authority is a cause: in males, overdependence on the mother, and in females, fear of a bullying father. The most constructive suggestion in recent years is that at least some homosexuality is not a positive urge towards one's own sex but a kind of phobia about the opposite sex. Young adolescents of both sexes are notoriously scared of each other, and in this view homosexuality is a projection of this kind of anxiety into adult life. It does not conflict with earlier theories but merely suggests a way in which early influences might work.

Attempts to treat homosexuality often fail. Unless the subject strongly wishes to change, they are bound to fail. Many adult homosexuals resent the suggestion that homosexuality calls for any treatment. They insist that it is a normal state, a simple alternative to heterosexuality. It is a difficult argument to follow, because it implies that sex is not primarily concerned with reproduction. This over-reaction to popular censure is understandable, but it may discourage youngsters who could be helped from seeking advice. Despite the propagandists, homosexuality is a handicap, and many of those affected never really come to terms with it. With young subjects (say, within 10 or 12 years of puberty) there is at least some chance that ◊ behaviour therapy may succeed.

Female sex hormones have been given to male homosexuals to suppress their sexual urges. This does not make them heterosexual. It is no more than a method of crime prevention to be used with people who, e.g. cannot stop themselves from assaulting children. The same treatment could be given to heterosexual rapists. Some German surgeons have performed minor operations on the brain to suppress certain reflex centres thought to govern homosexual behaviour, again in the hope of keeping persistent offenders out of prison. They claim that some of their patients are not only cured of their criminal tendencies but have become heterosexual. For the present, this cannot be regarded as more than an interesting experiment.

hookworm. A parasite of the duodenum, common in tropical countries more because of poor hygiene than climate. ◊ *worms.*

hordeolum = ◊ *stye.*

hormone. A substance released into the blood-stream by one organ to regulate the function of others. ◊ *endocrine.*

host. Animal or plant at whose expense a parasite lives.

humerus. The bone of the upper arm. The *head* is a smooth hemisphere, facing inwards and backwards to fit a shallow socket in the scapula at the shoulder. Below the head, the bone forms a straight cylinder, the shaft. The lower end is flattened, splayed out, and curled forwards like a scroll. It is widest just above the elbow, where on either side an *epicondyle* can be felt through the skin. The lower joint surfaces articulate with the radius and ulna (◊ *elbow*).

Three nerves lie directly on the bone: the *circumflex* nerve, running below the head of the humerus to reach the deltoid muscle, the radial nerve round the back of the shaft, and the ulnar nerve at the inner side of the elbow (the 'funny bone').

Several kinds of fracture are common. The tendons of the scapular muscles serve the shoulder as ligaments, and if the joint is wrenched they may be torn as sprained ligaments are torn. But they are strong, and sometimes it is not the tendon but the bone to which it is anchored that gives way. This is not as bad as it sounds, for broken bones heal better than ruptured tendons or ligaments.

Fractures of the humerus may be complicated by injury to any of the nerves mentioned; with fractures just above the elbow there is some risk to the brachial artery. Such complications are more troublesome than the actual fracture.

Fractures at the upper end of the humerus are often *impacted*, i.e. the fragments are driven together. Otherwise the scapular muscles twist the upper fragment so that it points outwards. It is too small and inaccessible to be manipulated, so the rest of the arm has to be brought into line with it by splinting with the arm raised. When the fracture is lower down the much stronger pectoralis major and latissimus dorsi pull the upper fragment inwards, and the arm has to be splinted in adduction, i.e. across the front of the chest.

Exact reduction of a fracture is much less important in the arm than in the leg. Angulation or shortening of a leg interferes with walking. In the arm, even fairly obvious deformity need not disturb function if the muscles are intact and the joints are mobile. A surgeon may settle for a poor-looking result, which would be unacceptable with a fractured femur, if striving for anatomical perfection means that the return to active movement will be delayed.

humours. Four fluids, supposed to permeate the body and determine the state of its health. This idea was the basis of medical theory from the earliest historical times until the 17th century of our era. It still survives in the language and perhaps in popular myth. The adjective *humoral* is still current as a term to describe chemicals such as hormones and antibodies that circulate and affect the functions of the body.

According to Empedocles (5th century B.C.) all matter consisted of four elements: earth, air, fire, and water. There were also four qualities: hot, cold, dry, and wet. Earth was cold and dry, air was hot and wet, fire was hot and dry, water was cold and wet.

In the body, four humours were thought to correspond with the elements: *black bile* with earth, *blood* with air, *yellow bile* with fire, and *phlegm* with water. Each had the qualities of the corresponding element.

Each element in turn corresponded with a temperament.

Black bile, hot and dry, was formed in the spleen (which in fact contains dark, tarry material formed by the destruction of spent blood cells), and the associated temperament is *melancholy* (or perhaps splenetic).

Blood, hot and wet, was associated with a *sanguine* temperament, and yellow or real bile, cold and dry, with a *choleric* temperament.

Phlegm (*pituita*; mucus), cold and wet, was supposed to be formed in the brain and especially in the pituitary body attached to the underside of the brain, and its temperament was *phlegmatic*.

The state of health depended on the balance between the four humours. A perfect balance of hot against cold, wet against dry (*eucrasia*) ensured good health. Illness was due to imbalance (*dyscrasia*) from excess of one of the humours, of which the most dangerous was black bile. The usual methods of treatment, such as emetics, purges, and blood-letting, were attempts to expel a harmful surplus of a humour.

There is a fairly close analogy between the humoral theory in Europe and the traditional medicine of China (◊ *acupuncture; Chinese medicine*).

hunch-back = ◊ *gibbus.*

hunger ◊ *appetite.*

Hunter, John (1728–93). Scottish surgeon and naturalist; he studied, taught and practised in London from 1748, first as pupil, later as partner, of his elder brother William.

If genius is a capacity for hard work then Hunter was a genius of the first water. He summed up his philosophy in the question ' *Why think? Why not try the experiment?*' ; he was a necessary antidote to the sterile theorizing that typified much of 18th-century science. As to theory, he simply accepted that Nature knew best. His task was to observe and record. He was a prodigious anatomist, dissecting every creature he could lay hands on, and collecting specimens to illustrate the nature of every kind of disease. He did not even stop at biology; he is regarded as the founder of scientific geology as well. His many contributions to medical science include the first satisfactory account of ◊ *inflammation*, a fine work on gun-shot wounds, and a brilliant but ill-fated study of venereal disease – to find whether syphilis and gonorrhoea were separate diseases he infected himself from a patient with gonorrhoea; unknown to him the patient had syphilis as well, and when Hunter developed both he concluded that they were two forms of a single disease.

hyaline-membrane disease. Respiratory distress syndrome, a common cause of death among new-born babies. The baby is born alive, and usually starts to breathe, but cannot keep his lungs filled with air. Unless breathing can be maintained artificially the baby is likely to asphyxiate.

The original name refers to a deposit (hyaline = glassy) on the lining of the air-passages, but this is now regarded as an effect rather than a cause of the infant's inability to breathe. Lungs are in effect a foam of tiny air bubbles. Because of surface tension a bubble tends to shrink. If the air can escape, a bubble collapses. Healthy lungs contain an agent that reduces surface tension so that they can remain full of air. Hyaline-membrane disease seems to arise from lack of this agent, which does not appear until shortly before the normal time of birth; the disease is therefore prevalent among premature babies. Since the surface tension remains high, the lungs collapse like pricked bubbles each time the baby tries to fill them, and the effort is too much.

Many of these babies are kept alive by artificial inflation of the lungs and supplementary oxygen until the natural mechanism takes over, but even with the best available treatment they do not all survive.

hydatid disease. Infection with a kind of tapeworm, *Echinococcus*. The adult worm is an intestinal parasite of dogs. Human hydatid disease is due to the larvae of the worm, which form cysts in muscle, liver and other tissues, sometimes needing surgical removal. The infection is acquired from food contaminated by dogs.

hydrocarbon. A chemical compound of hydrogen and carbon, e.g. paraffin, benzene (cf. *carbohydrate*, a compound of carbon and water, e.g. starch, sugar).

hydrocephalus. Enlargement of an infant's head by accumulation of cerebrospinal fluid, due to blockage of its normal circulation in and around the brain and spinal cord. Various surgical operations have been devised to relieve the pressure and prevent damage to the brain.

hydrogen peroxide. A potent antiseptic that is not inactivated by pus.

hydronephrosis. Distension of a kidney by retained urine, with progressive loss of function, due to obstruction to the flow of urine.

hydrophobia = ◊ *rabies*. The word 'hydrophobia' ('fear of water') refers to the patient's inability to swallow even fluids.

hydrops. Dropsy; excess of water in the tissues. ◊ *oedema*.

hymen. A membrane partly covering the opening of the vagina, torn when a woman loses her virginity. Rarely it closes the opening and has to be cut when the girl begins to menstruate.

hyoid. Small U-shaped bone in the neck, immediately below the jaw and above the larynx; it is an anchorage for numerous muscles.

The hyoid is important in forensic medicine, because a fracture of it is good evidence of manual strangulation.

hyoscine (scopolamine). A drug extracted from belladonna, hyoscyamus and other plants. It has similar actions to ◊ *atropine*, but is rather more narcotic and less liable to cause excitement.

hyoscyamine. A drug extracted from belladonna and stramonium; it is a form of ◊ *atropine*.

hyoscyamus (henbane). A plant related to ◊ *belladonna* (deadly nightshade), with similar poisonous and medicinal properties.

hyper-. Prefix = 'above'; 'too much'. Some of the uglier *hyper-* words in medical jargon are unnecessary or would be better with *over-*; e.g. hyperactivity, hyperventilation (overbreathing). Common words not listed separately include *hyperaemia* (congestion with blood), *-aesthesia* (abnormal sensitivity of nerve-endings), *-chlorhydria* (excess of acid in the stomach), *-metropia* (long-sightedness), *-pnoea* (needlessly deep or rapid breathing; overbreathing, a neurotic symptom), *-thyroidism* (over-activity of the thyroid gland; toxic goitre).

hyperemesis gravidarum. Severe vomiting in pregnancy, a kind of toxaemia, distinct from morning sickness which is a nuisance but seldom serious. Antihistamine drugs or tranquillizers may stop the vomiting, and pyridoxine (vitamin B_6) sometimes cures it promptly; but some of these patients need to be in hospital on a carefully controlled diet, or no diet with the necessary fluids given into a vein. The pregnancy may have to be artificially ended.

The cause is not known.

hyperpiesia. High blood pressure. This word has been offered in place of *hypertension* because it is all Greek instead of mixed Greek and Latin. But a vocabulary that admits *antibody, antigen,* and *roentgenoscopy* is unlikely to reject *hypertension.*

hyperplasia. Excessive or increased growth of tissue by multiplication of its cells (cf. ◊ *hypertrophy*). Hyperplasia is generally due to stimulation by hormones, e.g. the growth of the uterus and breasts during pregnancy, or overgrowth of the thyroid gland in response to excessive activity of the pituitary gland. It may also be a response to excessive demands on an organ such as the liver when part of it has been destroyed by disease. Hyperplasia differs from neoplasia (tumour formation) in that the new cells are perfectly normal.

hyperpyrexia. Extreme fever, where the body temperature is so high as to be itself a danger to life, regardless of its cause.

hypertension. High blood pressure, which may be a symptom of a recognized disease such as inflammation of the kidneys (*secondary hypertension*), or apparently a disease in its own right, i.e. one of which the cause is unknown (*essential hypertension*). Essential hypertension is divided into *benign* hypertension, with few symptoms and a prolonged course, and the much rarer *malignant* hypertension, with rapid deterioration unless treated.

These terms are necessarily vague, because nobody knows the limits of normal blood pressure.

◊ *blood pressure* (1).

hypertrophy. Excessive or increased growth of tissue by enlargement, without multiplication, of its cells (cf. ◊ *hyperplasia*). It is characteristically the response of muscle to work. Muscle cells (fibres) have little if any capacity for reproduction, but they are enlarged and strengthened by exercise, and shrink (*atrophy*) if they are not used.

hypnosis. State of mind induced by ◊ *hypnotism.*

hypnotic. 1. Related to hypnosis. 2. (Drug) used to promote sleep. How hypnotic drugs work, or whether they all work in similar ways, is not known, and is not likely to be understood until more is known of the nature of sleep.

A hypnotic is intermediate between a sedative and a narcotic. Sometimes the difference between the three categories is only the dose. Small doses of barbiturates are used as sedatives, i.e. to relieve agitation and worry. Larger doses are hypnotic. Still larger doses, for which only rapidly eliminated barbiturates are safe, are narcotic, i.e. they produce complete unconsciousness or anaesthesia and can be used for surgical operations.

Bromides, paraldehyde, and chloral hydrate have largely given way to the barbiturate drugs, but barbiturates are more habit-forming and the search for safer hypnotics goes on. But regular sleep is itself a habit, and when it is lost it is all too easy to make a habit of any kind of sleeping draught instead of re-establishing the natural habit.

A further objection to the regular use or abuse of hypnotics is that the quality of sleep suffers. The drugs suppress the natural periods of dreaming (REM sleep) which seem to be a necessary part of emotional health. The hypnotic *nitrazepam,* which is chemically unrelated to the others, seems not to have this defect.

Hypnotics have little effect on pain, and when sleeplessness is due to pain it is the pain that has to be dealt with.

hypnotism. Hypnotism is an extreme form of suggestion, where within limits the subject abandons his initiative to the operator. First, the subject must be willing to be hypnotized and to obey the operator. Second, the operator must hold the subject's attention absolutely. If either lets his thoughts wander, nothing happens. Many techniques are possible, but all are based on the same principle: the subject's attention is fixed by a simple, monotonous stimulus until he ignores all other sensation. It is rather like counting imaginary sheep in order to sleep; but the hypnotic state is not sleep. A susceptible subject with a good operator may go into a deep trance in which he is unaware of anything except the operator's voice; he can make no movement unless told to, and all his muscles are held as stiff as boards (a condition otherwise seen only in severe mental disorder). At a word from the operator the subject returns to normal consciousness, but is not aware of anything that has happened during the trance. Most subjects, however, cannot be hypnotized so deeply, and some cannot be hypnotized at all, perhaps because they do not wish to be. The hypnotist has no mysterious powers. Some are better at it than others but most people can learn.

During a hypnotic trance the subject's mind is closed to all incoming sensations except the operator's voice, and also to the countless distractions and inhibitions that circulate in the waking brain. Memory then turns out to be a much fuller store than one would have supposed. We do not forget the past, but we store it in a library with no index and the keys to half the rooms hidden. Under hypnosis, events long 'forgotten' are accurately recalled, if the operator asks for them. And new instructions can be learnt that in waking life would be confused in a welter of second thoughts; conditioned reflexes can be established because the instructions are not questioned. It is claimed that if the instructions are morally repugnant to him the subject will not obey.

The first practising hypnotist was the Austrian physician Mesmer (1734–1815). He thought hypnosis was a kind of celestial magnetism, and established a cult in Paris that earned him a great deal of money and probably cured some cases of hysteria.

Many painless surgical operations have been done on hypnotized patients, but the method has not been widely adopted, because quite apart from the personal objections of patients and doctors it is too unreliable. No surgeon would be happy with a substitute for anaesthesia that might or might not work.

Some kinds of neurosis respond quickly to hypnotism. The repressed memories that psychoanalysis brings into the open can be revived more quickly than by analysis, and the patient may accept suggestions that he would be unable to take in if he were wide awake. But again the method is unreliable. Even when it seems to work it does not always solve the patient's problem. Neurosis may be regarded as an unconscious, perhaps misguided, attempt at self-defence. A person who develops a stammer to cover a sense of inadequacy is no better off if the stammer is cured while the underlying

trouble is ignored; he will probably develop a new neurosis. But provided that the hypnotist is aware of this objection, hypnotism can be a valuable short cut in treating neuroses. Merely to suppress symptoms without considering their causes is bad practice in any branch of medicine, but that does not condemn all suppression of symptoms. Morphia would be poor treatment for a broken bone, but it can be a valuable adjunct to setting and splinting the fracture. Similarly hypnotism may not be the whole answer to illness due to emotional disturbance, but it is a useful tool.

hypo-. Prefix = 'below'; 'too little'. It is the converse of *hyper-* and most technical terms with *hyper-* have their opposites with *hypo-*.

hypochondria(sis). Undue preoccupation with one's real or supposed ailments; it is more of a hobby than an illness. It differs from malingering and hysteria. The malingerer may say he has a headache when he has none, in order to evade work or responsibility; the hysteric does something similar at an unconscious level and gets a real headache without physical cause; the hypochondriac spends a happy day trying new remedies for the headache that might come on.

⟷ *hypochondrium.*

hypochondrium (= below cartilage). The part of the abdomen covered by the cartilages of the lower ribs, once thought to be the seat of hypochondria, perhaps because it contains the liver on one side and the spleen on the other, respectively the supposed sites of biliousness and melancholy.

hypodermic. Under the skin; subcutaneous.

hypoglycaemia. Deficiency of sugar in the blood. Normal blood contains about 0·1 per cent of glucose. Numerous mechanisms interact to keep the level constant despite great variation of both intake and disposal of glucose. All carbohydrate absorbed from the diet is converted to glucose, which is then stored in the liver and muscles in the form of animal starch – *glycogen*. As glucose is consumed to provide energy, fresh supplies are released from the glycogen stores. Several hormones are concerned in keeping the balance between storage and combustion of glucose. The most important is insulin (⟷ *diabetes*), and the usual cause of hypoglycaemia is too much insulin. In diabetics this can arise from overdosage or wrong diet. In others, it is due to overactivity of the insulin-forming tissue of the pancreas. The excess of insulin removes glucose from the blood by increased combustion, and also increases the storage of glycogen at the expense of the blood.

The brain has no reserve of fuel; it depends entirely on a constant supply of glucose from the blood. Hypoglycaemia promptly impairs the efficiency of the brain. The symptoms vary greatly. They include uneasiness, hunger, sweating, and unaccustomed churlishness. If the blood-sugar is still further reduced, the patient may have an epileptic fit or simply lose consciousness; he may even die.

Rare causes of hypoglycaemia include failure to store carbohydrate with severe liver disease, and disturbances of other glands concerned with the distribution of glucose.

People who are prone to attacks of hypoglycaemia learn to recognize the symptoms and stop the attack by eating sugar.

hypophysis. The ◊ *pituitary* gland.

hypothalamus. A region of the brain below the third ventricle, i.e. in the floor of the front part of the brain between the cerebral hemispheres. It is connected by nerve fibres with most other parts of the nervous system, and its functions are bewilderingly diverse. They include:

1. Regulation of the autonomic nervous system, and so of the heart and abdominal organs, especially their response to emotion;

2. The emotions themselves, and mood (excitement, depression etc.);

3. Regulation of the body temperature;

4. Appetite and thirst;

5. The increased flow of blood through muscles during exercise, which is independent of the control of blood vessels in general to maintain the blood pressure – a function of the medulla oblongata;

6. Control of the pituitary gland, which in turn controls the output of the other endocrine glands and the kidneys.

Thus the hypothalamus is the link between the central and autonomic nervous systems and between the nervous system and the endocrine glands.

hyster(o)-. Prefix = 'of the uterus'; e.g. *hysterectomy*, surgical removal of the uterus.

hysteria. A kind of neurosis, most often affecting women and once thought to arise in the uterus. Sustained anxiety, usually with little foundation, expresses itself in physical symptoms vaguely resembling those of physical illness of the part of the body that the patient associates with her worries. The hysterical fit, simulating epilepsy, has been out of fashion for many years.

◊ *anxiety* (3).

I

iatrogenic. Caused by medicine: iatrogenic diseases are those that result from the treatment of other diseases. If the term is extended to all the possible ill-effects of medical and surgical treatment, the list becomes so long as to be meaningless, because effective medicines and operations have always entailed some risk. There is no need to give a special name to side-effects of a drug that are known to be the price of the cure. 'Iatrogenic' is best reserved for illnesses, often unrelated to the original illness or to the expected effect of the treatment, arising from treatment and sometimes persisting after the treatment has been stopped. Even with this limitation the list is formidable. Some can be regarded as unexpected poisoning, either because the patient is unusually susceptible to a drug or because the drug is more dangerous than anyone had suspected. For example, phenacetin was a household remedy for aches and pains, second only to aspirin in popularity, for three quarters of a century before it was found to cause irreparable damage to the kidneys. The most notorious case of this kind was that of ◊ *thalidomide*. Some drugs occasionally appear to cause metabolic diseases such as diabetes, gout, and porphyria. It is likely that the patient was predisposed and would have developed the disease sooner or later, but one cannot be certain. A serious complication of antibiotic treatment is ◊ *superinfection*, when the antibiotic cures the original infection but also kills useful bacteria that normally compete with yet other microbes: the field is then clear for these last to set up a new infection. A common type of iatrogenic illness is produced without the help of drugs. A patient who misunderstands what a doctor tells or does not tell him, may develop unfounded but serious anxieties about his health, a kind of iatrogenic neurosis.

Ibn-an-Nafis (1210–88). Arabian physician. He appears to have discovered that blood circulates through the lungs some centuries before anyone else, but his work attracted no attention.

icterus = ◊ *jaundice*.

icthyosis. A hereditary defect of the skin: the sweat and grease glands are fewer than normal and the skin has a dry, scaly appearance. Icthyosis in childhood sometimes improves at puberty. Greasy ointments help, but a complete cure is unlikely.

ictus. A sudden attack of illness such as a stroke or fit.

id. According to ◊ *Freud*, the instinctive element of the personality.
Id reaction: ◊ *ringworm*.

idiocy. The severest degree of mental deficiency, where the mental age is 2 years or less, and the subject cannot guard himself against common physical dangers. In English law the term was given up in 1960; idiocy is now included in 'severe subnormality'.

idiosyncrasy. This word is sometimes used in the limited sense of allergy to a particular substance. Since we already have the word *allergy*, it is better to keep *idiosyncrasy* for cases where the patient is abnormally susceptible to a drug for some other reason, such as deficiency of an enzyme needed for disposing of the drug or inability to excrete it.

idoxuridine (IDU) ◊ *virus* (2).

ileitis. Inflammation of the *ileum*; Crohn's disease (◊ *enteritis*).

ileostomy. Surgical operation to by-pass the large intestine by bringing the end of the ileum to the surface, used in treating severe ulcerative ◊ *colitis*. An ileostomy is managed in the same way as a ◊ *colostomy*.

ileum. The lower part of the small intestine.

iliac. Of the ◊ *ilium*.
Iliac arteries. The *aorta* divides in front of the 4th lumbar vertebra into left and right *common iliac* arteries. Each of these divides into an *internal iliac* artery, which supplies the pelvic organs, and an *external iliac*

artery, continued as the *femoral* artery, the main vessel of the lower limb.

Iliac fossa. Part of the abdomen immediately above the groin, of which the concave inner surface of the ilium, covered by the *iliacus* muscle, is the floor.

Iliac veins. The veins corresponding with the iliac arteries. They join to form the *inferior vena cava*.

ilium. The haunch-bone, a part of the ◊ *pelvis*.

imbecility. Mental deficiency where the mental age reaches a level of 3–6 years and the subject is likely to need special care, now classified in English law as 'moderate subnormality'.

Imhotep (27th century B.C.). The first physician named in history; he was also prime minister under the 3rd Egyptian dynasty and the architect of the Step Pyramid. Imhotep was later deified as god of healing.

immersion foot = ◊ *trench foot*.

immunity. Natural resistance to infection. All animals have to contend with natural enemies, and microscopical parasites are as dangerous as large predators. For a species to survive, it must evolve means of defence against both: not only teeth, horns, or the brains to devise weapons, but ways of dealing with infection by microbes.

Most parasites, including microbes, restrict themselves to one or two species of host. Bacteria that cause tuberculosis in birds cannot infect man; on the other hand leprosy, a disease closely related to tuberculosis, infects only man. Thus entire species can be immune to a parasite harmful to some other species.

Intact skin is a good barrier to infection. The outer layer is almost impermeable, and sweat is mildly antiseptic. The mucous membranes lining the various openings and passages of the body are more vulnerable. They cope with certain types of bacteria that normally colonize them, but unfamiliar types may penetrate intact mucous membranes. If either skin or mucous membrane is damaged any bacteria can get through.

Infection is more than just entry of microbes; it means that having entered the body they multiply. The human body provides a suitable environment for only a few species of the thousands that might acci-

dentally find their way in; these few are the only true 'germs'. The lining of the mouth teems with bacteria which must penetrate the surface when a tooth is pulled, and for a short time after the loss of a tooth bacteria can be found in the circulating blood. But trouble from this source is quite exceptional, because these microbes do not establish a foothold and multiply.

Phagocytes are mobile cells like amoebae, found in the blood as *white blood cells* and also at large throughout the body. They engulf any small particles in their path, including bacteria, and can usually destroy them, though they may be themselves killed in the process. Apart from the action of phagocytes, all body fluids (blood, urine, digestive juices, tears, sweat) contain substances poisonous to most bacteria. The immediate response to infection is discussed further under ◊ *inflammation*.

1. ANTIGENS AND ANTIBODIES

In the restricted technical sense, immunity is the presence in the body of specific chemical antidotes to infection, *formed in response to infection*. These substances – *antibodies* – react with some component of the infecting microbe and put the microbe out of action. They will not react with anything else, so unless two different species of microbe possess the same component or *antigen* (which is unusual) new antibodies have to be formed for each new kind of infection. Since it takes several days to form antibodies, infection is well established by the time they come into action. But when once an antibody has been formed the process can be repeated without delay. A second infection with the same microbe can be dealt with at once, before it takes a hold. In other words, the subject is *immune* to that disease. By no means all infectious diseases give lasting immunity, but most epidemic diseases do so – if they did not, the human race could hardly have survived.

The very earliest accounts of epidemics mention that the people who recovered did not catch the disease again. Many centuries ago the Chinese noticed that a particular outbreak of smallpox usually bred true. In one season most cases would be mild; in another most would be severe. Lucky people caught smallpox in a mild outbreak and were then immune during serious outbreaks. Chinese physicians therefore deliberately infected people who had not had smallpox from mild cases to protect them against severe infection. The practice spread through Asia, and in 1718 Lady Mary Wortley Montagu introduced it to England from Constantinople. It was not very reliable, because the smallpox virus does not breed quite true, and some people had fatal attacks of smallpox after inoculation. In 1796, Jenner introduced *vaccination*. This was inoculation with *cow-pox*, of which the virus resembles that of smallpox closely enough to provoke immunity to both diseases, but not closely enough to be dangerous to man. The relation of microbes to infection was still unknown.

As soon as Pasteur in France and Koch in Germany had shown how microbes cause disease (1860–80) bacteriologists began to study immunity. In Pasteur's laboratory, Emile Roux and Alexandre Yersin isolated a poison or *toxin* released by diphtheria bacilli and responsible for many of the dangerous symptoms of diphtheria (1888). In Koch's laboratory two years later Emil von Behring and Shibasaburo Kitasato isolated an antibody (*antitoxin*) against the toxin of tetanus, and soon it became possible to treat diphtheria and tetanus by injecting antitoxins. This kind of immunity (*passive immunity*) does not last, because the patient's own tissues have not 'learnt' to form antibodies of their own. It is used for treating an actual attack, or for short-term protection when there is a special risk.

Active immunity – by antibodies formed in the patient's own tissues – arises naturally from having the disease, or artificially from vaccination with a relatively harmless form of the infecting microbe, such as Jenner's cow-pox virus. Various methods of rendering microbes innocuous but preserving their ability to evoke antibodies have been found. Pasteur (1885) 'attenuated' the virus of rabies by infecting a succession of rabbits. In its passage from rabbit to rabbit the virus became less and less dangerous, and virus taken from the 25th successive rabbit and dried was a safe vaccine against a disease that had hitherto been almost invariably fatal. But most vaccines are prepared by killing the organism, which makes them safer but gives shorter-lasting immunity. 'Live' vaccines still in general use include those for smallpox (not now cow-pox, but *vaccinia*, a smallpox virus attenuated by Pasteur's method) and BCG, a vaccine against tuberculosis prepared from bacilli attenuated by cultivation for some years in an artificial medium. (◊ *immunization*.)

The new science of immunology does not stop at providing active immunity for prevention and passive immunity for treatment of infection. It also plays an important part in exact diagnosis of infection. If a laboratory animal is immunized with a given microbe, then serum from the animal's blood will contain antibodies that destroy microbes of that species, and can be used for identifying them. Conversely, a patient's serum can be tested against known species of bacteria. If the serum destroys a particular bacterium the patient must have been infected with it. If in successive tests this effect increases, the patient is still infected. This is a valuable method of identifying obscure fevers.

The reaction of antibodies with antigens can, under certain circumstances, be a cause of illness: see ◊ *allergy; autoimmunity; transfusion; transplantation.*

The nature and formation of antibodies are considered further under ◊ *antibody.*

Immunization. Production of immunity to an infectious disease by artificial means, i.e. other than by an attack of the disease itself.

Vaccination, the oldest established method in Western medicine, is the injection of live microbes, so modified that they are practically harmless yet still induce immunity. Vaccines are used against *smallpox, tuberculosis, yellow fever, rabies*, and *poliomyelitis* by preparing *attenuated* strains of microbes that have lost their virulence but still provoke antibody formation. An alternative to the attenuated tubercle bacillus (BCG) is a bacillus that causes tuberculosis in voles but not in man, yet confers immunity to human tubercle bacilli.

An alternative method is to use dead microbes, killed in ways that preserve their ability to confer immunity. Diseases with which this has been possible include *cholera, influenza, measles, poliomyelitis* and *rabies* (alternatives to the attenuated viruses), *typhoid*, and *whooping cough.*

Diphtheria and *tetanus* are dangerous not because of damage to tissue at the site of infection but because of highly poisonous toxins released into the circulation. The toxins can be modified with formaldehyde to innocuous forms that still cause antibodies (antitoxins) to be formed.

The degree and duration of immunity vary with different diseases. To avoid unpleasant reactions some vaccines have to be given in two or three doses, and a 'booster' dose may be needed after a time (usually several years) to sustain immunity.

The primary object is to protect the individual, but immunization of large numbers of people also protects the whole community: if a large proportion of a population is immune to a disease an epidemic cannot get under way. The exact proportion depends on the disease; usually if some three quarters of the people have been immunized a disease begins to die out. Those who are not vaccinated are protected by those who are. Here a social problem arises, because vaccination is not quite free of risk. Very rarely, someone has a dangerous reaction. But in many developed countries, smallpox itself is also very rare so rare that the risk of getting smallpox s comparable with the risk of vaccination. But if everyone stopped having vaccination because of the risk there is little doubt that smallpox would resume the hold that it had until the 18th century in Europe, and still has in many parts of the tropics.

immunology ◊ *immunity* (1).

impaction. A fracture is said to be impacted when the broken ends of bone are driven together and firmly interlocked. Colles' fracture above the wrist is usually impacted, but the fragments are nearly always far enough out of line to need resetting.

An impacted tooth is one that has grown out of line and become wedged in the jaw and unable to come through.

impetigo. Infection of the outer layers of the skin by staphylococci, forming clusters of small abscesses. It is contagious, especially among children, and from the original site other areas of the patient's own skin can be infected by contact. Antibiotics applied to the surface usually clear up impetigo in a few days, but with spreading infection and in the case of small children the drug may have to be given by mouth or by injection.

implantation. Embedding of an embryo in the lining of its mother's uterus, about 6 days after conception.

impotence. Inability to perform coitus; in the main it is a disorder of men from failure of erection, but it may also occur in women from structural anomalies or painful inflammation with spasm of the muscles around the vagina; the spasm can also be due to anxiety.

There are many possible physical causes, none of them except ageing very common, such as disorders of the sex organs and of the glands and nerves that control them. But more often than not there is no physical defect, and the problem is psychiatric. When a husband is impotent his wife naturally supposes that he has an aversion to her, but his real trouble is as likely to be lack of confidence in himself. Some men are potent with prostitutes but not with their wives because with prostitutes they have no worries but with their wives they are over-anxious to succeed. Worry suppresses sexual reflexes as readily as it suppresses appetite for food.

incision. Wound made by cutting, e.g. in a surgical operation (as opposed to *laceration*, a torn wound, or *abrasion*, a graze).

incisor. Chisel-like front tooth, of which there are two pairs in each jaw.

incontinence. Inability to control reflex emptying of rectum or bladder, sometimes because of a disorder of the organ itself but more often from loss of co-ordination in the nervous system, e.g. with brain damage or senility. The best treatment would be to deal with the cause, but that is not always possible. Even, however, when voluntary control is irretrievably lost the reflexes, controlled by the spinal cord, can often be educated so that they operate at reasonably spaced intervals and the patient knows when to take steps to avoid soiling himself.

incubation. The *incubation period* of an infectious disease is the interval between infection and the first symptoms. The period may be as short as a few hours with bacterial food poisoning or as long as several years with leprosy, but for a given disease its limits are fairly well defined. With a few diseases the incubation period hardly varies, e.g. smallpox (12 days); chickenpox (14 days). With most, however, there is some variation between cases.

The chart shows that virus diseases do not usually appear until more than a week after infection. A virus has first to find its target organ and then establish itself before it can multiply and cause symptoms (◊ *virus*). In the two exceptions shown, common cold and influenza, the portal of entry is also the affected tissue; the virus has no journey to make.

Bacteria do not have to establish themselves before they can multiply; they can start at once, and the incubation period is usually short. The chart shows several apparent exceptions. The symptoms of tetanus are due not to the growth of microbes in the wound but to poisons which travel from the wound up the nerves to the brain. The delay with whooping cough is less easily explained: it may simply be that symptoms are not noticeable until the infection is advanced, for many children are

	week			
	1st	2nd	3rd	4th
virus diseases				
common cold				
influenza				
measles				
smallpox				
chickenpox				
poliomyelitis				
German measles				
mumps				
hepatitis				
bacterial diseases				
food poisoning				
cholera				
gonorrhoea				
scarlet fever				
cerebrospinal fever				
diphtheria				
tetanus				
whooping cough				
typhoid fever				

average incubation periods·

certainly infected without ever showing obvious signs. Typhoid is a special case. It is in fact a typical bacterial disease, starting soon after infection, but for a time the trouble is confined to the depths of the small intestine. The fever and other symptoms do not begin until the microbes break

through to invade the blood-stream, which may take a few days or several weeks.

indigestion (dyspepsia). The term indigestion (dyspepsia) includes various symptoms arising from the stomach: discomfort or pain, flatulence, nausea. There is sometimes a recognizable cause such as gastritis or a gastric ulcer, but often indigestion is due to interference with the normal working of the stomach by overeating, eating when appetite has been suppressed by worry, anger, drugs, heavy smoking, unsuitable diet, the common habit of swallowing air, or hurried, unattractive meals.

Any number of drugs can be used to relieve the symptoms; an aperitif occasionally helps by imposing a few minutes' rest before eating, encouraging appetite, and allaying anxiety; but alcohol on an empty stomach would aggravate conditions such as gastritis or ulcer.

indomethacin. A drug used to relieve pain and inflammation. ◊ *analgesic*.

induction. *Induction of labour* is the use of artificial means to start the process of childbirth if there has been undue delay or the health of mother or child is at risk. The hospital routine of warm bath followed by enema, followed if necessary by injections of a pituitary hormone to stimulate the uterus, often works. If this fails, releasing a little fluid from the membranous bag surrounding the baby may set off contractions of the uterus. Successful induction may avoid Caesarean section.

infarct; infarction. Congestion and blockage of a blood vessel on which a part of an organ depends, with death and scarring of the affected tissue. It differs from gangrene in that there is no bacterial infection to spread the damage. The segment of lost tissue may be called an infarct. In general, if one artery is blocked, neighbouring arteries, with communicating branches, take over the work. Infarction occurs in places where small arteries do not communicate with each other, such as the kidney; or where the arteries together supply only enough blood for the whole organ, with little in reserve, as in the brain; or where alternative arteries to the blocked one are also unhealthy and cannot take over, as in many middle-aged hearts. If one were to simulate coronary thrombosis (clotting in an artery in the heart muscle) by artificially closing an artery in a healthy heart, probably nothing untoward would happen because the other coronary vessels would suffice. Postmortem studies have shown that people who have died from other causes have at some time had a coronary thrombosis without symptoms. In this disease it is the infarction that matters, and it can arise from narrowing of the vessels without actual thrombosis.

infection. Infection arises when microbes enter the body, establish themselves, and multiply. Entry by harmless microbes that do not multiply in their new surroundings is not strictly infection; nor is the presence of harmful microbes on an intact body surface. In fact most body surfaces are permanently contaminated by bacteria. 'Surfaces' include inner linings as well as skin. The bacteria of the intestine are *outside* the body in the sense that water in a domestic pipe is not *in* the house unless the pipe leaks.

True infection is followed after an interval (◊ *incubation*) by ◊ *inflammation* locally, and in most cases by the more wide-spread effects of poisons (*toxins*) formed by bacteria. (For the various types of microbe and their effects, see ◊ *bacterium; protozoon; fungus; virus.*)

Most microbes live harmlessly in the soil, on plants or animals, even on human skin, but do not infect man. Of the thousands of species of bacteria that normally leave man alone only one or two can cause serious illness, e.g. *tetanus*. Most harmful microbes (pathogens, germs) habitually live as parasites and cause disease. A few are harmful to some people but not to others.

To take a few examples: measles is due to a virus found only in people who actually have measles. Typhoid can be caught from patients or from 'carriers' who have recovered from typhoid, perhaps years before, without getting rid of the bacteria. Diphtheria can be carried by people who have never had the disease, to whom this happens to be a harmless species of microbe. For every patient with obvious poliomyelitis there may be as many as a hundred who have it so mildly that it is not noticed, yet they can transmit the disease to others while their symptom-free infection lasts, making it virtually impossible to trace the course of an epidemic.

Apart from a few tropical parasites, too large to be counted as real microbes, germs do not penetrate intact skin. Either they enter a wound (an invisible scratch or pinprick will do) or they are injected by the bites of insects etc. (◊ *insect*). The mucous membranes lining the mouth, air-passages, and digestive and urinary tracts are much more vulnerable, and many kinds of microbe pass through them without trouble. Particular species have their chosen portals of entry: typhoid and dysentery bacilli penetrate the lining of the intestine but not of the lungs, and they do not infect wounds; the natural inhabitants of the intestine seldom cause trouble there but will set up infection if they find their way into the urinary tract. Infection of the intestine is transmitted by food or drink, and infection of the nose, throat and lungs as a rule by droplets from coughs and sneezes. People with active tuberculosis of the lungs have been known to infect their own intestines by swallowing sputum.

How the nature of infection was discovered is summarized under ◊ *microbe*. Before Pasteur's work (1861 onwards) on the role of microbes in disease there could be no concerted attack against either wound infection (including the inevitable infection that made surgery so dangerous) or specific infectious diseases, though there were flashes of inspiration. A few surgeons had insisted on cleanliness, e.g. Henri de Mondeville (14th century) and Ambroise Paré (16th century); and in 1861 Semmelweis published his great work on the control of infection in childbirth. Jenner introduced vaccination against smallpox in 1796, and in 1854 Snow stopped an outbreak of cholera by tracing an infected water supply. The only effective drugs were mercury against syphilis (16th century) and quinine against malaria (17th century).

As soon as Pasteur had published his findings the English surgeon Lister began to apply them to operative surgery and to the treatment of wounds. Compound fractures, where the broken bone is exposed to direct contamination from a wound, had usually called for amputation, and even if the operation was done promptly half the patients died (without operation they nearly always died). In view of Pasteur's proof that fermentation, putrefaction, and infection were similar processes, and of the fact that carbolic acid rendered sewage innocuous, Lister dressed compound fractures with carbolic acid, and found that many cases recovered without amputation. If he still had to amputate, then carbolic dressings made the operation much safer. This work was published in 1867. Three years later, Lister introduced the carbolic spray. It squirted a mist of carbolic acid over the field of a surgical operation in order to prevent infection from bacteria in the air. For the first time patients could submit to major operations with no great risk of dying a week or two later from spreading infection, introduced by the surgeon or caught from the person in the next bed. And surgeons could safely operate in regions such as the abdomen where hitherto surgery had been unthinkable.

Since the other great obstacle to surgery had just been removed by the discovery of anaesthetics, surgery took one stride from antiquity into modern times.

Within a few years the spray was found to be unnecessary if everything that was to come into contact with the patient was sterilized before the operation; thus antiseptic surgery gave way to aseptic surgery. (◊ *surgery; antiseptic; wound*).

While the surgeons were revolutionizing their craft, Pasteur and other bacteriologists were applying to other diseases than smallpox the principle of vaccination. Early hopes that all infection might be controlled by vaccines were not fulfilled, but by the turn of the century people could be protected against several epidemic diseases, and there were effective antidotes to the bacterial toxins of diphtheria and tetanus (◊ *immunity*; *immunization*).

In the 20th century the most important development has been the discovery of drugs that will destroy bacteria in the body without harming the patient. In 1911 Ehrlich (who already had a Nobel Prize for his work on immunity) introduced an arsenic compound safe enough to be used against syphilis – salvarsan (606). Other drugs of the same type followed, then in 1935 Domagk discovered that sulphonamides cured a wide variety of infections. Penicillin and other antibiotics introduced since 1941 provide effective treatment for virtually all infections caused by bacteria.

The search for drugs effective against virus infections has met little success. The few 'viruses' that respond to antibiotics are probably not viruses but primitive bacteria. With true virus diseases, prevention by some form of vaccination is still the best hope. Poliomyelitis has become a rare disease in countries where vaccines are widely used, and measles is likely to follow suit.

Besides prevention and treatment of particular diseases, general hygiene has advanced greatly since the 18th century. Decent housing, sanitation, clean drinking water and clean and sufficient food all contribute to the reduced incidence of infectious diseases, even if the effect of any one factor cannot be assessed. Since 1950, when effective drugs against tuberculosis came into general use, the death rate from tuberculosis has fallen dramatically. But it had been falling gradually for many years. With good drugs, people who already have tuberculosis are less likely to die of it. With good general hygiene, they are less likely to catch it in the first place. Cure and prevention interact. If the sick are cured they can no longer infect the healthy.

infertility ◊ *fertility.*

inflammation. Inflammation (denoted by the suffix *-itis*, e.g. *meningitis*) is a defensive reaction to injury or irritation in any part of the body. It is most obvious as a response to infection by bacteria, but it may be evoked by anything that damages living tissue.

Celsus (1st century A.D.) described the signs of inflammation as *rubor et tumor, cum calore et dolore* – redness and swelling, with heat and pain.

When inflammation is due to infection, pus is often formed. Surgeons throughout the Middle Ages regarded inflammation as a sort of disease, and the formation of pus as something very desirable, to be encouraged by irritating and contaminating wounds. The horrible doctrine of 'laudable pus' survived almost into modern times.

John Hunter (18th century) gave the first clear account of inflammation as a means of protection and healing, with pus as an unpleasant by-product. He ascribed the symptoms mainly to increased flow of blood. There were, he said, three stages of inflammation: *adhesion*, an attempt to seal off the trouble; *suppuration*, the formation of pus from elements extruded from the blood; and *ulceration*, breakdown of the surface in order to shed diseased or dead tissue.

The process was explained in detail in the 19th century, mainly by the German pathologist Virchow and his pupil Cohnheim. Virchow was concerned mainly with the effects of inflammation on the tissues. To the four cardinal signs of Celsus he added a fifth: *disordered function.* The fact that inflamed organs do not work properly is especially important with regard to kinds of inflammation that are not useful, such as allergy.

Cohnheim demonstrated the actual processes of inflammation in living tissue by microscopy of living membranes in frogs. In response to chemical or other irritation the minute blood vessels in the region widened. The flow of blood increased at first, but after a short time it slowed almost to stagnation. With severe irritation the flow might stop altogether and blood tended to clot in the dilated vessels (*thrombosis*). White blood cells stuck to the walls of the vessels and then squeezed themselves through the walls into the tissue spaces, together with watery fluid from the blood. With very severe inflammation all the elements of the blood, including red cells, leaked out – i.e. there was actual bleeding into the tissues. If the process continued, enough fluid and white cells accumulated to form an obvious collection of pus – a 'gathering'.

1. MECHANISM OF INFLAMMATION AND HEALING

Inflammation is a means of dealing with causes of injury and also the first step in repairing the damage. Defence and healing are two aspects of a single process which is one of the most important factors in the struggle for survival. Damaged cells release a substance – probably ◊ *histamine* – that causes blood vessels in the neighbourhood to widen and also to leak. Even healthy capillary vessels allow water to escape, but it does not accumulate in the tissues because the protein in the blood draws water back into the vessels by ◊ *osmosis*. The osmotic effect is lost when inflamed capillaries allow protein to escape into the tissues. Three of the classic signs are thus explained: redness and heat from the excess of blood, and swelling from escaped fluid as well. The fourth sign, pain, is due partly to pressure from the swelling and partly to irritation of nerve-endings by substances causing or resulting from inflammation.

The fluid dilutes poisons, and is mildly antiseptic. The white cells from the blood are *phagocytes*, able to engulf and remove foreign particles. They can destroy bacteria but may be killed in the process. The blood cells are joined by other phagocytes resident in the tissue spaces; these cells remove and digest dead tissue, cleaning up the battlefield. Phagocytes of all types appear to be attract-

ed to the area by a chemical stimulus from a substance (unknown) released by damaged cells.

Since the fluid – *inflammatory exudate* – contains the same proteins as blood it has the same ability as blood to form a solid clot, and in this way to prevent the irritant from spreading. This is the *adhesion* that Hunter described. With a clean injury such as a surgical operation, or if infection is slight enough to be overcome in the early stages of inflammation, this clot is the start of healing. It sticks the edges of the wound together and firm new tissue grows into it. At first the scar consists of blood vessels and tough fibres. Later the characteristic tissue of the injured organ may grow across. Bone heals perfectly, with no trace of the injury. Skin does fairly well, but sweat glands and hair are not replaced. Muscle and nerve cells cannot reproduce themselves; they can heal but only with fibrous tissue. (A cut nerve may regain some function if it is repaired, because it is composed of conducting fibres from living cells in or near the spinal cord. If the body of the cell is intact its fibre may regenerate.)

If irritation persists, inflammation goes further, and healing has to wait. Pus begins to accumulate. It is generally a thick yellowish fluid, composed of inflammatory exudate, and disintegrating cells and bacteria. Some bacteria form pigments and give the pus a characteristic colour, and with others the pus may be watery or blood-stained.

A collection of pus is a foreign body and a barrier to healing. But if the damaged tissues cannot come together they can still form fibrous tissue in the same way as a healing wound, and so form a tough capsule around the pus. This is an ◊ *abscess*. The fibrous wall protects the rest of the body from spread of infection, but also protects the bacteria from the body's defences, and prevents the pus from being absorbed. The trouble therefore persists until the pus is released. When the pus has drained off the walls of the abscess can stick together and heal.

Local inflammation is accompanied by various reactions in other parts of the body. The bone marrow and other blood-forming tissues are stimulated to produce more white cells. An excessive number of white cells in the blood is good supporting evidence that pus is being formed somewhere in the body. The body temperature rises, and chemical processes in the body are accelerated. ◊ *Antibodies* are formed to deal with bacteria and their harmful products (◊ *immunity*).

Inflammation may be *acute* or *chronic*. The difference is firstly a matter of duration – acute conditions progress more rapidly than chronic – but there are other differences. The above account applies mainly to acute inflammation, such as pneumonia (lung), dysentery (intestine), or a septic finger. Some irritants, such as the bacteria of tuberculosis, act slowly and provoke a less dramatic response. With this chronic inflammation there is generally less exudation of fluid, the cells that collect are mainly lymphocytes instead of granulocytes (◊ *blood* (3)), and healing more or less keeps pace with damage, so that a good deal of fibrous tissue is formed round a focus of infection, sometimes enough to cut off the blood supply so that the centre of the affected tissue dies. If this happens internally a sort of chronic abscess, almost without symptoms, is formed; if it involves a body surface (skin or interior lining) an ulcer or persistent sore results. Such ulcers are difficult to clear up because healing needs a good blood supply. They may need surgical treatment.

A wound of which the sides stick together and join is said to heal by *first intention*. If a gap has to be bridged, healing is by *second intention*. First, the gap is filled with soft *granulation tissue*, consisting mainly of small blood vessels and easily damaged. Then a firm scar grows into the granulation tissue. Skin will grow only over a limited span of granulation tissue. Large defects have to be covered with skin grafts.

2. HARMFUL INFLAMMATION

As a rule inflammation is useful. Without it, injuries would not heal and trivial infections would end in death from blood-poisoning. But it has drawbacks, of which the most important is interference with function. A septic finger can put a hand temporarily out of action, partly because it hurts but partly because the inflamed finger does not work properly. When the lining of the nose is inflamed with a cold it pours out mucus and the sense of smell is lost. Inflammation is also destructive, and if it persists functional tissue tends to be replaced by inert fibrous tissue. While the liver is inflamed by a virus infection it allows bile to accumulate and produce jaundice, and it ceases to help digestion. It recovers when the infection is overcome. But if it is kept in a state of low-grade inflammation for long enough, for instance by continual irritation with alcohol, repair outpaces destruction until there is much more fibrous tissue than active liver.

The ill effects are an acceptable price for the defensive action. They are often the price of survival. But inflammation can also be due to harmless causes, and then it becomes a disease. An army has to accept casualties from its own weapons in wartime that it would not accept in peacetime. The reaction between bacterial poisons and the antidotes formed by the body, which is the basis of ◊ *immunity*, provokes inflammation. In the presence of acute infection this is a good thing. With chronic infection such as tuberculosis it is a mixed blessing and may give almost as much trouble as the infection itself (though not quite as much, for without this opposition the infection would be rapidly fatal). But when the process of immunity is applied to a perfectly harmless substance such as a face-powder or a particular food, then the resulting inflammation is wholly objectionable and becomes part of a disease (◊ *allergy*).

A number of diseases are characterized by chronic and sometimes destructive inflammation with no apparent cause. ◊ *rheumatic fever; autoimmunity.*

Various drugs can be used to suppress unwanted inflammation. Aspirin is the most widely used, and many of the newer pain-relieving drugs have the same effect. Thus they have a double action in diminishing the sensation of pain and also damping down its source. Corticosteroid hormones almost completely stop inflammation if enough is given, but complete suppression means that healing also stops and that the body cannot react to infection. These drugs have other undesirable effects, and the dosage has therefore to be very carefully regulated.

Inflammation is stimulated by warmth (hot-water bottles, poultices) or irritant drugs (mustard plasters, liniments, any application that reddens the skin), or simply by rubbing the skin. The value of these measures is probably more in relieving discomfort than in reinforcing natural defences (◊ *counter-irritation*).

influenza. A virus infection, primarily of the air-passages, but with effects on the whole body such as fever, headache, and weakness. The virus itself can be dangerous, but the special risk is added bacterial infection of the lungs. Of the estimated 20 million deaths in the pandemic of 1918–19, most were due to pneumonia to which the influenza made people highly vulnerable. Subsequent pandemics have been far less lethal.

An attack confers immunity to that strain of virus. Each successive wave of influenza, usually at intervals of some ten years, is due to a new strain of virus to which people are not immune. There are two explanations of the new strains, both probably valid. One is the evolution of modified forms of the virus; the other is infection of man by viruses that were previously confined to animals.

Effective vaccines can be prepared to give protection against known strains of influenza virus, but they will be useless against a new epidemic, when a new vaccine will be needed.

inguinal. Of the groin – the fold in front of the hip-joint where the muscles of the abdomen and thigh meet.

INH = ◊ *isoniazid.*

injection. Administration of a fluid such as a solution of a drug directly into a tissue or organ by means of a syringe. Related procedures include instillation (dropping fluid, e.g. into the eye), and infusion (allowing a fluid to flow into the body, e.g. saline solution to correct dehydration).

Intradermal injection, into the skin itself, is used to test the patient's reaction to a substance: if he is sensitive to it a red flare will appear. *Subcutaneous* injection, into the layer of fatty tissue, allows a drug to be absorbed into the circulation at a moderate rate. This route is not suitable for irritant substances. *Intramuscular* injections are given with a larger needle into the depths of a muscle at a selected point where there are no blood vessels or nerves to be injured, such as the upper and outer quadrant of the buttock. This is perhaps the commonest site for injections. *Intravenous* injection, directly into a vein, is used either for very rapid effect or to dilute an irritant drug with the large volume of circulating blood and prevent it from damaging the tissues.

In addition, drugs are sometimes injected straight into the affected part of the body, such as a joint.

innocent. Benign (of tumours that have no tendency to invade neighbouring tissues and are not cancerous).

innominate (Lat. = unnamed). Several anatomical structures are illogically so named.

Innominate artery. A large branch of the arch of the *aorta*; it divides into right *subclavian* and *common carotid* arteries (on the left these arteries are separate branches of the aorta).

Innominate bone. The hip-bone or *coxa*: ◊ *pelvis.*

Innominate vein. Large vein formed from the *subclavian* and *internal jugular* veins. The left and right innominate veins join to form the *superior vena cava.*

inoculation. Deliberate infection from a mild case of a disease in order to confer immunity, a method used against smallpox before the discovery of vaccination. ◊ *immunity* (1).

insect. A six-legged *arthropod.* Insects play an important part in human illness. Some arthropods that are not strictly insects (e.g. ticks and mites, related to spiders) also carry disease; in this context they need not be distinguished from true insects. Arthropods cause trouble in several ways.

Contamination. Flies are the main offenders. They are dirty feeders with sticky feet, and they cause much illness simply by carrying bacteria from one place to another. Intestinal infection is often transmitted in this way where sewage disposal is deficient. In hot countries one of the most useful health precautions is to protect food from flies.

Infestation. Sometimes the insect is itself the disease. Infestation with lice or fleas should count as a disease in its own right, and *scabies* is the presence of itch-mites in the skin. The tropical tumbu-fly produces grubs that hatch in the skin, causing an unpleasant but fairly harmless sort of boil.

Poisonous bites and stings. Bees (◊ *bee sting*), wasps and hornets inject minute doses of poisons resembling snake venoms, but the real danger is a severe allergic reaction in sensitized people (◊ *allergy*). ◊ *Scorpions,* ◊ *spiders,* centipedes, and many other arthropods have similar venoms, and a few species can inject enough to be dangerous to human victims, especially children.

Transmission. Numerous diseases are transmitted by insect bites. The responsible microbes can infect either the insect or man, sometimes in different phases of a complex life-cycle (e.g. malaria parasites undergo sexual reproduction in mosquitoes but not in man). An insect that transmits a disease is the *vector* of the disease. Common vectors include *mosquitoes* (malaria, yellow fever, filariasis); *fleas* (plague, typhus); *lice and ticks* (typhus, relapsing fever); and numerous tropical insects. Parasites have a strictly limited choice of victims, and particular vectors carry only particular diseases. Fleas, lice and ticks each transmit their own particular kind of typhus, and the mosquitoes of malaria are not those of yellow fever.

Most insect-borne diseases are tropical, and most tropical diseases are insect-borne. An important factor in the eradication of tropical disease is the control of insects, and the 1948 Nobel Prize for Medicine rightly went to the Swiss chemist Paul Müller for his work on DDT and other new insecticides.

insomnia ◊ *sleep.*

insulin. A hormone formed in the pancreas and released into the blood-stream. It promotes the uptake of glucose from the blood by the body cells; without it, glucose is neither consumed as fuel nor adequately stored, but simply accumulates in the blood until it spills over into the urine (◊ *diabetes*). An excess of insulin dangerously decreases the amount of glucose in the blood (◊ *hypoglycaemia*).

Insulin is thought to act by facilitating the passage of glucose through the outer membranes of cells. Chemically, it is a lightweight protein; its molecule is a chain of 51 amino-acids. F. Sanger received the 1958 Nobel Prize for Chemistry for establishing the exact structure.

intercostal (Lat. = between ribs). The space between any two ribs is bridged by two layers of intercostal muscles, and contains intercostal nerves and blood vessels.

intercurrent. (Illness) arising in the course of another illness; e.g. serious injury may lower a person's resistance so that he is an easy prey to intercurrent pneumonia.

interferon. A substance produced in cells infected with viruses; it prevents the growth of other kinds of virus, so that a person with one kind of virus infection is unlikely to develop another at the same time. It is theoretically possible that this process might be used in medicine by infecting with a relatively harmless virus to protect against a dangerous one.

intertrigo. Soreness where two areas of skin rub together and sweat collects, a particular nuisance to fat people. Most of the trouble is due to bacteria. Intertrigo is treated with dusting powders and mild antiseptics, and to some extent prevented by losing weight and keeping cool.

intervertebral disc ◊ *vertebra* (1).

intestine.

1. STRUCTURE

The intestine or bowel is the part of the alimentary canal or digestive tube beyond the stomach. It is a soft elastic tube of muscle, lined with a thick mucous membrane. The stomach ends in a narrow outlet, the *pylorus*, and from here the tube widens into the intestine. The first and longer section is the small (i.e. narrow) intestine; when examined *post mortem* it is about 20 ft long and 1½ ins. in calibre. The second part is the large intestine, about 5 ft long and 2½ ins. in calibre. In life, muscle tone shortens the intestine by about 20 per cent.

Small intestine. The first part of the small intestine is the duodenum. It is about 10 ins. long. The next section, about 8 ft long, is the *jejunum*. The remainder of the small intestine is the *ileum*.

Seen from in front, the duodenum is like a letter C embracing the pancreas, in front of the right kidney and below the liver. The liver and pancreas are offshoots of this part of the intestine. Their ducts (bile duct and pancreatic duct) open together into the duodenum. In addition to bile and pancreatic juice, the duodenum receives mucus from the small (Brunner's) glands in its walls.

While the duodenum is firmly plastered to the back of the abdomen by a layer of peritoneum, the rest of the small intestine hangs in a loose fold of peritoneum, the *mesentery*, and is draped to and fro across the central part of the abdominal cavity. The lining of the small intestine is like velvet; magnified, it somewhat resembles a rubber suede-brush. The little protusions or *villi* together have an enormous surface area for absorption, and electron microscopy shows that each villus is coated with minute replicas of itself – microvilli.

Large intestine. The first part, the *ascending colon*, runs straight up the right side of the abdomen. The ileum enters it at a T-junction an inch or two from its lower end. The blind end below this junction is the *caecum*, a loose pouch from which the *appendix* projects like a tail. Under the liver the large intestine makes a bend to the left, the *hepatic flexure*. From here it crosses below the stomach to the spleen and bends sharply downwards at the *splenic flexure*. The part between the two flexures is the *transverse colon*; it hangs loosely in a fold of peritoneum, the *transverse mesocolon*. From the splenic flexure the *descending colon* runs down the left side into the pelvis. The *pelvic colon* is slung in another fold of peritoneum. These folds are important to the surgeon because the mobile, suspended sections of intestine are much more easily accessible than the fixed sections.

The colon is continued in the pelvis as the *rectum*, which is firmly anchored to the front of the sacrum.

Vessels and nerves. The arteries of the duodenum, stomach, liver, pancreas, and spleen are branches of the *coeliac* artery. The *superior mesenteric* artery supplies the intestine as far as the transverse colon, and the *inferior mesenteric* artery supplies the rest of the colon. These are all branches of the aorta. The veins are tributaries of the *portal* vein, which carries blood from the intestine to the liver. The whole alimentary canal is well provided with lymph vessels. There are collections of lymphoid tissue in its walls, of which the most obvious are the tonsils and adenoids at the entrance to the pharynx. Similar collections in the wall of the ileum are known as Peyer's patches, and the appendix and caecum contain lymphoid tissue which may flare up as if in sympathy when the tonsils are inflamed, closely simulating appendicitis.

The intestine is stimulated by *parasympathetic* nerves (mainly the *vagus* nerve) and inhibited by *sympathetic* nerves. The only conscious sensation from the intestine is stretching, which may produce anything from a sense of repletion to severe pain. Any kind of inflammation makes the intestine much more sensitive. Intestinal pain is ◊ *referred* to the mid-line. But pain from the peritoneum – the lining membrane of the abdomen – may be felt at an actual site of inflammation; e.g. pain from the appendix itself is felt in the centre, and pain from the overlying peritoneum on the right side.

2. DEVELOPMENT

The digestive tube is derived from ◊ *endoderm*. At an early stage the stomach and whole of the intestine hang from a single mesentery, which lies more or less vertically. The intestine grows so fast that for a time there is not room for it in the abdomen, and most of it protrudes through the umbilicus as the *physiological hernia*. Later, when the growth of the rest of the embryo catches up with the growth of the intestine, the intestine returns to the abdomen. By this time it is very much longer than its line of attachment at the back, and the mesentery is gathered like a kilt with a short waistband and a hem several yards long.

3. FUNCTION

The workings of the intestine are considered under ◊ *digestion*. Briefly, the complex molecules of foods are broken down by *enzymes* to smaller molecules which can be absorbed through the lining of the intestine into the blood-stream and carried to the liver and elsewhere to be resynthesized. The intestine receives partly digested food and drink from the stomach together with the fluid secreted by the glands in the wall of the stomach. To this is added fluid secreted by the liver and pancreas and by the intestine itself. A very small amount of this fluid is passed in the stools. The rest is reabsorbed. If this reabsorption fails the stores of salt and water can be quickly depleted, for the daily turnover amounts to a fifth of the total amount in the body – to about $1\frac{1}{4}$ gallons of water and $1\frac{1}{2}$ oz. of salt. A baby with severe diarrhoea or an adult with cholera can die of dehydration within a day or two if the fluid lost from the intestine is not replaced.

The contents of the intestine are squeezed along by the contractions of the intestinal muscle. The normal transit time is a few hours in the small intestine and a day or more in the large intestine.

In health the small intestine is almost free from bacteria, but the large intestine teems with them. They are harmless where they are, but dangerous if they escape to other parts of the body.

4. EXAMINATION

Most intestinal diseases cause symptoms which point to the intestine as the affected organ; in other words one usually knows where to look for the trouble. Almost the whole of the intestine can be felt through the soft belly-wall.

The last 12 ins. of the large intestine can be inspected with a lighted tube (*sigmoidoscope*). A light anaesthetic is sometimes needed for this rather disagreeable examination, but it is the only certain way of identifying some important disorders of the large intestine. If the diagnosis is still uncertain after looking at the inside of the intestine a small specimen of the lining can be taken for microscopic study.

X-rays are used in the same way as for the stomach. The patient swallows fluid (barium meal) which is opaque to X-rays, such as a suspension of barium sulphate. The intestine can then be shown in silhouette as the fluid passes along it. Similar fluid injected into the rectum (barium enema) gives a picture of the large intestine.

A specimen of the fluid in the small intestine can be taken with a syringe attached to a long, soft rubber tube. The end of the tube is swallowed and passes along the stomach to the duodenum or beyond. Its position can be determined with X-rays. A small device for taking a sample of the lining of the intestine can be introduced in the same way.

Laboratory examination of the stools is an important guide to the state of the intestine. Chemical analysis reveals defective breakdown or absorption of foods. Intestinal parasites are identified by microscopy; in hot countries where this kind of infection is rife microscopic examination of the stools is a matter of routine. Bacteriological investigation of the stools is needed for the exact diagnosis of intestinal infection, for tracing the source of infection, and for the proper control of people whose work involves handling food or drinking water.

Sometimes the only way to make a diagnosis is to operate and look at the intestine. This is less drastic than it sounds. An exploratory operation carries little risk, and certainly less risk than the sort of suspected trouble that calls for it. Most abdominal operations are in a sense exploratory. What looks like acute appendicitis may turn out to be a leaking duodenal ulcer or a twisted ovarian cyst. These, and several other disorders with similar symptoms, could probably be distinguished without operation if there were time, but most of them require immediate surgical attention. The provisional diagnosis 'acute appendicitis' may be a convenient abbreviation of 'case for urgent abdominal operation, probably but not necessarily appendicitis'. Suspected cancer often needs the same approach: if the patient is kept waiting until the diagnosis is proved beyond doubt it may be too late to operate. Seen in this light, the risk of an un-

necessary operation seems reasonable enough. ◊ *abdomen* (1).

5. DISORDERS

There are many different ailments of the intestine, and the patient usually has symptoms to indicate *something* wrong in the intestine. But the symptoms alone may not show precisely *what* is wrong, because widely different causes produce similar effects. The intestine is a very simple apparatus in which only a few things can go wrong. Intestinal disease may impair the absorption of food (◊ *malabsorption*), or it may disturb the purely mechanical function of moving the contents along the tube: they can be moved too quickly, with ◊ *diarrhoea*; too slowly, with ◊ *constipation*; or not at all if the tube is blocked.

Pain from the intestine is felt when its nerve-endings are stretched. This will obviously happen when the intestine is distended with gas or overloaded with food. The pressure also increases if it is blocked or if its muscle is over-active. When the intestine is inflamed it becomes over-sensitive and the normal pressure changes become painful. In one way or another, then, almost any intestinal disorder may be painful.

Bleeding is a common symptom of many disorders. Blood undergoes chemical change in the intestine and becomes black. It is recognizable as blood only if the bleeding is from low down, e.g. from piles or cancer of the rectum. Otherwise it merely darkens the stools. Significant amounts of blood may be passed without being noticed: the loss of a teaspoonful of blood daily can cause serious anaemia in time. Anaemia of this type is very common (duodenal ulcer, hookworm disease, piles, regular use or abuse of aspirin), but perhaps intestinal bleeding is even more important as a warning sign. Most cancers of the intestine can be removed if they are recognized in the early stages, and a trace of blood may be the first sign.

The actual diseases are discussed under their own headings; what follows is no more than a crude attempt at classifying some of the important ones.

Emotion and mood play a large part. Fear or misery can cause sustained over-activity of the intestine. This does not always lead to diarrhoea. Often the activity is not co-ordinated and the result is constipation and discomfort. Symptoms ascribed to constipation such as headache and lethargy are more likely to be an accompaniment than a real consequence of constipation. The intestine reacts to any emotion, but it reacts most to emotion centred on itself. Some people seem to be obsessed with their digestive organs. This is perhaps because so much of an infant's earliest training has to do with the action of his bowels. Nothing is more likely to disturb this action than the constant fear that it might be disturbed. Finally, physical disease of the intestine can cause anxiety and so set up a vicious circle. It is sometimes impossible to distinguish cause from effect.

Malabsorption may occur simply because there is not time for complete absorption, either because the intestine is inflamed and over-active or because it is too short, usually as a result of surgical removal of an irreparably damaged section. Secondly, it may be due to a defect of the lining which reduces its ability to absorb, e.g. ◊ *sprue*, ◊ *coeliac disease*, intestinal tuberculosis. Thirdly, it may be due to the absence of digestive enzymes, e.g. with disease of the pancreas or with congenital defects such as ◊ *carbohydrate intolerance*.

Over-activity, apart from the emotional factors already discussed, is usually due to inflammation. Inflamed mucous membranes pour out fluid; therefore the contents of the intestine are increased. The muscles and their nerves are irritated, and the contractions are exaggerated. Both fluid and contractions contribute to diarrhoea. But violent contractions are not always co-ordinated. Instead of a smooth, orderly progress along the intestine, one section may contract before the following section has had time to relax: it is then pushing against an obstruction, which causes distension and pain. Inflammation of the intestine (*enteritis*) is most often due to infection. The agent may be a virus ('summer diarrhoea', 'gastric flu'), a bacterium (food poisoning, dysentery, cholera, typhoid and paratyphoid fevers), or a more highly developed creature (amoebic dysentery, worm infestation). Many poisons cause symptoms like those of bacterial infection. Purgative drugs may act by irritating the intestine to greater activity, by 'drawing' an excess of fluid into the intestine, by increasing the bulk of the contents, or (which may come to the same thing) by lubrication.

Crohn's disease and *ulcerative colitis* are instances of inflammation without infection; their causes are not known for certain.

Activity may be *impaired* in two ways. If the nerves fail, the muscle ceases to contract and there is stagnation. Or there may be a mechanical blockage. Lack of co-ordination of the intestinal muscles can cause constipation; this never amounts to a stoppage but only to impaired efficiency. When the peritoneum is inflamed (*peritonitis*) the intestine ceases to contract; it becomes an inert tube, unable to propel its contents. This condition, known as *ileus*, appears to be a reflex by which the nerves of the intestine are inhibited. The same thing may happen after a serious injury or operation. There is no need for the whole intestine to be paralysed. If only a short section goes out of action it acts as a barrier to the passage of the contents. This may follow interference with the blood supply, e.g. by thrombosis of an artery or pressure on the mesentery, or severe localized inflammation. In a rare congenital disorder, *megacolon*, certain nerves fail to grow into a section of the large intestine. Since the affected section cannot squeeze its contents along it is in effect a barrier, and the intestine above it becomes more and more distended.

Actual blockage (*intestinal obstruction*) can arise in several ways. Congenital defects include *atresia*, when a part of the intestine – usually the junction of the rectum with the anus – remains solid, without a canal; and faulty development of the mesentery can result in twisting or *volvulus* of the intestine. Volvulus can, rarely, occur even with a normal mesentery. It causes obstruction of the blood vessels rather than of the intestine itself, but either condition is equally lethal unless promptly relieved by surgery. Another cause of obstruction in early childhood (sometimes later) is *intussusception*: a section of intestine is sucked into the section beyond.

The commonest cause of obstruction is *hernia*, which arises where a weak point in the muscles of the abdomen allows a loop of intestine to slip between the muscle fibres. In most cases it comes to no great harm, but there is always a danger that it will be constricted. A similar condition arises within the abdomen if a loop of intestine is trapped behind a fibrous band (*adhesion*) joining two organs. The band may be a congenital anomaly or a result of scarring after inflammation, injury, or surgical operation.

All types of intestinal obstruction need surgical treatment.

Tumours are very rare in the small intestine but two types are common in the large intestine: *polyp*, which is usually harmless but occasionally leads to the other type, *cancer*. Most intestinal cancer, however, is without apparent cause apart from a tendency to run in families. Constipation used to be blamed, but without evidence. Piles most emphatically do not cause cancer. Their importance is that bleeding from a curable cancer is all too often ascribed to piles until the cancer has become incurable.

About a sixth of all cancers reported in Great Britain affect the large intestine, and in many countries the proportion is still higher. The usual treatment is to remove the affected section and repair the cut ends. When the rectum is involved normal function cannot often be restored without the risk of leaving some of the cancer behind, and an artificial anus (*colostomy*) has to be made. Even when a cure seems unlikely the operation is usually worth trying, if only to prevent the misery of obstruction. And in some 50 per cent of cases the disease can be cured. This figure is very much higher in cases where unexplained bleeding and above all a *change of bowel habit* have been investigated as soon as possible. The kind of change is immaterial; any change – more frequent motions, less frequent, less regular – calls for full examination. The cause may be entirely innocent, but it has to be ascertained.

Other important disorders of the intestine, not mentioned above but discussed under their own headings, are *duodenal ulcer* (◊ *peptic ulcer*), *appendicitis*, and *diverticulosis* – small pockets or diverticula in the lining of the large intestine, harmless in themselves but apt to become inflamed. These three are among the commonest causes of *perforation* of the intestine with leakage of its contents into the peritoneal cavity and peritonitis; this highly dangerous condition calls for immediate operation.
◊ *abdomen* (1); *stomach*; *rectum*.

intrauterine device ◊ *contraception*.

intussusception. A cause of blockage of the intestine: a length of the tube is telescoped into the next section, and drawn further and further in by the action of the intestinal muscles. It is rare in adults, but is not uncommon in the first year of life. The condition needs urgent attention, usually surgical.

involution. Shrinkage, in particular of the uterus after pregnancy: this organ takes several weeks to return to its former size. Also (mainly in psychiatry) the period of life when one has at last to accept that one is not getting any younger. In women, the menopause is an abrupt reminder.

involutional melancholia. Depression, severe and irrational enough to count as a form of insanity or psychosis, at the time of the menopause. ◊ *depression*.

iodine. A very small amount of this element is necessary to health because it is a component of thyroid hormone. In most places, the diet and drinking water supply enough, but in some areas there is hardly any in the soil and the inhabitants are subject to goitre – enlargement of the thyroid gland – showing as a rounded swelling of the front of the neck. This represents, so to speak, an attempt by the gland to make bricks without straw. If iodine is provided the swelling subsides.

A solution of iodine is a powerful antiseptic, suitable for sterilizing intact skin before a surgical operation but too corrosive for use in wounds.
◊ *isotope*.

ipecacuanha (ipecac). An extract of the root of a Brazilian shrub, containing the alkaloid emetine. Large doses cause vomiting, but small doses irritate the stomach just enough to stimulate the mucous glands in the lungs by reflex action, and so help to ease a dry cough.

iridectomy. Surgical operation on the eye: a small hole is made near the margin of the iris to allow fluid trapped in the front of the eye to circulate in case of *glaucoma*. The raised pressure is thus relieved and the danger to sight is overcome.

iris. Flat ring of pigmented tissue in the front of the eye, between the cornea and the lens. Its muscle fibres widen the hole in the middle, the pupil, in poor light and constrict it in bright light. The pigment, melanin, is the same in all eyes, but in brown eyes it is near the surface and in blue eyes it is obscured by overlying tissue.

iron. A healthy adult body contains 3–4 grammes of iron; enough for a 2-inch nail.

Most of it is combined with protein to form ◊ *haemoglobin*, the oxygen-carrying component of the red blood cells. Some is held in storage, in the reticulo-endothelial cells of the liver and other organs. Small amounts are needed by enzymes concerned with the use of oxygen throughout the body.

The outermost layer of the skin and mucous membranes is continuously shed (the extent is seen when a limb has been in plaster for a few weeks and the shed layer has had time to accumulate). In this way, the body loses about 1 mg. of iron daily, and in healthy men this is the only loss, and all that the diet has to replace. A balanced diet contains at least ten times this amount of iron, but only 10 per cent is absorbed. The amount absorbed can be increased to 30 per cent if the body is short of iron, or slightly decreased if there is a surfeit; but the mechanism, still unknown, cannot cope with large discrepancies. If the stores have been depleted they are only slowly replenished. If, as rarely happens, there is a gross excess of iron, the body dutifully stores it and it becomes a nuisance.

Normal menstruation costs about 30 mg. of iron per month, so that a woman loses and needs twice as much iron as a man. If her loss is at all heavy her intake may not keep pace; then she has not enough to replace the lost haemoglobin and she becomes anaemic (◊ *anaemia* (B.2)). Pregnancy makes special demands. A new-born baby has 300 c.c. of blood, containing 150 mg. of iron, and a further 250 mg. in store, all provided by the mother. To maintain her store during pregnancy, she needs three times as much iron as a man. Her milk also contains a little iron, but not much more than she would lose by menstruation if she were not feeding a baby.

Growing children have not only to maintain the store of iron; they must steadily increase it as the volume of blood grows.

In all these cases of extra demand there is unlikely to be much spare iron to meet emergencies, and any continued bleeding will cause anaemia. Even in grown men, the store can be depleted in time by quite trivial losses. 2 c.c. of blood – half a teaspoonful – contains 1 mg. of iron, and a daily loss of this amount doubles the requirement.

1. SUPPLY OF IRON

Most foods contain some iron. Liver is an excellent source; meat, eggs, and cereals are good; most vegetables are fair (spinach is commonly over-rated); milk is poor, which is why new-born babies need a large store. In societies where toddlers are breast-fed, e.g. parts of China and Africa, children are often anaemic. Vitamin C, present in fruit and vegetables, improves the absorption of iron from the intestine, and the anaemia of scurvy (lack of vitamin C) is partly due to poor absorption. Any mixed diet has enough iron for normal requirements, but a generally poor diet will not meet the extra demands described above. If the stores have been depleted even a very good diet will not replenish them. An artificial supply is needed.

In Greek mythology the seer Melampus treated impotence with a decoction of iron rust. But the first person to record the true value of iron, in the treatment of anaemia, was the English physician Sydenham (1624–89). Many salts of iron are suitable. Solutions are unpleasant to take, but coated tablets are generally acceptable. People whose stomachs are upset by one preparation may have no trouble with another. Overdosage is a mistake. Only a limited amount can be absorbed, and the percentage falls as the dose is increased. Impatient people who take two or three times the standard dose do not assimilate two or three times as much iron, and the unabsorbed portion upsets the digestion.

If the deficiency is due to inability to absorb iron, or if the iron is needed in a hurry, injections can be given.

2. IRON POISONING

The body has no natural means of getting rid of excess iron; it goes on storing it. In a very rare disease, *bronzed diabetes*, far too much iron is absorbed from the food and deposited all over the body. The skin becomes 'bronzed' with iron salts, and the damage to the pancreas causes diabetes. Ultimately the liver fails. A similar condition can affect people who have had scores or hundreds of blood transfusions (◊ *anaemia* (A.2)). This sort of chronic poisoning is very rare.

Although the proportion of a dose of iron which can be absorbed becomes smaller as the dose increases, enough is absorbed from a really massive dose to be dangerous. Furthermore a very high concentration of iron in the stomach has a corrosive action. A bottle of 50 tablets contains enough iron to kill a small child, and in fact a number of children have died after swallowing a handful of iron tablets. When children are around, these preparations have to be kept out of reach as carefully as any other drug.

The compound *desferrioxamine* readily assimilates iron to form a new compound, ferrioxamine, that can be excreted by the kidneys. This is an effective means of treating all forms of iron poisoning.

irritability. The ability of living tissues to respond to change, in particular the response of nerve and muscle to stimulation. Haller (1708–77), one of the founders of modern physiology, taught that irritability was the characteristic property of living matter.

ischaemia. Insufficient supply of blood to a part of the body, e.g. to the heart muscle, causing angina.

ischium. The rump-bone, a part of the ◊ *pelvis.*

islets of Langerhans. Clusters of cells scattered through the pancreas in which *insulin* is formed.

isoimmunity. Immune (allergic) response to tissue from another member of one's own species. An important instance is incompatibility between the blood of an unborn baby and that of its mother (◊ *rhesus factor*).

isolation. Patients may need isolation to prevent their infecting others or to protect them from infection. The latter reason has been recognized only in recent years; it can apply to premature babies, patients whose natural defences have been suppressed by drugs in order to prevent tissue grafted from another person (e.g. a kidney) from being rejected after the operation, and patients with certain blood diseases that make them unduly vulnerable to infection.

To be effective, isolation demands a complex ritual that needs a special hospital unit, where everything that has been in contact with the patient is disinfected on its way to the outside world and vice versa.

With many common infectious diseases the need for isolation is much less than it was before there were antibiotics to cure the diseases, but antibiotics have introduced a new class of disease that needs the strictest isolation: infection with newly evolved strains of microbe that resist the usual antibiotics. It is precisely in hospitals, where antibiotics are in constant use, that these strains are likely to appear.

isoniazid. Isonicotinic acid hydrazide (INH), shown by Domagk to inhibit the growth of tubercle bacilli; it has been used since 1952 for treating tuberculosis, usually with streptomycin. It is closely related to the vitamin nicotinamide, which also has some effect against tuberculosis in animals.

Many patients treated with isoniazid have found that it raises their spirits. As a result similar compounds in which this action is enhanced have been prepared for the treatment of ◊ *depression.*

isotope. One of two or more forms of a chemical element with similar chemical properties but different atomic weights. Isotopes are used in medical research for tracing the movements of chemical substances in the body. A substance can be labelled by incorporating in its molecules an unusual isotope which can later be identified. Radioactive isotopes are easily traced by recording their radiations. ◊ *scintigram.*

Radioactive isotopes can be used for diagnosis, and have a limited place in the treatment of disease. If diseased tissue has a special affinity for an element, a radioactive isotope of the element can be used to suppress or destroy the tissue. For instance, the thyroid gland collects nearly all the iodine in the body, and a dose of radioactive iodine should suppress cancer of the thyroid; unfortunately the cancer cells are abnormal and do not necessarily assimilate iodine.

itch. 1. = ◊ *scabies.*
2. A little understood sensation. No nerve-endings have been identified as 'itch endings' in the way that special endings for pain, touch, heat, and cold, and the pathways that carry these sensations to the brain, can be at least provisionally identified. There is evidence that itch may be carried by the same nerve fibres as pain, but it is not conclusive. Since 1830 it has been generally accepted that one nerve fibre does only one job, but it is possible that slight stimulation might cause one sensation and stronger stimulation another. Scratching temporarily replaces itch with slight pain. Why itch should so readily arise without any stimulation at all, merely from thinking about it, remains a mystery.

IUD. Intrauterine device; ◊ *contraception.*

IVP. Intravenous pyelography. ◊ *kidneys* (3).

Jacksonian fit. (J. Hughlings Jackson (1834–1911), British neurologist.) Focal ◊ *epilepsy*.

jalap. Drug extracted from a Mexican plant, strongly purgative.

Jarisch-Herxheimer reaction. An abnormal response, with inflammation and fever, to the injection of drugs against syphilis and perhaps other infections; variously explained as stimulation of the parasites by inadequate dosage, and as a sudden release of poisons by killing large numbers of parasites.

jaundice. Yellow discoloration of the skin and mucous membranes by excess of bile pigment in the blood.

Bile pigment is an end-product of haemoglobin, formed as worn-out red blood cells are destroyed. There is always a small amount in the blood. The liver disposes of it and excretes it into the bile, which passes down the bile ducts to the gall bladder and finally into the intestine. Bile pigment accumulates in the blood: (1) if too much is formed; (2) if the liver cells do not dispose of it; or (3) if the bile ducts are obstructed.

Too much pigment is formed with certain types of anaemia, due to excessive destruction of blood cells (◊ *anaemia* (A.2)).

The working of the liver cells is impaired by infection (◊ *hepatitis*), various poisons, and rare chemical defects.

Obstruction of the flow of bile from the liver cells, with reabsorption of pigment into the blood, may occur within the liver from inflammation (hepatitis again; reaction to certain drugs; congestion due to heart failure), or in the larger ducts leading from the liver (diseases of the gall bladder; gall stones).

When jaundice is due to obstruction, no pigment reaches the intestine, and the stools are therefore uncoloured. On the other hand, a large amount of pigment is filtered from the blood by the kidneys, and the urine is dark.

Of the symptoms that may be associated with jaundice, itching is actually due to jaundice, whereas nausea and inability to tolerate fatty food have the same causes as the jaundice itself.

Bile pigment stains connective tissue, and the yellow colour persists for some days after an attack of jaundice is really over.

A trace of jaundice is common in the first few days of life and is not a serious matter. But a severe and dangerous jaundice arises from incompatibility between the baby's blood and the mother's; ◊ *rhesus factor*.

jaw. ◊ *maxilla* (upper jaw); *mandible* (lower jaw).

jejunum. Part of the small intestine, from the duodenum to the ileum.

Jenner, Edward (1749–1823). English country practitioner, a pupil of John Hunter. He invented vaccination. For half a century, *inoculation* had been used to prevent dangerous attacks of smallpox. The principle, known for centuries in Asia, was to infect people deliberately from mild cases of smallpox, because as a rule the disease breeds true: mild cases cause mild cases. The person is then immune to all smallpox. Inoculation worked well as regards conferring immunity, but it meant having smallpox and there was no certainty that the attack would be mild or even that it would not be fatal.

Jenner took up a popular belief that people who had had cow-pox, a mild disease, were safe from smallpox. In enough cases to prove the matter, he found that: (1) people who had had cow-pox escaped smallpox during outbreaks in the area; (2) they could not be infected even by inoculation with smallpox; and (3) the same protection could be safely conferred by inoculation with cow-pox, which he called vaccination. The work was published in 1798.

joint. Joints between bones may be fixed (fibrous) or mobile (synovial). The bones of the skull are firmly bound together by fibrous tissue, and no movement between them is possible. The lower ends of the tibia and fibula are similarly joined by fibrous tissue, but this joint allows a small amount of play.

The bodies of the vertebrae are joined by

thick pads of fibrocartilage, which are flexible enough to allow some movement without impairing the stability of the column. A similar joint at the angle of the sternum allows the angle to be increased when a deep breath is taken. The symphysis pubis, also a fibrocartilaginous joint, does not move.

A much commoner type is the *synovial joint*. Where the bones touch each other they are coated with smooth and slippery cartilage. The joint is hermetically enclosed by the tough fibrous *capsule*, which is lined with the slippery *synovial membrane*. This membrane exudes clear, viscous *synovial fluid*, which keeps the joint surfaces moist. The capsule is a continuation of the periosteum, the fibrous sheath of the bones. It becomes considerably thicker than the periosteum, and where it is subject to particular stresses its fibres are arranged in stout bands or *ligaments*. Beyond these *capsular* ligaments, the joint may be strengthened by *accessory* ligaments spanning the bones. A ligament is effective only when it is taut. It serves to limit movement in a particular direction, rather than to support the joint in any position. For instance, the thrust from the hip in striding forwards would be less effective if the joint could be bent backwards as readily as it can be flexed. When the thigh is fully extended, the strong ligament down the front of the hip-joint is tightened and so ensures that the body is pushed forwards and not the thigh backwards. In other positions of the hip, this ligament is slack and does not support the joint. The stability of most joints depends more on muscles than on ligaments. A muscle acting on a joint is anchored to bone on either side of the joint. Its obvious function is to contract and

so bring its two points of attachment closer together. But even at rest a muscle exerts a gentle pull, and this pull is maintained in any position, and counteracted by the equal pull of muscles on the other side of the joint. Thus the muscles are adjustable guy-ropes. The principle can be seen at work in the 'Anglepoise' table lamp, which has a jointed skeleton supported by accurately balanced springs.

A ◊ *sprain* is the result of forcing a joint beyond the limit set by its ligaments, when a ligament becomes torn. A ◊ *dislocation* is an actual disruption of the joint; the joint surfaces become separated from each other. Any kind of inflammation in a joint is ◊ *arthritis*. Disorders of particular joints are discussed under the names of the joints (◊ *shoulder, knee* etc.).

jugular veins. Large veins of the neck. Most of the venous blood from the brain leaves the skull by an opening to each side of the foramen magnum, the *jugular foramen* (◊ *skull*), and enters the *internal jugular vein*. This very large vessel runs vertically down the side of the neck at the outer side of the carotid arteries and under cover of the sternomastoid muscle. It ends behind the sternoclavicular joint, where it meets the *subclavian* vein to form the *innominate* vein.

The *external jugular vein* is a much smaller vessel, receiving blood from the face and the side of the scalp, which runs down on the surface of the sternomastoid to the subclavian vein. The slight bulge of this vein can sometimes be seen through the skin at the side of the neck. A tributary, the *anterior jugular vein*, runs down the front of the neck.

K

kala-azar (Dumdum fever). A tropical fever due to a kind of ◊ *Leishmania* transmitted by sandflies. The infection is mainly in the bone marrow and lymphatic system. The symptoms include fever, anaemia, and enlargement of the spleen and liver. In untreated cases, the disease is commonly fatal, but there are several effective drugs, mostly compounds of antimony.

Kala-azar is confined to dry regions of north-east Africa and southern Asia.

kaolin. Powdered aluminium silicate, a bland substance used to absorb fluid and irritants from the intestine in the treatment of diarrhoea; also applied externally as a poultice because it retains heat.

keloid (cheloid). Tough lump of fibrous tissue at the site of a scar: it is like an ordinary scar but there is too much of it. Keloids are very unusual on fair skins, but dark-skinned people and especially negroes are prone to them. They are harmless but disfiguring, and although they are easily removed, the operation leaves a scar in which new ones may form.

keratin. A protein; the main component of finger-nails, hair, and the thin, tough outer layer of the skin.

keratitis. Inflammation of the *cornea* (round window at the front of the eye).

kernicterus. Jaundice of new-born infants so severe as to damage the brain. ◊ *rhesus factor.*

ketosis. Poisoning by ketones (acetone and related substances). These are intermediate products in the combustion of fat in the body. Normally they are quickly broken down to harmless substances – ultimately carbon dioxide and water. But when the chemical disposal of fat is disturbed, as in severe diabetes or starvation, ketones accumulate in the blood. They can then be identified in the urine as a sign that diabetes is not being controlled by treatment, and the breath may smell of acetone. The 'odour of sanctity' may have been the odour of ketosis, due to starvation from prolonged fasting.

kidneys. A pair of large excretory glands at the back of the abdomen, concerned primarily with regulating the amount of water in the body. All life is aquatic. The simplest animal, the amoeba, lives under water. Its cell-membrane is a leaky structure: it prevents the body-substance or protoplasm from escaping, but water can diffuse in and out of the amoeba, as can salts and other simple chemical substances dissolved in the water.

The amoeba takes up substances from its environment to be incorporated into its own body-substance, and the chemical processes of life create unwanted by-products which would poison the cell if allowed to accumulate. Foods and waste products are exchanged by simple diffusion, which depends on the tendency of molecules in a fluid to move from zones of high concentration to zones of low concentration. Provided that the water in which the amoeba lives contains the right substances in the right proportions, both supply and waste-disposal are passive and automatic.

The only problem is the water itself. Sea-water is rather too strong a solution of salts etc., and fresh water is much too dilute for the needs of a living animal. Simple diffusion has to be supplemented by active selection. Animals living in sea-water retain more water than simple diffusion would allow, and animals in fresh water reject it, so that the solution inside the cell is kept at the right strength. In either case this solution is equivalent to somewhat diluted sea-water.

Although a man does not live in water, each of the millions of cells of which he is built must do so. More than half of his body weight is water; most is inside the cells, a little in the blood, and some 12 litres or 2½ gallons is interstitial fluid (tissue fluid), which permeates every minute crevice and bathes every cell. This fluid is the real environment of our component cells, and although we have evolved from creatures which left the sea several hundred million years ago it is still dilute sea-water. Like amoebae, our cells get their supplies and dispose of their waste by diffusion from and to the surrounding fluid. As amoebae have special arrangements for actively conserving or rejecting water, so human cells have certain 'chemical pumps' for modifying the action of simple diffusion on particular substances – the most important of these keeps potassium inside the cells at the expense of sodium – but in principle our cells behave like their remotest marine ancestors.

heart, which is by no means 'heart' shaped). It is the size of a cupped hand, about $4\frac{1}{2}$ ins. from top to bottom and $2\frac{1}{2}$ ins. from side to side; it is 1 to $1\frac{1}{2}$ ins. thick. The concavity or *hilum* faces inwards, forwards, and slightly downwards.

The urine formed by the kidney enters the *renal pelvis*, a funnel-shaped structure in the hilum which narrows to a slender tube, the

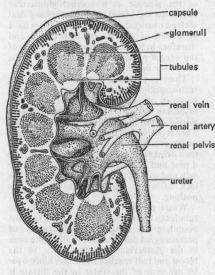

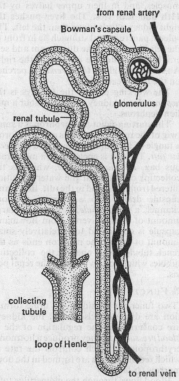

(Left) *Section of kidney.* (Right) *Enlarged diagram of nephron.*

No living cell can withstand much change in its environment. Even slight changes in acidity or concentration will kill a highly developed structure such as a human nerve cell. The organs mainly responsible for preventing such changes are the kidneys.

1. STRUCTURE

Man has two kidneys, one at each side of the backbone between the thick muscles of the back and the abdomen. A kidney is in fact 'kidney' shaped, like a bean (unlike the

ureter. The ureter passes straight down the back of the abdomen to the bladder, a distance of about 10 ins.

The principal artery and vein of the body, the aorta and the inferior vena cava, lie between the kidneys. From either side of the aorta a very large renal artery enters the renal pelvis; between them these arteries carry about a quarter of the total blood circulating when the body is at rest. (The flow through the kidneys, about 70 litres or 15 gallons an hour, remains constant during wide fluctuations of the total blood-flow.)

The blood returns to the vena cava by the renal veins.

The kidneys are embedded in a special kind of fat: ordinary fat is liquid at body temperature, but this is firm. Hence the tendency of the kidneys to slip downwards ('floating kidney') in people who have lost much fat.

Behind, the kidneys are well protected by muscles, and in their upper halves by the 11th and 12th ribs. The liver pushes the right kidney a little lower than the left. The spleen, pancreas, and stomach lie in front of the left kidney, and the duodenum and several loops of intestine in front of the right. An important gland (◊ adrenal) is perched on the top of each kidney.

The working unit of the kidneys is the nephron. Each kidney contains about a million nephrons.

The starting-point of a nephron is a small twig of the renal artery. This arteriole forms a tangle of fine capillary vessels, a glomerular tuft. The tuft is enclosed in a membranous bag, Bowman's capsule, which is the collecting chamber for the watery solution filtered from the blood in the tuft. Bowman's capsule drains into a narrow, tortuous channel, a renal tubule, in which the large amount of fluid delivered from Bowman's capsule is condensed to a relatively small amount of urine. The nephron ends as the renal tubule joins one of the collecting tubules which convey urine to the renal pelvis.

2. FUNCTION

(Two functions subsidiary to urine formation are discussed elsewhere: the kidneys are concerned in the regulation of the ◊ blood pressure, and they produce a hormone, erythropoietin, which controls the rate at which red blood cells are formed in the bone marrow (◊ blood).)

Blood flows through the glomerular tufts under high pressure. The first part of the nephron acts as a simple filter, with pores small enough to hold back blood cells and the large molecules of proteins but large enough to allow substances with a molecular weight below 70,000 to pass. The fluid entering Bowman's capsule – the glomerular filtrate – thus consists of everything in the blood except cells and proteins, namely water, salts, nutrients such as sugar (glucose) and the amino-acids of which proteins are built, and waste products. It is filtered at a rate of 120 c.c. per minute, which would dispose of all the water in the body in about 5 hours, together with a couple of ounces of sugar and half a pound of salt.

In the tubules this large volume of filtrate is changed to a small volume of urine. This is done by selective reabsorption. Of the 120 c.c. of water, all but 1 c.c. is returned to the blood. In general, nutrients are also reabsorbed. The tubules can return nearly all of the glucose in a normal glomerular filtrate to the blood, but they cannot deal with an overload. People with diabetes have an excess of glucose in their blood, and therefore in the glomerular filtrate; some of the excess passes along the tubules to be lost in the urine.

There is a special arrangement for salt: reabsorption is adjusted to need. If the body is short of salt, hardly any reaches the urine, but if there is an excess the concentration of salt in the urine can reach 2 per cent. This is an important figure, because sea-water averages 3 per cent. Therefore if a man drinks a pint of sea-water he must pass a pint and half of urine to get rid of the salt, and so runs a greater risk of dying from lack of water than a man who drinks nothing.

Waste products tend to remain in the tubules to be excreted in the urine. The most abundant is urea, an end-product of protein breakdown. About half of the urea in the glomerular filtrate returns to the blood and half reaches the urine. Since over 99 per cent of the water in the filtrate is returned, the net effect is that urea is concentrated 60-fold: in other words, 1 c.c. of urine contains as much urea as 60 c.c. of blood. There is only a very small amount of urea in the blood at any time; in a healthy person the total is about 1·5 grammes. Yet as much as 30 grammes may be passed in the urine in 24 hours. Some waste products can be concentrated even more than this. As the concentration of waste products in the tissues rises, the products diffuse into the tissue fluid in the same way as they would diffuse from an amoeba into a pond. The concentration is then higher in the tissue fluid than in the blood, and therefore there is further diffusion from the tissue fluid to the blood, of which a fraction is filtered off in the kidneys. The flow of waste products from the cells to the glomerular filtrate is thus passive. The only active process required is the selective reabsorption of water (or non-absorption of waste) from the tubules.

The kidneys also help to regulate the acidity of the body fluids. In health, this is very slightly alkaline (pH about 7·4). Small changes are harmful, and large changes are lethal. Because many by-products of body chemistry are acidic, a constant tendency to acidosis has to be overcome. The first line of defence is elimination of carbon dioxide, equivalent to carbonic acid, from the lungs (◊respiration (2)). But this mechanism is suitable only for immediate adjustments. It is soon exhausted if there is no other means of getting rid of acid. The kidneys provide two or three pathways. They form ammonia, which neutralizes acids to form ammonium salts. They receive alkaline phosphate (Na_2HPO_4) from the blood but excrete acid phosphate (NaH_2PO_4) into the urine; in effect the phosphate takes up acid. And there are probably other mechanisms.

Regulation of Urine. Under average conditions a man passes about 1·5 litres of urine daily, but this amount can vary greatly in accordance with demand. The amount of the glomerular filtrate – 120 c.c. per minute or 160 litres daily – is almost constant, but the proportion of this huge quantity of water reabsorbed in the tubules can be adjusted. Normally, over 99 per cent returns to the blood. Thus reabsorption need only be reduced by 1 per cent for the amount of urine to be more than doubled. A sensory organ in the hypothalamus, in the floor of the brain, responds to slight changes in the dilution of the blood. This organ governs the release of anti-diuretic hormone (A D H) from the pituitary gland. A D H promotes reabsorption in the tubules, thus conserving water and reducing the volume of the urine. By this means the rate of urine formation can be increased tenfold or more. People with the uncommon disease *diabetes insipidus*, who lack A D H, may pass as much as 20 litres of urine (about 4 gallons) in 24 hours, because instead of 99 per cent they can reabsorb only 90 per cent or less of the glomerular filtrate.

While the amount of urine can be increased to meet any likely excess of water, it cannot be safely reduced to less than about 600 c.c., say a pint, per day. This is the least amount that will carry away waste products.

Factors other than a relative lack of water can stimulate release of A D H and so diminish the volume of urine. These include severe emotional upsets, and normal sleep.

The amount of salt in the urine is determined by a hormone from the adrenal glands, *aldosterone*. This hormone increases the reabsorption of sodium in the tubules. It is released in response to lack of salt, and also to lowered blood pressure. Indirectly, it affects the volume of urine, because a large amount of salt excreted in the urine requires a large amount of water to dissolve it. Conversely, if an excess of salt is retained in the body, water is also retained. This is why abnormal collections of fluid in the body, e.g. with heart disease, can be dispersed by reducing the amount of salt in the diet.

3. EXAMINATION OF THE KIDNEYS

Little can be learnt about the state of the kidneys from ordinary clinical examination because they are so inaccessible. In people of average or slender physique it is just possible to feel the lower ends of the kidneys and judge whether they are enlarged, or sore from inflammation. The patient's symptoms and general condition are a better guide but still not a good one. Kidneys are best examined indirectly by testing the urine, for even minor disorders which cause no particular symptoms are usually indicated by some abnormality of the urine such as the presence of albumin or of blood cells (◊ urine).

The kidneys throw only a faint shadow on an X-ray plate, but there are two ways of getting very clear X-ray pictures. Iodine compounds are opaque to X-rays. Some iodine compounds are rapidly excreted by the kidneys – they pass into the glomerular filtrate and are not reabsorbed in the tubules. If one of these is injected into a vein it becomes concentrated in the kidneys and then passes down the ureters to the bladder, all of which thus cast clear shadows, and any deformity becomes obvious. The intensity of the shadow and the rate at which it develops roughly indicate the efficiency of the kidney. If a kidney is not working it cannot concentrate the 'dye' and does not show up. This method is known as *intravenous pyelography* (IVP). The second method is *retrograde pyelography*. By means of a ◊ cystoscope a fine tube is inserted into the end of each ureter in the bladder and an iodine-containing solution is injected. This gives a clear X-ray picture of the renal pelvis and ureter on each side, regardless of whether the kidneys are working.

The efficiency of the kidneys can be

roughly assessed by measuring the concentration of waste products in the blood. *Urea* is the most easily measured, and an excess of this relatively harmless substance indicates that other, more poisonous products are also being allowed to accumulate. But healthy kidneys can do more work than is ever required of them, so an excess of waste products in the blood implies fairly serious impairment of the kidneys. A more sensitive test is to measure the rate at which a given substance such as urea can be eliminated.

4. DISORDERS

One normal kidney is enough to maintain good health; two kidneys can tolerate a good deal of damage. Even with advanced kidney disease the symptoms are often mild and vague until a very late stage. If the kidneys stop working altogether the patient quickly succumbs to acidosis and poisoning by waste products unless he can be treated.

The effects of disease of the kidneys are more easily classified than the causes.

The flow of urine may be impeded at almost any point, e.g. by a misplaced artery crossing and kinking the ureter, by faulty development of one of the passages, by scarring after infection or injury, by pressure on the ureters from other organs in the abdomen, by a stone, or in men by enlargement of the prostate gland at the outlet of the bladder. Whatever its cause, obstruction leads to stagnation of urine, and stagnant urine sooner or later becomes infected by bacteria. Above the blockage, the passages are stretched by accumulated urine and the pressure in them rises. The distended renal pelvis encroaches more and more on the substance of the kidney, which works less and less efficiently against the rising pressure. The nephrons may suffer damage from distortion of their blood vessels or from infection, and in the final stage the kidneys stop working altogether. But this stage is not usually reached because the obstruction can nearly always be treated surgically.

Pain from a kidney is ◊ *referred* to the back or loin and may, if the ureter is involved, pass round to the groin. It is probably due to stretching or spasm of the renal pelvis or ureter; the common causes are acute infection (◊ *pyelitis*) and sudden obstruction, as by a stone passing from the wide pelvis into the narrow ureter.

The relation of the kidneys to the blood pressure is discussed under ◊ *hypertension*.

Briefly, persistently high blood pressure can damage the kidneys, and on the other hand diseases of the kidneys, especially those which interfere with their blood supply, can cause high blood pressure and create a vicious circle.

One of the commonest effects of kidney disease is ◊ *oedema* (dropsy), which is accumulation of water in the body. The principal reason for oedema with kidney disease is leakage of protein through the defective nephrons until the concentration of protein in the blood falls below the normal level, which causes leakage of water into the tissues by ◊ *osmosis*. Another mechanism is failure of the diseased kidneys to excrete enough salt. The concentration of salt in the body fluids is kept constant: if there is too much of it, an excess of water is retained to keep the solution at the right strength. Finally, kidney disease may lead to heart disease which is itself a cause of oedema, and this is a vicious circle because heart disease can damage the kidneys by reducing their supply of blood.

The commonest early sign of trouble in the kidneys is protein in the urine. By itself this proves nothing; it is occasionally found in perfectly healthy people. But it is a useful warning to investigate the kidneys further.

Congenital defects are commoner in the kidneys than anywhere else in the body. If neither kidney develops the baby does not survive. Underdevelopment or absence of one kidney does not matter if the other is healthy. In one person in a thousand the two kidneys are joined together; apart from making surgical operations on the kidneys more difficult this is of no significance. A defective renal artery is a rare cause of high blood pressure. Various structural defects can impede the flow of urine, leading to stagnation and infection. Many can be corrected surgically. In addition to these anatomical oddities, there are certain rare congenital disorders of the chemical functions of the kidneys in which the tubules are unable to reabsorb a substance which should be restored to the blood. Thus some people do not completely reabsorb glucose and regularly pass sugar in their urine; this harmless condition might be confused with diabetes. A similar excess of phosphate in the urine leads to deformity of bone (*renal rickets*). The *Fanconi syndrome* is a more serious defect of the tubules involving numerous substances.

Injuries are uncommon because the kidneys are well protected, but a heavy blow can bruise or tear a kidney. Bleeding is the danger. Usually it stops in good time, but a badly torn kidney may need surgical repair, and occasionally the safest course is to remove it.

Infection by bacteria, spreading to the kidneys from the bladder, is discussed under ◊ *pyelitis*. The only other important type of infection is ◊ *tuberculosis*; this was once a common disease, but in recent years tuberculosis of the kidneys has become comparatively rare.

Bright's disease (◊ *nephritis*) is inflammation of the kidneys not directly due to bacterial infection.

Several types of stone (◊ *calculus*) can arise in the kidneys. They can be a result of infection, but on the other hand a stone in the renal pelvis or ureter can obstruct the flow and so cause infection.

Tumours of the kidney are commonly harmless and discovered only by chance during an operation or a postmortem examination. But about 1 per cent of all cancer occurs in the kidneys. The only common symptom is bleeding into the urine; if this is observed early the affected kidney may be successfully removed. One of the few cancers of infancy, *Wilms' tumour*, arises in the kidneys. This kind of cancer grows fast, and distension of the child's belly is often the only symptom. The outlook is poor but not hopeless, because as long as the tumour is confined to the kidney it can be completely removed. Even very large Wilms' tumours may be curable.

5. TREATMENT OF KIDNEY DISEASE

The more important conditions are considered under their own headings. The following notes concern kidney disease in general.

Several reasons for operating on the kidneys are mentioned in the previous section. The surgeon can approach the kidney from in front, through the abdomen, or from behind, under the ribs. He gets a better view from in front, but for most purposes it is less complicated and safer to work from behind; if the 12th rib is in the way it can be removed without disabling the patient in any way. Since blood vessels do not cross from back to front of the kidney it can be cut open along its outer border, as if it were an oyster, with little loss of blood (e.g. to remove a stone).

The effects of poor function can be miti-

gated by reducing the load on the kidneys. If the amount and concentration of the urine can no longer be varied to meet variations of intake, the intake of water and salt has to be adapted to what the kidneys can manage.

Waste products in the urine are mainly derived from protein. The amount can be reduced by limiting the amount of protein in the diet. For severe cases the amount and constitution of the diet can be balanced with the body's requirements; this is a tedious process but it can keep people in fairly good health who would die if they took an uncontrolled diet.

If the kidneys fail completely their work has to be done by other means. Successful grafting of a healthy kidney from another person is the best way, but there are many problems to be overcome before this treatment can be at all widely used (◊ *transplantation*).

Patients can be kept alive without kidneys or with kidneys that no longer work by some form of *dialysis*, which amounts to selective filtration of unwanted matter from the blood. If blood is separated from water by a porous membrane through which small but not large molecules can pass, then cells and proteins will remain in the blood, while salts, glucose, amino-acids, and waste products will diffuse into the water, as in the glomerular filtrate of a normal kidney (section 2 above). The tendency for water to cross the membrane and dilute the blood is overcome if the blood is kept at a suitable pressure by a pump. This simple arrangement indiscriminately washes out waste products such as urea and essentials such as glucose and salt. The kidneys overcome the problem by selective reabsorption; our apparatus will do the same thing if instead of water on the other side of the membrane we use a solution of salt etc. in the same concentrations as in the blood. These essentials will then cross the membrane in either direction at the same rate, with the net result that none is lost from the blood, while waste products leave the blood.

The *peritoneum*, which lines the abdomen, is a membrane of the right type. If a suitable solution is run into the abdominal cavity through a hollow needle, waste products find their way from the blood-stream into the solution, which is then drained away. This technique, *peritoneal dialysis*, is safe and simple, and reasonably effective; but it is uncomfortable and many patients find repeated peritoneal dialysis hard to tolerate.

The *artificial kidney*, devised in Holland at the end of the Second World War, uses exactly the same principle with a synthetic membrane. In Kolff's original apparatus a cellophane tube was coiled round a beer can. Blood from an artery was pumped through the tube and returned to a vein. The system was immersed in a bath of dialysing solution. This type of apparatus is still in use. An alternative is to pump blood over sheets of cellophane with the solution on the other side. Elaborate and costly equipment is needed to ensure the correct concentration and temperature of the fluid and an even flow of blood at the right pressure. An important modification is the use of a synthetic tube joining one of the patient's arteries to a vein and left in place on the surface of his body. Each time dialysis is needed the apparatus is connected to this tube, which may not need replacement for a year or more, instead of to an actual blood vessel, which would have to be exposed surgically for each dialysis. A person without kidneys spends two or three nights a week connected to an artificial kidney and sleeps through the dialysis. Otherwise he can lead a fairly normal life.

knee. The knee joint is formed between the lower end of the *femur* and the upper end of the *tibia*. The *fibula* plays no part. The joint between the femur and the knee-cap (*patella*) shares the synovial membrane and capsule (◊ *joint*) of the knee. The surfaces are by no means a perfect fit, but the disparity is largely overcome by a cartilage or *meniscus* on each side of the joint. A meniscus is a flattened crescent of springy fibrous tissue, thick at the rim and wafer-thin at the inner edge.

The ligaments of the knee are very strong. They are at both sides, behind, and, most unusually, inside the joint. These last are the *cruciate* ligaments, stout bands from the tibia to the notch between the two condyles of the femur. In front, the knee is supported by the *quadriceps* muscle. This huge muscle, forming the front of the thigh, ends as a flat tendon spread over the knee and anchored to the front of the tibia. The patella is a disc of bone embedded in the tendon which slides up and down on the femur as the muscle acts.

The only deliberate movements of the knee are the pendulum-like flexion, by the hamstring muscles, and extension, by the quadriceps. But when the knee is straightened the ligaments are not all pulled taut at the same moment. Those which are still lax allow a slight inward twist of the femur; then all ligaments are tight and the knee is said to be locked. (Locking the knee has a second meaning, defined below.) The beginner on skis disobeys the instruction to bend his knees partly because he is unconsciously bracing them against a fall, but also because by 'locking' his knees he transfers the strain from his tired muscles to his ligaments.

Fractures of the tibia or femur which involve the joint surfaces often need operative treatment, for unless the fragments are exactly replaced the joint is bound to become stiff. Some fractures of the patella give little trouble, but after some bad fractures the patella has to be removed. This operation causes remarkably little disability.

Dislocation of the knee is very unusual, but torn ligaments are common. A complete tear of any of the main ligaments renders the knee unstable, and surgical repair may be needed.

The commonest disorder of the knee is a torn meniscus, usually at the inner side of the joint. A sideways jolt to the slightly bent knee is the usual cause. If the torn meniscus lies flat it gives no trouble, but the torn part tends to curl and block the joint. The knee is then painful and cannot be completely straightened. This limitation of movement is called 'locking' (see above). The patient often acquires a knack of twisting and straightening his knee to replace the tear, but the meniscus is still torn, and lacking a blood supply it cannot heal. The trouble therefore recurs, and the only cure is to remove the meniscus. A knee can function well without menisci, but the success of the operation depends largely on the condition of the muscles: indeed this is true of all surgery of the knee. The ligaments are very strong, but they are effective only when the knee is straight. In all other positions the strength of the knee is the strength of the quadriceps.

Koch, Robert (1843–1910). German physician and pathologist. If Pasteur laid the foundations of microbiology, Koch was the principal builder of this science. Much of his early work on bacteria was done while he was a busy general practitioner in Prussia. Pasteur had proved in general terms that bacteria could cause disease. Koch showed which types of bacteria caused particular diseases. He found methods of identifying and classifying bacteria, of growing them in pure culture (i.e. without contamination by other species), and above all of proving whether they were true causes of a disease or mere bystanders. ◊ *microbe* (1).

Kocher, Theodor (1841–1917). Swiss surgeon. His career is a bridge between the hazardous and limited surgery before Lister's use of antiseptics and present-day methods. He advanced many branches of surgery, but is especially remembered for his work on the nature and treatment of goitre, for which he received a Nobel Prize in 1909. In recent years, surgery has been more and more divided into specialties, and more and more a team effort. Kocher was for years undoubtedly the best surgeon in the world, a distinction that no one surgeon could claim today.

koilonychia. Thin concave finger-nails, due to lack of iron.

Koplik's spots. (H. Koplik (1858–1927), American physician.) Very small red spots with white centres, on the inner lining of the cheeks, a characteristic and early sign of measles.

Korsakow's syndrome. (S. S. Korsakow (1853–1900), Russian neurologist.) Deterioration of the function of nerves and brain, with loss of memory and poor mental coordination, sometimes with disturbed sensation or muscular action. Elaborate lies, perhaps to compensate for loss of memory, may be a symptom. The cause is deficiency of B vitamins, often due to chronic alcoholism.

kwashiorkor. A severe form of malnutrition first recognized among children in West Africa but now known to be widespread in the tropics. The condition sets in after weaning, which is sometimes delayed until the age of 2 years. An affected child does not look thin at first sight, because the skin and abdomen are distended with retained water. A swollen liver may add to the pot-belly. There is loss of pigment in the skin and often the hair, which becomes sandy and brittle. The skin changes have been confused with those of *pellagra*. These children have little resistance to other illness, and often die of what should be minor ailments. The digestive organs may become so impaired that the child can no longer absorb good food even if it is provided.

Kwashiorkor was formerly regarded as a pure protein deficiency, but it now seems that the limited supply of protein might suffice if there were enough other food to spare the protein from being squandered as fuel: hence the term *protein-energy malnutrition*. Why these very poor diets affect some children with kwashiorkor and others with the more predictable emaciation of *marasmus* is not clear. Failure to digest other foods than protein because of intestinal infection may be a factor.

kyphosis. Curvature of the spine producing convexity or arching of the back. The natural curve in the thoracic region of the spine is a slight kyphosis, as opposed to the *lordosis* or hollowing of the lumbar region below.

L

labial. Of the lips.

labium. Lip. *Labia majora, minora*: outer and inner folds of skin of the vulva.

labour. The process by which a pregnant woman is delivered of her baby. (The infant is considered under ◊ *birth*.)

The baby in the uterus is surrounded by watery fluid in a closed bag of membrane. He is nourished by the *placenta*, a thick disc attached to the inside of the uterus, where it draws supplies from the mother's blood, and joined to the baby by blood vessels in the *umbilical cord*. The uterus is a hollow muscle with a downward extension, the *cervix*, in the vagina. The cervix is a muscular ring, tightly closed during pregnancy.

In the *first stage* of labour the muscle fibres leading down to the cervix contract at intervals of a few minutes, while those of the cervix itself relax. The effect is to open the cervix and create a passage from the uterus into the vagina. The cervix is drawn up over the lowest part of the baby, normally the head. In advance of the baby's head, a pocket of fluid is trapped; after a time the membrane bursts and the fluid escapes. This may be a signal for the contractions to become stronger and more frequent. With a first baby, this stage can last all day, but it tends to be shorter with later pregnancies. It cannot be timed, because often it has no definite beginning. All through the latter part of pregnancy the uterus contracts and relaxes, and labour is only an intensification of the process.

The *second stage* is the descent of the baby and its actual birth. As soon as the cervix is wide enough the character of the contractions changes. They become more purposeful, and the woman instinctively helps by pushing. The muscle fibres of the uterus remain a littler shorter after each contraction, and the baby is pushed down the vagina. There are two obstacles: a sharp bend forwards from uterus to vagina, and the muscles, connective tissue and skin of the floor of the pelvis at the outlet from the vagina. which take some time to stretch.

After the birth of the baby, the *third stage* of labour is a few contractions to expel the placenta and leave the uterus as a tight knot of muscle. There may be waves of contraction (after-pains) for some time after delivery.

Nobody knows why, some 38 weeks after conception, labour should begin. It is probably set off by a chemical stimulus – a hormone, oxytocin, from the pituitary, but why the hormone should suddenly become active remains a mystery. The duration of pregnancy varies more in humans than in other animals, but more than a couple of weeks either side of the average entails risks for the baby. What really matters is not an exact number of days, but the stage of development of the baby at birth. A premature baby has difficulty in surviving as an independent being until it reaches the stage of growth at which it should have been born; and if labour is unduly late the baby may no longer be getting enough nourishment from the placenta, and labour has to be started artificially (◊ *induction*).

Contractions of the uterus in the first stage of labour are often no worse than rather uncomfortable. If there is pain, it is a sort of colic from stretching involuntary muscle; like other internal organs, the uterus does not transmit any other sensation (it is wholly insensitive to cutting or heat). The source of pain in the second stage is more obvious: a large baby is pushed through a narrow and sensitive passage, and although continued pressure tends to numb the skin of the outlet it cannot do so completely.

The amount of pain suffered by any individual woman in labour is partly dictated by her expectations and frame of mind. The uterus transmits signals up the spinal cord, but the interpretations of those signals is the function of the brain. They may be differently perceived by different people. Certainly a woman who expects to suffer (having been filled with tales of horror by relatives and friends) is likely to do so. Equally certainly, by setting up muscular tension which resists the process of birth, the suffering itself is likely to increase.

Training throughout pregnancy (it is useless to wait until confinement), usually by a physiotherapist, teaches women to relax the muscles of the outlet from the pelvis while pushing with their abdominal muscles, making labour quicker and easier. In good hands, this sort of training does much more: it helps to establish confidence and mental relaxation when the time comes. This method has sometimes been derided, perhaps because its merits had been exaggerated, but most women who have given it a serious trial have found it helpful.

When antenatal training achieves its object, 'natural childbirth', there is no need for drugs to relieve pain, but not all women have received this training and those who have do not all find that it works. The treatment of pain in childbirth is always a compromise. In the first stage, a large enough dose of an antispasmodic drug might take away all pain, but by taking away the spasm would bring labour to a halt. *Pethidine* is both pain-killing and antispasmodic and therefore perfectly suited to relieving the symptom, but it has to be used very cautiously in order not to prolong labour. The second stage brings a new hazard: if the baby is still under the influence of a narcotic drug when he is born, his breathing will be depressed, and his most urgent need in the first few minutes of life is a few deep breaths. Also, during the second stage the attendant needs the mother's cooperation. Hence the caution with which doctors and midwives give analgesic help such as gas and air. Unless the baby is to be delivered by forceps anaesthetics cannot be used until the last few contractions when they can guide the baby into the open air without help from the mother. Many women find the second stage of labour much less distressing than the last part of the first. Any pain brings with it the irresistible urge to push the baby towards its exit. The pushing, having something to do to help the birth along, makes the pain seem more tolerable: it is positive effort with a recognizable end in view.

Various types of spinal anaesthesia can be induced by injecting a local anaesthetic into the spine. Techniques of this kind can be used either throughout labour, the local anaesthetic being topped up whenever needed, or only in the second stage. Many obstetricians (and mothers) believe that this is the ideal form of childbirth analgesia, giving, in expert hands, a totally pain-free labour to a fully conscious woman. But there are technical problems to killing pain without killing muscular effort, and

thus slowing labour down. And the method demands skilled anaesthetists. Only a few hospitals can as yet offer this method to any woman who wants it.

By far the greatest hazard used to be infection ($\Diamond$ *puerperal* fever). Now that this is a rarity, labour is usually a safe venture. The remaining dangers are largely mechanical. Most babies are born head first, with the back of the head to the mother's front. Any other position is more difficult, and if possible the baby is manipulated into the natural position before birth.

Delay in the first stage does not matter if the baby's heart beat indicates that it is well; but if either mother or child is distressed Caesarean section may be needed. Delay in the second stage may be due to mechanical obstruction: the baby is too big for the passage, or in the wrong position. If the disparity is obvious, the trouble can be avoided by Caesarean section before labour begins. The *obstetric forceps*, giving a firm but gentle grip on the baby's head, can be used to ease the baby's head past the outlet. Although the midwife tries to prevent injury to the mother's skin and muscles if she can do so without delaying the birth, it is sometimes necessary to make a deliberate cut (*episiotomy*) that can be neatly stitched after the birth; this does much less harm than allowing the tissues to be torn.

Ergometrine, a drug derived from *ergot*, stimulates contraction of the uterus. It is often given at the end of labour to tighten the uterus and prevent bleeding.

labyrinth. The inner ear, embedded in the temporal bone of the skull, consisting of the organs of balance and hearing.

laceration. An irregular, torn wound (as opposed to an incision or cut).

lacrimal. Of tears, e.g. *lacrimal gland*, where tears are formed, under the upper lid. (There is no need for the fussier spelling *lachrymal*, which seems to have crept into English usage by mistake. At least in technical senses, *lacrimal* has international sanction and a proper pedigree.)

lactation. Formation of milk. $\Diamond$ *breast*; *milk*.

lactose. Milk sugar, a compound of the simple sugars *galactose* and *glucose*, to which it is broken down in the intestine. After assimilation, galactose is converted to glucose.

Laënnec, René-Théophile-Hyacinthe (1781–1826). French physician with an unsurpassed genius for diagnosis, a pupil of Corvisart. He wrote admirable studies of numerous disorders of the heart and lungs, in particular of tuberculosis, about which he left little to be said until the discovery of the causative microbe at the end of the century. His own early death was due to this disease.

Laënnec is best remembered as the inventor of the ◊ *stethoscope*, with the help of which he was able to recognize disorders in the chest much more accurately than anyone before him – indeed quite as accurately as anyone since, given the same equipment. Improvements since his time are due to better understanding of the nature and causes of disease and to the use of laboratory investigations, X-rays and the like; not to better clinical technique. The great diagnosticians of the 19th century, of whom Laënnec may be counted the first, used their eyes, ears, and hands to make correct and confident diagnoses that seem to us almost impossible without elaborate technical methods.

The most remarkable feature of Laënnec's discovery was that he himself said practically all that was to be said about its use: his descriptions of normal and abnormal sounds from the heart and lungs might have been written yesterday.

Lamarck, Jean-Baptiste (1744–1829). French naturalist; remembered more for two theories which were discredited (spontaneous generation, and inheritance of acquired characters: ◊ *Pasteur*; *evolution*) than for the fact that he was the first man to put forward a theory of evolution.

laminectomy. Surgical operation: removal of a plate of bone (lamina) at the back of one or more vertebrae to expose the spinal cord.

lanolin. Wool fat, a bland substance used on its own to soften hard skin, or mixed with more active ingredients as the basis of various ointments.

laparotomy. Literally: cutting the flank or loin. The accepted meaning is any surgical operation in which the abdomen is opened, especially in the sense of *exploratory laparotomy*, when the exact diagnosis is still in doubt until the abdominal organs are inspected.

lardaceous disease = ◊ *amyloid disease.*

laryngitis. Inflammation of the larynx caused by spread of infection either downwards from the nose and pharynx or, less often, upwards from the lungs or trachea. Sore throat, dry cough, and hoarseness are the symptoms; apart from infection they can arise from any irritation of the vocal cords such as excessive smoking or shouting. An attack of laryngitis seldom lasts more than a few days, and since there are various other causes of hoarseness (◊ *larynx*) persistent symptoms need to be investigated.

Inhaled air is normally warmed and moistened in the nose before it reaches the larynx. When the nose is blocked, e.g. by a common cold, air breathed through the mouth is still cold and dry when it reaches the larynx. This seems to irritate inflamed vocal cords, and is a good reason for staying indoors with laryngitis. Inhaled steam helps because it is moist and warm. Menthol, friar's balsam and other traditional adjuncts to the steam have a medicinal aroma which assures the patient that the treatment is doing him good. Perhaps the more important effect of the inhalation is on the nose; it may clear the airway.

There is no evidence that gargling has any effect on laryngitis.

laryngoscope. Instrument for examining the inside of the larnyx. For *direct laryngoscopy* an illuminated tube or half-tube is passed behind the tongue, and behind the epiglottis: this is possible only if the parts have been anaesthetized and the patient is in exactly the right position on an operating table, because the epiglottis is very sensitive and the axis of the larynx is at right angles to that of the mouth.

The usual and older method is *indirect laryngoscopy*. A dentist's angled mirror is held against the soft palate and used to reflect light into the larynx and an image of the larynx to the surgeon. The lamp can be worn on the surgeon's forehead or placed beside the patient and reflected into the patient's mouth by a mirror with a hole through which the surgeon peers. This method gives an excellent view of the parts behind the tongue, including the vocal cords. If the mirror is turned upwards the nasopharynx, above and behind the soft palate, can be examined.

Manuel Garcia, a teacher of singing who studied the movements of his own vocal

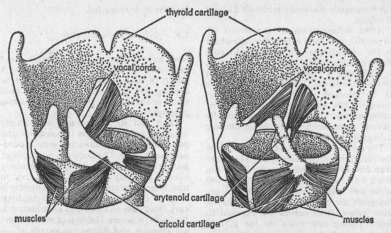

Larynx, dissected from behind to show closure and opening of vocal cords.

cords, is usually credited with the invention of laryngoscopy (1854), and the Hungarian surgeon Czermak with introducing it to medical practice (1858). But the method had already been discovered, and ignored, at least three times: by Levret (Paris, 1743), Bozzini (Frankfurt, 1807), and Senn (Geneva, 1827).

larynx. The voice-box at the entrance to the windpipe (*trachea*) in the front of the neck. The trachea and lungs arise in the embryo as an offshoot from the pharynx, which is a part of the digestive tube. At the entrance to the trachea from the pharynx a valve has been evolved, to be closed during swallowing. The voice is a secondary function; birds have a larynx but their voices come from the *syrinx* further down the trachea.

The larynx is enclosed by cartilages. Below it is supported by a firm ring, the *cricoid cartilage*, which is the entrance to the trachea proper. The much larger *thyroid cartilage* is perched on top of the cricoid. It is shaped like a snow-plough, with its two halves widely separated behind and meeting in front to form the Adam's apple. From inside the Adam's apple two fibrous ridges run back; these are the *vocal cords*. Each cord is attached behind to a small, mobile triangle of cartilage (*arytenoid cartilage*). The arytenoids slide on the cricoid, between the two halves of the thyroid cartilage.

The cartilages of the larynx have a complex set of muscles to move them. At most times the arytenoids are kept apart and the vocal cords, joined in front, form a V-shaped opening, the *glottis*, through which one breathes. For swallowing, the arytenoids are drawn together and the gap is closed. At the same time a flap of cartilage behind the tongue, the *epiglottis*, drops like a hinged lid over the larynx. For speech, the arytenoids are also drawn together, but the epiglottis stays up. The thyroid cartilage is tilted on the cricoid to vary the length and tension of the vocal cords and so adjust the *pitch* of the voice. The *volume* of sound depends on the amount of air delivered from the lungs (◊ *respiration* (1)). The *timbre* or quality of sound, which makes the difference between the vowels, depends on the configuration of the upper air-passages, including the nose and its sinuses. It is adjusted by changing the shape of the mouth.

1. DISORDERS

A blow on the Adam's apple can fracture the thyroid cartilage. This is a serious injury because it jeopardizes the airway. An artificial inlet for air in the trachea (tracheo-stomy) may be needed at once, and the fracture itself may need surgical repair.

The vocal cords can be damaged by the strain of shouting or singing; the usual injury is rupture of a small blood vessel. This may cause a swelling (*polyp*) like a small berry on the cord. A polyp causes hoarse-ness or even temporary loss of the voice, but fortunately it is easily removed without ill effects.

Acute inflammation of the larynx (◊ *laryngitis*) often follows infection elsewhere in the air-passages, e.g. a common cold above or acute bronchitis below the larynx. ◊ *Diphtheria* is especially dangerous if it involves the larynx, for the airway is liable to be blocked. When diphtheria was common this was the usual reason for tracheostomy. Tuberculosis occasionally spreads from the lungs to cause chronic laryngitis.

The muscles of the larynx are supplied by the recurrent laryngeal nerves. These are branches of the vagus nerves. They run down into the root of the neck – the left nerve well into the thorax – and then up, alongside the trachea, to enter the larynx from below. Both nerves are exposed to injury during operations on the thyroid gland, in which they are practically embedded as they run upwards, and the left nerve may be involved in disease such as cancer of the left lung, causing paralysis of the left vocal cord and hoarseness.

A cancer of a vocal cord the size of a pin's head is enough to cause hoarseness. At this stage the chance of removal and complete cure is extremely good. If the cords are not involved, cancer of the larynx is less obvious and the outlook is less good. The necessary operation can be anything from a nick in the vocal cord which heals completely to removal of the whole larynx. Even after the most drastic operations patients can learn to speak at least enough to make themselves understood by swallowing air and talking in controlled belches.

◊ *pharynx; laryngoscope.*

latissimus dorsi. Large flat muscle of the back; its fibres arise from the spines of the vertebrae from the 7th thoracic downwards, and from the back of the pelvis. They converge on a small flat tendon attached to the humerus a little below the shoulder.

The muscle forces the arm down and back, as in swimming or climbing.

laudanum. Tincture of opium; an alcoholic extract of opium formerly much used as a narcotic.

Laveran, Alphonse (1845–1922). French army doctor. He discovered the parasite of ◊ *malaria.*

laxative = ◊ *purgative.*

LE = ◊ *lupus erythematosus.*

lead. Salts of lead, e.g. lead acetate, have been used as astringents on the skin. A lotion of lead acetate is supposed to be cooling and good for sprains, but cold water probably does as well without being poisonous.

Lead and its compounds have many industrial uses, and in the 19th century lead poisoning was a common and serious occupational disease. The body has no means of getting rid of lead. Small amounts regularly inhaled or swallowed accumulate, and in time large amounts may be stored, mostly in bone in the place of calcium. Symptoms vary from case to case. The commonest is *lead colic*, a severe abdominal pain; others are anaemia, and damage to nerves or the brain. The precautions now used in all industries involving lead have made poisoning a rarity. Large supplements of calcium in the diet help to displace lead from the bones, and the chelating agent EDTA forms an inert compound with lead that is excreted in the urine.

Leeuwenhoek, Antony van (1632–1723). Draper, of Delft, Holland; in his spare time the most celebrated of all microscopists.

The compound microscope, invented some years before Leeuwenhoek's birth, had technical faults that were not overcome until the 19th century; it was then less efficient than the simple magnifying glasses that Leeuwenhoek ground for himself. With the aid of a tiny biconvex lens, Leeuwenhoek accurately observed and described details that a beginner with an expensive modern microscope can easily overlook.

He showed that muscles are composed of fibres, and recorded the alternating light and dark bands or stripes across the fibres (the bands are about 1/20,000 inch wide). He gave the first descriptions of spermatozoa, studied the flow of blood through capillary vessels (first seen by Malpighi), studied red blood cells of various species, noticing that those of fish had nuclei whereas human red cells had none, and in 1675 observed microbes (protozoa) in water. In a report published by the Royal Society, London, in 1683, he described bacteria from his mouth (◊ *microbe*).

leg. In descriptive anatomy the leg is only the part of the lower limb between the knee and the ankle, as distinct from the *thigh*.

The skeleton of the leg is the ◊ *tibia*, which carries the weight, with the slender ◊ *fibula* attached at each end to its outer side. Unlike the radius and ulna in the forearm, these two bones are rigidly joined to each other; there is no significant movement between them.

There are three groups of muscles: the *extensors* of the ankle and foot between the two bones in front, the *flexors* behind, forming the bulge of the calf, and the *peroneal* muscles at the outer side. At the inner side the flat surface of the tibia – the shin – is covered only by skin and fibrous tissue. The actions of the muscles are described under ◊ *ankle* and ◊ *foot*.

The nerves are branches of the ◊ *sciatic* nerve. The ◊ *popliteal* artery runs behind the knee, below which it divides into anterior and posterior tibial arteries. These are deeply buried in the extensor and flexor muscles, but they emerge near the ankle and their pulses can be felt on the top of the foot and immediately behind the lower end of the tibia. The veins accompanying these arteries are rather small, and much of the blood returns by the ◊ *saphenous veins* just below the skin.

In comparison with other parts of the body the circulation of blood in the legs is precarious, and very little interference with it can be tolerated. Gravity resists the return of blood and can be overcome only if the valves in the saphenous veins are competent. If they fail, blood collects in the veins and stagnates, and the nutrition of the skin is impaired (◊ *varicose veins*). Widespread disease of the arteries usually shows itself first in the legs and feet. Elsewhere the reduced flow of blood does not cause symptoms for a long time, but here there is little margin of safety.

Leishman, Sir William (1865–1926). British army doctor; a pioneer of tropical medicine.

Leishmania. A microscopical parasite similar to that of sleeping sickness; transmitted by sandflies, and causing either localized infection (Delhi boil or ◊ *oriental sore*) or a dangerous fever (Dumdum fever or ◊ *kala-azar*).

lens. The lens of the eye is a flexible structure the size and shape of a lentil. Most of the refraction is done by the rounded *cornea* at the front of the eye, which is a fixed component. The lens itself adjusts the focus as the surrounding muscle increases or decreases its curvature.

Leonardo da Vinci (1452–1519). Florentine artist and scientist. Modern medicine begins with the accurate observation of how the human body is constructed, and the first men to reject the anatomical dogma and superstition of the Middle Ages were not the doctors but the artists. Foremost among these was Leonardo, perhaps the first man in 13 centuries to dispute the doctrines of Galen and trust the evidence of his own eyes. He left incomparable drawings of his dissections of every part of the body, in which he corrected many of the fallacies that had prevented medical science from advancing. As an engineer he was especially interested in the action of muscles, and he came as near as anyone before Harvey to understanding the circulation of blood.

Leonardo's discoveries were not directly helpful to medicine, because they were not published; but the example of the artists encouraged doctors to study anatomy in the only rational way: from the human body and not from ancient texts.

leprosy (lepra). A disease once found in all countries but now almost confined to the tropics, due to *Mycobacterium leprae*, a microbe almost indistinguishable from that of tuberculosis. The infection is confined to the skin and nerves.

One form, *lepromatous* leprosy, causes raised blotches and lumps on the skin (including the well-known leonine facies or lion-face). The surfaces of the blotches may break down to form ulcers. The other common form, *tuberculoid* leprosy, affects nerves, causing patches of skin to lose all sensation, or sometimes only the sense of pain. There are also visible changes in the skin, more or less coinciding with the loss of sensation; they include loss of hair and, in dark skins, of colour. These areas of paler than normal skin are as near as one gets to the 'white as snow' of biblical lepers.

There are also *indeterminate* and *borderline* cases, which may develop into either lepromatous or tuberculoid forms.

The crippling deformities of advanced leprosy are due to the involvement of nerves. They include damage to joints by paralysis of muscles, and loss of tissue (notably fingers and toes) from both paralysis of blood vessels and unnoticed burns or other injuries.

Only the florid lepromatous form of leprosy is infectious, and even this is difficult to contract. Leprosy is very rare except among people who live in the closest contact with lepers. It is quite exceptional even for doctors and nurses in leprosaria to catch the disease.

Until about 1947 the standard drug for leprosy was chaulmoogra oil, which was not very effective. But research to find a sulphonamide to cure tuberculosis produced *dapsone* and other sulphone drugs. They do not cure tuberculosis, but they work well against leprosy. The drawback is that treatment has to be prolonged (two years or even longer), and the patient's bacteria may develop resistance to the drug. The answer then is to use another drug. *Thiambutosine* is as effective as dapsone, and often the two drugs complement each other, organisms resistant to one yielding to the other. Several drugs used mainly for tuberculosis, e.g. *rifampicin*, also arrest leprosy. But these alternative drugs are expensive, and it is in poor countries that leprosy is common.

Even if current drugs do not always cure leprosy they at least check its progress, and they make the patient non-infectious, thus protecting the next generation. If the ten million or so lepers scattered through many of the warmer parts of the world could have even an incomplete course of drugs this disease could probably be eradicated, and the campaign to do so is high on the list of priorities of the World Health Organization. The traditional leprosarium where lepers live and work and marry away from the world is already giving place to dispensaries where lepers attend for treatment while living safely with healthy people.

Leptospira. A *spirochaete* or spiral bacterium. Several species cause disease in animals that occasionally spread to man; the best known is ◊ *Weil's disease.*

lesion. Disturbance of the structure or function of a part of the body, such as a wound, abscess, tumour, or chemical abnormality.

leuc(o)-; leuk(o)-. Prefix = 'white' (blood cell, matter in the brain, as opposed to grey matter, etc.).

leukaemia. Leukaemia is a cancer-like disease of the white blood cells. Whereas most cancer grows and spreads from a single focus, leukaemia is a wide-spread affection of the bone marrow and other blood-forming tissue. The essential disorder seems to be failure of developing white cells to mature. Fully developed, effective white cells cannot reproduce themselves; after a life-span of a few days or weeks they are replaced by new cells. But leukaemic cells retain the ability to multiply, and they do not develop to a stage at which they can function as a defence against infection. As the disease progresses, these useless immature cells displace normal white cells, and the patient is as much at the mercy of infectious diseases as someone with no white cells at all. The abnormal activity in the bone marrow also encroaches on the formation of red blood cells and platelets, so that the patient becomes anaemic, and his blood does not clot properly. Although in some very acute cases the patient may live only a few months, it may be many years before serious symptoms appear – in the most chronic cases, 20 years or more. Unhappily, it is often in children that leukaemia progresses most rapidly. This is one of the forms of cancer that is becoming commoner, especially in the most developed countries.

The term leukaemia is a Greek rendering of 'white blood', Virchow's description of a case in which there were so many white cells that the blood had a milky appearance. In health, the number of these cells is not more than 10,000 per cubic millimetre. With leukaemia, counts up to 300,000 have been recorded.

Leukaemia is easier to study than other forms of cancer, because so much can be learnt from a drop of blood. Even with the recent increase, leukaemia is not very common, but many of the lessons learnt from it can be applied to cancer in general.

In some animals, leukaemia can be caused by a virus; this form of the disease can be transmitted to other animals. There is a growing suspicion that virus infection may also play a part in human leukaemia.

Leukaemia is slightly commoner among the relations of people with leukaemia than in the general population, but the difference is not enough to prove a hereditary basis. On the other hand, structural changes in one of the ◊ *chromosomes* are regularly found, but these could be a result rather than a cause of the disease. The affected pair of chromosomes (no. 21) is the pair which is abnormal in ◊ *mongolism* – a disorder often associated with leukaemia.

Complete recovery used to be reported from time to time, but it now seems likely that these were really cases of glandular fever, which has many of the symptoms of leukaemia at the height of the attack, but clears up completely. Present forms of treatment do not cure the disease. They may prolong life (a difficult thing to prove when the course of a disease is so unpredictable), and they certainly prolong useful life, i.e. they postpone until the very end the stage in which the patient actually feels ill. The object is to suppress the division and reproduction of cells. The rapidly dividing leukaemic cells are more susceptible than healthy cells, so that the treatment can be adjusted to suppress their activity without greatly damaging healthy cells. One method is by radiation. A gross excess of radiation stops the formation of all blood cells, but a small dose affects only abnormal cells. Radiation can be given either from outside with X-rays or from inside with radioactive phosphorus. Numerous drugs, such as nitrogen mustard and aminopterin, prevent cell division by blocking an essential enzyme. In the end, leukaemic cells may adapt themselves to the treatment, but it may be many years before this happens, and in the meantime the patient remains fit; the healthy elements of his bone marrow have a chance to maintain a complement of normal blood cells.
◊ *cancer.*

leukocyte. White blood cell. ◊ *blood* (3).

leukoderma. Patches of skin without pigment; ◊ *vitiligo.*

leukoplakia. Small white patches on a mucous membrane; they are areas where the outer layer is unduly thick. Leukoplakia in the mouth follows prolonged irritation, e.g. from heavy pipe-smoking, poor dental hygiene or chronic infection. A similar condition of the female genital organs is apparently due to deficiency of sex hormones after the menopause. The former condition is treated by removing the cause; the latter by supplying appropriate hormones.

Leukoplakia needs attention because it may be a precursor of cancer.

leukorrhoea. Excess of white or colourless secretion from the vagina; it may be only an exaggeration of the normal secretion, or a symptom of irritation anywhere in the genital organs, such as the common infections with *trichomonas* or *candida.*

leukotomy. A surgical operation devised in 1935 by Egas Moniz (1874 1955), a Portuguese neurosurgeon, for the relief of certain severe and progressive mental disturbances. The nerve cells of the prefrontal lobes at the very front of the brain are disconnected from the rest of the brain by cutting the underlying fibres. Moniz had remarkable success with otherwise hopeless cases, and won a Nobel Prize in 1949.

Since brain tissue cannot heal, the operation is irrevocable. People who have had it have altered personalities: they tend to be irresponsible. But most of us would rather be carefree than suicidal. With the discovery of drugs that act selectively on disordered areas of the brain (or disordered processes), leukotomy has fallen from favour, and in time it is likely to become obsolete.

levallorphan. An antagonist of ◊ *morphine.*

LGV = ◊ *lymphogranuloma venereum.*

libido. Freud's term for the instinctive sexual drive, which may conflict with civilized behaviour, causing emotional tension.

lichen. Several skin diseases with raised blotches: with *lichen planus* the blotches have a violet sheen, and itch. The cause is unknown, but emotional upsets seem to play some part.

ligament. Fibrous band between two bones at a ◊ *joint*. Ligaments are flexible but inelastic; they come into play only at the extremes of movement, and cannot be stretched when they are taut. Any intermediate position of a joint is held entirely by the muscles, which in any case are its main supports. The ligaments set the limits beyond which no movement is possible. 'Double-jointed' simply means that the ligaments are longer than usual and allow a larger range of movement.

A joint can be forced beyond its normal range only by tearing a ligament; this is a *sprain*. Fibrous tissue heals reluctantly, and a severe sprain can be quite as incapacitating as a fracture.

limb. All vertebrates have two pairs of limbs slung from the backbone. The pattern of two fore-limbs and two hind-limbs attached respectively to pectoral and pelvic girdles must have been laid down early in evolution. In birds, reptiles, and mammals even the components of the limbs correspond closely between species, although the proportions are adapted in ways that make external appearances widely different (◊ *skeleton*).

Excepting modifications to do with walking upright, human limbs have evolved little from the basic pattern: a girdle composed of three bony elements on either side (fused in the shoulder-blade and hip-bone); an upper segment with one long bone (*arm* with humerus, *thigh* with femur); next a segment with parallel long bones (*forearm* with radius and ulna, *leg* with tibia and fibula); next a cluster of small bones (*carpus, tarsus*); five straight bones protruding (*metacarpals, metatarsals*); and from each of the five a digit, four digits preserving the primitive four segments and one (thumb, big toe) with only two segments. Because the limbs are twisted during early growth out of their lizard-like position, the back of the arm finally corresponds with the front of the thigh, and the radius and thumb with the tibia and big toe. Most of the muscles correspond fairly closely between the limbs, and the nerves and vessels are roughly alike.

linctus. Medicine to be licked or sipped; a syrupy cough mixture.

lingual. Of the tongue.

liniment. Liquid preparation rubbed into the skin to relieve stiff muscles or aching joints, mainly by ◊ *counterirritation*, but perhaps also by some local effect of drugs absorbed through the skin.

lip(o)-. Prefix = 'fat'.

lipid; lipoid. Fat-like substance such as cholesterol. ◊ *fat*.

lipoma. A harmless tumour composed of fat cells, easily removed if it becomes unsightly.

liquorice. The root of the plant *Glycyrriza*, mentioned as a drug by Dioscorides in the 1st century A.D. and in use ever since as a digestive, laxative, and flavouring agent. A fairly recent suggestion that liquorice might promote the healing of gastric ulcers was fully confirmed by 1965. A pure substance extracted from the root, carbenoxylone, seems to increase the resistance of the lining of the stomach to erosion by acid, and some other drugs with a similar effect have also been extracted.

Lister, Joseph (Lord Lister) (1827–1912). English surgeon; professor of surgery in Glasgow (1860), Edinburgh (1869), and London (1877); perhaps the most important figure in the history of surgery. By preventing bacterial contamination (◊ *infection*), Lister converted surgery from something hardly less dangerous than the diseases it tried to cure into a relatively safe form of treatment: a medieval craft into a modern science. It was no chance discovery. From his student days Lister had studied the processes of inflammation, and he had already established himself as one of the great surgical investigators before 1867, when he published his first paper on antiseptic surgery. Almost as soon as Pasteur showed how infection took place, Lister showed how it could be avoided.

In addition, Lister made numerous advances in operative technique, including the introduction of satisfactory catgut ligatures.

lithium. Metal of the same class as sodium, with the ability to displace sodium from compounds in solution. Some types of mental disorder are associated with an excess of sodium in the brain cells. These disorders are relieved by giving the patient lithium carbonate, presumably because lithium replaces some of the sodium. The treatment is used mainly with *manic-depressive psychosis*, especially in the manic phase, but good results have also been claimed in some cases of schizophrenia.

lithotomy. Removal of a stone (calculus) from the urinary bladder, one of the oldest surgical operations, prohibited in the Hippocratic Oath (because it was to be done only by specialists). Before the discovery of antiseptics made abdominal surgery safe, the operation had to be done by approaching the bladder from below, between the thighs. The patient lay on his back with hips and knees flexed, like a trussed fowl. The position is still called the *lithotomy position*; it is used mainly for gynaecological examinations and operations.

Little's disease. Cerebral palsy (◊ *spastic paralysis*).

liver.

1. STRUCTURE

The liver, like the salivary glands and pancreas, is an outgrowth of the digestive tube: it is a very large gland opening off the beginning of the small intestine (*duodenum*). In the embryo it is at first a mid-line organ, but its right side soon outpaces the left. At birth, three quarters of the liver is to the right of the mid-line, and in an adult, seven eighths. The liver completely fills the part of the abdomen that is covered by the right side of the diaphragm and rib-cage.

All the blood from the spleen and from the stomach and intestine is passed to the liver by the *portal vein*. It seeps through the substance of the liver and returns to the general circulation by way of the *inferior vena cava*. In the process the liver cells take up materials digested and absorbed from the food.

The blood from the portal vein is the raw material on which the liver works. In addition, fresh blood is supplied by the *hepatic artery*.

The digestive secretion of the liver, the *bile*, flows through small channels to the common bile duct, which opens into the duodenum. Bile is formed continuously but is most needed when there is a meal to be digested. Between meals most of it is stored in the *gall bladder*, a bag projecting from the bile duct and stuck to the underside of the liver, able to contract and eject bile when stimulated by food in the duodenum.

2. FUNCTION

The liver is an organ of *digestion*, and of *excretion* (◊ *bile*).

Its many other functions include *synthesis* of proteins and other substances needed elsewhere, such as glucose, amino-acids, and the proteins of the blood; *storage*, especially of glucose (in the form of *glycogen*); and *neutralization* of poisons. These are functions of living cells in general, but many of the tissues of the body have become so specialized that they are no longer self-supporting in these respects. In several ways the liver is essential to life. The most urgent is keeping a steady concentration of glucose in the blood to replace what is consumed as fuel. The brain keeps no stores at all, and quickly dies if supplies from the liver are cut off.

3. DISORDERS

Injuries of the liver are dangerous. It is well protected by the ribs, but a heavy blow (e.g. from the edge of a steering-wheel in a car collision) may tear it. A neglected injury of this kind is almost bound to cause fatal bleeding. Some kind of surgical repair is imperative, but even immediate operation does not always succeed.

Infection of many kinds can involve the liver. Bacteria seldom invade the liver without first establishing themselves in the intestine or gall bladder, from which they can keep up a steady attack. Some viruses, on the other hand, attack the liver directly (◊ *hepatitis*). The liver is commonly involved in diseases due to more highly developed parasites, e.g. amoebic *dysentery*, *bilharzia*, *hydatid disease*, *malaria*, and *Weil's disease*.

Poisoning of the liver is common, because anything absorbed from the stomach is carried first to the liver, which therefore gets a higher concentration than other organs and is often damaged in the process of neutralizing poisons to protect the rest of the body. Much the commonest poison is alcohol, and many drugs and industrial chemicals can damage the liver.

Impaired circulation in the liver is a common effect of heart disease; it can also arise from disorders of the liver itself.

Tumours of the liver are common for the same reason as poisoning: they are carried from the stomach and intestine. Cancer in these organs sooner or later spreads to the liver unless it is checked. Cancer that begins in the liver is rare in most countries, though it is very common in tropical Africa; the difference is probably due to diet, not heredity.

The *effects* of liver disease are comparatively few. A healthy liver has much more capacity than is ever needed at one time: nothing goes wrong until at least three quarters of its cells are out of action. The minor upsets popularly ascribed to the liver – biliousness, feeling liverish, and the *crises de foie* of French drug advertisements

– are usually upsets of the stomach and not of the liver.

If the liver is damaged enough to cause symptoms the symptoms are wide-spread. With acute hepatitis, ◊ *jaundice* usually suggests the diagnosis. But with chronic liver disease the symptoms are often vague – feeling unwell, indigestion, perhaps loss of weight – and the liver may not come under suspicion for some time.

But the liver has great power of recovery. If the disease is neither progressive nor so severe that it overwhelms the patient, lost or damaged liver cells regenerate. This is as well, for medical treatment does not greatly affect the liver. As a general rule, treatment is designed to keep symptoms at bay and reduce the demands on the liver to a minimum while it restores itself.

The liver is a much more complex organ than the heart or kidneys, and nobody is likely to devise a machine to take over its many functions. There is a much better chance of overcoming the technical problems of transplanting a whole liver, and the preliminary experiments are well advanced.

Surgery has only a small place in the management of liver disease, apart from repair of injuries and drainage of abscesses. But ◊ *cirrhosis*, an effect of several kinds of disease, sometimes obstructs the flow of blood through the liver, with damage by back-pressure. This can be overcome by an operation to divert some of the blood to the vena cava or some other large vein leaving enough flow through the liver for its work to continue. These are hazardous operations, but they can be life-saving.

4. EXAMINATION

The functions of the liver are so diverse that a complete assessment is seldom practicable. Because of the considerable reserves of functional capacity, minor disturbances cause few if any symptoms and are difficult to detect.

Ordinary clinical examination will detect an excess of bile pigment in the blood sufficient to cause jaundice, and show whether this is accompanied by leakage of bile pigment into the urine; but jaundice does not appear until the blood contains several times the normal amount of bile. Chemical study of the blood is needed to reveal a small excess of bile pigment, and whether the excess is due to over-production or defective excretion.

An enlarged liver can be felt through the abdominal wall, and one can usually get some impression of the texture. The patient's symptoms may suggest the diagnosis, but special tests are often needed. The gall bladder can be examined by X-rays: a drug is given that is excreted in the bile and is opaque to X-rays, and the gall bladder then throws a shadow. The portal blood vessels can be shown by an analogous method.

There are many chemical tests of liver function, each measuring a single process. Usually several are done at the same time, because one function can be depressed while others remain normal.

When other methods have failed to give an answer, a minute specimen of liver tissue can be taken for microscopical examination through a hollow needle passed between the ribs into the liver.

A new and elegant technique for locating damage to the liver is *scintigraphy*. A radioactive form of a substance for which the liver has an affinity is given, and a scanner then shows which parts of the liver have taken up the substance and are working normally, and which have not taken it up and are not working. The resulting map is of great value to a surgeon who has to deal with a condition such as an abscess of the liver.

loa. A kind of threadworm (◊ *filaria*) in West Africa, transmitted by the bite of a fly. It causes severe itching by burrowing under the surface of the skin.

lobar ◊ *pneumonia.*

lobectomy. Surgical removal of one the lobes of a lung, e.g. for cancer or localized chronic infection. Each lobe of a lung is a structural unit that can be removed without disturbing the rest of the lung and with the minimum of risk.

lobeline. An alkaloid drug from *lobelia*; it has been used to stimulate breathing and ease spasm of the air-passages. Lobeline is related to nicotine, and might serve as a temporary substitute for people trying to give up tobacco; but the results of this treatment have been disappointing.

local anaesthetic ◊ *anaesthetics.*

lockjaw = ◊ *tetanus.*

lordosis. Curvature of the spine convex towards the front, e.g. the natural lordosis in the lumbar region which produces the hollow of the back. (Cf. *scoliosis, lateral curvature*; *kyphosis*, the opposite to lordosis.)

louse. A kind of small insect; several species are parasitic to man. Given decent living conditions and ordinary cleanliness, infestation is not usual, but a louse may transfer itself to anyone and where there is overcrowding or lack of hygiene it may be difficult to prevent lice from thriving. Warfare and natural disasters produce such conditions.

Two of the six 'formidable' epidemic diseases that are notifiable to the World Health Organization are transmitted by lice: typhus, and relapsing fever.

LSD ◊ *hallucinogen.*

Ludwig's angina. A kind of abscess in the floor of the mouth.

lumbago. Persistent ache in the small of the back, often associated with pain down the leg (*sciatica*). When these two occur together they are generally due to pressure on nerves by a 'slipped disc' (◊ *vertebra* (1)). Lumbago alone may have the same cause, or any of the other structures of the back may be strained by faulty posture. ◊ *backache.*

lumbar. Of the part of the back between the lowest pair of ribs and the top of the pelvis. The lumbar region is supported by the five lumbar *vertebrae.*

lumbar puncture. Insertion of a hollow needle between two of the lumbar vertebrae (usually the 3rd and 4th) into the spinal canal. The method is used to take a specimen of cerebrospinal fluid for the diagnosis of meningitis and other disorders affecting the brain or spinal cord, or to inject drugs into the spinal canal – e.g. antibiotics for treating meningitis, or anaesthetics for operations on the lower half of the body.

lung.

1. STRUCTURE

The two lungs fill most of the ◊ *thorax*, which is a smaller cavity than it appears to be. The heart, which separates the lungs,

encroaches more on the left lung than the right. The lower surfaces of the lungs are concave to fit the dome of the ◊ *diaphragm.* The lowest limit of the lungs is some 4 fingers' breadth above the margin of the ribs. The narrow apex of each lung rises above the level of the clavicles into the neck. The root or *hilum* of a lung faces inwards to the heart. It contains an array of tubes: the air-passages (main bronchi) and numerous blood vessels. Deep fissures divide the right lung into three *lobes* and the left into two.

The main *bronchus* divides into a branch to each lobe; these divide into segmental bronchi, ten on the right and nine on the left. A *segment* of the lung is roughly a pyramid with its apex to the hilum. The segmental bronchus divides and subdivides into smaller and smaller tubes. The narrowest and most numerous – comparable with the twigs of a tree – are the *bronchioles.* The terminal bronchioles open into small cavities, the air-sacs, each with several compartments called *alveoli.* The whole surface of the alveoli is some thirty times that of the skin.

2. FUNCTION

The bronchi serve merely to carry air to and fro. Their walls are strengthened with rings of cartilage, and contain muscle fibres which adjust their calibre. Their lining membrane secretes mucus; it keeps itself clean by the undulation of hair-like processes (*cilia*) which sweep any fine particles that are breathed in towards the trachea and away. Larger particles set up a cough reflex and are removed more rapidly.

The lining of the terminal bronchioles and alveoli allows gases to pass between the inspired air and the blood in the pulmonary capillaries. This exchange of oxygen and carbon dioxide is the primary function of the lungs; ◊ *respiration.*

In addition to respiration, the lungs have certain minor functions. Nearly half a litre of water is lost daily by evaporation into the expired air, an important factor in the fluid balance of the body. This evaporation causes the loss of about 250 Calories, a significant amount of heat but one that cannot be adjusted (◊ *temperature*). Animals which do not sweat, such as dogs, depend on this type of heat loss to keep the body temperature down after exertion. When a dog pants, water evaporates from the surface of the tongue, and excess heat is eliminated. Certain volatile substances such as alcohol, and of course carbon dioxide, are excreted through the lungs. A sudden excess of acid in the blood, such as the acid formed in working muscles, can be eliminated as carbon dioxide by deeper breathing.

3. PLEURAL CAVITY

Each lung is wrapped in two layers of thin membrane, the *pleura*. The outer, *parietal*

ate and free to slide. They are lubricated by tissue fluid. There is thus no friction between lung and ribs. In health the pleural cavity does not really exist, but with disease or injury the layers may be separated, e.g. by watery fluid (*effusion*), air (*pneumothorax*), or pus (*empyema*).

4. EXAMINATION

Common symptoms such as shortness of

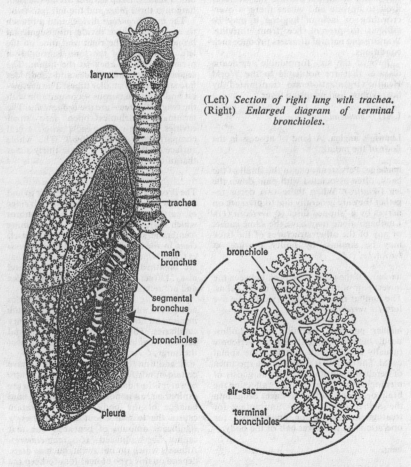

(Left) *Section of right lung with trachea.*
(Right) *Enlarged diagram of terminal bronchioles.*

larynx

trachea

main bronchus

segmental bronchus

bronchioles

pleura

bronchiole

air-sac

terminal bronchioles

layer lines the inside of the thorax. The inner, *visceral* layer coats the outside of the lung. The two layers merge at the hilum of the lung; elsewhere they are quite separ-

breath, cough, and pain in the chest can all arise from causes beyond the lungs. The symptoms of a few conditions – pneumonia, bronchitis, asthma – are sometimes almost unmistakable, but more often than not the exact diagnosis of lung ailments needs various objective tests.

A complete study of the lungs needs the resources of a research laboratory, but much can be discovered by simpler means, e.g. testing resonance (◊ *percussion*) and listening to the sounds of breathing (◊ *stethoscope*). But these methods do not always suffice. The stethoscope is still a most useful instrument, but for many purposes X-rays are more reliable.

X-rays pass freely through air, less freely through liquids and soft tissues, and hardly at all through bone. In a healthy chest the backbone and ribs throw heavy shadows, and the heart is massive enough to be opaque, but the lungs are transparent apart from the tree-like pattern of their blood vessels. In nearly all disease of the lungs air is displaced by liquid or solid matter which is less permeable to X-rays and therefore throws a shadow.

Direct examination of a part of the lungs is possible by *bronchoscopy*: a lighted tube is passed down the trachea into a bronchus. This method is no part of the routine examination of the lungs, but occasionally it is valuable for establishing a diagnosis. Sometimes minor surgery can be carried out through the bronchoscope, e.g. removal of a fragment of tissue for microscopical examination.

The mechanical efficiency of the lungs can be studied in a laboratory, but few tests are simple enough for general use. Chest expansion means little, for the most important muscle of respiration, the diaphragm, does not move the ribs. A much more useful measurement is the volume of air which can be blown out in one second; time is as important as quantity because the important factor is the rate at which air can be exchanged. ◊ *respiration*.

5. DISORDERS

No precise classification can be simple enough to be useful. What follows is merely a guide to some other entries in this book.

Injuries. The lungs may be injured by penetrating wounds or by a fragment of a broken rib. Bleeding into the pleural cavity (*haemothorax*) may be severe, but continued bleeding is usually from other structures than the lung. A punctured lung loses air and, since it is elastic, collapses like a balloon. As the lung shrinks the bleeding stops. In fact, the air in the pleural cavity may be a greater embarrassment than the blood (◊ *pneumothorax*).

Infection. Even in health the air-passages carry potentially dangerous bacteria, and the lungs are continually exposed to infection by microorganisms in the air. Nothing happens unless resistance is lowered, as by illness, or an unfamiliar organism to which the subject has never acquired resistance arrives or perhaps a familiar one in unusually large numbers. In such circumstances the lungs are very vulnerable. Infection primarily of the trachea and bronchi causes ◊ *bronchitis*; infection in the remoter parts of the lung causes ◊ *pneumonia*. An ◊ *abscess* may be formed in the lung as a result of stagnation beyond a blocked bronchus. Most lung abscesses respond to antibiotics, but surgical drainage is sometimes needed. Certain types of microbe are peculiarly liable to attack the lungs, e.g. ◊ *tuberculosis*.

Mechanical disorders. ◊ *Asthma* is cramp in the muscles of the bronchi, obstructing the free passage of air. ◊ *Bronchiectasis* is abnormal distension of the bronchi. ◊ *Emphysema* is loss of the elasticity of the alveoli, resulting in over-distension of the lungs. ◊ *Atelectasis* is failure of the lung or some part of it to take in air after birth, or loss of air with collapse of the lung. ◊ *Hyaline-membrane disease* is a cause of death of new-born babies.

Occupational diseases. Several diseases are due to inhaling dusts associated with particular jobs: ◊ *pneumoconiosis; farmer's lung.*

Tumours. Benign tumours of various kinds are found. They usually have to be removed because there is no other way of telling that they are not cancerous. Much the commonest tumour is ◊ *cancer*, either originating in the lung (*primary*) or seeded off from a cancer elsewhere (*secondary*). The enormous increase in primary lung cancer during the 20th century has made it a leading cause of death in many countries: it is generally ascribed to cigarette smoking (◊ *tobacco*). The only effective treatment is removal, which may be impossible by the time the disease is recognized, for in the early, curable stages there may be no symptoms. But as many as half of the cases found by chance at an X-ray examination are operable – a strong argument for routine chest X-ray. ◊ *pleura.*

lupus erythematosus (LE). One (or probably more than one) of the ill-understood disorders loosely known as collagen diseases or connective-tissue diseases; the group also includes rheumatoid arthritis. There are grounds for regarding all these diseases as instances of ◊ *autoimmunity*, a sort of allergic reaction to one of one's own tissues.

Discoid LE is a degeneration of connective-tissue elements of the skin. It takes the form of red, often scaly patches on exposed skin, aggravated by strong sunlight. Screening ointments against ultraviolet light help to prevent it, and chloroquine (a drug more often used against malaria) may clear up the skin trouble. Most cases improve with time.

Disseminated (systemic) LE may affect connective tissue anywhere in the body. The skin changes resemble those of discoid LE, and in addition there may be symptoms identical with those of rheumatoid arthritis. The kidneys and other organs can be involved. This is one of the diseases in which *corticosteroids* can be life-saving. The treatment may have to be maintained indefinitely, but on the other hand many of the patients have only occasional attacks, subsiding with little or no treatment, and long periods between – sometimes many years – without trouble.

Further research is likely to show that discoid LE does not really belong to this group of diseases, and that systemic LE includes more than one disease.

lupus vulgaris. Tuberculosis of the skin, mainly of the face, formerly a common and disfiguring disease but now rare. It responds well to the drugs used for tuberculosis in general.

luxation. Dislocation of a joint.

lymph. Part of the ◊ *tissue fluid*, which instead of returning to the blood in the capillaries enters the lymphatic vessels (◊ *lymphatic system*). The small amount of protein in the tissue fluid is concentrated in the lymph; otherwise the two fluids are alike. In the intestine, fat is absorbed into the lymphatic vessels and not the blood capillaries. This gives lymph from the small intestine a milky appearance, from which these lymphatic vessels are known as *lacteals*.

In addition to molecules (e.g. protein) too large to return to the circulation by the capillaries, particles such as bacteria leave the tissue spaces in the lymph, to be filtered off in the lymph nodes.

Lymph nodes (also called *lymph glands*, or simply *glands*) are small bean-like bodies in the course of the lymphatic vessels. Several small vessels enter the periphery and a single larger vessel leaves the concavity of the node. The distribution is described under ◊ *lymphatic system*.

The *lymphoid tissue* of which the nodes are mainly composed forms lymphocytes (a type of white blood cell) and also ◊ *antibodies*. Similar tissue is found in the *tonsils* and *adenoids* and along the rest of the digestive tract, and in the *spleen*.

lymphadenoma = ◊ *Hodgkin's disease.*

lymphangiitis. Inflammation of lymph vessels from spread of infection, usually from a septic wound, seen as red lines in the skin between the wound and the nearest lymph nodes, e.g. from a sore finger to the armpit. It is generally due to infection by *streptococci*. Lymphangiitis (often misnamed *blood-poisoning*) is not to be neglected, because if the infection has spread so far it may pass the barrier of the lymph nodes and set up a real blood-poisoning or septicaemia. A sulphonamide or antibiotic drug usually suppresses it promptly.

lymphatic system. A network of thin-walled vessels found in all parts of the body except the central nervous system. The vessels carry ◊ *lymph* from the tissue spaces. Small vessels unite to form larger vessels until finally the lymph is drained into the *innominate veins* at the root of the neck by two large lymphatic vessels: the *right lymphatic duct* from the upper half of the right side of the body and the *thoracic duct* from the rest. The vessels have valves like those of the veins, which prevent back-flow.

The vessels are interrupted by ◊ *lymph* nodes which filter off bacteria and other foreign particles, and contribute lymphocytes and antibodies.

If the lymphatics are obstructed protein is not drained from the tissues, and fluid collects (◊ *oedema*) because the osmotic pressure falls (◊ *tissue fluid*).

The lymph nodes are a barrier, preventing bacterial infection from spreading from the tissue spaces into the blood-stream. Unless a focus of infection is contained and eradicated by local defence mechanisms (◊ *inflammation*) the lymph nodes for the area

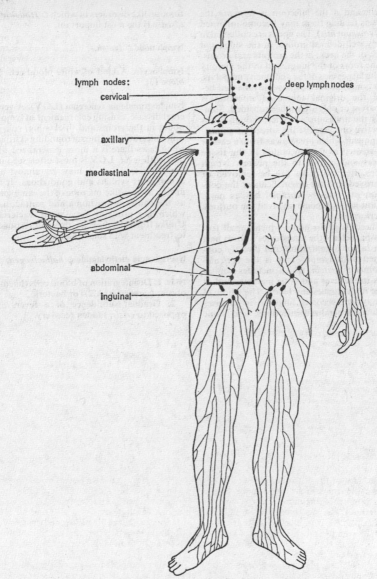

lymph nodes:

cervical

deep lymph nodes

axillary

mediastinal

abdominal

inguinal

Principal groups of lymph nodes.

swell, and if the infection is ◊ *acute* the vessels feeding them may become inflamed (◊ *lymphangiitis*). The nodes are collected in fairly well-defined groups, at the sides and back of the neck, in the armpits and groins, at the roots of the lungs, and in the vicinity of the large veins of the abdomen and pelvis. The lymph nodes may become inflamed before the original source of infection is apparent or only after it has subsided. Similarly the nodes are a barrier, though a less effective one, against the spread of cancer. Fragments which break away from a cancer are treated as foreign bodies in the tissue spaces and carried to the nearest lymph nodes. If these nodes can be removed or destroyed with the original cancer the condition may still be curable, but as more distant nodes become involved the outlook deteriorates.

The cells in the nodes which engulf foreign particles – the phagocytes – form part of a larger organization, not directly concerned with lymph. This is the *reticulo-endothelial system*, which includes similar cells in the liver and bone marrow, and at large in the tissues and blood. The whole of this system becomes involved in diseases such as generalized infections, and some tumour-like disorders of which ◊ *Hodgkin's disease* is the most important.

lymph node ◊ *lymph.*

lymphocyte. A kind of white blood cell. ◊ *blood* (3).

lymphogranuloma venereum (LGV). A venereal disease, causing enlargement of lymph nodes in the groins and thickening, sometimes ulceration, of the surrounding skin; in some cases there is a more generalized illness with fever. LGV is most often seen in the tropics, where it may be almost as common as syphilis and gonorrhoea. It is due to a virus-like microbe of the same sort as the causes of trachoma and psittacosis, which are probably very small bacteria. Unlike true virus diseases, these all respond to treatment with sulphonamides.

lysergic acid diethylamide ◊ *hallucinogen.*

lysis. 1. Disintegration of blood cells (haemolysis; ◊ *anaemia* (A.2) : or bacteria.

2. Gradual subsidence of a fever, as opposed to *crisis*, sudden recovery.

M

Mackenzie, Sir James (1853–1925). General practitioner in Burnley, later a heart specialist in London. With the help of a device that he called a ◊ *polygraph*, which made simultaneous recordings of the heart beat and of pulses in veins and arteries, he was able to explain all the common disturbances of the heart beat (◊ *arrhythmia*). Einthoven's invention of the electrocardiograph drew attention from Mackenzie's work rather too soon, for the possibilities of the polygraph were never sufficiently explored.

macro-. Prefix — '(*unusually*) large'; e.g. *macrocyte*, abnormally large red blood cell; *macrophage*, large scavenging cell in the tissues; *macroscopic*, seen with the naked eye.

macule. Spot or blemish, level with the surrounding skin; as opposed to *papule*, a raised spot.

maduromycosis (Madura foot). A fungus (mould) infection spreading through the tissues (including bones) of the foot, seldom seen outside the tropics. The newer antibiotics are worth a trial, but as a rule the affected tissue has to be removed surgically.

Magendie, François (1783–1855). French physiologist. Anticipating his still greater disciple Bernard, he rejected the academic speculation and near-mysticism that still clouded scientific thought, insisting that the human body obeyed the same natural laws as everything else in nature. He was the first to describe the separation of nerves joining the spinal cord into sensory and motor roots, and the pathway of reflex action from a sensory organ along a nerve, to the spinal cord by the sensory (posterior) root, then from the spinal cord by the anterior root and lastly to the responding (effector) organ.

Magendie's experiments with diet established the main ingredients needed, in particular the very different food value of different proteins. He was also a founder of modern pharmacology; he isolated the active principles of many plant drugs and described their actions.

magnesium. Small traces of this metal in the body fluids seem to be essential to the working of the nervous system. Deficiency may occur in some other mammals but has not been described in man.

Magnesium *trisilicate, carbonate, hydroxide* and *oxide* (magnesia) are used as antacids. Magnesium *sulphate* (Epsom salt) is a saline purge.

malabsorption. Failure to assimilate essential ingredients from the diet, leading to symptoms of malnutrition.

In a normal person, each of the chemical ingredients of the food is broken down by particular enzymes to small, simple molecules. Only these can pass through the lining of the intestine into the circulation, to be resynthesized and incorporated into the tissues.

If an enzyme is lacking, the corresponding food substance cannot be broken down and is not absorbed. Examples are ◊ *cystic fibrosis*, where several enzymes from the pancreas are lacking and several kinds of food are affected, and ◊ *carbohydrate intolerance*, where a particular sugar (usually milk sugar) remains in the intestine.

Alternatively, the intestine may fail to absorb the products of digestion although the enzyme system is intact. After drastic operations on the intestine, food may pass through too quickly to be completely absorbed, and with defects of the mucous membrane of the intestine absorption may be delayed. Undue haste and poor absorption are combined with chronic inflammation of the intestine (◊ *enteritis*). ◊ *Coeliac disease*, a kind of malabsorption in childhood, is due to a defect provoked by the protein *gluten*, found in certain cereals. ◊ *Sprue*, a similar disease affecting adults in the tropics, may be caused by damage to the lining of the intestine by vitamin deficiency (but cause and effect are difficult to distinguish).

Malabsorption can lead to malnutrition, amounting in the worst cases to starvation. It may also cause diarrhoea, because unabsorbed fats and sugars in the intestine have a purgative action. With sprue and coeliac disease, diarrhoea is the leading symptom. With chronic inflammation of the intestine, the diarrhoea of malabsorption is added to that of the primary disease.

malaria. An infectious disease due to a minute animal parasite (protozoon) transmitted by mosquitoes, one of the commonest causes of sickness and death in the world.

A mosquito sucks blood from an infected person. The parasites breed in the stomach of the mosquito, and after about 10 days their offspring invade the salivary glands. The mosquito is then infectious, and everyone she bites gets an injection of parasites in a droplet of saliva.

The young parasites are carried in the patient's blood to the liver and other organs, where they multiply without causing symptoms. After a variable incubation period – often a fortnight but sometimes much longer – parasites return to the blood-stream and invade red blood cells, where they multiply rapidly. The infected red cells are soon destroyed, setting free countless parasites to invade other red cells. When this happens the patient has an attack of fever. The attack commonly begins with headache and violent shivering (*rigor*). After anything from an hour to a day the symptoms vanish until the next batch of parasites is released, with further destruction of red cells. All types of malaria cause attacks of fever at more or less regular intervals, and increasing anaemia from loss of blood cells.

There are four known types of malaria parasite, all species of the protozoon *Plasmodium*. *P. malariae* causes quartan fever with attacks every 3 days (the 'four' implied by *quartan* are counted from 1, not 0). These parasites may hibernate in the liver for many years and cause occasional attacks long after the patient has left a malarial region. Quartan malaria is common in subtropical countries.

P. vivax causes tertian fever, with attacks on alternate days. It, too, may persist for some time after the original bout. This type of malaria used to be common in the temperate zone, as far north as Finland.

P. ovale causes tertian malaria in parts of Central Africa.

P. falciparum causes subtertian (malignant tertian, MT) fever, the most dangerous kind of malaria. The attacks are frequent and irregular, at intervals from a few hours to two days; or the fever may simply persist. All types of malaria can cause diverse symptoms, and MT is notorious for imitating every other acute illness. Many of the symptoms are due to congestion of the blood vessels in an affected organ by masses of damaged blood cells. MT malaria can cause a kind of *dysentery*, and also *cerebral malaria* (invasion of blood vessels in the brain), which kills many thousands of children. A rare but equally dangerous complication, *blackwater fever*, seems to be an abnormal response to treatment of MT malaria with quinine. This parasite does not hibernate in the body; when a bout is over it does not recur. But the patient can start a new attack if another infected mosquito bites him. MT malaria is the commonest type in tropical Africa and also occurs in the hotter parts of Asia and South America.

If malaria – even MT – is untreated, most patients recover after anything from two or three to a dozen episodes of fever. The complications of MT malaria are often fatal, but much of the large death rate (and far larger sickness rate) is due to the anaemia and sheer exhaustion of repeated infection. Children in the tropics die of what should be trivial complaints because they no longer have any natural resistance.

An attack of malaria does not confer immunity, but after repeated attacks with the same strain of parasite the attacks become less and less severe, in those who survive.

There are many drugs for treating malaria, all highly effective. The oldest, quinine, is seldom used because of its toxic effects. Any of the newer and safer synthetic drugs (chloroquin, pyrimethamine, proguanil etc.) promptly stops an attack, and cures MT malaria. With the other types, the parasites hibernating in the liver are not killed by these drugs, and relapses occur unless they are eliminated with another drug such as primaquine.

In some parts of Asia, strains of malaria parasite have evolved that resist the usual drugs, and new drugs are having to be sought.

Ideally there should be no need for treatment, because malaria can be prevented and, in time, eradicated. If every case could be treated, mosquitoes could not become infected and their bites would be harmless. This is the situation in most of Europe: mosquitoes of the right sort are not uncommon but there is nobody to infect them. Small outbreaks can still occur when someone imports active malaria.

Hippocrates advised people recovering

from malaria to retire to the hills, where the disease did not occur, and a close association between malaria and a wet environment must have been obvious from early times. But until recently marshes were supposed to exude noxious vapours that caused the disease (*malaria* = 'bad air').

It became possible to cure individual cases in the Old World when Jesuit missionaries brought cinchona bark (quinine) from the New World in the 17th century. But the first step towards prevention was Laveran's discovery of the parasite in 1880. In 1894 Manson suggested that the infection might be transmitted by mosquitoes (which of course flourished in the places where malaria was commonest, the marshes); and in 1897 Ross proved Manson's theory.

All malaria is carried by mosquitoes of the genus *Anopheles*. These can be distinguished by their posture when they settle. Other mosquitoes settle with their bodies level; *Anopheles* at an angle, head down. They can breed only where there is standing fresh water, in which they lay their eggs and their larvae develop.

If the cycle is broken at any point, malaria disappears. The first method has been mentioned: it is to treat all the patients.

Secondly, the mosquitoes can be prevented from biting. Houses are cleared of adult mosquitoes with insecticides. People in malarial regions avoid sitting out of doors in the early evening when the mosquitoes bite most; they may be able to cover their windows with gauze; they sleep under nets.

Mosquitoes are prevented from breeding by attention to their breeding places. This includes anything from drainage of vast swamps to proper disposal of discarded cans where rain might collect, clearing the banks of streams and stagnant backwaters (running water is no danger), and spreading a film of oil over the surface of pools to suffocate the larvae. Prevention of breeding is the most effective means of malaria control, but it can be very expensive.

Finally, people exposed to infection can protect themselves by taking regular small doses of an antimalarial drug.

By such methods many circumscribed areas have been freed from malaria. Even in heavily infected regions most large towns are now safe. But rural areas, especially the huge and sparsely populated plains of Africa, present special problems. To deal with breeding places – and it must be done regularly – would need more money and staff than could be found. The only hope is to apply long-acting insecticides to every dwelling and offer treatment to every patient. It will take a long time.

malignant. A term used to distinguish severe or progressive forms of a disease from mild or self-limiting (*benign*) forms. A malignant tumour is cancerous, whereas a benign tumour is a simple growth that does not invade other tissues. Malignant malaria is the subtertian form associated with the highly dangerous blackwater fever and with fatal involvement of the brain; benign malaria is tertian or quartan and does not have these complications.

malingering. Deliberate feigning of illness; doubtless a common condition, but a diagnosis that can seldom be made with certainty. A man may claim to have hurt his back at work in the hope of compensation. It is one thing to prove that he has broken no bones, but quite another to say that he is lying about what he feels.

malleolus. Knob of bone at either side of the ankle.

malleus. One of the three small bones that conduct sound from the ear-drum to the organ of hearing in the inner ear.

malnutrition. Deficiency of any essential component of a proper ◊ *diet*. Malnutrition can be due either to illness where food is not assimilated (◊ *malabsorption*) or, much more often, to poor diet. Anyone whose health could be improved by more or better food is suffering from malnutrition, and this is surely the state of more than half the people in the world.

Some effects of particular deficiencies are mentioned under ◊ *vitamins* and ◊ *kwashiorkor*; but single deficiencies are not as common as general malnutrition. If a diet is inadequate in one respect it is likely to be so in others. The commonest picture is a negative one: failure to thrive, failure to resist trivial infection, lack of energy or initiative.

Even in wealthy communities where the average diet is more than enough (and a surplus contributes nothing to health) there can be under-nourished individuals. The great risk is to lonely old people who cannot be bothered to feed themselves properly even when they can afford to. It is a vicious circle, for malnutrition makes them more apathetic than ever.

Civilization tends to spread malnutrition by enlarging the population without increasing the production of food. One dose of quinine will save a child from dying of malaria, but it may take years to grow new crops for him to eat. Scientific medicine is a doubtful blessing without scientific agriculture and, above all, education in the uses of both.

malocclusion. Faulty alignment of the teeth, causing an inefficient bite.

Malpighi, Marcello (1624–94). Physician and anatomist; professor at Bologna and Pisa; the first professional anatomist to work with a microscope. He greatly extended the science of embryology, which had of necessity been rather crude while such a small object as an early embryo could be studied only with the naked eye. Here, his work was a direct continuation of that of Harvey a generation before him. A still more important extension of Harvey's work was Malpighi's discovery of capillary blood vessels, of which Harvey could only infer the existence when he proved that blood must find some pathway between arteries and veins. Malpighi left accurate descriptions of most of the organs and tissues of the body, and half a dozen or more of the minute structures of the body are still named after him.

Malta fever. A kind of ◊ *undulant fever*, primarily an infection of goats but often transmitted to man.

maltose. A compound sugar obtained from starch; its molecule consists of two units of glucose.

malunion. Healing of a fracture with the broken ends of the bone out of their true line. If the deformity is enough to interfere with function the bone may have to be broken again and reset.

mandelic acid. An antiseptic drug: it is excreted by the kidneys and kills bacteria in the urine in cases of cystitis (inflammation of the urinary bladder).

mandible. Lower jaw; a single bone loosely jointed with the skull at the temporo-mandibular joints in front of the ears. Its movements are described under ◊ *mastication*. The upper jaw, the *maxilla*, is a component of the skull proper.

The development of jaws from the forward gills was one of the decisive steps in evolution; with jaws an animal is better equipped for self-defence and for extending its diet, two cardinal factors in the struggle for survival. But as regards evolution the human jaw served its purpose long ago. The hands have taken on many of its primitive functions, and the modern human mandible is a poor thing in comparison with that of less advanced creatures.

mandragora (mandrake). A plant of the same family as belladonna and with similar effects as a drug; used as a narcotic in ancient Egypt and, until recently, in Western Europe. During the Middle Ages its forked root was thought to resemble a man and to imprison a lost soul. The plant was uprooted by tying it to a dog's tail, so that nobody should die from the horror of hearing it scream.

mania. Mental disturbance with aimless and ungovernable excitement.

manic-depressive psychosis. One of the two common types of severe mental disturbance (the other is schizophrenia); also called *affective psychosis*, because the apparent disorder is of ◊ *affect* – the patient's ideas and emotions and their expression are all of a piece, instead of being incongruous as in schizophrenia.

The illness may take the form of *mania*, when the patient is endlessly busy, talks for the sake of talking, seems full of ideas that he never pursues because he is so soon involved in the next pointless task; he may be too busy to eat or sleep. These symptoms would pass for *hypomania*, a sort of harmless eccentricity, except that the absurd over-activity of true mania is neither rational nor open to discussion, and interference may be violently opposed.

Or the patient may be profoundly melancholic, in extreme cases to the point of mute immobility.

The two kinds of attack do not at first appear to have any similarity but the common factor is that the patient is helplessly at the mercy of his confused emotions.

After an attack, which without treatment may last weeks or months, most patients are perfectly normal, though they may have further attacks later. In some cases, attacks of mania and depression alternate.

With either type of attack the patient may need a spell in hospital. Mania can now be treated with large doses of tranquillizers – too large to be given without constant supervision – and melancholy with various drugs (◊ *depression*). This psychosis can also be treated with ◊ *lithium*. When drugs fail, electro-convulsive therapy often cuts an attack short. Neither type of patient is often dangerous to others, though neither is easy to live with. But they can be a great danger to themselves. An untreated maniac can exhaust himself with his unceasing activity, and he can starve for lack of time to eat. A depressive can also starve for lack of any wish to eat or even live. At the depth of his attack he may lack the determination to kill himself, but there is real risk of suicide when he is recovering and can find the energy to do it.

The outlook is much better than one might suppose from seeing a patient at the height of an attack. The personality does not deteriorate, even after repeated attacks; and with modern treatment most attacks can be shortened or controlled. ◊ *depression*.

manipulation. Replacing dislocated joints and setting broken bones must be among the oldest of medical procedures, and in principle the methods described in Egypt 3,500 years ago have not changed. Dislocated joints are manipulated to replace the moving parts of the joints and restore their function. Fractures are manipulated to put the broken ends in the best position for healing. Thus far, there is no disagreement. The manipulative treatment of supposed partial dislocations does, however, arouse differences of opinion, because more often than not the dislocation or displacement cannot be demonstrated. Two systems of treatment outside medical practice make much use of this kind of manipulation. *Chiropractic* is based on the theory that diseases are caused by pressure on nerves and are cured by manipulating the backbone. *Osteopathy* holds that partial dislocations (osteopathic lesions) interfere with the circulation of blood. Neither theory is accepted by orthodox medicine, but it may be in order to manipulate joints for the purpose of breaking down adhesions, though when it comes to demonstration the adhesions are apt to be as elusive as osteopathic lesions or the

compressed nerves of chiropractic. In a given case, practitioners of all three schools might offer the same treatment for three different reasons. Perhaps this need not worry the patient if he is relieved of his symptoms.

It has often been argued against chiropractors and osteopaths, not to mention untrained bone-setters, that they could endanger a patient's life by failing to recognize a condition such as a tuberculous joint, and causing a violent reaction by manipulation; but trained chiropractors and osteopaths are well aware of this, and are taught to avoid such mistakes.

Even such a seemingly clear-cut diagnosis as a slipped disc can be a matter of conjecture. In some cases there is no doubt at all. but in others it is by no means clear what, if anything, is going on between the vertebrae to cause symptoms such as pain round the shoulder or stiffness of the neck. Some of these cases respond well to manipulation, though opinions differ about what the manipulation actually does.

In the treatment of stiff joints after injury or operation, manipulation takes second place to active movement by the patient himself.

Mantoux test. Injection into the skin of a minute dose of *tuberculin*, a substance extracted from tubercle bacilli; a reaction indicates that the subject has at some time been infected with tuberculosis or immunized against it. The test is used to show whether immunization is needed, and less often as a help in diagnosis.

MAO = ◊ *monoamine oxidase.*

marasmus. Extreme emaciation, particularly in infancy. Marasmus is now taken to mean wasting as a result of gross malnutrition in infancy. It has been ascribed to lack of fuel (Calories), but recent evidence suggests that like ◊ *kwashiorkor* it is a form of *protein-energy* malnutrition.

March fracture ◊ *foot* (1).

marihuana ◊ *hemp.*

marrow. 1. *Bone marrow*; the soft core of a bone. At birth, all the bones are filled with *red* marrow, a highly active tissue in which most blood cells originate. In adult life, the red marrow of the limbs is replaced by *yellow* marrow, consisting largely of fat; in the rest of the skeleton the red marrow persists.

2. *Spinal marrow* = ◊ *spinal cord.*

masseter. A powerful muscle of mastication at the side of the jaw.

mastectomy. Surgical removal of a breast. It is a fairly simple operation because the breast lies wholly in the layer of connective tissue under the skin. When the operation is done for cancer it includes removal of the lymph nodes from the armpit, because that is the direction in which the cancer might have begun to spread. Sometimes the pectoral muscles have to be included in the operation, and this weakens the shoulder.

mastication. The lower jaw (*mandible*) is slung by powerful muscles from the base of the skull, with which it forms a loose joint in front of the ear.

In biting, the jaws are pulled together by the powerful *temporalis* and *masseter* muscles, arising respectively from the sides of the skull and the cheek bones. The muscles below the chin which open the mouth are weak: gravity does most of the work. In carnivores, the jaws can carry out only this hinge-like movement. In other mammals, including man, the mandible is free to slip backwards and forwards and from side to side, which makes the rotary action of chewing possible.

Mastication breaks up food and mixes it with saliva to facilitate swallowing. It may also stimulate the flow of saliva. Otherwise it is not very important from the point of view of digestion. But it seems to preserve the teeth, and much dental decay is ascribed to the soft diet of Western civilization.

mastoid. Breast-shaped; the *mastoid process* is the knob of bone projecting down from the skull behind the ear, to which is attached the front part of the sternomastoid muscle. The *mastoid antrum* is a cavity in the bone above the process and a finger's breadth from the surface. It communicates by a small opening with the cavity of the ear-drum or middle ear (◊ *ear* (2)) which lies in front of it, and the mastoid process is honeycombed with small air-cells which open off the antrum. The mucous membrane lining the antrum and air-cells is a continuation (by way of the Eustachian tube and middle ear) of the mucous membrane of the nose.

Acute inflammation of the mastoid antrum was a common and serious complication of infection of the nose or throat, such as measles or tonsillitis, until the discovery of sulphonamides and antibiotics. It is now rarely seen. If an abscess does form in the antrum the bone has nearly always to be opened surgically. Without operation the pus may find its own way out, and the path of least resistance is to the inside of the skull. Meningitis and brain abscess are uncommon but very dangerous complications of untreated mastoid infection. The more usual outcome is chronic infection with a steady trickle of pus through a hole in the ear-drum and increasing deafness. In this chronic state, which may last indefinitely, pain is unusual but a continuous hissing or ringing sound (*tinnitus*) can be almost as disturbing as pain. Treatment is aimed not only at relieving these tiresome symptoms but also at reducing the danger of a sudden flare-up with further spread of the infection. Antibiotics and patient cleansing may serve, but a fairly extensive operation is often the only cure. The thick bony cover of the antrum has to be removed, together with the small conducting bones of the middle ear and the membrane of the ear-drum. The ear often works surprisingly well after this rather drastic treatment, and in any case the operation does less to restrict hearing than untreated infection, which would end in complete deafness.

masturbation. So many children and adolescents play with their own genitalia at times that the practice cannot seriously be called abnormal. Nor is there the least evidence that it is dangerous or harmful. At the worst, persistent masturbation may be a symptom of insecurity, when it is comparable with, say, nail-biting. Because of a misinterpretation of Genesis xxxviii, where the Lord slew Onan for failing to impregnate his brother's widow, masturbation has been branded as a sin; and the uninhibited masturbation of certain mentally deranged people has been mistaken for a cause of their madness.

materia medica. Substances used to treat illness, i.e. drugs in the widest sense. Also the study of drugs, pharmacology.

maxilla. Upper jaw; a component of the skull extending from the orbit to the roof of the mouth. It is the principal element of the skeleton of the face. The bone is hollowed out by the *maxillary sinus* or *antrum*, which opens into the nose.

measles (rubeola; morbilli). One of the most wide-spread and contagious of all infections; due to a virus spread from case to case by air-borne droplets. Major outbreaks are to be expected every two or three years.

After an incubation period of 7–14 days, the attack begins with fever and running nose and eyes, followed by sore throat. A day or two later small red spots with white centres (Koplik's spots) can be seen on the lining of the mouth. The typical blotchy skin rash appears about the fourth day and spreads down from the face. In an uncomplicated case the temperature soon begins to subside. The whole attack lasts about a week.

By itself, the measles virus is not often dangerous; but during the attack the patient is abnormally vulnerable to all sorts of bacteria. Most deaths from measles are in fact due to secondary bacterial infection. The commonest complications of this sort are pneumonia and infection of the middle ear. Antibiotic drugs have no effect on the virus, but greatly reduce the danger from bacteria.

An effective vaccine against measles was not discovered until 1960, and a suitable one for routine use only in 1964.

meatus. Canal or passage; e.g. *external auditory meatus*, ear-hole.

mecamylamine. A drug used for ganglion-blockade. ◊ *ganglion-blockers.*

Meckel's diverticulum. (J. F. Meckel (1714–1774), German anatomist.) A protrusion from the small intestine; it is a vestigial structure representing the yolk-stalk, found in about 2 per cent of people. It resembles the *appendix*, and can be inflamed with symptoms like those of appendicitis.

meconium. Greenish fluid, mostly bile and mucus, in an infant's intestine, passed soon after birth (or before birth if labour is difficult and the infant is distressed).

medial. Towards the mid-line (in anatomical description).

median. 1 (anat.). In the mid-line. The *median plane* divides the body into left and right halves.

2 (statistics). The middle value of a series, e.g. the 3rd of 5 or the 11th of 21. The median is sometimes a more useful 'average' in medical statistics than the usual arithmetic mean.

Median nerve. A branch of the brachial plexus; it is motor to most of the flexor muscles in the forearm and to the small muscles of the thumb, and carries sensation from the radial (thumb) side of the hand. It lies superficially at the wrist, and is liable to injury when the wrist is cut, as by pushing the hand through a pane of glass. ◊ *carpal tunnel.*

mediastinum. Compartment between the lungs, containing the heart, major blood vessels, trachea, oesophagus etc.

medicine. 1. Drug or mixture of drugs.

2. Any science or practice concerned with sickness and health.

3. In England, also the more specialized field of practice that excludes surgery and obstetrics, formerly called *physic* and practised by physicians whose social status was higher than that of the surgeons. Elsewhere, this specialty is called *internal medicine*, and its practitioners are *internists*.

medulla = ◊ *marrow*, or the central zone of a gland or other organ.

medulla oblongata. The lowest part of the brain; in other words, the upward continuation of the spinal cord into the skull. It contains the *vital centres* which govern the reflexes for breathing, heart rate, and blood pressure. If the impulses from these centres stop, the heart can still beat at its own rate, but breathing is impossible; serious injury to the medulla oblongata is immediately fatal.

megacolon (Hirschsprung's disease). A congenital defect of the large intestine, where the network of nerves in a segment of the intestine is incomplete and therefore the muscles do not work. The contents of the intestine are held up at this point, and the intestine becomes enormously distended. The child is cured by removing the affected length of intestine and joining the cut ends.

Meibomian glands. (H. Meibom (1634–1700), German anatomist.) Sebaceous (grease) glands at the edges of the eyelids. Inflammation of one of these glands causes a kind of *stye*. Simple blockage causes a *Meibomian cyst*, a painless round lump that is easily removed.

melaena. Blackened faeces, from the presence of iron compounds (usually derived from blood, e.g. from a bleeding gastric ulcer).

melancholia. Severe ◊ *depression.* (= black bile, one of the four ◊ *humours* of the classical theorists.)

melanin. The dark brown pigment of the hair, skin, and eyes, present in blue or brown eyes (◊ *iris*) and, in different amounts, in the skin of people of all races. Chemically, it is derived from the same raw material as adrenaline.

An ◊ *albino* is unable to synthesize melanin.

melanoma. Pigmented tumour, containing melanin, such as a mole; also a rare kind of cancer.

menarche. Onset of menstruation at puberty.

Mendel, Gregor (1822–84). Austrian monk; Abbot of Brünn (Brno). By numerous experiments in cross-breeding, mainly with pea plants, Mendel founded the science of ◊ *genetics.*

Ménière's syndrome. (P. Ménière (1799–1862), French neurologist.) An affection of the inner ear, with disturbance of both its functions – hearing and balance. Typically, the patient has attacks of deafness with *tinnitus* (a ringing or hissing sound in the ear), accompanied by giddiness which may be severe enough for him to fall down or to vomit.

Ménière's syndrome resembles migraine in the periodic attacks, the frequent absence of demonstrable cause, the number of theories to explain it, and the various forms of treatment offered. A disturbance of blood-flow, with altered pressure, seems the likeliest explanation of most though not all cases.

Several different kinds of drugs are used, and the most suitable for a particular case is found by trial and error. Incapacitating one-sided attacks can be treated, as a last resort,

by an operation to put the inner ear out of action. Loss of the balance organ is unimportant, because balance is maintained by several other mechanisms. A selective operation that preserves the hearing organ may be possible. Such drastic treatment is not often justified. If the disease is progressive it will itself paralyse the affected balance organ, and the attacks cease without treatment. Otherwise, most cases tend to improve with time, except that hearing may be permanently impaired.

meninges (pl. of *meninx*). Membranes enclosing the ◊ *brain* and ◊ *spinal cord.* Three layers are described. The innermost, the *pia mater*, is like tissue paper stuck to the outside of the brain and cord, dipping into the various folds and crevices. The outer layer, the *dura mater*, is a parchment-like membrane applied to the inside of the skull and spinal canal. Folds of dura mater partly separate the cerebral hemispheres and the cerebrum from the cerebellum; there is a smaller fold between the cerebellar hemispheres. Otherwise the dura mater does not leave the bone. The intermediate layer, the *arachnoid mater*, is a filmy membrane attached to the inner surface of the dura mater. The arachnoid and pia are joined by fine threads (arachnoid = 'like a cobweb'). The *subarachnoid space* between arachnoid and pia is filled with cerebrospinal fluid (CSF).

Inflammation of the meninges, usually from bacterial infection, is known as ◊ *meningitis.*

meningismus. Stiff neck and other symptoms resembling those of meningitis, such as may occur at the start of many kinds of fever although the meninges are not involved.

meningitis. Inflammation of the *meninges* from infection by viruses or bacteria.

According to the type of infection, meningitis ranges from a mild, fleeting disturbance to a rapidly fatal disease. Common to all types are fever and a disproportionately severe headache. Inflammation anywhere causes reflex tightening of surrounding muscles, and with meningitis spasm of muscles in the neck and back is usual. With the more severe types, there may be convulsions, vomiting, and delirium.

The diagnosis is confirmed by examining the *cerebrospinal fluid*, which shows characteristic chemical changes, often with turbidity from the presence of numerous white blood cells. The infecting microbe can usually be identified.

Many of the common viruses occasionally cause meningitis. Except in rare cases where the brain is also infected, there is little danger – fortunately, for drugs have no effect on viral meningitis.

The commonest bacterial meningitis is ♢ cerebrospinal fever, caused by the meningococcus. Many other bacteria can infect the meninges, generally by spreading from another infected organ, e.g. as a complication of pneumonia. These are dangerous diseases, but as a rule they respond to treatment with antibiotics.

Tuberculous meningitis was invariably fatal until the discovery of streptomycin in 1944. It is a fairly unusual complication of tuberculosis elsewhere in the body. Treated early, it is now a curable disease; but it starts so insidiously that serious harm can be done before it is recognized.

meningococcus. Neisseria meningitidis, the cause of epidemic meningitis (cerebrospinal fever).

meningocoele. Bulging of meninges through a gap in a defective vertebra (♢ spina bifida).

meniscus. A slip of cartilage at either side of the ♢ knee joint, separating the joint surfaces.

menopause (change of life; climacteric). The time when a woman's ovaries cease to set free an ovum every 4 weeks and she is no longer fertile. Menstruation stops because there is no stimulus from the ovaries. The usual age is in the middle or later forties, but there is much individual variation.

The accompanying changes are due to readjustment of pituitary and ovarian hormones.

The onset is often gradual, the periods becoming less and less regular, or it may be quite sudden.

Although many women accept unpleasant symptoms as inevitable, by no means all women suffer. Some, especially when the onset is gradual, have no symptoms except lack of menstrual periods.

Many of the symptoms blamed on the menopause are not due to it, and there is a very real danger of neglecting other disorders that could and should be treated, by putting them down to the change of life.

Disorders of blood vessels, digestive organs, joints and other organs may well happen to start at about the same time as the menopause. More perhaps than any other symptom, depression is wrongly, or no more than half rightly, regarded as a direct result of the menopause. The altered balance of sex hormones may well cause some emotional instability and so prepare the soil for depression, but the immediate causes are only coincidental. A man is allowed to age gradually and adapt himself to the inevitable changes, but a woman is suddenly, perhaps brutally confronted with middle age at a time when children leave home and husbands no longer look forward to promotion. The blackest of all moods is a sense of being unwanted.

The direct symptoms of the menopause are relatively few. With luck, there may be none at all. Disturbed reflexes of blood vessels can cause hot flushes, palpitations or other odd sensations. Mucous membranes, especially those of the sex organs, may become dry and inflamed. Later effects include weakening of bone and hardening of arteries. These are all controlled by small doses of sex hormones: it is simple replacement therapy, comparable with giving insulin for diabetes or vitamins for malnutrition.

menorrhagia. Excessive bleeding with menstruation.

menses. Menstrual (monthly) periods.

menstruation. Periodic bleeding in women of childbearing age. When a girl is born her ovaries contain the rudiments of up to half a million eggs (ova), which lie dormant until puberty. From then until the menopause some 30 years later, an ovum is released each month from one or other ovary (ovulation), and finds its way to the adjacent Fallopian tube. Before it is released an ovum ripens in a sort of shell, the Graafian follicle. Only the ovum, a single cell, is released. The follicle remains in the ovary and grows into a small endocrine gland, a corpus luteum.

The corpus luteum produces a hormone, progesterone, that stimulates the lining of the uterus to form a thick layer, with an abundant circulation of blood, ready to receive an embryo if the ovum becomes fertilized.

An embryo forms a hormone that keeps the corpus luteum in being and so preserves the enriched lining of the uterus. But if the ovum is not fertilized, the corpus luteum withers in 2 weeks, and the uterus, deprived of progesterone, sheds its lining. The process is spread over a few days. The raw surface left behind bleeds a little: the average loss during a menstrual period is about 2 ounces (60 c.c.) of blood.

As soon as the bleeding is over the lining of the uterus regenerates, and some 2 weeks later the cycle begins again with the release of another ovum.

The interval between ovulation and menstruation – i.e. the life-span of the corpus luteum if there is no pregnancy – is nearly always 2 weeks. But the interval between menstruation and the next ovulation varies from person to person, and also from month to month in the same person. The whole cycle may last from 3 weeks to 5 or more.

⋄ *dysmenorrhoea.*

mental deficiency. The Mental Health Act of 1959 replaced the term 'deficiency' with 'subnormality', defined as a state of incomplete or arrested development of mind. It is quite different from mental illness, where the working of the mind is disturbed.

An international classification distinguishes *idiots*, whose mental age reaches only 2 years or less; *imbeciles*, with mental ages from 3 to 6; and *morons*, from 7 to 9. In English law, the Mental Health Act (1959) limits subnormality to cases needing special care or training, and severe subnormality to cases needing protection. The Education Acts recognize children who cannot be educated in the ordinary sense (though they may benefit from various forms of training), and children who are *educationally subnormal* (ESN) and have to be taught in special classes.

Among normal people, intelligence varies as widely as muscular strength. If subnormality meant 'below average' then half of the population would count as subnormal, and even if it meant 'well below average' it would still include people who were not abnormal, but at the bottom of the normal range. A child of this last type may well be ESN if his home life is unsatisfactory, but with careful teaching he may later hold his place in an ordinary class of school-children.

Many children of average – even above-average – intelligence are thought to be subnormal because of an unrecognized handicap such as defective hearing or eyesight, or word-blindness.

True subnormality implies that the mind has not developed as it should have done because of some defect. Rarely, the trouble starts some time after birth from some such cause as tuberculous meningitis, but nearly always the defect arises at birth or before.

Congenital syphilis, once the commonest cause, is now very rare. But German measles, a more innocent-looking infection acquired before birth, has been recognized as a wide-spread cause of mental and physical defects.

Premature birth, poor nutrition from a defective placenta, or serious difficulties during labour can affect the brain cells. Harmful disorders of body chemistry include severe jaundice in infancy, lack of thyroid hormone (cretinism), and phenylketonuria.

Mongolism is due to a fault in the fertilized ovum at the time of conception.

None of these defects is very common. There are many others that are extremely rare.

Some types of mental deficiency, e.g. cretinism, can be cured, and others, e.g. German measles, poor nutrition, severe jaundice (⋄ *rhesus factor*) and difficult labour can often be prevented with good ante-natal supervision. For the rest – admittedly still the majority – treatment means making the best of what the child has. The outlook is generally better than it appears to be. Only a small minority of defectives are really incapable of learning anything useful; these will always need protection. The majority can be taught at least to look after and occupy themselves, and many can earn a living. In particular, mongols are often *better* than other people at caring for animals; and any subnormal person gets a sense of achievement from work that better-endowed people would find boring. It is difficult for a normal person, anxious to help, to imagine what would keep a subnormal person happy. What seems tragic to a normal parent or teacher may be nothing of the kind to the subnormal child.

mental illness. Illness, as opposed to deficiency, of the mind cannot be defined except as abnormal working of the mind, of which normal working cannot be defined. Serious illness is at least recognizable, but minor disorders merge imperceptibly into normality; where the line is to be drawn is purely a matter of opinion.

Some general patterns are more or less recognizable.

Various physical diseases affect the brain. A patient who is delirious at the start of a fever is for the time being insane. Similarly, acute intoxication with alcohol or any of a large number of drugs and poisons causes temporary insanity. More lasting injury to the mind can be due to gradual and continued poisoning, e.g. with alcohol (*Korsakow's syndrome*), mercury, or lead. Degeneration of arteries in the brain with diminished flow of blood is among the commonest causes of mental deterioration in middle age and later.

But no physical cause can be shown in most cases of mental illness. They fall roughly into three groups: *neuroses, psychoses,* and *personality disorders.*

The common view that a neurosis is less serious than a psychosis is no more than half true. The essential difference is that neurosis does not affect ordinary reasoning, and however disturbed the emotions may be, the conscious mind keeps touch with reality; whereas psychosis distorts conscious reasoning. The neurotic is fully aware of his abnormality (though he may not be able to identify it), but the psychotic is not, because he cannot distinguish fantasy from reality.

Two examples may illustrate the difference. First, a clerk in a large firm is over-anxious about his work and afraid of being dismissed. He disapproves of his own weakness and tries to suppress his fears, but instead of tackling them at source by ensuring that he satisfies his employer, he pushes them to the back of his mind – sweeps them under the carpet. Although he is no longer consciously aware of fear as such, his emotional tension remains to affect his behaviour or his bodily health. He is all too aware that he is unwell. He may complete the circle by regarding his poor health as the cause of his inefficiency – real or supposed – as a clerk. This man is *neurotic.* The fears at the root of his trouble may have been ill-judged, but they were not nonsensical. Like anyone else he must have had his faults, and bad clerks can lose their jobs. His neurosis is an exaggeration of normal responses.

Second, another clerk is delighted with his work but is unshakeably convinced that the management committee meets solely to discuss plans for getting rid of him. This man is *psychotic.* His belief is irrational, yet he sees nothing wrong with it, and is not open to argument.

Neuroses are considered further under ◊ *anxiety,* ◊ *depression,* and ◊ *psychosomatic disease.*

A psychosis may be either *organic,* where the brain is physically damaged, or *functional,* where the mind is disturbed without any recognizable physical cause. Organic psychoses include those due to injury, arterial disease, infection (e.g. syphilis), and poisons such as alcohol and numerous drugs. The two common types of functional psychosis are ◊ *schizophrenia* and ◊ *manic-depressive psychosis.* The distinction between organic and functional psychosis does not mean much. In this context, 'functional' means no more than that the cause is not yet known, but it seems more and more likely that physical causes for these diseases will be found.

Some of the conditions described as *personality disorders* should not really be counted as mental illnesses. Nobody achieves perfect harmony with his neighbours and surroundings, but some do better than others. The ones who do less well are said to have personality disorders, but there is no clear dividing line.

Some types of personality are associated with particular types of mental illness – e.g. a cold, withdrawn type with schizophrenia, or an easy-going, rather irresponsible type with manic-depressive psychosis, or emotional instability with various forms of neurosis – but these are no more than pointers to what *might* happen if the person should ever become mentally ill.

But one group of personality disorders – *psychopathic personalities* – amount to diseases, though it is the neighbours rather than the patients who suffer. These are the social misfits, a most varied collection of drug addicts, alcoholics, drifters, perverts, and habitual criminals. Psychopathic behaviour of one sort or another can be a symptom of mental deficiency or illness, but the term ◊ *psychopath* is usually restricted to people who seem normal apart from their behaviour. In some 'problem families' it is difficult to say whether heredity or upbringing is the main factor.

mental subnormality ◊ *mental deficiency.*

mepacrine. A synthetic drug introduced as an alternative to quinine for treating malaria, also effective against some intestinal worms. For many years it was the standard anti-malarial drug, but less toxic substances have largely superseded it.

mercury. The metal itself, and its chlorides *calomel* (HgCl) and *corrosive sublimate* (HgCl₂) are fairly ancient remedies. Until the present century they were the only drugs with any effect on syphilis; and calomel and grey powder (mercury and chalk) were widely used purgatives until very recent times.

Compounds of mercury still in general use include diuretics such as mersalyl, and numerous antiseptics.

Mercury is as poisonous as ◊ *lead*, with similar symptoms and treatment. Its industrial uses are now carefully controlled, but mercury poisoning was once common in some trades, including the preparation of felt: 'mad as a hatter' and 'hatter's shakes' are reminders of the effect of mercury on the nervous system.

mersalyl. A ◊ *diuretic* drug (i.e. a drug for increasing the flow of urine), containing mercury.

mesenteric. Of the *mesentery*.

The *mesenteric arteries*, branches of the aorta, supply blood to the intestine. Since there are no effective communicating vessels between their small branches, there is no alternative supply if a branch is blocked by a clot (*thrombosis*), and the affected segment of intestine is deprived of blood. This is a dangerous situation requiring prompt surgery.

The *mesenteric veins* carry blood from the intestine to the *portal vein* and so to the liver.

mesentery. A pleated membrane in which the intestine is loosely slung from the back of the abdomen, with the mesenteric blood vessels and lymph nodes between its two layers.

Mesmer, Anton (1734–1815). Austrian physician. ◊ *hypnotism*.

mesoderm. Layer of cells in an ◊ *embryo* from which muscle, bone, blood, connective tissue and some other structures grow.

metabolism. The chemical changes by which foods are converted into components of the body or consumed as fuel, the chemical structure of the tissues is modified, and

waste-products are broken down to substances that can be eliminated. Metabolism consists of *catabolism*, the breakdown of large, unmanageable molecules into small components (e.g. proteins to amino-acids), and *anabolism*, the reconstruction of large molecules.

metacarpus. The middle of the hand, from wrist to fingers. The 5 *metacarpal* bones radiate from the wrist (*carpus*); their rounded ends form the knuckles.

metastasis. Migration of disease (infection, cancer etc.) from its original site to another part of the body by carriage of bacteria, diseased cells etc. in blood or lymph.

metatarsus. Part of the foot corresponding with the *metacarpus* of the hand.

Metchnikoff, Ilya (1845–1916). Russian biologist in Paris; he did much to elucidate the mechanism of immunity against infection, in particular the role of the white blood cells in destroying bacteria. He shared a Nobel Prize with Ehrlich in 1908.

meteorism. Painful distension of the intestine with gas.

methadone. A synthetic substitute for morphine.

methanol. Methyl ◊ *alcohol*; wood spirit.

methotrexate. A drug chemically related to folic acid. Folic acid is a reagent in the growth of tissue by multiplication of cells. Methotrexate interferes with this action, and is used to discourage abnormal cells from proliferating in some types of cancer and also in certain skin diseases.

methyl-dopa. A drug used to suppress the synthesis of noradrenaline. ◊ *blood pressure* (1); *dopa*.

methyl salicylate. Oil of wintergreen, derived from various plants or synthetically. It is among the oldest and most popular of external applications for stiff or painful muscles or joints. It acts mainly by ◊ *counter-irritation*, but it may be that enough is absorbed through the skin to act in the same way as other salicylates such as aspirin.

It is too strong an irritant to be applied to injured or very young skin, and is a corrosive poison if swallowed.

microbe. A microbe or microorganism is a living creature too small to be seen with the naked eye. A germ or *pathogen* is one of the relatively few types of microbe that can cause disease by ◊ *infection* of an animal or plant. It is with these that medicine is directly concerned.

Some microbes, the *protozoa*, are animals. The pathogens of this type include the parasites of malaria and amoebic dysentery. Others, such as the microscopic *fungi* which cause ringworm, are plants. The *bacteria* resemble plants in some ways and animals in others; at this very low level there is no clear boundary between animals and plants. Lower still, the *viruses* are on the border between living and inanimate matter. These four groups are discussed separately under ◊ *protozoon*, ◊ *fungus*, ◊ *bacterium*, and ◊ *virus*. But even with this broad classification there are doubtful cases. The cause of actinomycosis is a microbe which could be an underdeveloped fungus or an advanced bacterium. The 'bacterium' of typhus and the 'virus' of trachoma both fall somewhere between bacteria and viruses.

1. HISTORY

The discovery of microbes and the gradual recognition of infection as a cause of disease are two separate chapters which did not come together until the middle of the 19th century.

No medical writer before the 16th century went beyond a vague idea that some diseases might be spread by contagion, though many described epidemics in great detail. Thucydides, describing the pestilence of 430 B.C., says that people were afraid of catching the disease from each other but that those who had recovered were in no danger of catching it again – surely the first mention of immunity in history. In the 2nd century A.D. Galen ascribed fevers to disorders of the 'humours', blood, phlegm, yellow bile, and black bile, without mentioning the possibility of contagion; he nevertheless removed himself from plague-stricken areas on two occasions. During the Black Death (1346–9) Guy de Chauliac reported that many physicians would not visit patients for fear of catching the plague, and Boccaccio, in the introduction to the *Decameron*, said that the plague was caught not only by associating with the sick but by touching anything that they had touched. But in general, infectious disease was not recog-

nized as such; rather it was supposed that a stricken region was subject to some climatic or other influence, and when people fled from epidemics it was from these influences that they fled. Since environmental factors are important in the spread of infection, the theory was reasonable. Its greatest exponent was Hippocrates, who accurately described conditions which would favour particular diseases. Malaria prevailed in low-lying regions (where as we now know the mosquitoes that transmit the disease are found), and diarrhoea in hot places (where there are most flies and not enough rain to wash the place clean).

The first general account of infection was by Fracastorius of Verona. In *De Contagione* (1546) he correctly ascribed numerous diseases to infection, and said that the 'seeds of contagion' could be transmitted by direct contact with a patient, by contact with articles that the patient had touched, or at a distance. He recognized that the seeds of a particular contagion could produce only that disease, and that infection and putrefaction were similar processes.

The first suggestion that germs might be small living creatures came from a German priest, Athanasius Kircher, in about 1650; he claimed to have seen plague germs with his microscope, but since he advised killing them by lighting fires to burn off their wings and feet it seems unlikely that he saw actual bacteria.

Microbiology really began in Holland with the work of Leeuwenhoek, published in 1683. Protozoa and bacteria of various kinds are easily recognized from his descriptions and drawings. But no microbe was shown to cause disease until 150 years later.

In 1835 Bassi showed that a minute fungus caused muscardine, a disease of silkworms, and suggested that human diseases such as smallpox and plague had similar causes. The first of these to be identified was the fungus which causes favus (a kind of ringworm), by Schönlein in 1839. In the next few years many other microbes were associated with different diseases.

A great problem was that an *association* of a microbe with a disease did not prove that the microbe was the *cause* of the disease, and it was later found that many of the microbes blamed for diseases were innocent bystanders. The bacterium still known as *Haemophilus influenzae* was discovered in 1892; 40 years later it was shown that influenza was in fact due to a virus. Koch (see below) showed how to avoid such misattribution.

Worse still, there was little proof that microbes were ever the cause of disease, how ever strong the circumstantial evidence, while there was still a possibility that the disease produced the microbes. Many good biologists believed in spontaneous generation – in the formation of new life in decaying matter. In their view the bacteria found in diseased tissues had appeared as a result of the disease, just as maggots in rotting organic matter were a result of the rotting. In fact, the Italian physician Francesco Redi had disposed of the maggots in 1668 by showing that if meat was shielded with gauze from egg-laying flies, no maggots would grow, but his work was ignored. An English priest, John Needham, published in 1745 the results of careful experiments which seemed to show that all living matter was able to generate microbes, but he had not managed to prevent his specimens from being contaminated by bacteria in the air. An Italian priest, Spallanzani, refuted this theory by heating the air surrounding his specimens and excluding other air: no bacteria appeared. Needham replied that Spallanzani's rough treatment had spoiled the specimens and invalidated the experiment. For a century scientists were divided between the two schools of thought. The question was argued most fiercely in France, where Buffon and later Lamarck supported Needham, and Spallanzani found an unexpected ally in Voltaire; and it was a French chemist, Pasteur, who found the answer.

Pasteur proved that fermentation of wine and beer, souring of milk and similar processes depended on living microbes – yeasts (fungi) or bacteria. If the microbes in a specimen were destroyed by heat there would be no fermentation and no new microbes would appear unless the specimen was then contaminated by untreated air. He devised a simple trap which allowed air to reach his specimens, but not microbes; still there was no fermentation. As soon as the trap was removed microbes found their way in and multiplied, and fermentation began. Pasteur then showed that fermentation, putrefaction, and infection were all due to contamination by microbes – that the microbes were the cause and not the effect of these processes. One of the first doctors to see the importance of Pasteur's work was the English surgeon Lister, who took steps to exclude bacteria from wounds and so initiated safe surgery ($\diamond$ *infection*).

The relation of microbes to disease was finally and fully established by Pasteur's German contemporary Robert Koch. If Pasteur had proved that microbes in general could cause disease, it was still necessary to show which particular microbe was responsible for a particular disease. For instance, sputum from a case of tuberculosis would contain half a dozen or more different kinds of bacteria, and the specimen might be contaminated by still other types on its way to the laboratory; but only one type had anything to do with the disease, and in practice it was usually outnumbered by harmless types. Before anything could be proved the different types had to be separated and studied individually. To this end Koch prepared a solid medium, originally of gelatin, later of agar jelly with added nutrients. A specimen wiped over the surface of the medium left a trail of bacteria, each free to multiply on its own. After incubation for a day or two the medium was peppered with visible colonies, each composed of the progeny of one bacterium from the original specimen. By sowing a sample of a colony on a fresh medium 'a pure culture' of one species of bacterium could be established.

Koch then set out the following rules to be observed before ascribing a disease to a particular microbe:

1. The microbe must be regularly associated with the disease;

2. It must be isolated in pure culture;

3. Microbes from the pure culture must reproduce the disease in animals and be recovered from the infected tissues.

These rules were a restatement of rules proposed as early as 1840 by the anatomist Henle, but it was Koch who showed how they could be fulfilled. They are known as *Koch's postulates*, and they established medical bacteriology as a proper science with Koch as its founder. In the two decades between Koch's announcement of his postulates and the end of the 19th century most of the bacteria involved in common diseases were identified by Koch or one of his many pupils.

There remained the problem of diseases that were obviously due to infection for which no microbe could be found. Bacteria will not pass through the finest filters (hence the use of filters to purify drinking water). Fluid extracts from tissues infected by these obscure diseases were still infectious after filtration; therefore the agents had to be smaller than bacteria and too small to be seen with the microscopes then available. The name 'filterable virus' was coined for them; later they became known simply as viruses. They could not be demonstrated; their existence had to be inferred from the infectivity of the extracts. Nor could they be grown in pure culture, because, as we now know, a virus can multiply only when it is incorporated into a living cell. Therefore Koch's postulates could not be met, and the study of viruses had to be based on circumstantial evidence. The first disease to be ascribed to a virus in this way was the mosaic disease of tobacco plants (Ivanowski, 1892), and the next was foot-and-mouth disease of cattle (Loeffler and Frosch, 1898).

In 1931 Goodpasture evolved a method for making pure cultures of viruses in chick embryos. This work, carried out at Nashville, Tennessee, was a development of a method suggested 50 years earlier by Ogston, the discoverer of staphylococci. More recently other methods of tissue culture, by which fragments of tissue removed from living organs can be kept alive almost indefinitely, have been used for growing viruses. Since 1938 it has been possible to make detailed photographs of viruses with the electron microscope. With very few exceptions the earlier inferences about virus diseases have been confirmed in accordance with Koch's postulates, and many unsuspected virus diseases have been identified.

Although the 'germ theory' of infectious disease has been proved beyond doubt, a microbe is not necessarily the sole cause of a disease associated with it. Like other accidents, infection has not only an immediate cause – the specific microbe – but also, as often as not, contributory causes. Tuberculosis is directly due to the tubercle bacillus, but poor standards of living, other sorts of illness, and even mental stresses can all make an actual attack more likely. Hereditary factors probably count as well; they are difficult to assess because members of a family are liable to infect each other. The essential point is that nearly everyone is exposed to infection by tubercle bacilli at one time or another, but most people escape the disease. Some contributory causes of infectious disease are evident from individual cases, but others are recognized only from the statistical study of large numbers of cases, which is *epidemiology*.

Some of the tributaries of microbiology have become almost as important as the main stream. The study of *immunity* to infection has provided effective vaccines against many of the most dangerous microbes, and also shed light on certain processes of disease such as *allergy*. Successful transplantation of organs from one person to another depends on controlling the 'immune response' by which the body rejects transplanted organs as though they were microbes.

The development of *antibiotics* for the treatment of infection is among the most valuable contributions of microbiology to medicine.

microbiology. The study of microbes, until recently generally called bacteriology; but since bacteriologists have to deal with all kinds of minute creatures, not only bacteria, the term microbiology is more appropriate.

microcephaly. Abnormally small head, with incomplete development of the brain and mental deficiency.

microorganism = ◊ *microbe*.

microscope. The founders of medical microscopy, Leeuwenhoek (1632–1723) and Malpighi (1628–94), used *simple* microscopes, i.e. powerful magnifying glasses, yet they managed to describe most of the structures that a present-day medical student is expected to see with an elaborate modern instrument. The *compound* microscope now used was invented by Galileo some years before Malpighi's birth, but the technical problems of lighting and correcting distortion of the image were not overcome until much later.

Objects smaller than the wave-length of light cannot be seen, because the waves pass them by. This limits the useful magnification of an optical microscope to about 1000 diameters. Cross-lighting may reveal smaller objects, rather as a shaft of sunlight in a shaded place reveals particles of dust in the air. But to show detail at higher magnification, something smaller than light waves must be used. The electron microscope gives several hundred times the magnification of an optical microscope.

◊ *histology; microbe.*

microsporum. A minute fungus, causing *ringworm* of the scalp.

micturition. Urination; act of passing urine. ◊ *bladder.*

midbrain. Part of the brain-stem, between the *pons* and the *hypothalamus.* Its primitive function, to control the movements of the eyes, is retained in the human brain, but most of it is occupied by enormous bundles of nerve fibres connecting the cerebral cortex with lower centres. The most interesting structure in the midbrain is the *reticular formation,* a collection of nerve cells interspersed among a network of nerve fibres; it extends downwards from the midbrain to the upper end of the spinal cord. It appears to be a switching station in which sensations from the periphery are diverted either to consciousness or to reflex paths, and impulses to suppress or to stimulate muscles are sent to the periphery. Consciousness is an active process depending on impulses from the reticular formation. Sleep is a passive state in which these impulses are reduced.

midwifery = ◊ *obstetrics.*

migraine. A common and distressing kind of headache, with no evident cause. Attacks last a few hours. They may be frequent, but some people have only one or two typical attacks in a lifetime. Warning symptoms such as a sense of flickering before the eyes are common; during the attack the patient cannot stand bright light. Most patients feel nauseated during or after the attack, and some actually vomit. The classic accounts of migraine describe the headache as one-sided: this is quite common but by no means the rule.

The site of the trouble seems to be the arteries inside and outside the skull, but the nature and cause of migraine are still unknown. It has no lasting effects, and the attacks become less frequent with time. Over-activity of substances such as histamine and serotonin that affect the relaxation and contraction of arteries is the likeliest explanation of migraine; one must then account for the over-activity. Emotional upset, perhaps acting through such substances, plays some part but is not the main factor.

Many different kinds of treatment work in particular cases, suggesting that migraine might have various causes. When antihistamine drugs work, for example, this is a strong hint that the attacks may be allergic. Drugs derived from ergot are perhaps more often effective than any others, but until the causes are better understood the treatment of migraine will remain a matter of trial and error.

miliaria = ◊ *prickly heat*; minute sweat-blisters like *milia* – millet-seeds.

miliary tuberculosis. Small, widely scattered points of tuberculous infection.

milieu intérieur. Internal environment; the tissue fluid, a watery solution derived from the blood, in which the cells of the body lead their aquatic existence. ◊ *Bernard, Claude.*

milk. Human milk differs considerably from cow's milk in the proportions of its main ingredients: it contains about the same amount of fat, but twice as much sugar (lactose) and half as much protein. Human milk contains only just enough calcium and iron for the baby's needs.

For a few days after the birth of a baby, a woman forms a special kind of milk known as *colostrum,* corresponding with the beestings of cows. Colostrum contains about 8 per cent of protein, 2·5 per cent of fat, and 3·5 per cent of sugar (compared with 2 per cent, 4 per cent, and 8 per cent in ordinary human milk).

The vitamins in milk depend on the mother's diet, but the other components are maintained, if she is underfed, at the expense of her tissues, at least for a while. But after a few weeks the supply of milk fails if the mother has a poor diet or is ill, or even if she is emotionally disturbed.

A few drugs can affect the baby by way of the milk, but most, including alcohol, pass from the mother's blood-stream into the milk only in very small amounts.
◊ *breast.*

minim. In the apothecaries' measures, 1/60 drachm or 1/480 fluid ounce; roughly one drop.

miosis. Contraction of the pupil of the eye; *miotic* is a drug to cause this.

miscarriage ◊ *abortion.*

mite. A kind of small insect, e.g. *Sarcoptes scabei,* the itch-mite, which burrows into the skin and causes scabies.

mithramycin. An antibiotic, too poisonous

to be used for treating infection, but (like actinomycin) more poisonous to certain cancer cells than to healthy tissue. It may therefore find a place in the treatment of cancer.

Mithridates(*fl.* 100 B.C.). King of Pontus. As a precaution against murder (for which he gave cause in plenty) he built up a resistance to poison, probably arsenic, by taking a small daily dose.

mithridaticum. The universal antidote, a favourite medieval remedy with scores of unpleasant and useless ingredients. Its name is derived from ◊ *Mithridates*.

mitosis. Reproduction of a cell, with duplication of the chromosomes so that each of the two new cells has all the properties of the original one; it is the normal process by which tissues grow.

mitral stenosis. Narrowing of the *mitral valve* by inflammation; the cause is nearly always rheumatic fever. As a result of scarring, the valve is both tight and leaky, and the efficiency of the heart is impaired. In some cases the heart muscle compensates for the defect by pumping harder, but this may not be possible if the muscle itself has also been damaged by rheumatic fever or if the valve is much affected, and the condition then leads to disability.

A narrow mitral valve can be much improved by plastic surgery.

mitral valve. Passage between the left atrium and left ventricle of the heart. ◊ *valve.*

Mittelschmerz. Pain mid-way between menstrual periods, at the time of ovulation.

mole ◊ *birth-mark.*

molecule. The smallest complete unit of a substance; a molecule can be broken down to smaller molecules or to its component atoms, but the substance then loses its identity.

Mondino de Luzzi (d. 1326). Anatomist at Bologna; the 'restorer of anatomy'. ◊ *anatomy.*

mongol (mongoloid). Affected with *mongolism* or *Down's syndrome*, a congenital defect of physical and mental development. The physical characteristics include a flat, round face, a fold of skin over the inner corner of the eye, and coarse, straight hair, which are said to confer a Mongolian appearance. The numerous other signs include short stature, squat hands with a characteristic arrangement of the skin creases, a small skull, and a gruff voice. These signs are important mainly as pointers to the diagnosis; what matters is the mental retardation. The affected children are usually friendly and cheerful, and although they can cope with only a very limited education they can generally learn to look after themselves and to occupy themselves usefully. Many of them have a gift for caring for animals.

It was discovered in 1959 that the body cells of mongols each have 47 instead of the normal 46 chromosomes. Normal chromosomes occur in matched pairs, one derived from each parent (◊ *genetics*), since the ovum and sperm each contain 23 single chromosomes instead of 23 pairs. Occasionally one of the smallest pairs fails to split when an ovum is formed; the resulting ovum then has 22 single chromosomes and one intact pair. If this ovum is fertilized, the child of the union will have 22 normal pairs of chromosomes and one triplicated chromosome. This child becomes a mongol. The tendency to form abnormal ova of this type increases with age: more than 50 per cent of all mongols are born to women over 40. A second, much less common cause of mongolism, is an abnormal arrangement of the chromosomes in either parent, of which the only effect is a predisposition to form abnormal ova or sperms, regardless of age. The two types are distinguished by investigating both parents. With the first type there is an excellent chance that a subsequent child will be normal, but with the second type the risk of producing another abnormal child, either a mongol or a carrier of the parent's anomaly, is high.

By means of ◊ *amniocentesis* it is possible to say early in pregnancy whether or not the child will be born a mongol, while there is still time to consider an abortion.

Monilia ◊ *Candida.*

Moniz, Egas ◊ *leukotomy.*

monoamine oxidase (MAO). An ◊ *enzyme*

which promotes the oxidation of adrenaline and similar substances (pressor amines), rendering them inactive. These substances transmit impulses from certain nerve fibres to adjoining nerve cells; if they were not promptly destroyed they would set off unwanted nervous activity. ◊ *Depression* appears to be associated with a deficiency of some pressor amine in the brain. Drugs which suppress MAO activity (MAO-inhibitors) and so prolong the life of the amines relieve depression. Special precautions are needed with these drugs, because MAO is needed for inactivating various substances that are dangerous if they are allowed to accumulate. Patients taking MAO inhibitors have to avoid numerous other drugs and also certain foods including cheese: ◊ *depression*.

monocyte. A large white blood cell. ◊ *blood* (3).

mononucleosis ◊ *glandular fever.*

Monro, Alexander (1697–1767). Scottish anatomist. He studied under Boerhaave at Leyden, a school that had become the leading centre of medical science. Monro returned to Edinburgh and brought its medical school into the front rank, where it has remained. He was succeeded in the chair of anatomy by his son (1733–1817) and grandson (1773–1859). These three Alexanders held the chair from 1720 till 1846.

morbilli = ◊ *measles.*

Morgagni, Giovanni-Battista (1682–1771). Professor of anatomy at Padua from 1715 until his death; the last of a dynasty of geniuses that had begun in 1538 when Vesalius, the founder of scientific anatomy and therefore of modern medical science, was appointed to this chair. Morgagni's fame rests not on any particular discovery, but on a new approach to the problem of disease. He applied the detailed knowledge of his illustrious predecessors to the symptoms of disease, and related symptoms to the alterations of normal anatomy that could be found either by clinical observation or by postmortem examination. His masterpiece *De Sedibus et Causis Morborum* is a series of accurate case-histories with the patients' symptoms related to the site and nature of the disease.

morning sickness. A common, tiresome, but seldom serious condition in the early part of pregnancy. The cause is not known. A very light snack (e.g. a few biscuits) before rising may be enough to allay the symptoms. Antihistamine drugs, mild tranquillizers, and vitamin B_6 have been successfully used for some years. A newer drug, *metoclopramide*, is also effective. The trouble usually clears up in a few weeks.

More serious and persistent vomiting (*hyperemesis gravidarum*) is probably a different kind of disorder.

moron. A feeble-minded person; one with slight mental deficiency, attaining a mental age of 7–9 years.

morphia; morphine. The main active principle of opium. The alkaloid morphine is used in the form of compounds such as the hydrochloride or the sulphate. The term 'morphia' includes all these. Their effects are identical.

Morphine and its derivatives (heroin etc.) suppress pain better than any other drugs except general anaesthetics. Very large doses of morphine actually induce anaesthesia, but they are too near to lethal doses to be safe.

Small doses probably do not interfere with the transmission of pain impulses to the brain, but they so alter the state of mind that these impulses cause little distress. Whether this is the same as suppressing pain depends on the definition of pain; according to the point of view taken here (◊ *pain*) it is the same. Without the element of distress, pain has little meaning.

Larger doses depress the whole brain, and especially the vital centres for the regulation of breathing and circulation. Slight depression of the cough reflex is sometimes useful; for this purpose *codeine* (methyl morphine) is better and safer than morphine itself.

Morphine causes spasm of some involuntary muscles, e.g. in the intestine, and in this way can aggravate colic. Constipation is a tiresome side-effect. A few people complain of nausea. Continued administration of morphine inevitably induces ◊ *addiction.*

For all its drawbacks, morphine is among the most valuable drugs. Apart from synthetic drugs closely related to morphine (e.g. pethidine) there is nothing to take its place, and Sydenham's dictum that nobody ought to be a physician without opium still holds good.

Morphine antagonists (nalorphine; levall-orphan) are drugs chemically related to morphine but lacking its depressant action on the brain. Nerve cells take them up instead of morphine, and cannot then take up morphine, because they can accommo-date only a limited amount of either. These drugs have some value in treating over-dosage of morphine, and especially in protecting new-born infants from narco-tics given to the mother during labour.

morphology. Comparative anatomy; the study of similarities and differences between species. The word was coined by Goethe; it took on new significance half a century later with Darwin's theories of evolution.

mosquito. Kinds of flying insect; the females of several species transmit infectious mic-robes by sucking blood. *Anopheles*, the carrier of malaria, can be distinguished from other mosquitoes by its slanting pos-ture when it settles.

Other mosquito-borne diseases include *dengue* and *yellow fever* (*Aëdes* mosquitoes), and some types of virus *encephalitis* and *filariasis* (*Culex* mosquitoes).

Since mosquito-borne diseases are not contracted in any other way they can be eradicated by control of mosquitoes (◊ *malaria*).

motion sickness = ◊ *travel sickness.*

motor neurone disease. An uncommon and mysterious degeneration of groups of nerve cells in the spinal cord and brain, with loss of function in the corresponding muscles. Neither cause nor remedy has yet been discovered.

mouth. Entrance to the digestive tract. In lower animals, the mouth is often no more than a hole at the front. In all vertebrates, one of the gill-openings is modified to form a movable jaw, and this is one reason for the dominance of these animals over other types. With this kind of mouth an animal can choose its food instead of merely accept-ing what comes, and the mouth can also be a weapon of defence or attack. Man has to rely much less on his mouth than other vertebrates, because he can do even better with his hands.

The mouth extends from the lips to the back of the tongue where the pharynx be-gins. The roof (hard palate) and the arch of the lower jaw are rigid; otherwise the mouth is surrounded by muscles. These muscles act in concert with the tongue during the mastication and swallowing of food, and they are essential to articulate speech.

The whole of the cavity is lined with a mucous membrane. Small mucous glands are scattered throughout the membrane except on the outer surface of the lips. The mucus from these glands, together with the saliva, keeps the mouth clean and lubri-cated.

Specially modified nerve-endings, the taste-buds, are found on the surface of the tongue and palate.

In the embryo, the tissues of the mouth grow from each side into the gap between the brain and the heart and meet in the mid-line. Incomplete fusion results in various degrees of harelip and cleft palate (◊ *palate*).

The mouth teems with bacteria, yet al-though minor injuries to the lining are very frequent, serious infection is quite uncom-mon. Most of the bacteria, but not all, are harmless, and there seems to be far more resistance to infection than most mucous membranes have. Even severe wounds of the mouth generally heal without much trouble – whereas human bites on the skin, which must be contaminated with the same bacteria, nearly always develop serious infection and are notoriously slow to heal.

But if the general health is poor because of malnutrition or chronic poisoning (e.g. alchohol, lead), or especially with fevers when the flow of saliva is reduced, infection of the mouth is very common. Keeping the mouth clean and moist is an important part of general nursing with any severe illness.

moxibustion. Treatment of disease by burn-ing a *moxa*, a small heap of dried mugwort, on the skin to raise a blister. The method differs from the use of poultices in that the moxa is not necessarily applied over the affected organ, but at some point from which the organ is said to be influenced. ◊ *Chinese medicine.*

mucopus. Mucus contaminated with pus, e.g. sputum with bronchitis.

mucosa. Mucous membrane.

mucous. Associated with *mucus*. A *mucous membrane* is a delicate skin-like layer con-taining glands that secrete mucus, e.g. the linings of the air-passages and digestive tract.

mucoviscidosis = ◊ *cystic fibrosis*.

mucus. A clear viscous fluid, forming a protective barrier on the surfaces of lining membranes.

Müller, Johannes (1801–58). German philosopher and medical scientist; a physiologist with whom only Claude Bernard (1813–78) stands comparison. Müller was a late product of the Renaissance: Bernard, with his insistence on arguing from nothing that had not been demonstrated, was a specialized scientist of our own time. Most of the current concepts of normal and abnormal bodily function can be traced directly to the work of one or the other.

Müller put every known science to the service of medicine, and himself contributed a most versatile imagination. He is best known for his theory of *specific nerve energies* – a given sensory nerve conveys only a single kind of sensation, regardless of how it is stimulated, and our awareness of the world therefore depends on the properties of our nerve-endings. This has the profoundest implications for psychology as well as for the mere mechanics of the nervous system. Possible exceptions to the theory (◊ *taste*) do not affect its value as a working hypothesis, a starting-point for research.

His studies embraced far more than one man could develop in a lifetime, but fortunately he was among the greatest of teachers, and there was no shortage of younger men to extend his work. Müller's pupils included the physicist Helmholtz, who explained the mechanisms of vision and hearing, Henle and Schwann, who brought microscopic anatomy up to date, and the greatest of pathologists, Virchow.

multiple sclerosis (disseminated sclerosis). A chronic disease of the central nervous system in which small, scattered areas of the brain and spinal cord degenerate and nerve fibres lose their insulating myelin sheaths and their ability to conduct impulses. The *sclerosis* resembles scarring after a virus infection such as poliomyelitis; but there is no evidence of infection or any other cause.

The symptoms depend entirely on where the patches of sclerosis appear, and they can therefore mimic those of almost any disorder of the nervous system. This is an episodic disorder: symptoms come and go, and between episodes the patient may be well for months or years. As a result, the most extravagant claims have been made for all manner of remedies; but at present no treatment is of proven value.

mumps (epidemic parotitis). A common virus disease to which most people acquire immunity through a childhood attack.

The virus, which resembles that of influenza, is air-borne. An attack begins 2–4 weeks after exposure with mild fever, followed by painful swelling of the parotid salivary glands lasting a day or two. As a rule the symptoms then vanish, but sometimes the infection spreads to other salivary glands or, less often, to the testes or pancreas. Like other virus diseases, mumps can involve the nervous system, but the symptoms are nearly always mild and short-lasting.

In grown men, mumps occasionally causes sterility; and a few cases of diabetes from involvement of the pancreas have been recorded.

murmur. Any sound from the heart additional to the normal heart sounds. ◊ *stethoscope*.

muscarine. A highly poisonous alkaloid from the mushroom *fly agaric* (*Amanita muscaria*); both chemically and in its effects it resembles *acetyl choline*. The effects are abolished by atropine.

muscle. Muscle is the most abundant tissue in the body; it accounts for some two fifths of the body weight. The specialized component is the *muscle fibre*, a long slender cell or agglomeration of cells which becomes shorter and thicker in response to a stimulus. These fibres are supported and bound together by ordinary connective tissue, and are well supplied with blood vessels and nerves.

The chemical components include *actomyosin*, a protein responsible for the actual contraction; *myoglobin*, which resembles the haemoglobin of blood and maintains the store of oxygen; *phosphates* for transferring energy; and glucose, stored as *glycogen*, for fuel.

There are 3 types of muscle: striated, smooth, and cardiac.

Striated (= striped, voluntary, skeletal) muscle is the flesh or lean meat. The 'stripes' are bands across the fibres about 1/1000 mm. wide produced by regular alternation of the actin and myosin components of actomyosin. Nearly all striated muscle is under conscious control, but also takes part in unconscious reflexes (◊ 'Mechanics', below).

Smooth (= plain, involuntary, visceral) muscle is found in the walls of the digestive and urinary tracts and other hollow organs, and of the blood vessels. Its fibres, each a single cell, are much shorter than striated fibres. All smooth muscle is controlled unconsciously through the ◊ *sympathetic* and ◊ *parasympathetic* nervous systems, usually together, one stimulating and the other inhibiting.

Cardiac muscle, the substance of the heart, can be regarded as an enormously developed involuntary muscle in the wall of a blood vessel, but it differs from any other muscle. Its fibres are short and thick, and form a dense mesh. They contract rhythmically without any nervous impulse; the nerves only modify the rate of contraction (◊ *heart*).

1. NATURE OF MUSCLE CONTRACTION

Within a muscle fibre threads of the two proteins actin and myosin are arranged in interlocking bundles. When the protein actomyosin is formed the bundles of actin are drawn further into the bundles of myosin, so that the fibre is shortened. The energy for this chemical reaction is provided by the breakdown of adenosine triphosphate (ATP) to adenosine diphosphate (ADP) (◊ *energy*). Myosin is itself the enzyme which promotes this breakdown.

Energy is then needed to convert ADP back to ATP. The ultimate source is the combustion of glucose (stored in the muscle as ◊ *glycogen*) with oxygen to form carbon dioxide. But oxygen may not be immediately available – it is quite usual to hold the breath during brief exertion such as a short sprint where the deep breathing comes after the race. The conversion of glucose to lactic acid provides some energy without using any oxygen at all: $(CH_2O)_6 \rightarrow 2(CH_2O)_3$. This mechanism cannot, however, be used for long, because if lactic acid accumulates muscle quickly tires. It simply delays the moment when oxygen must be brought in to complete the conversion to carbon dioxide, with further release of energy: $2(CH_2O)_3 + 6O_2 \rightarrow 6CO_2 + 6H_2O$. In the meantime there is a state of *oxygen debt*.

The motor nerve joins the muscle fibre at the motor end-plate. An impulse in the nerve causes release of *acetyl choline*, which triggers off the conversion of ATP to ADP. How this 'pulls' the bundles of actin and myosin together is not yet known.

Some impulses to smooth muscle are transmitted by noradrenaline instead of acetyl choline. Heart muscle gets energy from fat rather than glucose and so is undisturbed by variations in the amount of glucose in the blood.

2. CONTROL

Smooth muscle fibres are so arranged that some bundles encircle the organ and others run the length of it. The former squeeze while the latter shorten a segment of the organ, pushing the contents forward to the next segment, which is relaxed to receive them. Waves of contraction flow along the organ. This activity is called *peristalsis*. Most smooth muscle has a double nerve supply: one causes contraction and the other actively promotes relaxation.

Striated muscle has only one set of motor nerves, originating in the spinal cord, and relaxation is merely the absence of contraction. But the motor nerve cells in the spinal cord are connected with other nerves of which some stimulate (for instance those under conscious control from the brain) and others inhibit.

The conscious will determines the kind of movement to be made, *and no more*. Even a simple movement needs several muscles to contract, not all by the same amount, and other muscles to relax. This is all reflex action. A man decides to drive a screw home. Having placed the screwdriver he must grip it and turn it clockwise. He grips with the flexor muscles to his fingers, but most of them arise in the forearm and also flex the wrist. The wrist is kept straight by simultaneous action of its extensors. He twists mainly with his biceps. The muscles for twisting the forearm anticlockwise must be inhibited. On its own, the biceps would also bend the elbow; therefore its antagonist the triceps also contracts to steady the elbow. To prevent the thumb side of the hand from being turned outwards away from the screw the whole limb must be rotated inwards by the shoulder muscles. If the man has to exert pressure on the screw the muscles joining the shoulder-blade to the trunk come into play. All this

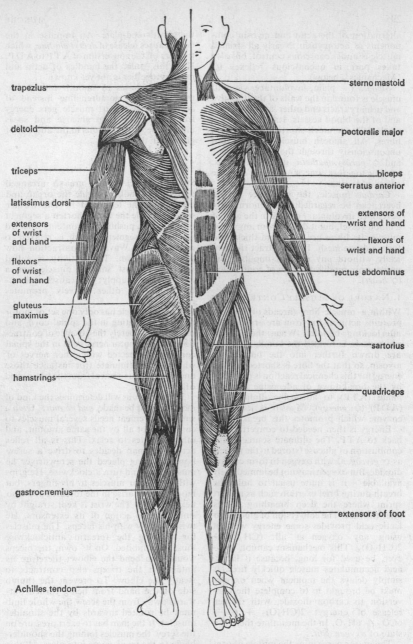

Superficial muscles, back and front.

activity is unconscious and reflex except the intention to turn a screw.

3. MECHANICS

Even at rest a muscle is not completely flabby. Continuous activity of the nerve cells maintains a slight tension or *tone*, which causes no movement because it is balanced by the tone of the opposed muscles. The engine is kept permanently ticking over, never switched off. If anything tends to stretch a muscle, the tone is automatically increased to resist the tendency. An increase of tone without shortening is called *isometric* contraction. In the example of the screwdriver, the triceps contracts isometrically. If on the other hand a muscle pulls, i.e. shortens, against a steady resistance, the tone is constant while the length changes; this is *isotonic* contraction. In practice most activity is a mixture of the two.

The action of a particular muscle is usually described in terms of the movement when it contracts isotonically – its attachments to the skeleton are brought closer together. Thus the quadriceps muscle in front of the thigh straightens the bent knee by pulling the front of the tibia up towards the femur, a kicking movement. But when the opposing hamstring muscles bend the knee, the quadriceps is stretched. The reflex of muscle tone would resist this, and has to be suppressed by a contrary reflex action.

A man standing at the alert with his knees slightly bent uses the isometric contraction of quadriceps to hold the position against gravity. This kind of static or postural action is the most important function of many muscles, especially in a precariously balanced animal such as man.

4. DISORDERS

There are few common diseases of muscle. Tumours are very rare excepting an innocent tumour of the uterus (◊ *fibroid*). Primary infection of muscle is also rare (the muscle abscesses seen in tropical Africa are thought to arise from malnutrition).

Several hereditary diseases affect the growth and function of muscles (◊ *myopathy*). Apart from familial periodic paralysis, a disturbance of potassium balance, they are little understood.

The balance of potassium and sodium is upset by loss of salt from severe sweating

or diarrhoea, and this interferes with the transmission of impulses in muscle.

Some bacterial toxins and chemical poisons appear to affect muscle directly, but the motor nerves are much more vulnerable. In ◊ *poliomyelitis* motor nerve cells in the spinal cord are destroyed, and all activity in the corresponding muscles ceases as though the nerves had been cut. On the other hand ◊ *tetanus*, like strychnine poisoning, stops inhibition of the motor cells, throwing the muscles into uncontrolled contraction.

Calcium plays some part in muscle action, perhaps in triggering the breakdown of ATP (◊ 'Nature of Muscle Contraction', above). If the calcium balance is disturbed, e.g. by ◊ *rickets*, ◊ *parathyroid* disease, or ◊ *alkalosis*, the muscles become irritable and over-active, a state known as *tetany*.

Impulses from nerve to muscle are transmitted by the release of acetyl choline. ◊ *Myasthenia gravis* is a disease in which this mechanism fails from time to time. Poisoning with ◊ *curare* prevents acetyl choline from acting on the muscle fibres; this is a useful means of relaxing muscles to facilitate surgery.

muscle relaxants. Drugs that prevent nerve impulses from being transmitted to muscle fibres. The muscles are thus as effectively paralysed as an electric light with a blown fuse.

The principal use of temporary paralysis is for surgical operations, where the complete relaxation makes the surgeon's work easier (and therefore safer), and reduces the dose of anaesthetic. The same principle can be applied to diseases in which violent muscle spasm is a threat to life, such as tetanus. The original drug of this type is ◊ *curare*.

Some tranquillizing drugs relax muscle spasm, at least under experimental conditions, and this effect on physical tension may account for some of their effect on the symptoms of emotional tension.

muscular atrophy ◊ *myopathy*.

muscular dystrophy ◊*myopathy*.

muscular rheumatism ◊ *fibrositis*.

mushroom. Kinds of large fungus. The mushroom itself is the spore-bearing or reproductive part of the fungus.

There are many species, some edible and some poisonous, and the differences are not always obvious. The only safe rule is to eat no fungus that one cannot positively identify. Accidents are uncommon, but when they do happen they are serious.

Some poisonous varieties are made relatively safe by their disgusting taste. The two most dangerous kinds of poison are *muscarine* and *phallin*. Muscarine occurs in several species, notably *Amanita muscaria*, a red toadstool with white spots. It resembles ◊ *acetyl choline*, and has similar effects: diarrhoea, vomiting, and depression of the heart. Atropine is an effective antidote. Phallin behaves like a snake venom. The symptoms are delayed for some hours. They include severe dysentery, and damage to the nervous system, blood cells, liver, and kidneys. Many of the patients die a few days later from liver failure and general exhaustion. The main source of phallin poisoning is *Amanita phalloides* (death cap), which bears a superficial resemblance to the common mushroom.

Edible mushrooms are an attractive garnish and flavouring, but the food value is negligible.

mutation ◊ *genetics* (4).

myasthenia gravis. An uncommon disease, affecting voluntary muscles. The characteristic symptom is rapid weakening of muscles when they are made to work, with slow recovery at rest. An affected muscle does not respond to stimulation by the trace of acetyl choline released from its controlling nerve, exactly as though it were poisoned with curare. The drug *eserine* increases the effect of acetyl choline and restores a normal response.

Myasthenia gravis is often associated with disease of the thymus gland, and there is evidence that at least some cases may be due to ◊ *autoimmunity* to both thymus and muscle cells.

Often the muscles recover when the thymus is removed.

-mycin. Suffix to names of antibiotics obtained from fungi of the genus Streptomyces.

Mycobacterium. A genus of bacteria slightly resembling minute fungi, including the bacilli of tuberculosis and leprosy.

mycosis. Disease caused by a ◊ *fungus.*

myelin. A greasy substance forming an insulating sheath around nerve fibres. In many diseases of the nervous system the fibres lose their myelin sheaths and fail to conduct impulses.

myelitis. Inflammation of marrow: an ambiguous term because *marrow* can mean bone marrow or the spinal cord.

myelocoele. Protrusion of spinal cord through a defect in a vertebra. ◊ *spina bifida.*

myelography. X-ray examination of the spinal cord.

myeloma. A tumour of bone-marrow cells, with a tendency to appear simultaneously in several places. There are several types, corresponding with the various types of cell in bone marrow. Some are comparatively harmless, but some are progressive in the manner of *leukaemia*. All are rare.

myocardial infarction. Blockage of blood supply to part of the *myocardium* (heart muscle). ◊ *coronary thrombosis.*

myoglobin. Oxygen-carrying pigment in muscle, similar to *haemoglobin* in blood.

myoma. Tumour of muscle; a very rare condition (because muscle cells cannot normally multiply), except for the innocent tumours of the uterus known as ◊ *fibroids.*

myopathy. Literally, any disease of muscle; in practice, any of a group of rare diseases of which inadequate function of voluntary muscles is the principal or only symptom.

The various myopathies affect different parts of the *motor unit.* This consists of a *nerve cell* in the spinal cord or brain, with a long thread-like extension, a *nerve fibre*, leading to a muscle. There is a small gap between the end of the nerve fibre and its subordinate *muscle fibres*, which complete the unit. A defect anywhere in the unit has much the same effect: the muscles are inefficient.

Numerous types of myopathy have been described, according to the part of the motor unit that is defective or, less logically, to the groups of muscles that are weak. The rarest types have the longest names.

A muscle without a nerve does not thrive. Myopathy of this type is known as *muscular atrophy*. With congenital types where the original number of nerve cells is defective, the corresponding muscle fibres never develop. Where groups of nerve cells degenerate in adult life (*motor neurone disease*) the affected muscles waste. With different types of muscular atrophy the disability may be anything from trivial to incapacitating. No effective treatment has been found because lost nerve cells do not regenerate.

◊ *Myasthenia gravis* is a defect of transmission across the gap between nerve and muscle.

Muscular dystrophy is apparently a defect of muscle fibres and therefore myopathy in the most literal sense. Muscles waste as though they had lost their nerve supply, but the nerves remain normal. Like muscular atrophy, the condition may be trivial or serious, and no means of cure or prevention has been found.

Myotonia is abnormal tension of resting muscles. It is seldom a serious affliction.

Familial periodic paralysis behaves as the name suggests. The periodic attacks of paralysis are due to inability to keep a constant concentration of potassium in the blood; they are treated by adjusting the intake and output of potassium.

Lastly, some disorders of endocrine glands, especially over-activity of the thyroid, may cause a kind of myopathy, treated by treating the primary disorder.

myopia. Short sight. ◊ *vision.*

myositis. Inflammation of muscle. Bacterial infection is not usual in muscle, but one type – gas gangrene – is extremely dangerous if it does occur. Natives of tropical Africa commonly suffer from large abscesses in muscle (*pyomyositis*) without evidence of infection.

Myositis ossificans is a very uncommon disorder where bony deposits appear in muscle.

Some rheumatic diseases may affect muscles as well as joints, and this can be regarded as a sort of myositis (or fibrositis).

myotonia ◊ *myopathy.*

myringotomy. Surgical perforation of the ear-drum to release pus from the middle ear with *otitis media.*

myxoedema. Coarsening of the skin with other symptoms of failure of the thyroid gland in adult life. ◊ *thyroid* (2).

N

naevus ◊ birth-mark.

nagana. A disease of cattle in tropical Africa, carried by tsetse flies and closely related to human sleeping sickness. ◊ trypanosome.

nail-biting. This very common habit appears to be a symptom of insecurity.

nails. A nail grows from a tuck in the skin. It is composed of keratin like that of the outermost layer of the skin and the hair. The small patch of skin covered by the tuck forms the matrix from which the nail grows. The rest of the nail-bed – under the exposed part of the nail – does not contribute. If the matrix is seriously damaged, the whole nail is lost.

Ill health, especially when there is an element of malnutrition, commonly affects the growth of the nails. Iron deficiency causes softening and concavity of the nails. But the commonest defect – splitting – has no apparent cause.

Small injuries at the side of a finger-nail are easily infected, and the infection may get between the nail and its bed to form a kind of whitlow (paronychia). Acute paronychia is a painful condition, often needing a minor operation to release a bead of pus. If the infection has already spread for any distance part of the nail may have to be removed.

Chronic paronychia is common among housewives, because constant immersion in hot water makes the skin of the finger-tips soggy and vulnerable to mild infection. There is little swelling or pain, but the trouble persists and the nail may become deformed. Antibiotics are used to overcome the infection, but the most effective treatment is keeping the hands dry.

Ringworm of the nails, usually associated with 'athlete's foot', is a minor but tiresome complaint. In the past an affected nail had usually to be removed before the infection could be eradicated, but the antibiotic griseofulvin now provides an effective remedy without surgery.

Psoriasis, a common disease of the skin, often causes small blemishes on the finger-nails.

nalorphine. An antagonist of ◊ morphine.

narcolepsy. A rare disorder: the patient is normal except for fits of uncontrollable sleepiness and sudden waves of muscular weakness. The cause is unknown. Amphetamine and similar drugs generally ward off the attacks.

narcosis. Dulling of consciousness ('a drowsy numbness'); also = anaesthesia.

narcotic. Any drug producing narcosis, especially morphine and similar drugs of addiction.

The word narcotic illustrates the difficulty of classifying drugs. Many drugs conventionally placed in other categories act as narcotics, and their classification depends on the dose. Hemp (cannabis) is a true narcotic, but its devotees take it not so much for this effect as for the mental derangement, including hallucinations, which releases them from reality. Hence this drug is often classified as a hallucinogen, along with other drugs that excite rather than benumb the brain. Hyoscine is an antagonist of the parasympathetic nervous system, like ◊ atropine, but unlike atropine it has a narcotic action that has been used to produce 'twilight sleep', a state of incomplete anaesthesia. All ◊ anaesthetics are narcotic, and in current German usage narcotic and anaesthetic are practically synonymous. To increase the confusion, the term narcotic is sometimes applied to drugs of addiction in general, though some of these have little or no narcotic action.

In this book, narcotic refers to a group of drugs used to relieve pain, that also sedate and, in larger doses, stupefy the patient. Drugs that relieve pain without this narcotic effect are classed as ◊ analgesic.

The prototype of narcotic drugs is ◊ morphine, extracted from opium, and the other members of the group have similar actions to morphine. Codeine, also found in opium, is intermediate between the narcotics and the simple analgesics. Heroin was first synthesized from morphine in the hope that it would be less addictive, but in fact it is even more so.

The numerous synthetic narcotics include *pethidine*, which does not depress respiration as much as morphine, and relieves rather than aggravates colic; *methadone*, sometimes given as an alternative to morphine or heroin as a first step in the treatment of addiction; and *pentazocine*, which is said to be less addictive than some of the others.

All drugs of this class are potentially lethal, and all must be regarded as addictive.

nasolacrimal duct. Passage for drainage of tears into the nose. The eyes water with a cold in the nose or hay fever, when the duct is blocked by swelling of the mucous membrane at its outlet.

nasopharynx. Region behind the nose, above and behind the soft palate. ◊ *pharynx.*

naturopathy. A system of preserving health by means of a simple diet, regular exercise, and the avoidance of drugs or anything that seems artificial. It is based on the principle that natural processes will keep the body in health if they are given a fair chance instead of being constantly thwarted by unnatural foods, customs, and medicines.

Naturopathy has no need to justify itself – that is amply done by the known results of overeating, smoking, lack of exercise and the rest. The difficulty arises from not knowing what is natural. People who think it natural to wear no clothes forget that *Homo sapiens* is a subtropical species that has adapted itself to other climates by having the ingenuity to dress. Other species depend for survival on physical attributes, but man lives by his wits. He avoids starvation by farming – which is systematic interference with Nature – and by cooking and preserving some of his food. Muck-spreading is no more 'natural' than spreading accurately measured chemical fertilizers.

Purists in this cult avoid all drugs or medicines. They miss the chance of curing some eminently curable diseases, but they also avoid dangers such as poisoning their stomachs with aspirin, their kidneys with phenacetin, or their intestines with purgatives. It is harder to justify a belief that some medicines are natural and good,

while others are artificial and bad. All effective medicines are potentially dangerous, and in fact the chemists have yet to produce anything as lethal as the 'natural' poisons of some medicinal plants. All chemicals must be made from naturally occurring raw materials, and many synthetic drugs are only slight modifications of substances found in living matter. Cinchona bark is a natural remedy for malaria. It has the disadvantage that different samples contain different amounts of the active principle, quinine. Therefore quinine, unnaturally extracted from cinchona, is a better drug: the dose can be measured exactly. Even refined quinine is neither as safe nor as effective as the newer synthetic drugs of the same chemical family. The raw material is coal tar. But coal tar is itself derived from plants; it is as natural as cinchona bark.

To object, as the strictest naturopaths do, to all medicines, and even to food grown with the aid of artificial fertilizers, is to deprive man of the one thing that has enabled him to survive – his ability to devise methods of adapting his environment to his needs, which he has evolved while other creatures have wings or claws or long legs as their means of survival. But only fools would argue with naturopaths about walking rather than driving, and moderation in diet, and escaping from large towns whenever possible, and eating fresh vegetables rather than slimming pills.

nausea. Sensation of being about to vomit; either an inborn ◊ *reflex* from irritation of the vagus nerves in the stomach, or a conditioned reflex from stimulation of the same nervous pathways, e.g. by disgusting sights or smells, when a sort of overspill of nervous activity triggers off impulses in the brain that are usually associated with over-activity of the stomach muscle.

navel = ◊ *umbilicus.*

necator. A kind of hookworm. ◊ *worms.*

neck. The core of the neck is the column of 7 *cervical vertebrae* encased by a complex system of muscles which move the vertebrae or maintain their posture. The neck serves to direct the main sensory organs and weapons without the need for cumbersome movements of the whole body. Man lives more by his hands than by his ears, nose, and teeth, and in this sense has less use for a neck than other animals. On the other hand his highly developed, stereoscopic vision requires a mobile neck, as anyone knows who has tried to play tennis with a stiff neck.

In an early human embryo only the mouth separates the head from the heart. At about 3 weeks a set of gills begins to appear in the mouth region, pushing the head and heart further apart. Most of the face and neck, and also the lungs, arise from these gills. The heart and lungs migrate to the ◊ *thorax*, dragging with them the various structures still joining them to the head and neck. Thus there are two groups of organs in the front of the neck: structures in transit to the thorax, and structures properly belonging to the neck.

1. STRUCTURES IN TRANSIT

In the mid-line the ◊ *pharynx* lies immediately in front of the vertebrae. It is the continuation of both nose and mouth, and starts as a channel common to breathing and eating. At the level of the Adam's apple the air-passage becomes separated from the digestive tube as the ◊ *larynx*. The pharynx continues downwards behind the larynx; here it is concerned only with swallowing, and the larynx with breathing and speaking. Below the thyroid cartilage the pharynx continues as the ◊ *oesophagus* – still lying on the vertebral column – and the larynx as the ◊ *trachea*.

At either side of the pharynx, mostly under cover of the sternomastoid muscle, the ◊ *carotid artery* runs up to the head with the internal ◊ *jugular vein* beside it. The ◊ *vagus* nerve accompanies the artery, and the ◊ *sympathetic* nerve chain runs behind, on the transverse processes of the vertebrae.

Spinal nerves emerging from the sides of the vertebrae between the muscles of the neck are distributed to the neck itself and to the upper limbs (◊ *brachial* plexus).

Since the ◊ *diaphragm* first arises in this region and migrates with the heart to the thorax, it derives its nerve from the neck.

The vertebral column protects the ◊ *spinal cord* and the two *vertebral arteries*, which share the supply of the brain with the internal carotid arteries.

2. LOCAL STRUCTURES

The salivary glands (◊ *saliva*) at the rim of the lower jaw are on the boundary of neck and face. The ◊ *thyroid* gland is at the front and sides of the larynx and trachea. The 4 ◊ *parathyroid* glands are behind the thyroid gland.

Lymph nodes are widely distributed in the neck. One chain encircles the neck from nape to chin; another runs down alongside the internal jugular vein.

3. DISORDERS

With so many vital structures at risk, *injuries* are obviously more serious than in most parts of the body. Fractures and dislocations (◊ *vertebrae*) may cause paralysis or, if the uppermost part of the spinal cord is torn, death. The fractures are not in themselves important; what matters is the extent to which the cord is involved.

The neck is crowded, and *swellings*, whether from bleeding, inflammation, or tumours, may interfere with swallowing or breathing.

The *gills* disappear long before birth, leaving only the structures derived from them (e.g. jaws, tongue, thyroid, parathyroids, ear, larynx). But occasionally a gill remains, either as a cyst or as an opening at the side of the neck. These anomalies can be corrected surgically. *Torticollis* (wryneck) may be due to injury of a sternomastoid muscle at birth.

Other disorders are discussed under the names of the various structures.

necropsy. Postmortem examination.

necrosis. Death of some portion of an organ, e.g. from damage to its blood supply or poisoning by bacteria.

Neisseria. A genus of bacteria, including those of cerebrospinal fever and of gonorrhoea. They are fragile organisms, difficult to grow in the laboratory, and unable to survive long in the open air.

nematode. Roundworm. ◊ *worms*.

neoarsphenamine. A compound of arsenic used for treating syphilis, introduced by Ehrlich as an improvement on his earlier discovery arsphenamine (606; salvarsan).

neomycin. An antibiotic extracted from the

fungus *Streptomyces fradiae*. Since it is rather toxic it is seldom injected, but only an insignificant amount is assimilated if it is taken by mouth and it can therefore be used against intestinal infection. It is most used in ointments and creams for the skin.

neonatal. Of new-born babies, conventionally limited to the first 4 weeks of life.

neoplasm. New growth; a useless proliferation of tissue (= ◊ *tumour*).

nephrectomy. Removal of one kidney. Provided that the other kidney is healthy, the operation does not cause disability; a single kidney has enough functional reserve to take on the work of two.

nephritis. Inflammation of the kidneys. The two kidneys have a rich supply of blood, from which a watery fluid is rapidly filtered off by the *glomeruli*. From the glomeruli the filtrate passes into the *tubules*, where most of the water is returned to the blood together with useful substances such as glucose. This leaves a concentrated solution of unwanted waste products, the *urine*. Urine flows into a receptacle at the outlet of the kidney, the *renal pelvis*, down a long tube, the *ureter*, and into the *bladder* where it is stored until it can be passed.

Inflammation is the normal response to bacterial infection. Bacteria can reach the kidney by way of the ureters from the bladder; then the first part of the kidney to become inflamed is its pelvis (◊ *pyelitis*), and the inflammation resulting from spread to the kidney proper is called *pyelonephritis*. Or bacterial infection such as tuberculosis may be carried to the kidneys by the blood-stream.

Poisons affecting the kidneys begin by attacking the tubules, because the tubules concentrate waste matter to be eliminated in the urine, and so poisons may reach dangerous concentrations in them. The changes represent degeneration rather than inflammation, and this type of disorder is loosely called *nephrosis*, which means no more than an affection of the kidney. Nephrosis can be due to bacterial poisons from elsewhere in the body (e.g. typhoid fever, pneumonia), to chemical poisons, including certain drugs, and to severe injuries to any part of the body (here, failure of the circulation of blood is an important factor but probably not the only one). The tubules are

often completely restored if the patient can be tided over a period when his kidneys are not working (◊ *kidneys* (5)).

Unfortunately, *nephrosis* also applies to a type of Bright's disease (see below) with gross waterlogging of the tissues.

A kind of inflammation due neither to bacterial infection nor to any recognized poison starts in the glomeruli (*glomerulonephritis*). The natural history of this condition can take several courses, and it is probably a group of diseases, some better understood than others.

Acute glomerulonephritis starts suddenly with fever, and leakage of protein and blood cells from the inflamed glomeruli into the urine. Because the volume of urine formed is reduced, excess water and salt are retained in the blood and leak into the tissues, often causing visible swelling under the skin (e.g. puffiness about the eyes). As with many other kidney diseases, the blood pressure may rise. The attack usually lasts a couple of weeks but may last much longer. The great majority of patients recover completely. A few develop the chronic form of the disease (see below). Rarely, a patient may die of the acute attack; this has become much less likely since the invention of artificial kidneys (◊ *kidneys* (5)). Although bacteria cannot be directly incriminated, nearly all cases follow an infection with streptococci such as scarlet fever or tonsillitis. Acute nephritis appears to be related in the same way as rheumatic fever to streptococcal infection. The type of inflammation suggests a kind of allergy. It may be that the streptococci produce something which alters a protein in the kidneys, and that the altered protein is then treated as a 'foreign' substance and destroyed by the body's defences, or that antibodies formed to destroy certain streptococci are also harmful to the kidneys (◊ *immunity*).

Chronic glomerulonephritis is a slow, insidious process of deterioration of the kidneys – so slow that the patient may well die of other natural causes before the kidneys fail. Sometimes it begins with an attack of the acute illness described above, which subsides, but not completely. Or it may begin with heavy loss of protein in the urine and gross accumulation of water (*oedema*) in various parts of the body – this is the condition sometimes described as nephrosis but more often as 'nephrotic syndrome'. Or there may be no symptoms at all for months or years, except abnormalities of the urine found by routine examination. These various beginnings all lead to the same condition – Bright's disease – with leakage of protein, some (but seldom much) oedema, inability to concentrate or dilute the urine as needed, and often high blood pressure. A very similar condition is a *result* of high blood pressure. The cause of chronic nephritis is unknown, apart from the association with streptococci of the cases which begin as acute nephritis. ◊ *Auto-immunity* has been suggested, but nothing has yet been proved.

Since the cause is unknown, no completely rational treatment of chronic nephritis is possible; the various symptoms have to be treated as they arise and on their own merits. In fact, much can be done to adapt the patient to living with defective kidneys (◊ *kidneys* (5)), although in the long run the disease is still not curable.

nephroblastoma (Wilms' tumour). Cancer of the kidney in infancy. ◊ *kidneys* (4).

nephrolithiasis. Stone in the kidney; renal ◊ *calculus.*

nephrosis. Any disease of the kidney with *oedema* (dropsy, retention of water in the body) as the main symptom. The term *nephrotic syndrome* is more usual, because it implies that the condition is a symptom of something else and not a definite disease.

Nephrosis is commonly a phase in the evolution of ◊ *nephritis* (Bright's disease). It can also occur as a complication of diabetes and other generalized diseases, as a result of damage to small blood vessels.

nerve. A nerve is a bundle of conducting fibres, a cable. Motor fibres conduct impulses *from*, sensory fibres *to* the brain or spinal cord. Nearly all nerves include both kinds.

Twelve pairs of ◊ *cranial nerves* arise from the brain and pass through the skull, and 31 pairs of ◊ *spinal nerves* arise from the spinal cord and pass between the vertebrae. All other nerves are branches of these; some are formed from the union of several branches.

The conducting fibres are projections (axons) of cells in the brain or cord. A nerve fibre in the foot is part of a cell which has its nucleus at the level of the lowest ribs. Since lost nerve cells cannot be replaced, and nerves are easily injured, it is well that

the vital part of the cell is out of harm's way.

Each fibre is enclosed in an insulating tube of myelin, an arrangement like a telephone cable. If a nerve is injured these tubes must first heal before the conducting fibres can be restored. With a crushing injury the tubes may still be intact although the fibres within are broken, in which case healing is no problem. New fibres can grow down the tubes from the nerve cells. This regeneration may take many weeks but it is likely to be complete. When a nerve is cut the ends can be sewn together and will heal, but the thousands of fibres cannot all be expected to grow down the right tubes. A fibre from a motor nerve cell which grows down a tube leading to a sensory organ in the skin cannot function. Thus even after prompt and careful surgery a cut nerve seldom recovers completely, but with luck the results can be surprisingly good. The brain seems to learn to interpret signals arriving by new paths.

Nerve fibres within the brain and spinal cord are equipped with a simpler kind of myelin sheath which is not restored when it has been cut, and here injured fibres do not recover.

Conduction in nerves can be interrupted in several ways. Cold, lack of oxygen, pressure, and local anaesthetic drugs all block nerves. They are effective wherever along the course of the nerve they are applied. A local anaesthetic may be injected at the root of the neck to paralyse the nerves of the hand during an operation, and the pressure of a bone or tendon in the same region may cause numbness of the fingers.

◊ *nervous system; neuralgia; neuropathy.*

nervous system.

1. CENTRAL NERVOUS SYSTEM

Even the simplest animal – a protozoon made of a single cell – responds to a stimulus by withdrawing itself. In more advanced creatures some of the cells in the outer layer of the body are adapted to receive stimuli and transmit them to other cells adapted for movement. Cells that transmit impulses to other cells are called nerve cells or *neurones*. In all higher animals the neurones are gathered together to form an anatomical unit, the *nervous system*, derived entirely from the outermost layer of the embryo (*ectoderm*), which also forms the outer coat of the skin.

In the embryo of a vertebrate (such as man) the future neurones are gathered in the mid-line of the surface of the back. This strip, running the length of the embryo, is first depressed to form a groove and then submerged, as the tissues of the back close over it, to form a tube. Later this *neural tube* is surrounded by the skull and vertebrae, to form the ◊ *brain* and ◊ *spinal cord*, together making the *central nervous system*.

A neurone consists of a cell-body with several thread-like projections or *processes*. There are generally several branched processes, *dendrites*, and a single long process, the *axon*, which is the main conducting fibre. An axon may be very long – extending, for instance, from a cell-body in the spinal cord at the small of the back to a muscle in the foot. Similarly, sensory processes extend from the periphery to their parent cells in the nerve roots (◊ *spinal nerves*). The nerves of the body are simply bundles of conducting fibres, each with its parent cell in the central nervous system. Each fibre has a coat of *myelin*, a fatty insulating substance. The myelin sheath accelerates conduction and is essential to repair if the fibre is damaged. Fibres within the central nervous system have rudimentary myelin sheaths and no power of healing (◊ *nerve*).

Twelve pairs of ◊ *cranial nerves* spring from the under-surface of the brain and 31 pairs of ◊ *spinal nerves* from the spinal cord. Their parent cells are only the outer links of complex chains of neurones within the central nervous system. A group of muscle cells is activated by a single motor neurone in the spinal cord, but this neurone may receive impulses through its dendrites from hundreds of other neurones, of which some stimulate and others inhibit. Only a few of these, in the upper part of the brain, are involved in conscious activity or sensation. The rest operate ◊ *reflex* actions.

Herophilus (Alexandria, 3rd century B.C.) recognized that nerves had to do with sensation and movement, and he described the brain in some detail. His contemporary Erasistratus taught that the nerves were hollow and acted by transmitting vital spirit, a belief that was not seriously challenged until late in the Renaissance. Vital spirit flowed through nerves into the muscles and caused them to swell and shorten. Two thousand years later Descartes was expounding the same theory – he even described and drew valves within the 'hollow' of the nerves. Swammerdam dis-

proved the theory in the 17th century, but his work was not published until 1737. The first modern account of the nervous system was by Albrecht von Haller in 1766. Having shown the tendency of muscle fibres to contract in response to stimuli, Haller proved that some nerve fibres carried impulses from the central nervous system which stimulated the muscles, while others carried sensory impulses to the brain. Although the idea that nerves might be sensory or motor was very ancient – it was put forward by Herophilus and elaborated by Galen (2nd century A.D.) – sensation as a property of the brain and not of the organ stimulated was a revolutionary concept. A pricked finger does not feel pain; it only transmits an impulse along a nerve to be interpreted in the brain.

The nervous system functions largely by ◊ *reflex* action. Descartes was the first to suggest this. It was a lucky guess with no shred of evidence behind it. Descartes was concerned not with the workings of the body but with the human soul. Having denied the existence of a soul in animals he had to postulate something like reflex action to explain animal behaviour. Descartes's theory was confirmed by the experiments of Hales, published in 1761, showing that the withdrawal of a limb when the skin was pricked was determined by the spinal cord. Marshall Hall (1833) described spinal reflexes and their modification by impulses from the brain. The current view of the nervous system as an integrated whole is largely due to Sherrington's work around the turn of this century.

Johannes Müller's discovery (*c.* 1830) that a given nerve fibre, however stimulated, can produce only one kind of effect was the first step towards understanding the nature of nervous impulses, though it now appears that there are exceptions to Müller's rule. In 1852 Helmholtz recorded the speed of conduction in a nerve. Later knowledge is due largely to Lucas, Sherrington, Dale, Adrian, Hodgkin, and Huxley in England, and to Erlanger and Gasser in America. Excepting Lucas, all these physiologists have been awarded Nobel Prizes.

2. Autonomic Nervous System

In all vertebrates a special system of nerves regulates the organs of blood-circulation, respiration, digestion, excretion, and reproduction. Since its activity is wholly reflex and appears to be independent of the brain it was named the autonomic system by J. N. Langley (Cambridge, 1898). Functionally the system is in two parts: the ◊ *sympathetic* system, arising from the thoracic and upper lumbar spinal nerves, and the ◊ *parasympathetic* system from certain cranial nerves, of which the most important is the ◊ *vagus*, and from the sacral nerves. The autonomic motor nerve cells are in groups or *ganglia* outside the central nervous system. The sympathetic ganglia form a chain at either side of the backbone, and the parasympathetic ganglia are actually on the organs supplied.

When the neural tube is formed in the embryo (see above) some of the developing neurones are stranded between the tube and the back of the embryo. They form the *neural crest*. These neurones migrate, some to become the autonomic nerves and the medulla of the ◊ *adrenal* gland (which is a modified sympathetic ganglion) and others to the sensory ganglia of the spinal nerves.

Despite appearances the workings of the autonomic and central nervous systems are intimately related. Autonomic activity is determined partly by the ◊ *vital centres* in the brain-stem and partly by centres in the floor of the forebrain which are also concerned with emotion – the outward signs of emotional changes such as blushing, pallor, sweating, palpitation, are autonomic reflexes.

Galen described the vagus nerve as part of a single nerve comprising the 9th, 10th (vagus) and 11th cranial nerves. The error is to his credit because it proves that he had studied the matter: the three nerves are quite distinct in the neck, but if they are traced back to their origin in the brain-stem they are seen to be intimately related. Galen also gave some account of the sympathetic nerves and their ganglia, but the first accurate description of this system was by Eustachius in the 16th century. Numerous physiologists, notably Claude Bernard, studied the autonomic system during the 19th century; the first to recognize it as a co-ordinated system was W. H. Gaskell of Cambridge, who named it the *involuntary nervous system*. More recent studies have been mainly concerned with the connections of the system in the ◊ *brain*, where autonomic and central nervous systems are no longer distinct.

3. THE NERVOUS IMPULSE

A living nerve fibre at rest is electrically charged. The potential difference between the inside and outside of the fibre is about 80 millivolts. It depends on the different concentrations of potassium inside and outside: the ratio is about 30:1. The two elements potassium and sodium are more or less interchangeable in a dead structure. If a nerve fibre were inert, both would diffuse freely until their concentrations were the same inside and out. But the living fibre actively rejects sodium by some unknown mechanism (the 'sodium pump'). The chemical stability of the cell requires one or other element – which one does not matter – and since sodium is lacking, potassium is retained and with it an electric potential.

If the electric potential is lost the nerve is said to be *depolarized*. This happens if the lining membrane becomes freely permeable: sodium then enters and the surplus of potassium is released. A nerve impulse is simply a wave of depolarization, started by various kinds of stimulus, e.g. an electric current, heat, pressure, or certain chemicals. Once the process has begun, the depolarization of any part of a neurone is a sufficient stimulus to depolarize the next segment. Thus the impulse travels to the end of the nerve fibre. This is quite different from ordinary electrical conduction, and much slower. The thickest fibres conduct at a rate of 100 metres per second, and some very slow fibres at only about 1 metre per second. This is easily demonstrated because pain is conveyed in fast and slow fibres. A mildly painful stimulus such as a pinprick or touching a hot kettle causes an immediate rather indefinite sensation, followed a second or so later by a slowly conducted but precise sense of pain.

When the impulse reaches the end of the fibre it has to be passed to the next nerve cell (for all activities depend on more than one neurone) or to an effector organ such as a muscle (◊ *reflex*). This is done by releasing a *chemical transmitter* from the nerve-ending. The gap between a nerve-ending and its target is a *synapse*. Some chemical transmitters are known. Muscle fibres and most autonomic nerve cells respond to *acetyl choline*. Sympathetic nerve-endings usually release *noradrenaline*. Within the central nervous system there are certainly other transmitters as well as these. *Serotonin* appears to be one. And since there are inhibitory nerves there are presumably inhibitory transmitters. None is definitely known, but gamma-amino-butyric acid (GABA) has been suggested.

Two kinds of mechanism control bodily functions: nervous activity, and chemical activity by *hormones* released from glands such as the pituitary and thyroid. The distinction is convenient, but less clear-cut than it appears to be, for the function of a nerve is to release a chemical transmitter when it is stimulated. The difference between a nerve and a gland is that a nerve releases its chemical transmitter at a given point, where it is destroyed as soon as it has acted, whereas a gland releases its transmitter into the blood-stream to act throughout the body. The adrenal medulla is a collection of sympathetic nerve cells behaving as a gland; it releases adrenaline into the blood-stream to activate other sympathetic nerves in distant organs.

A nerve cell returns to its resting state almost immediately after transmitting an impulse. Within one or two milliseconds its charge is restored and ready to be fired again. The process can be repeated indefinitely. Waking or sleeping, the nervous system is constantly active throughout life. No fresh cells, it seems, are formed after birth. The original stock serves for a lifetime, and the cells that wear out and die are not replaced.

4. SUPPORTING STRUCTURES

The central nervous system is protected by the skull and backbone and their lining membranes, the ◊ *meninges*, which enclose the ◊ *cerebrospinal fluid*. The fluid acts as a shock-absorber.

A neurone is the most helpless of living cells. It is like the legendary genius, pre-eminent in his chosen specialty but incapable of looking after himself. A neurone keeps no stores. If it is deprived of blood, and so of glucose and oxygen, for more than a few seconds it dies. If the blood stops flowing, the stagnant blood in the vessels carries enough supplies to keep nerve cells alive for a few minutes.

There is no ordinary connective tissue in the nervous system. Instead the neurones are supported by a network of spidery cells, the *neuroglia*, which appears to do for them most of the routine chemical work that less delicate cells in other tissues do for themselves.

Nerve fibres are insulated with a layer of myelin. In the actual nerves, outside the brain and spinal cord, the myelin is formed by *Schwann cells*, which wrap each fibre in layer upon layer of myelin. If a nerve fibre is cut, the Schwann cells can form a new tube into which a new fibre can grow, provided that the cell-body of the neurone is intact. But in the brain and spinal cord the myelin is laid down by the neuroglia, which does not lay down new paths for damaged fibres. Here, then, any damage is permanent.

5. DISORDERS

Localized disorders are discussed elsewhere (◊ *brain; spinal cord; nerve*). ◊ *Mental illnesses* are presumably disturbances of the brain (a few are known to be), but this is open to dispute because nobody can say where or what the mind is.

Disease of the nervous system is usually disease of its supporting structures. Since nerve cells cannot divide they cannot form tumours. Apart from the tumours of embryonic nerve cells, occurring very rarely in infancy, tumours of nervous tissue arise from the neuroglia.

Diseases as different as syphilis, arteriosclerosis, and diabetes affect the nervous system by injuring its small blood vessels (diabetes probably has other effects as well).

If the myelin sheaths are damaged conduction is impaired. Many disorders are of this kind, including damage to nervous tissue by diphtheria, alcohol, and multiple sclerosis. The actual nerve cells remain healthy, but they are ineffective unless the myelin recovers.

All parts of a neurone are vulnerable to pressure. Even slight pressure on a nerve disturbs sensation and causes tingling or 'pins and needles', and if the pressure continues the fibres cease to conduct – everyone has experienced numbness in a limb after sitting awkwardly. Nerve fibres recover when the pressure is relieved, but the cell-bodies in the central nervous system can be killed by pressure. Normally the cerebrospinal fluid is kept at a constant pressure, but a part of the brain or spinal cord may be compressed by bleeding, abscess, tumour, or fractured bone. If the compression is not relieved there is liable to be permanent damage.

neuralgia. *Neuralgia, neuritis,* and *neuropathy* have become almost synonymous, though they should mean different things. All refer to affections of *peripheral nerves.*

Neuritis is inflammation of a nerve.

Neuropathy means any disorder of a nerve, or perhaps any disorder other than inflammation. *Neuralgia* is a pain originating in a nerve. For instance, the pain of sciatica, arising in the roots of the sciatic nerve, is neuralgic, but the pain of a decaying tooth, which is merely conducted by a nerve, is not.

Trigeminal neuralgia, or *tic douloureux*, is a severe pain on one side of the face, in an area corresponding with a branch of the trigeminal (5th cranial) nerve. A typical attack is severe for a minute or so, but it is soon over and the patient is completely well until the next attack, which may not be for several weeks. In more advanced cases attacks become more frequent, and adequate treatment is imperative.

Trigeminal neuralgia is permanently cured by cutting the nerve near its origin. This is a drastic remedy, but a priceless refuge if milder treatment should fail. An injection of alcohol into the nerve usually stops the symptoms for a year or more. Some cases are cured by an operation to allow more room for the nerve as it passes through the floor of the skull. Such methods as these have been necessary because the usual pain-killing drugs have so little effect, but a new drug, *carbamazepine*, has a curious affinity for the trigeminal nerve, and often relieves the symptoms.

neurasthenia. A kind of neurosis, with tiredness as the main symptom; also a convenient label for lassitude not due to anaemia, infection, malnutrition or other recognized disease.

neuritis. Inflammation of a nerve (mononeuritis) or several nerves (polyneuritis). Most of the conditions called neuritis do not involve inflammation, and are better classified as ◊ *neuropathy* (◊ *neuralgia*). True inflammation can be due to infection by viruses (e.g. herpes) or bacteria (e.g. leprosy), but often the cause is obscure.

neurodermatitis. Atopic ◊ *dermatitis*; atopic eczema.

neurofibromatosis (von Recklinghausen's disease). A rare hereditary disorder, with fibrous swellings of nerves and dark blotches on the skin.

neuroglia. The connective tissue of the ◊ *nervous system*.

neurology. Study of the nervous system and its disorders.

neuroma. Tumour of nerve tissue. A mature nerve cell, unlike most other cells in the body, cannot reproduce itself. A rare kind of neuroma is made of embryonic nerve cells; most tumours of the nervous system arise from the *neuroglia*, the connective tissue that supports the active nerve cells.

neurone (neuron). A nerve cell with its conducting fibres. ◊ *nervous system*.

neuropathy. Any disorder of peripheral nerves (cf. ◊ *neuralgia*), especially one without inflammation. The symptoms of disturbed function are much the same whatever the cause: tingling, numbness, sometimes pain, muscular weakness, sometimes poor condition of the skin (from deficient regulation of its blood vessels), all in the area to which the affected nerve is destined. The commonest cause is *pressure*, which impairs conduction; e.g. ◊ *carpal tunnel* syndrome and 'slipped disc' (◊ *vertebra* (1)). Other common causes include diabetes, disorders of the circulation (both, probably, by decreasing the supply of blood to nerves), and numerous poisons including lead and other metals and some drugs. Lack of vitamins, especially of B_{12} (pernicious anaemia), niacin (pellagra) and B_1 (beri-beri), can cause severe neuropathies, advancing to paralysis of the affected regions if they are untreated. Vitamin B deficiency is the immediate cause of neuropathy with chronic alcoholism.

neurosis. A large and ill-defined group of mental disturbances, merging on the one hand with normality and on the other with real derangement of the mind. Probably no boundary can be drawn between normality and neurosis: one man's due regard for detail is another man's obsession. There is a clearer distinction between neurosis and derangement (psychosis): the neurotic is all too aware that something is wrong, and the psychotic is not; and the neurotic's reason is not impaired.
 ◊ *anxiety*; *mental illness*.

neutrophil. The most numerous of the white blood-cells. ◊ *blood* (3).

niacin; nicotinamide ◊ *vitamin B*.

nicotine. An alkaloid in tobacco. Small doses stimulate nerve-endings in the sympathetic and parasympathetic systems, with reflex effects such as constriction of blood vessels, nausea or vomiting, alteration of the heart beat. With novices to smoking, parasympathetic reflexes (slow pulse, faintness, nausea) often predominate; with habitual smokers, sympathetic reflexes (quick pulse, raised blood pressure, impaired appetite and digestion). Larger doses suppress these reflexes and then cause convulsions, paralysis, and death.

The worst effects of smoking are due to tobacco tar. Nicotine accounts for the headache, and probably for the liability of smokers to diseases of the arteries. Above all, it is nicotine that causes the dependence on tobacco that causes sane people to smoke although they fully understand the risks (◊ *tobacco*).

nikethamide. A drug used to stimulate the vital centres in the brain in certain states of collapse. Its main effect is on breathing.

nipple ◊ *breast.*

nit. A louse's egg, firmly adherent to the hair or clothing of an infested person.

nitrite. A salt of nitrous acid (HNO_2). Nitrites are used medicinally to dilate small arteries, e.g. in treating ◊ *angina*. Some compounds that are not strictly nitrites but have the same effect, such as glyceryl trinitrate (nitroglycerin), are included in the group. Although these drugs have been given for many years to dilate narrowed coronary arteries they probably work by relaxing other arteries, lowering the pressure and taking the load off the overworked heart muscle.

nitrogen. The principal component of air; an essential element in all living matter. No animal can use the pure nitrogen of the air, but bacteria in the soil and in certain plants synthesize nitrogen compounds that other creatures can assimilate. By far the most important nitrogen compounds are the *proteins*, the basic stuff of a living organism. Nearly all the nitrogen of the diet is in animal or vegetable proteins, which are broken down by digestion to *amino-acids* and then resynthesized. Waste nitrogen in the body is excreted by the kidneys, mainly as *urea.*

nitrous oxide (laughing gas). N_2O; the first general anaesthetic and still one of the most useful. ◊ *anaesthetics* (2).

noma. *Cancrum oris*; a dangerous infection of the mouth leading to gangrene, usually a complication of some other illness in severely under-nourished children. It was often fatal until the discovery of antibiotics. These drugs generally cure the disease rapidly, but there is nearly always severe malnutrition to be treated at the same time. Noma is still common in the poorer parts of the tropics.

noradrenaline. Arterenol; nor-epinephrine ◊ *adrenaline.*

normal. Since medical practice aims to prevent or correct departures from normal functioning of the body we should be able to recognize normal people when we see them. We cannot in fact do so with any confidence, and common sense may be as good a guide as science.

For many purposes, normal means average. A normal man weighs 70 kg., has 5 litres of blood and a body temperature of 37°, and an intelligence quotient of 100. His blood contains 0·1 per cent of glucose, and his kidneys produce 1·5 litres of urine every 24 hours. Figures such as these are needed whenever one has to generalize, but nobody supposes that they are anything more than typical values. Absolute values belong to physics, not biology. Nearly all biological measurements follow a Gaussian or normal distribution, i.e. most individuals are clustered around the average value for the whole population, and the further one gets from the average, the fewer individuals one finds. Thus most healthy adult men are found to weigh, say, between 60 and 80 kg.; some weigh as little as 55 and some as much as 85; and a few are outside these limits. None of them is necessarily abnormal. If a man is seven feet tall *and* has a pituitary tumour to explain his unusual size, then his height is truly abnormal. But if he has no tumour and no sign of illness then his height can only be called unusual.

But the average can be misleading. For many years medical students learnt that normal women had less haemoglobin in 100 c.c. of blood than normal men – about 13·5 grammes against nearly 16. It now seems that so many women are anaemic that the average is depressed. If iron lost by excessive bleeding is replaced there is little difference between the sexes. When the amount has been brought up to a maximum between 15 and 16 grammes iron does no further good. This, then, is apparently the ideal value, and it is a more realistic normal than the average. Similarly, a peasant in a poor tropical country is average if he has malaria, worms, and malnutrition, but it will be a bad day for humanity if he is counted as normal.

This kind of thing leads to very serious difficulties. In Western society it is widely considered normal to have a smoker's cough, to put on weight in middle age, or to need aspirin. Medical diagnosis is confused because normal values are not the same for everyone. Among healthy people, blood pressure may vary by as much as 20 per cent either side of the average for the population, and it may be impossible to say whether a rather high pressure is at the upper limit of the normal range or the lower limit of hypertension, i.e. of disease. In this as in many other cases (e.g. the instance of the very tall man) normal and abnormal are not set figures but ranges of values, and they may overlap. This, of course, is one of the great advantages of the family doctor over the consultant: the family doctor may know what the patient's blood pressure was a couple of years ago, and an increase is much more significant than today's high reading.

More than anything else it is the uncertainty about what is normal that makes medicine a very inexact science and sets experience at such a premium. Even such apparently precise investigations as X-ray films and blood chemistry have to be judged and often their interpretation is open to argument. If it were not so, there would be little need of specialists, and doctors could be trained in half the time. We are still with Hippocrates in 400 B.C.: 'Life is short, and the Art is long; the occasion fleeting; experience fallacious, and judgement difficult'.

nose. The projection on the front of the face is only a small part of the nose. That the human nose projects at all does not mean that it is important but that the upper jaw has receded in the course of evolution.

The bridge of the outer nose, between the eyes, is supported by the nasal bones. The cavity, extending to the back of the hard palate, is completely divided into left and right halves by the nasal *septum*. This is a thin sheet of bone behind and of cartilage in front. The cartilaginous septum supports the outer nose below the nasal bones.

At the back of the hard palate the two halves of the nose open into a single cavity, the nasal part of the ♢ *pharynx*. At each side the *maxilla* forms the wall of the nose; the floor is the *palate*, and the roof is the base of the skull. Three small flaps of bone, each with its lower edge curled under, protrude from the side-wall into the cavity of the nose. These *conchae* (turbinate bones) increase the surface area of the cavity, and shield the openings of the sinuses.

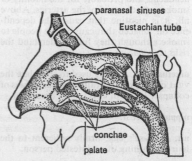

Side wall of the nose. The conchae are partly removed.

The bones surrounding the nose are hollow. Their cavities, the (paranasal) *sinuses*, communicate with the nose by small openings in the side-wall. Two other openings are important: that of the *nasolacrimal duct*, by which tears flow down (hence blowing the nose to get rid of a foreign body in the eye), and the *Eustachian tube*, connecting the middle ear with the pharynx immediately behind the nose proper.

The mucous membrane of the nose also lines the various extensions of the nasal cavity. It is a lax membrane, easily distended by blood and tissue fluid; when inflamed by infection (e.g. common cold) or allergy (e.g. hay fever) it can quickly swell until the nose is blocked. In health it is kept moist by mucus, secreted by its many tiny glands. Its surface is covered with *cilia*, microscopic hair-like structures which undulate and keep the mucus moving towards the back of the nose. When the membrane is inflamed the cilia can no longer cope with the excess of mucus which is formed, and in any case the sinuses could not be cleared because their openings are blocked by the swollen membranes. This gives a simple mechanical explanation of the watering eyes, headache, faceache, and earache which may accompany a severe cold in the nose. This stagnation brings a risk of more serious infection of the sinuses or ear (◊ *sinusitis; ◊ otitis*).

The nose warms and moistens the inhaled air. Even on a cold day the air is saturated with water and within a few degrees of body temperature when it reaches the trachea. To some extent the nose also acts as an air-filter. The sense of smell is discussed in section 2 below.

1. DISORDERS

The commonest disorders – common cold, hay fever, and sinusitis – have been mentioned and are further discussed under their own headings.

Inflammation of the nasal mucous membrane, of which the common cold and hay fever are acute instances, is called *rhinitis*. Chronic rhinitis, with a more or less permanently running nose, is usually associated with a stagnant focus of infection: sinusitis, a polyp, or, in children, tonsillitis with swollen adenoids. A nasal polyp is a soft, round protusion from the mucous membrane, looking rather like a pearl. It is a result of inflammation which then keeps the inflammation going. A large one may completely block its side of the nose. The removal of nasal polyps is a simple and satisfactory operation. Less often, rhinitis may be dry or *atrophic*. The mucous membrane is then shrunken and does not secrete enough mucus; the patient is troubled by dry crusts which collect in the nostrils. Such patients are often subject to hay fever.

Nose-bleed (epistaxis) may be caused by an obvious injury or by an utterly trivial injury to an exposed vessel weakened by past inflammation. It is a common symptom of many fevers, including the fevers of childhood and typhoid. Sometimes it is due to high blood pressure or to disorders of the blood. The bleeding vessel is most often near the front of the septum, just inside the nostril, and the bleeding can be stopped by pinching the nose for a few minutes. In most cases, of course, the bleeding stops on its own; but a nose-bleed has to be treated with some respect. If it continues,

the loss of blood can be serious. Skilful packing of the nose with gauze will stop almost any bleeding, but unskilful attempts are more likely to make matters worse.

A broken nose is a common sporting injury. The fragments are replaced by gentle leverage through the nostril, under local or general anaesthesia.

The shape of a nose can be changed by plastic surgery, approaching the supporting cartilage and bone through a nostril. New bone can be grafted in, or excessive bone or cartilage removed. This kind of operation can greatly improve the appearance after serious accidents. In countries where leprosy is common a cured leper may be rejected by the community because his collapsed nose marks him out. Many such patients have been made acceptable by operations to restore the lost tissue. This kind of surgery has been practised for centuries in India. In modern times many healthy people have operations to change the shape of the nose.

2. SENSE OF SMELL

The nerve-endings for perceiving smells are confined to a small area at the top of the nasal cavity. The nerves pass through small holes in the ethmoid bone to join the olfactory (1st cranial) nerves. The part of the brain concerned with smell (rhinencephalon) is prominent in lower vertebrates, but in man it is completely overshadowed by recently evolved structures.

Although carried in quite different paths the senses of smell and *taste* are closely related. Taste is a very crude sensation; all subtleties of flavour depend on smell. This is evident when the narrow slit at the top of the nose is obstructed with a cold, and the tongue (which is not really affected) seems to lose most of its sensibility.

The mechanism of smell is unknown, and it is difficult even to suggest a working theory. The nose can distinguish more smells than the ear can distinguish sounds. But all sounds are simply vibrations. They differ only in the rate and the amount of vibration, and it is easy enough to suppose that different nerves respond best to different frequencies. Taste and vision are even simpler. Only four tastes can be distinguished, and colour vision can be explained in terms of only three types of nerve-ending, each responding to a particular range of wave-lengths. But the nerve-endings in the nose, which appear to be all alike, convey thousands of distinct sensations from the stimuli that do not appear to be related as sounds or colours are related. Yet there must be a common factor; one cannot suppose that the nose contains 10,000 different kinds of sensory organ. The size and shape of the incoming molecules seem to affect their odour, and it has been suggested that the character-istic vibrations of molecules are what the sense of smell actually records.

nosology. Nomenclature and classification of diseases (Gk *nosos* = 'disease').

notifiable diseases. In all countries certain diseases have to be reported to the public health authority, in order that preventive measures against spread can be taken, or to provide statistics from which the behaviour of diseases in the community can be studied. The diseases specified are not necessarily the same in all countries or at all times. In Britain, notifiable diseases are reported to the Medical Officer of Health either by the attending doctor or by the head of the family (in practice, nearly always the doctor). The MOH sends a weekly return to the Ministry of Health, and informs the Ministry at once of any-thing as serious as, say, smallpox.
International rules. Six 'formidable' epi-demic diseases are notified to the World Health Organization: *cholera*, *plague*, *relapsing fever*, *smallpox*, *typhus* (not typhoid), and *yellow fever*. Doctors all over the world have to notify these to their national authorities which inform WHO in Geneva by telegram.
National rules. Other infectious diseases are notifiable within a country. In Britain they include the more serious childhood fevers, and tuberculosis, pneumonia, puerperal fever, and infections liable to be carried by food or drinking water, in all some 20 diseases. In the United States about 40 diseases are notifiable in addition to the 6 international ones. In many other countries the lists are much shorter.
Regional and other rules. In many countries state or provincial authorities draw up additional lists in accordance with local conditions. In Britain, a County Council can make any disease temporarily noti-fiable. For instance, if a case of smallpox is reported, chickenpox may be made a notifiable disease while there is a risk of further cases, because mild smallpox could

be mistaken for chickenpox, and notific-ation enables the MOH to have the diag-nosis confirmed.
The Factories Act requires notification to the Ministry of Labour of certain diseases arising from the patient's work, including *anthrax* (also notified to the Ministry of Health) and numerous indus-trial poisons.
Hospitals in Britain inform the Regis-trar-General of all cases of cancer and their progress. This information provides a national register from which the various types of cancer and the effects of treatment can be studied.

notochord. The simplest form of backbone, found in some primitive fish-like creatures; it is a rod of connective tissue to give the muscles purchase. In all vertebrates a notochord appears in the embryo, to be replaced by a vertebral column. Small remnants of the notochord persist in an adult human in the centres of the inter-vertebral discs; ◊ *vertebra* (1); *skeleton* (1).

nucleic acids ◊ *genetics* (1).

nucleoprotein. A compound of a nucleic acid with a protein.

nucleotide. A link in the chain of a nucleic acid molecule, composed of a purine or pyrimidine base, the sugar ribose, and phosphoric acid.

nucleus. The kernel of a living cell; it is composed largely of nucleoprotein, the structure of which determines what proteins the cell can make and thus determines the biological properties of the cell.

nursing. The general care of sick people, as opposed to medical attention to their diseases, was not suddenly invented during the Crimean War. Hippocrates had plenty to say about what is now called nursing, and even when medical practice fell to its lowest ebb in the Middle Ages several religious orders provided and staffed hos-pitals. After the Renaissance new orders were founded especially for the care of the sick and needy. The greatest of these was St Vincent de Paul's order, the Sisters of Charity, founded in Paris in 1634. But the Renaissance coincided with the Reform-ation and in Protestant countries there was nobody to take the place of the monks and nuns, and the care of hospital patients was left to untrained domestic servants.

Even the few nurses that there were – lay or religious – had no special training. The doctors prescribed medicines of which the patients' attendants understood nothing. The first person to act on the principle that spiritual care was not enough was Theodor Fliedner, a German clergyman, who established the world's first school of nursing at Kaiserswerth in 1833. In 1851 Florence Nightingale took a course of training at Kaiserswerth. Three years later she led a team of nurses to the Crimean War and transformed military hospitals from squalid prisons into decent places where the wounded stood a reasonable chance of recovery.

In 1860 Florence Nightingale established at St Thomas's Hospital, London, the school that became the model for schools of nursing everywhere. After three years of properly supervised training and experience, her nurses were entitled to regard themselves as members of a new profession, no longer the well-meaning amateurs of earlier times. In the 20th century, laws have been passed in nearly all countries to regulate the training and registration of nurses.

Nursing was defined in Florence Nightingale's *Notes* (1859):

'I use the word nursing for want of a better. It has been limited to signify little more than the administration of medicines and the application of poultices. It ought to signify the proper use of fresh air, light, warmth, cleanliness, quiet, and the proper selection and administration of diet – all at the least expense of vital power to the patient.'

Even at that time, accurate observation could have been added to the list, and today a nurse has to be skilled in the use of all manner of scientific apparatus for diagnosis and treatment, in addition to the duties that Miss Nightingale laid on her.

nutrition ◊ *diet; digestion; malnutrition.*

nux vomica. The seed of a tropical tree from which the poisonous alkaloid *strychnine* is extracted. It has a long history as a tonic: since large doses cause violent and fatal convulsions, small doses are supposed to stimulate the nervous system in a more modest way. In fact it has no medicinal value.

nystagmus. A reflex scanning movement of the eyes to keep moving objects in view. It can be observed when someone watches the scenery from a moving vehicle. The reflex is partly under control of the balance organ of the middle ear. If co-ordination between this organ and the eyes is disturbed, e.g. by alcohol, disease of the inner ear, work in a cramped position and a poor light (miner's nystagmus), or certain disorders affecting the brain, nystagmus occurs when the eyes should be still. The subject may have the illusion that everything is spinning round him (vertigo), but some people are unaware of their nystagmus. ◊ *ear* (3,ii).

nystatin. An antibiotic from the mould *Streptomyces noursei*, used to treat *thrush*, i.e. infection of mucous membranes with the fungus *Candida*.

O

obesity. Excess of body-fat; it is almost but not quite the same as corpulence or over-weight. It is hard to define without first knowing how much fat is normal for a given person. Professional boxers know within a pound or two how much they should weigh: above their ideal weight they lose speed, and below it they lose strength. Other people can judge their ideal weight from the statistics provided by insurance companies, bearing in mind that the statistics give average values for healthy people, and that the ideal weight for an individual of a given height may differ by as much as 10 per cent from the average.

The ideal weight for a boxer or anyone else is the weight at which his body is most efficient. In an affluent society almost everyone's weight is either correct or too much; only the sick are too thin. According to some estimates almost half the adult population of countries such as Britain and the United States carry too much fat. Even the very poor can be obese, though under-nourished, because a cheap inadequate diet can still be fattening.

The proportion of fat in the body should provide an objective definition of obesity. It should not exceed 25 per cent in men or 30 per cent in women. By this definition it is possible to be too fat without being too heavy in terms of average weight for height – a person with poor muscular development may make up a 'normal' body-weight with fat instead of muscle. The term 'adiposity' has been suggested to distinguish this condition from ordinary obesity. Conversely an athlete may be well over average weight for his height because of large muscles, without any excess of fat.

It is highly significant that most of the statistics of obesity come from insurance companies, which have to bet on probable life-span. The figures amply confirm Hippocrates' aphorism: 'Persons who are naturally very fat are apt to die earlier than those who are slender'. The risks are numerous. Although no disease is confined solely to fat people, many dangerous conditions are far commoner among the fat than the thin. Those related to the excess of *fat* as such include diabetes, gall-stones, and degenerative diseases of the kidneys, heart, and arteries. Those related to excessive *weight* include arthritis from undue strain on joints, hernia, varicose veins, and broken bones. Above all, a slightly defective heart may manage well with a normal body weight but fail if it has to provide for a mass of useless ballast.

Of more practical importance than the association of these risks with obesity is the fact that they are greatly reduced if the weight can be brought down to normal. If this were not so – if fat people were liable to diseases because of constitutional defects that remained after slimming – there would be little point in shedding excess fat. But all the evidence shows that people who tackle obesity improve their health and prolong their lives.

Fat people – especially fat young people – often think they have something wrong with their glands. Fatness from this cause is exceedingly rare – a busy doctor might go through his career without seeing a case. To all intents and purposes, obesity is the result of eating too much, or too much of the wrong food. The three types of fuel in the diet – protein, fat, and carbohydrate – are to some extent interchangeable. Any unburnt fuel can be converted to fat and stored in the tissues. In practice, the excess is nearly always carbohydrate and not fat or protein. Too much fat in the diet is difficult to stomach, and too much protein looks after itself because protein increases the rate of combustion and the excess is burnt and not stored. But carbohydrate is easily assimilated, and if the intake is not balanced by an equivalent output of energy – of muscular work – the excess is converted to fat and remains in the body.

There is little justice about obesity. Some people seem able to eat any amount without putting on weight. Others are chemically less adaptable and have to be strong-minded if they are to keep their body weight within reasonable bounds. These differences have not been explained.

Overeating is a common neurosis, in some way due to a sense of insecurity. In such cases the patient is not likely to reduce his diet without skilled attention to the emotional problem. Or it may be a habit acquired in early childhood and hard to break later on. The popular belief that fat babies are healthy is fostered by advertisers of baby foods and judges of baby shows. It is a dangerous belief. Fat babies grow into fat children and fat adults. Exertion is a trial to fat children, so they take less than enough exercise and grow still fatter.

A tendency to fatness is partly inherited and partly acquired by living with fat parents who tacitly approve of their own well-fed image.

There are only two certain ways to lose weight. One is to eat less, in particular less sugar and starch. The other is to use more energy without eating more, but exercise promotes appetite and very little extra food cancels a great deal of exercise. Fruits, salads and special 'reducing' breads help by filling the stomach and taking the edge off appetite without providing much fuel. It is also possible to lose weight without reducing the total amount of food by taking more protein but less carbohydrate. Many drugs have been given to help patients to lose weight. For a time, *thyroid extract* had a vogue. By producing the symptoms of a toxic goitre, including abnormally rapid consumption of fuel in the body, it made people thinner, but the price was extreme nervous tension and a threat of heart failure. When this treatment had fallen into total disrepute, *amphetamine* came into use, followed by allegedly safer derivatives. These drugs, by quite different means, had the same ill effects as thyroid extract, with the added risks of addiction and, on occasion, of grave mental disorder. Their intended effect was to suppress appetite and make dieting easier. Newer drugs for suppressing appetite, such as *fenfluramine* and *diethylpropion*, appear to be much safer, but a planned, controlled diet without drugs is safer still.

A final point: ill-informed slimming also has its dangers. The dictators of fashion are not concerned with health, and when fashion decrees that girls should look like starving boys the girls run a slight risk of malnutrition and a serious risk from drugs supposed to suppress appetite.

obstetric forceps. Tongs ending in curved loops, shaped to hold a baby's head firmly but safely; used to ease the head past a resistant outlet when birth is delayed at the final stage; invented in about 1600 by an English obstetrician, Peter Chamberlen,

and kept as a family secret for more than a century.

obstetrician. Specialist in the management of childbirth.

obstetrics. Midwifery; medical care in pregnancy and childbirth. Progress was much hindered in the past by superstition and taboo. Only a century ago most Englishwomen had misgivings about allowing a physician – a man – to attend them in labour, and the midwives had little or no training. Although physicians had studied obstetrics since the time of Soranus (2nd century B.C.) their knowledge did not often reach the patients. In many parts of the world the old taboos live on: men are excluded from midwifery, and few women are trained.

Many surgeons in the 17th and 18th centuries wrote good accounts of the mechanics of labour, but the turning-point for obstetrics did not arrive until the 19th century when Semmelweis overcame the great hazard, infection (◊ *puerperal* fever). This work was soon followed by the discovery of anaesthetics. In the 20th century, the midwives have become an organized profession with prescribed courses of training and examination.

◊ *labour; pregnancy.*

occipital. Of the back of the head; the *occipital bone* is the back of the floor of the skull. It forms a movable joint with the backbone. The brain-stem passes through a large hole in the occipital bone (*foramen magnum*) to become the spinal cord.

The *occipital lobe* is a part of the brain at the back of the skull above the cerebellum. It records and interprets vision.

occupational disease. Paracelsus, in the 16th century, seems to have been the first physician to recognize a trade as the cause of a disease. He described chronic inflammation of the lungs in miners, and poisoning by heavy metals in smelters.

The systematic study of occupational disease began with Ramazzini, whose *De morbis artificum diatriba* was published in 1700. He correctly identified most of the typical ailments of the trades of his time and suggested ways of avoiding them, such as cleanliness, ventilation, and better posture. To the questions that doctors had been asking since the time of Hippocrates he added: *What is your job?*

The Industrial Revolution introduced new kinds and conditions of work, and with them many new diseases. The pioneer of modern industrial medicine was C. T. Thackrah (1795–1833) of Leeds, whose work was the inspiration of a series of Factories Acts for protecting the health of workers.

If many of the old hazards have been overcome by safer machinery, better designed factories, protective devices and so on, new hazards are always likely to arise; and even when safeguards are available there is no guarantee that they will always be used.

Injuries and skin troubles are by far the commonest of occupational hazards (◊ *accidents; dermatitis*). Others are lung diseases from inhaled dust (◊*pneumoconiosis*), and many kinds of poisoning.

People working with animals or animal products are exposed to kinds of infection that other people escape, such as anthrax and undulant fever. Doctors and nurses can get diseases such as tuberculosis from their patients – less often than one might expect because they acquire immunity to most common infections during their apprenticeship.

occupational therapy. A valuable method of treating various chronic and disabling illnesses. The original idea was surely to relieve boredom, but reading to patients and bringing them jigsaw puzzles is more than simple kindness: it is a positive factor in their recovery. A patient who is bored and miserable does not recover as quickly as one who is interested in life. He may even abandon a course of treatment or discharge himself from hospital before he is ready to go. An occupational therapist, though, is much more than a reliever of boredom with a box of embroidery wool and raffia. She is a *therapist*, i.e. she has an active part in the treatment of patients, and a detailed knowledge of their abilities and handicaps. Finding suitable diversions and recreations, which may range from gardening to drama, is only a part of the work. This new profession overlaps two others. On the one hand, a patient who will be left with a lasting physical or mental disability may need either to re-learn lost skills or to acquire new ones so that he will be ready for a job in keeping

with his abilities. Here, occupational therapy merges into industrial therapy (some long-term hospitals have elaborate workshops where patients are taught to earn a living again), and vocational training. On the other hand, occupational therapy overlaps physiotherapy by giving the patient interesting or rewarding tasks that also restore the function of muscles, nerves or joints. It has lately been suggested that these two professions might unite.

Any patient facing a long spell of confinement in hospital or at home is likely to find occupational therapy helpful. Those who need it most are the mentally sick. When the symptoms of a severe disorder such as schizophrenia have been controlled with drugs, occupational therapy becomes the most important part of the treatment. When the patient can take a pride in what he is doing, he is well on the way to resuming his place in society.

oculist. Eye specialist; opthalmologist.

oculomotor nerve. Third cranial nerve, controlling movements of the eye.

odontology. Study of the teeth.

oedema. Excess of tissue fluid, either throughout the body (dropsy) or around some local disturbance. About 60 per cent of the body weight is water, making some 40 litres. The water is divided between the blood (3 litres of plasma), the body-cells (25 litres), and the *tissue fluid* (12 litres). The tissue fluid permeates all the minute spaces and crevices of the body; it is the environment in which the cells live like fish in the sea.

Tissue fluid is derived from the blood. The arteries and veins are waterproof, but the microscopical capillary vessels that carry blood from the arteries to the veins allow water to leak from blood to tissue fluid and back. The pumping pressure from the heart drives water out of the capillaries. But protein dissolved in the blood cannot easily escape from the capillaries, and it draws water in, from the tissue fluid, by ◊ *osmosis*. These two opposing forces balance, so that the amount of tissue fluid remains more or less constant. Oedema or waterlogging of the tissues occurs either when the mechanical pressure in the capillaries is too high, or when the osmotic pressure is too low. In either case the balance is upset and water is forced out of the blood faster than it can return. (The blood does not become depleted, because its volume of water is maintained by the balance between the amount drunk and the amount passed in the urine.)

1. MECHANICAL OEDEMA

High blood pressure in the ordinary sense does not cause oedema, for only the pressure in the arteries is high. It is kept high by constriction of the smallest arteries; beyond them, in the capillaries, the pressure is normal. If you tread on a hose-pipe the pressure rises between you and the tap, not beyond you. It is when the veins beyond the capillaries are congested that the pressure in the capillaries rises and oedema develops.

Thus tight garters cause swollen feet, and so do *varicose veins*, in which the flow may be severely impeded.

By the time blood reaches the veins, the impetus of the heart beat is spent. The squeezing action of the leg muscles is needed to push the blood up the veins of the legs towards the heart. The imperceptible automatic movements of keeping the balance are usually enough, but if one stands perfectly still for long periods the feet may swell because of stagnation and raised pressure in the leg veins. Soldiers kept standing at attention are taught to work the muscles of their calves without appearing to move, and stationary household chores might be less tiring if housewives learnt the same trick. These forms of oedema are due only to gravity. They are promptly corrected by raising the feet. Five minutes of lying down with a pillow under the feet does more than an hour in a chair.

A good example of mechanical oedema can be seen at the end of an all-night journey by air. The passengers take off their shoes and sleep. Their legs are relaxed and still, and the seat-fronts gently compress the veins of their thighs. In the morning they can hardly get their shoes on, but the oedema subsides quickly when the blood-flow in the veins has been restored by working the leg muscles – wiggling the toes, stretching, walking down the cabin.

A more serious type of mechanical oedema is due to ◊ *heart failure*. The essence of heart failure ('failure' means inefficiency, not collapse) is that instead of emptying the veins that enter it the heart allows them to become engorged. This creates back-pressure on the capillaries and causes oedema. The excess of tissue fluid will collect wherever gravity is added to the back-pressure from the veins, not only in the legs but also in the cavity of the belly (◊ *peritoneum*), where there is almost unlimited space for water to accumulate. Oedema within the peritoneum is known as *ascites*. Obstruction to the veins in the liver, e.g. with cirrhosis of the liver, causes severe ascites without much oedema elsewhere.

The oedema of heart failure is not all mechanical; it is partly osmotic as described below.

2. OSMOTIC OEDEMA

Water can pass freely in and out of the capillaries, but only small amounts of protein get through, and these are carried away in the lymphatic vessels. Thus tissue fluid is a very weak solution of protein, whereas blood is a concentrated solution. The difference in concentration determines the amount of osmotic pressure for drawing water back into the blood from the tissue fluid.

If there is either too much protein in the tissue fluid or too little protein in the blood, the osmotic pressure is no longer high enough to oppose the mechanical pressure from the heart beat, and an excess of water remains in the tissue fluid as oedema.

Damaged capillaries allow too much protein to escape into the tissue fluid. The causes include infection, allergy (nettlerash), and physical injury such as scalding or bruising.

If the lymphatic vessels are obstructed, the normal traces of protein are not removed from the tissue fluid, and their concentration rises until the osmotic pressure is impaired. This type of oedema may follow surgical operations for cancer, where lymphatic vessels are closed to prevent spread of the disease. A tropical parasite, *filaria*, lives in lymphatic vessels and occasionally causes massive swelling (*elephantiasis*) of the legs or scrotum.

The oedema of starvation is due to lack of protein: there may not be enough in the diet to supply the blood proteins. And lack of vitamin B_1 causes oedema through heart failure. With severe liver disease the synthesis of blood proteins is deficient. With kidney disease, protein is lost in the urine.

A different kind of osmotic oedema is due to retention of *salt*. In health, the kidneys remove any excess of salt from the blood and pass it into the urine. But if the kidneys are defective, or if the circulation of blood through them is sluggish, salt begins to accumulate. Instead of going into the urine, it passes into the tissue fluid, and it 'draws' water with it. This is the main cause of oedema with kidney disease (◊ *nephritis*), and one of the causes with ◊ *heart failure*. The rate at which salt is passed in the urine (given properly functioning kidneys) is determined by hormones from the adrenal glands. The balance of these hormones is altered by menstruation and by pregnancy, and much of the associated discomfort, e.g. premenstrual tension, is probably due to slight oedema from salt retention.

3. TREATMENT OF OEDEMA

With so many possible causes there can be no one form of treatment. In general, oedema disappears when the cause is removed. For example, digitalis was long considered a specific remedy for dropsy. So, in a sense, it is – if the 'dropsy' is due to heart failure. Digitalis removes oedema only by improving the efficiency of a defective heart.

Some of the fluid can be drawn off through hollow tubes, but this once popular method is now seldom used except for releasing fluid from the abdomen to relieve pressure.

Drugs which increase the flow of urine (◊ *diuretics*) relieve oedema. Most diuretics act by removing salt, which automatically takes water with it. Sometimes one can get the same result by reducing the amount of salt in the diet, but a salt-free diet is extremely dull. It is very seldom necessary to reduce the amount of water drunk, for unless the kidneys are in serious trouble they can get rid of reasonable amounts of water. Indeed they cannot get rid of salt unless there is water to go with it.

oesophagus. The gullet; it is the downward continuation of the ◊ *pharynx*. The oesophagus is a strong muscular tube, flattened from front to back when empty. In the neck it lies behind the trachea immediately in front of the backbone. Behind the heart, it crosses in front of the aorta from right to left and passes through the diaphragm to widen out into the ◊ *stomach*.

The sole function of the oesophagus is to convey food and drink from the pharynx to the stomach, which it does by means of waves of muscular contraction along its walls. In man, gravity usually helps, but the oesophagus can easily maintain a flow against gravity, as when a quadruped drinks. The action is controlled by the ◊ *vagus nerves*.

Blood is supplied by the nearest vessels along the course of the oesophagus; at the lower end these are branches of the gastric vessels of the stomach. The blood in the gastric veins flows to the ◊ *portal vein* and so must traverse the liver before reaching the heart. Blood from the rest of the oesophagus flows straight to the heart by tributaries of the superior vena cava. The two systems communicate, and thus the oesophageal veins offer a by-pass for blood from the stomach if the portal vein is obstructed.

1. DISORDERS

Congenital defects arise mostly from incomplete development: at some point the passage may be too narrow (*stricture*) or completely absent (*atresia*). A stricture can often be stretched, but complete atresia is always serious, because it needs a major operation on a baby which may be in no condition for heroic surgery. There may be other congenital defects, or the baby may develop pneumonia from inhaling milk. Nevertheless, operations for atresia offer a 70 per cent chance of complete recovery as against no chance without operation.

Stricture later in life may be a congenital defect which at first gave no trouble, or the result of injury (e.g. by swallowing corrosive liquids) or of pressure by a tumour. *Cardiospasm* causes the same difficulty with swallowing as a stricture. Though the word implies tightening of the outlet to the stomach (cardiac sphincter), the fault is probably not a tight sphincter but a lax oesophageal wall due to a congenital defect of the nerve endings. The oesophageal muscles are thus unable to push food past the normal resistance of the sphincter.

With ◊ *cirrhosis* of the liver the portal vein may be obstructed; the veins of the oesophagus (see above) are then overloaded and liable to bleed.

oestrogen. A kind of female *sex hormone*. *Oestradiol* is the most important natural oestrogen. For medicinal use it has the

disadvantage that it is ineffective when taken
by mouth; but closely related synthetic
drugs can be so used. Synthetic oestrogens
that are not derived from oestradiol include
stilboestrol and *dienoestrol*. ◊ *sex hormones*

olecranon. Upper end of the *ulna*, forming
the point of the elbow.

olfactory. Concerned with the sense of
smell. ◊ *nose* (2).

olig(o)–. Prefix = 'few', 'little'; e.g. *oli-
gaemia*, insufficient volume of blood (cf.
anaemia, defective quality of blood); *oli-
gophrenia*, mental deficiency; *oliguria*,
diminished flow of urine.

omentum. A loose fold of membrane
(peritoneum), heavily impregnated with
fat, hanging from the stomach and colon
in front of the small intestine.

onchocerca. A kind of parasitic worm (◊
filaria).

oncology. Study of tumours.

onychia. Infection under a finger-nail. The
nail often has to be removed so that the
infection can be cleared up to allow a fresh
nail to grow. Otherwise the infection may
destroy the growing tissue under the base
of the nail so that the nail is permanently
lost.

oophor(o)– (oöphor(o)–). Prefix = 'of the
ovaries'; e.g. *oophorectomy*, removal of an
ovary.

ophthalmia. Conjunctivitis (inflammation of
the covering membrane of the eyelids and
front of the eye). The term is generally
confined to certain types of conjunctivitis.
Ophthalmia neonatorum, conjunctivitis of
the new-born, is due to contamination
during birth. When it is caused by *gonorrhoea* it can lead to blindness, but with the
use of antibiotics this has become a rare
complication.
Sympathetic ophthalmia is inflammation
of an eye due to injury to the other eye.
Sometimes it can be prevented only by
removing the injured eye. It is fortunately
very uncommon.
Egyptian ophthalmia = ◊ *trachoma*.

ophthalmic surgery; ophthalmology. Medi-

cal and surgical care of the eyes; ophthal-
mologists are medical practitioners specializing in disorders of the eyes (cf. *optician*).

ophthalmoscope. Instrument for inspecting
the inside of the eye. Its primary use is the
diagnosis of eye diseases; but the lining of
the eye is the one part of the body where
blood vessels can be directly inspected, and
the ophthalmoscope gives valuable evidence
of disorders as various as high blood pressure, diabetes, and Bright's disease. Also,
the optic nerve is the only part of the nervous system that can actually be seen.
Since the patient's own lens acts as a
powerful magnifying glass the structures
can be seen in great detail.

opiate. Narcotic; drug that dulls the senses
especially drugs derived from opium.

opisthotonos. Muscle spasm with extreme
arching of the back, from wide-spread
irritation of the nervous system e.g. by
tetanus.

opium. Drug extracted from the seeds of a
kind of poppy, *Papaver somniferum*. In the
past it was given as a crude powder or as an
alcoholic solution, *laudanum*; but as with
most vegetable drugs the purified active
principles are now preferred. The most
important of these, on which the effect of
opium largely depends, is ◊ *morphine*.
Opium also contains ◊ *apomorphine*, ◊
codeine (methyl morphine) and ◊ *papaverine*.

opposition. Action of turning the thumb to
face the other fingers and provide a firm
and sensitive grip, much better developed in
man than any other animal; it is one of the
features that has enabled the human race
to evolve beyond other species. ◊ *skeleton*
(4).

opsonin. A substance in blood that enables
white blood cells to engulf bacteria.

optic atrophy. Degeneration of the optic
nerve, with loss of vision. It can be due to
injury or poisoning of the nerve, or interference with its blood supply.

optician. Designer or maker of optical
instruments, especially spectacles and other
aids to vision. A *dispensing optician* makes
lenses to the prescription of an ophthal-

mologist (oculist). A *sight-testing* (ophthalmic) optician prescribes and supplies glasses.

optic nerve. Bundle of nerve fibres, carrying impulses from the *retina* – the light-sensitive lining of the eye – to the base of the brain. The optic nerves join inside the skull to form a cross, the *optic chiasma*, whence impulses from the right halves of both sides are transmitted to the right side of the brain and from the left halves to the left side.

oral. Of the mouth.

orbit. Eye-socket. ◊ *skull.*

orchi(o)–. Prefix = 'of the testicle (testis)'; e.g. *orchidectomy*, removal of the testis; *orchiopexy*, surgical fixation of an undescended testis in the scrotum; *orchitis*, inflammation of the testis, a painful complication of mumps and sometimes of gonorrhoea; *orchis* = testis.

orciprenaline. Drug related to adrenaline, used as a ◊ *bronchodilator.*

organ. A distinct, more or less separate structure in the body, serving particular functions; e.g. the brain, a kidney, a muscle. Organs are composed of various *tissues* (which may be similar in different organs). The supporting structure of an organ is its *stroma*. The elements that give it its special function are its *parenchyma.*

organic. Related to organs or to living creatures (organisms) in general. *Organic chemistry* was at first thought to be the chemistry of organisms: the carbon compounds with which it dealt could be made only by some vital process. This was found not to be strictly true, and the term *biochemistry* had to be coined. But in fact the raw materials of organic chemistry – coal tar and the like – were formed in the first place by the decay of animal and vegetable matter.

Organic diseases are those in which structural changes in organs can be found. They are contrasted with *functional* diseases, in which function is disturbed without apparent alteration of structure. This is an unfortunate division, because it too easily implies that if a disease is not organic it is probably imaginary.

organotherapy. Treatment of disease with substances extracted from organs, usually from endocrine glands; now almost entirely superseded by treatment with purified or synthetic hormones.

oriental sore (Baghdad button; Delhi boil; etc.). Infection of the skin with a protozoon, *Leishmania tropica*, transmitted by a sandfly. A boil at the site of inoculation is followed by an open sore that may take several months to heal. The condition is fairly common in many of the drier regions of the tropics.

ornithosis. A kind of pneumonia transmitted to man by several species of bird: the term includes *psittacosis*, transmitted by parrots and budgerigars. It is a fairly dangerous disease, but the agent – formerly regarded as a virus but now as a ◊ *Bedsonia* – can generally be overcome with sulphonamide or antibiotic drugs.

oropharynx. The lower part of the pharynx, below the *nasopharynx*, behind the tongue.

orthodontics. Correction of faulty position of the teeth.

orthopaedics. Literally, the correction of deformities of children, such as abnormal curvature of the spine and club-foot; as now used, the term embraces the whole surgery of bones and joints, including the treatment of injuries (fractures; dislocations).

orthoptics. Training of eye-muscles, e.g. for the correction of squint.

os (oris). Mouth.

os (ossis). Bone.

osmosis. Selective migration of molecules through semipermeable membranes. Most living membranes – animal or vegetable – behave as molecular sieves. Small molecules pass through; large ones do not. Such membranes are called *semipermeable*.

The molecules of a liquid are in constant, rapid and haphazard motion like a cloud of gnats. Because their motion is haphazard they tend to become evenly distributed, as a drop of ink will spread itself evenly through a bucket of water, given time. This tendency of a solution to become uniform persists when a semi-permeable membrane separates a strong solution from a weak one. If water can pass through and the substance dissolved cannot, the traffic is in one direction: water from the weak solution passes through the membrane to dilute the stronger until both are of the same strength, and in so doing can build up a considerable pressure. The process is called osmosis, and the pressure is called osmotic pressure. This is one of the ways in which plants draw water from the soil.

The semipermeable membranes of the human body, e.g. the walls of the cells, generally give free passage to water, salts, sugars, and the amino-acids of which proteins are built, but they block the large molecules of completed proteins. Thus the proteins exert osmotic pressure.

Blood is pumped from the heart at an average pressure of about 100 mm. of mercury (0·13 atmosphere). By the time it reaches the minute capillary blood vessels the pressure has fallen to 32 mm., and at the further end of the capillaries it is about 12 mm. This pressure tends to force water etc. out of the capillaries into the tissues. But the proteins of the blood exert osmotic pressure at about 25 mm. in the opposite direction. Therefore water leaks out of the capillary at one end and in again at the other. The cells get a regular supply of their chemical needs from the blood, but the total volume of the blood is kept constant.

ossification. Deposition of new bone. ◊ *bone* (2).

osteitis. Inflammation of bone. True inflammation of bone is almost always a result of bacterial infection, involving the marrow: ◊ *osteomyelitis*.
Osteitis deformans = ◊ *Paget's disease*.
Osteitis fibrosa is thinning of bone from loss of the hard calcium salts, due to over-activity of the *parathyroid* glands.

osteoarthritis (osteoarthrosis). Degeneration of joints, with some loss of the almost frictionless cartilage linings and formation of rough deposits of bone. Since there is no inflammation, 'osteoarthrosis' is the better term. It is one of the seemingly inevitable processes of ageing, affecting mainly the joints subject to most wear and tear from weight-bearing – those of the legs and spine.

Joints that have been subjected to abnormal stresses by faulty posture, injury, or deformity are especially vulnerable and may develop osteoarthrosis before middle age.

Much osteoarthrosis is discovered by chance from X-ray pictures made for some other reason, the joint having given no trouble. In such cases the condition is ignored for osteoarthrosis is no threat to health. Its symptoms – if any – are strictly confined to affected joints. They are discomfort or pain, and limitation of movement.

Since this is in no way a dangerous condition, treatment need go no further than the patient's comfort requires. Mild analgesic drugs, warm applications, or support for aching joints may be enough.

Surgery has much to offer in advanced cases. Becauses the pain comes from movement, a completely fixed joint is better than one with very limited and painful movement. Surgical fixation of the hip used to be the best treatment of severe osteoarthrosis of the joint. Later, various methods of realigning the joint were devised. But the best results at present follow replacement of the joint with a metal ball and socket.

osteoblast. Bone-forming cell (◊ *bone* (2)); cf. ◊ *osteoclast*.

osteochondrosis (osteochondritis). Defective growth of part of a bone. Numerous types have been named, e.g. Perthes' disease (hip), Scheuermann's disease (one or more vertebrae), Schlatter's disease (below the knee), and others. At least some of these disorders arise from minor fractures; perhaps they all do.

osteoclast. Bone-absorbing cell (◊ *bone* (2)). (Bone grows and is maintained by simultaneous deposition of new bone by osteoblasts and absorption of old bone by osteoclasts.)

osteoclastoma. Kind of bone tumour. ◊ *osteoma*.

osteoma. Tumour of bone. The term could be applied to any tumour arising from bone, but is generally restricted to benign, i.e. non-cancerous tumours. A true osteoma is an uncommon tumour, most likely to arise from the skull and jaw. Benign tumours in other bones are usually mixed tumours of bone and cartilage, osteochondromas.

Commoner than either is an *exostosis*, which is a superflous lump of bone near a joint or at the attachment of a muscle; this is not a real tumour but an overgrowth of normal bone. All these conditions are cured by simply removing the lump.

Osteosarcoma (osteogenic sarcoma) is a cancer of bone-forming cells with a tendency to form deposits in the lungs. There are several uncommon types of bone cancer. They include *myeloma*, a tumour of bone marrow affecting the blood-forming tissue.

Osteoclastoma is a tumour arising from osteoclasts, the cells responsible for removing old bone to make way for new. They destroy bone substance in their neighbourhood, but have little or no tendency to disseminate themselves. They can nearly always be cured by scraping out the abnormal tissue or destroying it with X-rays.

osteomalacia. Softening of bones from lack of vitamin D in adult life, a similar disease to *rickets* in childhood, but rickets also impedes growth. Osteomalacia affects mainly the weight-bearing bones: the vertebrae are compressed and the legs bowed.

Since enough vitamin D is formed in the skin under the influence of sunlight, osteomalacia does not affect people who are able to get into the open, and is unknown in sunny regions. Except during and after pregnancy adults do not need much vitamin D in the diet, even if they live indoors, and deficiency is most often due to intestinal disease, with failure to assimilate the vitamin from the food.

The condition is cured with supplementary vitamin D.

osteomyelitis. Infection of bone, with abscess formation in the marrow. Since bone is rigid, the pus of the abscess has no chance to escape and therefore spreads along the length of the bone. The pressure interferes with the circulation and may deprive parts of the bone of their blood supply. A fragment of dead bone (sequestrum) will harbour bacteria indefinitely, because it is no longer accessible to the defence mechanisms (or drugs) carried in the blood. Established osteomyelitis usually needs surgery to open the cavity and remove dead bone.

The infection can follow a compound fracture (a fracture with the broken ends of bones exposed to contamination), but it is more often carried by the blood-stream from a site of infection elsewhere, such as a septic throat. The warning symptoms are pain and tenderness, fever, and more or less severe general illness. X-rays do not show any change in the early stages, and the diagnosis has to be made by inference.

Since the discovery of antibiotics, osteomyelitis has become much less common because the primary infection can be arrested before it spreads to bone; and the condition itself has become much easier to treat. The infection can usually be controlled before the need for surgery arises.

Chronic osteomyelitis used to be a common sequel, with a persistent leakage of pus from an ulcer in the overlying skin and slow deterioration of the patient's health; several operations were sometimes needed. Few cases now reach this stage, and although they all need surgery to clear away dead and infected bone, antibiotics greatly hasten their recovery.

The usual microbes are streptococci and staphylococci. Tuberculosis and syphilis used often to cause kinds of smouldering infection of bone, but all tuberculosis other than that of the lungs is now rare, and syphilis is seldom allowed to reach this late stage.

Typhoid and relapsing fevers occasionally lead to a mild, persistent osteomyelitis.

osteopathy. A system of medical practice, founded by A. T. Still (1828–1917), an American country doctor. Its principles are that the body will look after its own ailments if it is given a chance, and the usual hindrance is a structural defect such as a displaced bone that can be corrected by manipulation. The defect or *osteopathic lesion* is said to affect neighbouring organs by disturbing their blood supply. Still taught that all disease was caused in this way, but present-day osteopaths regard osteopathy as an addition to orthodox medicine rather than an alternative to it.
    ⟫ *manipulation.*

osteoporosis. Thinning of the texture and weakening of bone; a condition so common in old people that it seems an inevitable process of ageing. There is evidently some association with decreased production of sex hormones: women whose ovaries have had to be removed may develop osteoporosis at any age unless artificial hormones are given. An excess of adrenal hormones has the same effect; osteoporosis is one of the complications of ◊ *corticosteroid* treatment if it is prolonged. Any bone that is completely immobilized develops osteoporosis in time, and the whole skeleton is weakened after a long period in bed.

One factor is loss of calcium from bone, and it has been suggested that old people would be less liable to osteoporosis if they took more calcium in their food. Milk is the most convenient source.

otitis externa. Inflammation of the skin or the external ear (including the canal of *meatus*), due to infection with bacteria or fungi. The irritation of wax in the canal seems to facilitate infection. The ear-drum is an effective barrier to spread into the middle ear, but if the drum is perforated by previous injury or infection the middle ear is likely to become involved.

Some people are prone to otitis externa after swimming, and have to protect their ears with plugs or bathing caps.

The condition generally responds quickly to simple cleansing; antibiotic drugs are sometimes needed.

otitis interna. Inflammation of the inner ear (labyrinth), from spread of infection either inwards from the middle ear or outwards from within the skull. In other words it is a possible complication of either otitis media or meningitis. The treatment with antibiotics of the primary disorder also deals with the otitis interna, but there is a danger of permanent damage to the hearing organ.

otitis media. Inflammation of the middle ear, from infection within the ear-drum. The infection nearly always comes from the back of the nose by way of the Eustachian tube, a direct passage from the ear to the nose. The usual sequence is a virus infection of the nose (e.g. measles, common cold) making the mucous membrane vulnerable to bacteria that would normally do no harm, with spread of bacterial infection up the tube to the middle ear.

Acute otitis media causes violent earache, often with fever and other constitutional symptoms of infection. Unless the attack is cut short with antibiotic drugs the earache persists until the pus in the middle ear escapes. The drum may perforate spontaneously; otherwise it has to be punctured

surgically. When the infection has cleared up the drum generally heals and there is no further trouble. Occasionally the pus, instead of escaping safely to the outer ear or down the Eustachian tube, seeps into the mastoid bone behind the ear or, still worse, into the skull-cavity. These complications need urgent operation. They used to be common, but thanks to sulphonamide and antibiotic drugs are now rare.

Chronic otitis media represents a kind of stalemate between acute infection and natural resistance: the severe symptoms of an acute attack are overcome, but the infection smoulders for months or years. The perforation of the drum fails to heal, there is a slight discharge of pus, and hearing is usually affected. With patient cleansing the infection can often be controlled, but if the bone is involved a surgical operation may be needed. Large defects in the drum, with serious loss of hearing, can often be repaired by grafting when the infection has been successfully treated.

Serous otitis is a common cause of attacks of deafness. The middle ear becomes filled with clear, sticky fluid which prevents the transmission of sound. This form of otitis may follow minor infection such as a cold, but by the time symptoms arise there is generally no sign of infection. As a rule, the fluid drains itself through the Eustachian tube. Antihistamine drugs hasten the process. It is occasionally necessary to puncture the drum and wash the fluid away.

otolith organ. The balance mechanism of the inner ear. ◊ *ear* (3, ii).

otology. Study of the ears.

otorhinolaryngology. Branch of medicine dealing with ear, nose and throat (ENT).

otosclerosis. A hereditary defect of the middle ear, with formation of superfluous bone that may prevent the slight movements of the small bones that transmit vibration from the drum membrane to the sensory organ of the inner ear. In most cases the condition is harmless, but if the abnormal bone blocks transmission to the inner ear hearing is lost. This kind of deafness is treated surgically. *Fenestration* – making a new opening to the inner ear – has now been superseded by replacement of the immobilized conducting bone by a synthetic substitute. On the whole, the results of surgery are good, but some patients still need hearing aids even after operation.

ouabain. A drug from the strophanthus plant with similar effects to digitalis.

ovary. The primary female sex organ, homologous with the male testis. A woman has two ovaries, one at each side of the uterus immediately below the opening of the Fallopian tube. The ovary is the only organ in the abdomen and pelvis that has no coating of peritoneum. Instead, it is covered with germinal epithelium, of which some cells form *ova* (eggs). The cells destined to form ova pass from the surface into the substance of the ovary where each is surrounded by a membrane to make a primitive (primordial) follicle. When a girl is born, her ovaries contain some hundreds of thousands of primordial follicles, of which only a few hundred will ever mature.

After puberty, a single follicle matures every month. The surrounding membrane grows rapidly and bursts on the surface of the ovary. The ovum – a single cell – is released and enters the Fallopian tube, where it may become fertilized. The rest of the follicle continues to grow into a small gland, the corpus luteum. If the ovum is fertilized, the corpus luteum continues to grow and secrete hormones that maintain pregnancy. If the ovum is not fertilized the corpus luteum withers, and menstruation occurs. The cycle continues until the menopause, some thirty years after puberty.

In addition to forming ova, the ovary serves as an endocrine gland, secreting the *sex hormones* that determine various female sex characters.

The activities of the ovary are governed by hormones of the pituitary gland. Sterility from failure to release ova for fertilization is more often due to deficiency of a pituitary hormone than of the ovaries themselves.

The common disorders of the ovaries are various types of abnormal growth. These swellings are often filled with fluid, and are then known as *ovarian cysts*. Many of these are practically harmless in themselves, but any ovarian cyst is liable to bleed, or to become twisted at its base and therefore congested and painful. Some ovarian swellings grow so large as to be a nuisance. A few are found to be cancers when they are examined by surgical operation. For these reasons it is standard practice to remove a defective ovary, regardless of the kind of disorder – it is seldom possible to identify the disorder without operation. Removal of one ovary has no ill effects. If both have to be removed the patient is then sterile, but in such circumstances she is likely to have been already sterile before the operation, because an ovary that needs removal has usually ceased to provide ova. Menstruation ceases after removal of both ovaries. Symptoms associated with this artificial menopause are controlled in the same way as those of the natural menopause, by regular small doses of oestrogens to replace the lost hormones.

oxalic acid. Oxalic acid and its salts (*oxalates*) are found in sorrel, rhubarb tops and other plants, and are synthesized for various industrial uses. Oxalic acid is extremely poisonous in two ways. It corrodes the lining of the mouth and stomach; and it interferes with the working of nerve and muscle fibres by neutralizing the active calcium of the body fluids, which is essential to nerve conduction and muscle contraction. Calcium compounds – e.g. chalk – are used as antidotes.

oxygen. One of the most widely distributed elements; it constitutes about one fifth of the air. All known forms of life except a few bacteria depend on a constant supply of oxygen to provide energy by combustion of glucose or other fuel. Some tissues can work for a short time without oxygen, but the deficit has to be made up later (◊ *muscle* (1)).

Oxygen is taken into the lungs and combined with the haemoglobin of the blood to be carried to every part of the body (◊ *blood* (2); *haemoglobin*; *respiration*).

Oxygen has many medicinal uses. It is given to enrich the air when either breathing or circulation is impaired. This is of the greatest value when the lungs are unable to take up enough oxygen from the air, e.g. with severe bronchitis, but cannot help much if the lungs are healthy but oxygen is poorly distributed because the flow of blood is limited, e.g. with heart failure. But oxygen still has a place in the treatment of heart failure, because some of the trouble is due to congestion of the lungs. Oxygen is a necessary adjunct to many anaesthetics.

Oxygen under high pressure (hyperbaric oxygen) is under trial for resuscitation from severe shock and other states of collapse, and the promotion of healing. It is an effective remedy against infection with bacteria that live without air (gas gangrene; tetanus).

oxyntic. Acid-forming; the oxyntic cells in the lining of the stomach secrete hydrochloric acid.

oxytocin. A hormone of the ◊ *pituitary* gland; it stimulates contraction of the uterus, which is especially sensitive to its action at the end of pregnancy. Oxytocin can be synthesized. It is used to start

contraction of the uterus if labour is delayed.

oxyuris. Pin-worm, an intestinal parasite.

ozone. An unusual form of oxygen, with molecules of 3 instead of 2 atoms. Its characteristic smell can be recognized near an electric motor. Ozone is a powerful antiseptic, and high concentrations are poisonous to all forms of life. The healthy ozone of seaside air is a myth.

P

pacemaker. The natural pacemaker of the heart is the *sinu-atrial node*, from which a wave of contraction spreads through the heart muscle with each beat (◊ *heart* (3)).

When the natural heart beat fails with certain types of heart disease the beat can be started again with an artificial pacemaker if one can be provided within a very few minutes. This apparatus delivers small regular electric shocks. It can be life-saving, e.g. when a patient who has had a coronary thrombosis has a second, potentially fatal attack in hospital where a pacemaker can be applied at once.

Patients in whom the conducting mechanism of the heart has broken down (heart block, ◊ *arrhythmia*) used to be in considerable danger, but they can now live normal lives when a small battery-driven pacemaker has been attached to the heart. The simplest and most reliable type acts at a fixed frequency of 70 beats per minute. Other types, not suitable for all cases, pick up the natural impulse from the sinu-atrial node and deliver it to the ventricles. With this type the rate is regulated by the patient's own nervous system.

Pacinian corpuscles. (F. Pacini (1812–83), Italian anatomist.) Minute round organs at the ends of some nerve fibres in skin and tendons, receiving the sensation of pressure.

paediatrics. Medical care of children. Paediatrics was a recognized specialty before the era of medical specialization began in the latter part of the 19th century. Some of the classical writers (e.g. Celsus; Soranus) drew attention to important differences between children and adults in their responses to illness and its treatment. The first book entirely devoted to paediatrics, by Paolo Bagellardo, appeared in Padua in 1472. But this, like other medical books of its time, was little more than an appraisal of ancient authorities. Paediatrics really began with the publication in 1765 of a treatise on children's diseases and their treatment by Nils Rosen von Rosenstein of Uppsala in Sweden. It is a record of careful observation and sensible inference. For instance, when Rosen described the ill effects of teething (which he overstated), he started with a stern warning against putting other ailments down to teething, instead of making 'a diligent inquiry into the real cause of the disease'. Today's paediatricians still have to sound the same warning, for it is all too easy to blame on teething any illness that happens to arise at the same time. Older children may find their ailments blamed on 'growing'. (For a similar danger in later life, ◊ *menopause*.)

Paget's disease. (Sir James Paget (1814–99), English surgeon.) Two diseases are named after Paget.

1. *Osteitis deformans* is a disorder of the skeleton. The normal processes of absorption and renewal of bones become disturbed and no longer co-ordinated. Some bones may lose calcium and with it their rigidity, and as a result they are deformed by weight-bearing. Later too much calcium is deposited and the bones are thickened. Paget's disease can be confined to a single bone or affect several, e.g. legs, skull, vertebrae. It is a very slow process and comparatively harmless. The cause is unknown. Most cases are discovered by chance, e.g. after a routine X-ray examination. Sometimes the affected bones ache, and in advanced cases the patient's activity may be restricted. X-ray treatment often relieves pain, and the hormone ◊ *calcitonin* has recently been used with success.

2. *Paget's disease of the nipple* looks like a harmless eczema of the nipple, but is in fact associated with an uncommon type of breast cancer and needs prompt surgical treatment.

pain. Pain is distinct from other sensations (except, perhaps, itch) and is carried by its own nerve fibres. These fibres follow two pathways: one, with fast conduction, carries a 'sharp' sensation; the other, a slower and duller sensation. The two components can be distinguished when the hand is pricked or pinched.

It is worth insisting that pain is not an event in the part of the body that is hurt, nor in the nerves that conduct impulses from the part, but in an area of the brain where the impulse is translated into a conscious feeling. If no feeling is aroused, one cannot say that there is pain. On the other hand, if the feeling *is* aroused there is pain. Whether or not pain is felt does not depend only on the nature and extent of the stimulus. It also depends on frame of mind. A man who is preoccupied may hardly notice an injury that he would find painful at another time. Another man who is expecting an injury and anxious about it may feel more pain than the injury would normally be worth. 'Imaginary pain' is almost meaningless. All pain is in the mind; it has no other existence. Colours, sounds, smells, textures and other things of which we are aware are our interpretation of real, measurable events around us. Pain has no such counterpart in the outside world.

The use of pain as a warning is obvious: it can prevent further injury by discouraging the activity that aroused it. But as often as not, pain is unpleasant to no good purpose.

The first aim in treating a disease is to remove its cause; to relieve pain is often a close second. The two may go together. Setting and splinting a broken bone deals with the injury itself and also stops painful movement of the broken ends. But in this as in many other instances there may be delay before definitive treatment, and the treatment itself is painful. With many other conditions, pain persists during the cure. For the patient himself the strict medical priorities are often reversed: treatment of causes takes second place. Many painful conditions resolve themselves, and some cannot yet be cured. In either case the sole object of treatment is to relieve pain.

The humane motive is the principal reason but not the only one for treating pain, for there is more than mental suffering at stake. Severe or protracted pain has physical effects. It provokes various reflex actions, of which sweating, nausea, and faintness are familiar examples. By disturbing the heart and circulation, pain contributes to *shock* (failure of the circulation), a sometimes fatal complication of extensive injury or severe acute illness. Anaesthetics have made surgery safer as well as less unpleasant.

Most pain arises from direct mechanical injury to the specific nerve-endings, such as a blow, a wound, or a burn, but pain can also be due to chemical irritation. When the flow of blood through a muscle is restricted, e.g. the heart muscle in angina, by-products of incomplete combustion accumulate and cause pain.

Not all tissues are sensitive to pain. In the skin and its underlying connective tissue many kinds of stimulus cause pain; in muscle, pressure or defective blood supply; in most abdominal organs, distension or muscle spasm. The linings of the abdomen and chest (peritoneum and pleura) and the membranous coating of bone are very sensitive; bone itself is not, nor is the interior of solid organs such as the liver, nor, surprisingly, the brain. The majority of the internal organs can be cut or burnt without sensation.

For drugs used against pain ◊ *anaesthetics; analgesic; morphine.*

◊◊ *counter-irritation; referred pain.*

palate. Roof of the mouth, divided into the hard palate in front and the soft palate behind the back teeth. Most of the hard palate is formed by the floor of the maxilla (upper jaw-bone); behind it are small *palatine* bones. The soft palate is a fibrous arch equipped with muscles which draw it up to close the back of the nose during swallowing. Behind the tongue the pillar at each side of the arch of the palate divides to embrace the *tonsil*. The downward projection from the centre of the arch, the *uvula*, does not appear to be useful. An unduly long one may cause a child to cough when lying down; it can be removed without ill effects.

The mucous membrane coating the soft palate contains a few taste-buds; they are much less important than those of the tongue.

The palate develops in two halves which normally fuse in the mid-line. Cleft palate, a common congenital defect, is incomplete fusion of the two sides. It is often associated with *harelip*, which is a similar failure of the two halves of the upper lip to join. The extent of the defect can be anything from a groove at the edge of the lip or in the uvula to complete separation of the two sides of palate and lip. Some degree of cleft is to be expected in 1:750 of babies, but if an immediate relation is affected the chance is about 1:20.

These defects can always be greatly improved and often made completely good by plastic surgery. Timing the operation can be more difficult than doing it. If the operation is likely to be prolonged it may have to be postponed until the baby is older and stronger. On the other hand if the defect makes it impossible for the baby to suck some kind of repair has to be done. If the operation is delayed until the child has learnt to speak the speech defect may be difficult to correct. The compromise is an early operation to establish the function of the palate or lip and a later operation to improve the child's appearance.

palliative. Treatment to suppress symptoms rather than the underlying disease. The word is often given a rather derogatory sense, as though palliation were bad practice; but this is not justified unless treatment of causes is neglected. It would be deplorable to suppress the cough of pneumonia or the pain of appendicitis and do nothing to control the infection, but the relief of symptoms is an important adjunct to curative treatment. And with many diseases the whole treatment is palliative – for instance, no known treatment will shorten a cold, but much can be done to make it less unpleasant while it lasts.

pallor. The pale complexion of sick people is usually due to constriction of blood vessels in the skin, which conserves heat by preventing blood from being cooled on the surface of the body. Pallor may also be due to a shortage of the red blood-pigment haemoglobin, i.e. anaemia.

palpitation. Awareness of the heart beat, either because the heart is in fact beating more forcibly than usual or because the subject pays undue attention to it.

palsy. Paralysis.

paludism. Malaria (*palus* = swamp, where mosquitoes are likely to breed and carry malaria).

panacea. Greek goddess of healing; cure-all.

pancreas. A broad strip of soft glandular tissue across the back of the abdomen, mostly under cover of the stomach. It is broadest on the right where it nestles in the curve of the duodenum, wrapped round the portal vein and closely applied to the arteries of the liver and the bile duct. From here it tapers away, upwards and to the left, between the stomach and the left kidney to reach the spleen. The pancreas receives blood from the coeliac artery (which also supplies the stomach, liver, and spleen), and returns it to the portal vein.

This is a dual-purpose organ. It is an offshoot of the intestine, and primarily a digestive gland. In this respect it is analogous to the salivary glands – in German it is known as the abdominal salivary gland. Most of its cells are arranged around branches of the pancreatic duct, into which they secrete the pancreatic juice. The duct enters the duodenum in company with the bile duct; in other words the pancreas and liver share the same opening into the intestine, and are both apt to suffer if the opening is blocked (e.g. by a gall stone or a tumour). The pancreatic juice is alkaline, and neutralizes the acid entering the intestine from the stomach. It contains numerous digestive enzymes – catalysts by which complex substances in the food are broken down to simple chemicals which can be absorbed from the intestine into the blood-stream (◊ *digestion*).

Apart from its primary digestive function the pancreas is concerned with the chemical control of sugar in the body. Scattered through the gland are small clusters of specialized cells which do not communicate with the duct and contribute nothing to the pancreatic juice. These are the *islets of Langerhans*. They produce two hormones, *insulin* and *glucagon*, which are released directly into the blood-stream. Their functions are complementary. Insulin promotes the uptake of sugar from the blood by the tissues, for storage and combustion. Glucagon promotes the release of sugar from the tissues (mainly the liver) into the blood. (◊ *carbohydrate; diabetes*).

1. Disorders

By far the most important disease involving the pancreas is *diabetes mellitus*. Diabetes is discussed under its own heading; it is not a single disease but a collection of symptoms due to failure to use insulin, either because the pancreas is not making enough or because the demand is abnormally great. Some diabetes is caused by disorders of the pancreas, but in many cases the pancreas is healthy.

Pancreatitis – inflammation of the pancreas – may be mild and transient, but at its worst it can be very dangerous with a clinical picture suggesting either severe disease of the gall bladder or perforation of a duodenal ulcer. Sometimes the diagnosis can be made only by surgical operation. If digestive enzymes leak into the abdominal cavity they set up a violent peritonitis with the same symptoms as peritonitis from any other cause. Most cases are due to, or associated with, obstruction of the pancreatic duct as it enters the duodenum, for instance by a gall stone blocking both pancreatic and bile ducts, or by swelling of the mucous membrane from heavy drinking.

Mild attacks of pancreatitis sometimes complicate mumps, not surprisingly because the virus of mumps has a predilection for the salivary glands which closely resemble the pancreas.

Chronic pancreatitis is an uncommon cause of poor digestion and pain. Its origin is usually obscure, but since the islets of Langerhans escape damage while the digestive part of the gland is slowly destroyed the trouble probably begins in the pancreatic duct, with which the islets are not concerned. The loss of pancreatic enzymes leads to ◊ *malabsorption*.

About 2 per cent of all cases of cancer arise in the pancreas. Some of these tumours are cured by surgical removal, but neither the diagnosis nor the operation is easy.

pancreatitis. Inflammation of the ◊ *pancreas*.

pandemic. Outbreak of infectious disease, more wide-spread than an epidemic (e.g. over a whole continent or even, as in some outbreaks of influenza, around the world).

pannus. Opaque inflamed membrane spreading over the front of the eye and obscuring vision; a complication of ◊ *trachoma*.

papaverine. An alkaloid extracted from opium, not related to morphine; it relaxes involuntary muscle and has been used for treating spasm in blood vessels and other organs. Its action is brief and not very reliable, and it has been superseded by synthetic drugs.

papilla. Small projection from the surface of a tissue, such as one of the minute structures that cover the tongue.

papilloma. Abnormal growth of papillae; wart.

papule. Pimple; raised spot on the surface of the skin.

Paracelsus (Philipp Theophrastus Bombast von Hohenheim (1493–1591), nicknamed Aureole; he does not appear to have adopt- ed the name Paracelsus before about 1540). Paracelsus was born at Einsiedeln of a Swabian father and a Swiss mother. He was brought up in Austria and later travelled throughout Europe, never settling for more than a year or two. He studied with equal enthusiasm theology, chemistry, and medicine, and their shadier counterparts necromancy, alchemy, and quackery. He had the learning and imagination to be one of the great reformers of all time, yet he achieved little. He has been called the medical Luther, but he was nothing of the kind. At the outset, Luther asked no more than that the established church should set its own house in order, and almost by accident found half Europe at his feet. Paracelsus set himself to reform the whole of medicine (and much besides), but converted nobody and changed nothing. His greatest opportunity came in 1526 when he was appointed town physician and professor in Basle. From this eminent post he could have influenced all Europe, but he so alienated his colleagues that he had to leave Basle after only a year. Publicly burning the works of Galen and Avicenna was good theatre, but tactless. Paracelsus might just have been forgiven for this, but not for claiming precedence over all other doctors, including his contemporaries.

Paracelsus intended to 'purify medicine of errors' by accepting only rules that had been proved by experiment. Here was the true scientific method; unfortunately Paracelsus did not follow it. He demolished the old, unproven theories, only to replace them with wilder fantasies of his own. He wrote a curious mixture of Latin with his native dialect. When he was short of a word he invented one, often without defining it. Throughout, his brilliant observations lie half submerged in mystical jargon.

His attitude to theology throws some light on this weird genius. He was a fiercer critic of orthodoxy than Luther. Men were being burnt at the stake for less – Paracelsus may have escaped because he was so unlikely to influence anyone else. Yet when leaders of the new Reformation approached him as a possible ally, he rudely told them that he was a good Catholic and had no time for their heresies.

Nobody need blame the doctors of his time for rejecting Paracelsus; he compelled rejection. But his patients loved him. With them he was considerate and even courteous.

Some of Paracelsus's discoveries were acceptable in the 16th century. He was the first man to describe miner's lung (◊ *pneumoconiosis*), the relation of cretinism to goitre, the distinction between mental defect and insanity, and the proper use of opium. He introduced chemistry to medicine with compounds of lead, iron, copper, and mercury, and he was the first to use sulphur and antimony as drugs. He believed in simple, clean dressings for wounds.

In other matters Paracelsus was centuries ahead of his time. Surgery was still considered an ungentlemanly craft, but Paracelsus believed that surgeons should have the same status as physicians and work closely with them. He insisted that anatomy should be studied and taught in relation to the living body – a view only now being adopted by medical schools. He detested polypharmacy, the giving of half a dozen remedies in the hope that one would work, for he maintained that one drug was as likely to cancel as to reinforce another. He said that talking to a patient and letting him talk might be the best treatment. None of these doctrines could hope to be accepted at the time. For this was the voice of Hippocrates, calling across 20 centuries. Men still shaking the dust of the Middle Ages from their ears could not possibly hear it.

paracentesis. Release of fluid from a tissue or body cavity by insertion of a drainage tube.

paracetamol. A drug closely related to phenacetin. ◊ *analgesic*.

paraesthesia. Abnormal sensation without external cause, e.g. tingling, 'pins-and-needles', a common symptom of compression or irritation of a nerve. ◊ *neuropathy*.

paraffin. A series of compounds of carbon with hydrogen, including gases, liquids and solids.

Liquid paraffin is a clear, inert, almost tasteless fluid; it is not absorbed from the intestine and therefore passes through as a lubricant. It has been much used as a mild laxative.

Soft paraffin (petroleum jelly; petrolatum) forms a good barrier to protect superficial injuries of the skin such as burns; it prevents dressings from sticking to raw areas. It is the basis of many ointments.

paraldehyde. A clear liquid with an aromatic smell and a disagreeable taste; it is an effective and relatively safe hypnotic.

paralysis. Loss of voluntary movement; failure of nervous impulses to reach muscles; it can be a symptom of almost any disorder of the nervous system. *Infantile paralysis* = ◊ *poliomyelitis*. *Paralysis agitans* = ◊ *parkinsonism*.

parameter. A fairly recent addition to medical language, borrowed from geometry. It is used of quantities that can be measured and compared in different individuals, such as body weight, blood pressure, or the concentration of sugar in the blood.

paranoia. A kind of mental disorder, with delusions of persecution and self-importance. On its own it is rare – some psychiatrists deny that there is such a disease. But paranoid symptoms are common in schizophrenia.

paraplegia. Paralysis of the lower part of the body, usually from injury to the spinal cord (cf. *hemiplegia*, paralysis of one side of the body).

parasite. A creature that lives at the expense of another living creature, its *host*. Human parasites include *viruses*, *bacteria*, *fungi*, *protozoa*, and *worms*. Nearly all parasites injure the health of the host to some extent, and many cause serious illness. Harmless parasites, such as the bacteria of the healthy intestine, are called *commensals*.

parasympathetic. One of the two divisions (cf. ◊ *sympathetic*) of the autonomic or vegetative nervous system, which are responsible for the automatic, unconscious regulation of bodily function. Most parts of the body receive twigs from both of these divisions, generally with opposite actions.

Two groups of nerves form the parasympathetic system. The *cranial* outflow arises from the lowest part of the brain. Several cranial nerves include parasympathetic fibres; the *vagus* (10th cranial) nerve carries most. The *sacral* outflow arises from the lower end of the spinal cord as the two sacral nerves (nervi erigentes).

Parasympathetic nerves have the following actions:

Fibres in the 3rd cranial (ophthalmic) nerve constrict the pupil and focus the lens of the eye.

Fibres in the 7th (facial) and 9th (glosso-pharyngeal) nerves stimulate the salivary glands. These nerves also carry the sense of taste, making a simple pathway for the reflex by which the taste of food stimulates the flow of saliva.

The vagus nerves are widely distributed. In the *heart* they slow the beat and reduce its force. The various reflexes that accelerate the heart act more by withdrawing the inhibition by the vagus than increasing stimulation by sympathetic nerves. In the *lungs*, they reduce the flow of air. They increase the activity of the *digestive* organs.

The pelvic nerves stimulate emptying of the bladder and rectum. They are also responsible for erection of the penis (but orgasm depends on sympathetic nerves).

To some extent, autonomic nerves act independently of the brain – hence their name – but the activity of the whole system is modified and co-ordinated in the brain, mainly in and around the hypothalamus. This part of the brain is also concerned with the emotions, which have their physical expression in reflexes of the autonomic system (widening of the pupils, sweating, quickened pulse, blushing, blanching, digestive disturbance etc.).

All the actions of parasympathetic nerves are due to the substance *acetyl choline*, which is released from the nerve-endings and activates the 'target organs'. The effects of an impulse in a particular nerve are confined to its own area, because acetyl choline is very rapidly destroyed.

Drugs such as *carbachol* that imitate acetyl choline, or *eserine*, that prevent its destruction, have similar actions to the parasympathetic nerves. Drugs such as *atropine* that interfere with acetyl choline suppress parasympathetic action.

parathyroid. One of several (usually 4) small glands behind or embedded in the thyroid gland. The parathyroids produce a hormone, *parathormone*, which regulates the concentration of calcium in the blood. If this concentration falls the parathyroids are thereby stimulated to release more of the hormone, which increases the solubility of calcium in the bones and so restores the amount in the blood.

Deficiency of the parathyroids is rare. It may occur for no known reason, or may follow injury to the parathyroids during surgery of the thyroid gland. The result is *tetany* – over-excitability of nerve and muscle, with twitching, cramp, and tingling sensations. Tetany is controlled by injecting either calcium or the hormone.

A tumour of a parathyroid may produce an excess of parathormone. Too much calcium is then withdrawn from the bones, which become fragile. The surplus of calcium in the blood is excreted in the urine; it may form stones in the kidneys. These tumours are not malignant. They can be removed surgically and usually cured. If after the operation there is too little para-thormone the deficiency can be made up by injections, but this is seldom necessary.

The ◊ *thyroid gland* produces a hormone (*calcitonin*) to combat excessive calcium in the blood, as a counterpart to parathormone.

paratyphoid fever. A group of infectious diseases related to ◊ *typhoid* fever but generally milder. Of the three types, only para-typhoid B is common in Western Europe. A and C occur mainly in the tropics and subtropics.

Most outbreaks are spread by contamination of food or drinking water by infected people, who may have long recovered from the illness. In hot, dry climates infection may be spread by dust or flies. Hygienic water supplies and food-handling greatly reduce the incidence.

Symptoms are of two kinds. Some cases are like typhoid fever: the patient is obviously ill without signs to incriminate any particular organ, and the diagnosis depends on identifying the bacteria in the laboratory. In other cases the trouble is confined to the intestine, and the main symptom is diarrhoea.

The bacteria of paratyphoid fever are species of *Salmonella*, a group that includes the bacteria of typhoid fever on the one hand, and of bacterial food poisoning on the other. Paratyphoid is intermediate between the two, or rather can take either form. ◊ *food poisoning* (5).

Paré, Ambroise (1510–90). French surgeon; one of the greatest figures in the history of surgery. Inspired by the anatomical work of Vesalius, he more than anyone else led surgery out of the Middle Ages. Vesalius had said that one of the main reasons for the decline of medical practice between the 2nd and 16th centuries was that by delegating all surgical work to uneducated barbers the physicians had lost touch with anatomy as the basis of rational medicine.

Paré founded his practice and teaching on Vesalius's anatomical studies. He was a barber-surgeon who raised himself to the highest ranks of the scholarly medical profession – without learning to write Latin.

Paré was the first to treat serious bleeding by finding the cut artery and tying a ligature round it, instead of burning it. He also abolished the use of boiling oil to take the 'poison' from gun-shot wounds. The cruelty of it horrified him. It chanced that in 1536, when attending a French force sent to relieve Turin, Paré had no oil. Instead he applied a bland dressing of egg-yolk, oil of roses, and turpentine. In the morning his patients were comfortable and their wounds not inflamed. Other patients, treated with boiling oil, were in great pain from their festering wounds.

The most famous sentence in Paré's extensive works summed up his principle of letting well alone: 'I dressed him. God healed him' (*Je le pansai. Dieu le guérit*).

paregoric. Compound tincture of camphor; camphorated tincture of opium. Paregoric contains about 1 per cent of morphine. It was a favourite household remedy in the 19th century, much used to calm fretful children – an undesirable practice, for children would have been better off without opium, and doping them must often have masked symptoms of illnesses that needed attention.

parenchyma. The working tissue of an organ. All organs have a framework (*stroma*) of unspecialized connective tissue, supporting the specialized tissue that gives the organ its distinctive character (*parenchyma*), e.g. the contractile cells of a muscle or the secreting cells of a gland.

paresis. Partial paralysis.

parietal. 1. Of the wall of a body cavity as opposed to its contents. The parietal pleura lines the inside of the thorax; the continuation of this membrane over the surface of the lungs is the *visceral* pleura. Similarly the abdomen is lined with the parietal peritoneum, and the abdominal organs are coated with the visceral peritoneum.

2. Of the side of the cranium or brain-box. The parietal bones cover about the same area as a cardinal's skullcap. The *parietal lobes* are the corresponding part of the brain. The front part of these lobes, immediately behind the part of the frontal lobes concerned with movement, records conscious sensation.

parkinsonism (shaking palsy; paralysis agitans). A disturbance of voluntary movement: muscles become stiff and sluggish, movement becomes clumsy and difficult, and uncontrollable rhythmic twitching of groups of muscles produces the characteristic shaking or tremor, which may be widespread or limited to one group of muscles. Mental faculties are not affected; they may seem to be if the patient cannot control the muscles of speech.

The site of the disorder is the *basal ganglia* – groups of cells in the centre of the brain where deliberate impulses to move, from conscious areas of the brain, are transmitted to nerves that direct the appropriate muscles. The basal ganglia can be affected in many known ways (poisoning, injury, stroke), but these are all rare. The pandemic of ◊ *encephalitis* lethargica that began in 1917 was complicated by parkinsonism. But in most cases, no cause for the degeneration of the basal ganglia can be found; the term Parkinson's disease is confined to these cases.

Voluntary movement is co-ordinated by a balance of opposing nerve actions, some exciting movement and some inhibiting it. In parkinsonism, it is as though these two actions were not equally impaired – unwanted excitation of muscle is not inhibited as it should be, and muscles contract without any conscious intention that they should do so. The inhibiting nerve cells in the basal ganglia have degenerated and cannot be repaired, while many exciting cells are still intact.

The effect of most forms of treatment of parkinsonism is to put all the nerve cells of the affected region equally out of action; then some kind of balance is restored. The drugs used probably act in some such way. Belladona (atropine) is the prototype, but it has many other actions, some of them unpleasant. Synthetic drugs with a more selective action are available. Surgery gives more lasting and generally more reliable results. Stereotactic surgery – a sort of three-dimensional geometry – makes it possible to coagulate a minute cluster of cells in the centre of the brain without other damage. It is a negative and destructive approach to a disease of which the cause is still unknown, but in many cases the results justify it. Surgery is especially effective against the tremor, but it usually has some effect on' the other symptoms, and has enabled many patients to write legibly again, or handle a knife and fork.

As with several other disorders involving the brain (◊ depression, schizophrenia) chemical anomalies that cannot be called causes are at least associated with parkinsonism. There appears to be a deficiency of dopamine, a chemical precursor of adrenaline, in the basal ganglia. Most of the drugs used act indirectly to counteract such a deficiency, but L-dopa (◊ dopamine) probably has a direct action in replacing the missing dopamine. This drug is especially useful for improving muscular coordination. It is not only a valuable form of treatment, sometimes complementary to surgery, but its effect sheds much light on the nature of the disease.

Parkinson's disease. (James Parkinson (1755–1824), London physician.) The commonest form of ◊ parkinsonism.

paronychia. Small abscess at the side of a finger-nail. ◊ nails.

parotid gland. Salivary gland behind the jaw. ◊ saliva.

parotitis. Inflammation of the parotid gland. It is occasionally due to bacteria, in which case an abscess may form and need surgical treatment, but the usual cause is the virus of ◊ mumps (epidemic parotitis).

paroxysm. A fit or convulsion, or any sudden, violent attack of illness.

parturition. Childbirth. ◊ labour.

PAS. Para-amino-salicylic acid; a valuable adjunct to streptomycin in the treatment of tuberculosis. Like the sulphonamides (which are ineffective against tuberculosis) it is chemically related to para-amino-benzoic acid, an essential foodstuff of many bacteria.

Pasteur, Louis (1822–95). French chemist; professor in Strasbourg, Lille, and Paris. His most important chemical discovery was that certain compounds exist in two forms, the molecules of one being mirror images of those of the other. Many ingredients of the body – e.g. glucose, amino-acids, adrenaline – are of this type, and although the two forms seem identical by ordinary chemical tests only one form is active in the living body.

Pasteur's greatest work was in biology, where he established the relation of microbes to fermentation, putrefaction, and infectious disease, as described under ◊ microbe (◊◊ infection). This discovery was one of the major turning points in medical history.

pasteurization. Pasteur's method of preventing the transmission of disease by infected milk (tuberculosis, typhoid etc.).

The milk is heated either to 65°C. (149°F.) for 30 minutes or to 72°C. (162° F.) for 15 seconds and then rapidly cooled. This does not sterilize the milk, but it kills the kinds of bacteria liable to cause disease.

Pasteurization is obviously useless unless the treated milk is protected from contamination.

patella (kneecap). A thick disc of bone set in the tendon of the ◊ quadriceps muscle in front of the knee. There is a general tendency for small bones to be formed in tendons which are pressed directly against bare bone; several of these sesamoid bones are found in the hand and foot. The patella is simply a large sesamoid. It may slightly increase the mechanical efficiency of the quadriceps by acting as a fulcrum, but the knee functions well without it.

The pull of the quadriceps is some degrees off vertical. Its tendency to dislocate the patella sideways is overcome by muscle fibres attached to the inner side of the patella. If these fibres are injured, or weakened by inflammation in the knee joint, the patella is unstable. Occasionally, repeated dislocation of the patella becomes such a nuisance that an operation is needed to repair the damaged fibres.

Sudden and powerful contraction of the quadriceps may snap the patella across, but a direct blow is more likely to break it into several fragments. If the fragments are held in place by the tendon, these fractures heal well in a plaster cast. But if the tendon is badly torn the patella must either be held together with sutures or, if there are several small fragments, removed. The loss of the bone is less disabling than a roughened joint surface.

patent. Open. Patent ductus: ◊ ductus arteriosus.

path(o)-. Prefix = 'disease'; 'suffering'.

pathogen. Microbe capable of causing disease.

pathogenesis. The processes by which a disease develops.

pathognomonic. (Symptom etc.) peculiar to a particular disease, sufficient in itself to establish the diagnosis.

pathology. Natural history of disease; study of abnormal changes in the body and their causes. While clinical medicine deals mainly with the effects of disease, pathology deals with the underlying processes.

Of necessity, pathology is a modern science: abnormalities in the body cannot be usefully discussed until normal structure and function (anatomy and physiology) are understood, and no clear idea of function was possible until 1628 when Harvey discovered the circulation of the blood. Diseases had previously been described in terms of their symptoms, and attributed to disordered balance of the ◊ *humours*. The humoral theory was so deeply ingrained that few people even looked for evidence of disease beyond the obvious outward signs. Two who did so were Antonio Benivieni of Florence (1443–1502), apparently the first man to do necropsies (post mortem examinations) in search of the true causes of disease, and Jean Fernel of Amiens (1497–1558), who broke new ground by devoting a section of his medical text-book to pathology.

Scientific pathology really began in 1761 with the publication of Morgagni's *De sedibus et causis morborum*, a large collection of case-histories in which patients' symptoms are related to disorders of particular organs found by necropsy.

John Hunter (1728–93) applied the experimental method to pathology and amassed a store of accurate observations, including thousands of specimens of diseased organs, many of them still preserved. But even at the end of the 18th century pathology had progressed no further than showing where in the body the trouble lay with various diseases. The actual processes remained a mystery, and the humoral theory was hardly less credible than some of the rival theories that sprang up. Hunter did, however, produce a substantially correct account of inflammation, one of the

fundamental processes of disease. Under the influence of scientists such as Hunter, pathology came to rely more and more on observed facts and less on philosophical speculation. One other pioneer of the 18th century must be mentioned: Bichat focused attention not on whole organs but on their constituent *tissues* as the sites of disease. Although Bichat himself was not a microscopist it was his doctrine that led others to study disease with the microscope. The flood of pathological discovery in the 19th century came largely from microscopical examination of diseased tissues.

Full-time professional pathologists began to appear early in the 19th century. One of of the first was Hodgkin in London. The busiest was Rokitansky in Vienna. By this time, complete postmortem examination was the rule when the cause of death was in any doubt, and Rokitansky attended some 70,000. His procedure for these examinations is still standard. More important, his unequalled experience and accuracy enabled him to leave precise descriptions of most of the known diseases. This great scientist suddenly clouded his reputation with a general theory that might have put pathology back into the Middle Ages if it had been accepted. When medicine had at last broken away from sweeping, unfounded generalizations, Rokitansky revived the old humours in a new guise. All diseases were affections of the circulating blood – crasis or dyscrasis, terms that seem to mean no more than normal or abnormal tendencies – and they were as ill-defined as the humours of 500 B.C. To be fair, Rokitansky may have meant no more than that chemical abnormalities determined the processes of disease; if this is so he was quite right regarding some diseases, and only putting the cart before the horse regarding others.

The greatest of all pathologists was Rudolf Virchow, a pupil of the physiologist Müller. As a young man, Virchow demolished Rokitansky's theories and set pathology back on the path of observation and experiment. His colleague Schwann had taken anatomy one step further than Bichat and shown that the fundamental unit was not the tissue, but the *cells* that composed it. Virchow showed that diseases were best explained in terms of changes that took place within the cells. This was almost as important to medical science as was the study of molecules rather than substances to chemistry. Excepting some very recent discoveries, most current ideas of pathology spring from the work of Virchow and of his contemporaries who discovered the nature of ◊ *infection*.

Pathology has come to deal with smaller and smaller units: from a vague concept of the whole person with the classical study of humours to the study of particular organs, then tissues, then cells, and, finally, molecules. In Virchow's day, only a few diseases such as diabetes and gout, involving the simple molecules of glucose and uric acid, could be studied chemically. But all processes in the body – normal or abnormal – are in a sense chemical, and in theory all disease might be expressed in terms of disturbed chemical reactions. Pathologists are now beginning to study these disturbances, and Rokitansky's theories seem rather less absurd than they did a century ago.

In the past, postmortem studies were the only possible way of learning about the nature of disease, and they are still very important for both research and teaching. But they reveal disease at a stage where it is beyond the help of medicine, and they reveal established, static conditions, not the dynamic processes that concern practical medicine. For all its great achievements, 19th-century pathology often seemed remote from the problems of living patients. It described in great detail what had gone wrong with a patient's anatomy, but it had little to say about his physiology – the workings of affected cells, tissues, and organs.

In the 20th century pathology has been coming to life by dealing more with active processes and less with fixed states. Techniques such as X-ray examination and biopsy – the study of small samples of living tissue – show what is going on while the patient is still alive and perhaps curable, instead of waiting until he is dead to find out what is wrong. The chemistry of the living body can also be studied in detail. A department of pathology now accomodates half a dozen different sciences, all involved not only in research but in the investigation and treatment of patients. Like other sciences, pathology is becoming on the one hand more specialized, and on the other hand more closely integrated with its neighbours.

Pavlov, Ivan Petrovich (1849–1936). Russian physiologist. He was originally concerned with the physiology of digestion, in particular the regulation of flow of saliva and digestive juice in the stomach. During his experiments, mainly with dogs, he found that salivation was induced not only by stimuli directly concerned with eating, but by any stimulus (e.g. the ringing of a bell) that the dog had learned to associate with food. These learnt responses he called *conditioned reflexes* (◊ *reflex*). In 1904 Pavlov received a Nobel Prize for his work on digestion. But his discoveries have a much wider significance; they shed new light on the whole study of learning and behaviour. If it is true, as many psychiatrists hold, that neuroses are ill-formed conditioned reflexes, then Pavlov helped to elucidate one of the commonest of all ailments (◊ *anxiety*).

pectoral. Of the chest. The pectoral muscles are *pectoralis major* and *pectoralis minor*. Pectoralis major is a large fan-shaped muscle covering much of the front of the chest, and converging on the humerus a little below the shoulder. It swings the arm across the body, and is highly developed in birds as a muscle of flying. In man it acts with *latissimus dorsi*, a large muscle of the back, to pull the arm down as in swimming breast stroke, or pull the body up as in climbing. Pectoralis minor is an unimportant muscle covered by pectoralis major.

pediculus. Louse. *Pediculosis* = infestation with lice.

pellagra. A form of malnutrition, very common among people whose staple diet is maize, due primarily to deficiency of *niacin*, a vitamin of the B group.

The tissues mainly affected are skin, mucous membranes, and nerve. Exposed areas of skin develop a sort of eczema with roughening and darkening of the surface (*pellagra* = 'rough skin'). Changes in the mucous membranes cause a sore tongue and, more seriously, chronic diarrhoea. Various symptoms of disturbance of the nervous system can arise, including severe mental derangement.

As with other vitamin deficiencies, the symptoms vanish with a mixed diet and supplements of the appropriate vitamin.

The association of pellagra with a maize diet is so common that a positive toxic action of maize has been sought. The explanation may be that the amino-acid *trytophan*, found in most protein, much reduces the need for niacin. Maize contains very little trytophan. Therefore maize-eaters need more niacin than other people, while as often as not they get less because the rest of the diet is poor.

pelvis. Lower limb-girdle, composed of the lower part of the backbone and the two hip-bones. (Also *renal pelvis*: the outlet of the ◊ *kidney*.)

The pelvis is a firm ring of bone. The centre-piece is the *sacrum*, consisting of 5 vertebrae fused into a single bone, broad and massive in its upper part and tapering to a point below, to which the rudimentary tail (coccyx) is attached. The hip-bones (haunches) are attached to either side of the sacrum at the rigid *sacroiliac joints*. In front the hip-bones meet at the *symphysis pubis*, where they are bound together with tough fibrous tissue. In the male, these joints are practically rigid; in the female they allow slight adjustment of the pelvis during childbirth.

Each hip-bone consists of three elements. The largest, the *ilium*, forms a barrier between the abdomen and the muscles of the buttock and thigh, and supports the sides of the abdomen. The *ischium* is the rump, on which one sits. The smallest element, the *pubis*, meets its fellow in the mid-line to complete the ring of bone in front. These three elements all contribute to the *acetabulum*, the socket of the hip-joint at the side of the pelvis. In contrast with the mobile shoulder-girdle, the characteristic of the pelvis is its great stability.

In the middle of the pelvis is a large opening spanned by a flexible diaphragm of muscle, through which the outlets of the reproductive, digestive, and urinary systems pass. The region below this diaphragm is the *perineum*.

1. PELVIC ORGANS

The cavity of the pelvis is merely the lower part of the abdomen, and the attempt to distinguish abdominal from pelvic organs is not very useful. For instance, the urinary bladder is within the pelvis when it is empty but mainly in the abdomen when it is full.

The large intestine enters the pelvis on the left side and crosses to the mid-line where its penultimate segment, the rectum, lies on the front of the sacrum and passes through the pelvic diaphragm to become the anal canal.

The urinary bladder rests on the pubic

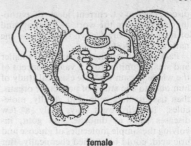

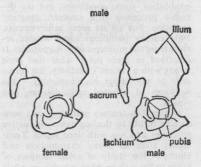

Front and right side of pelvic bones.

bones at the front of the pelvic cavity. In the female, the vagina and uterus are between the bladder and the rectum.

The principal nerves and blood vessels of the pelvis lie close to the bone. The femoral nerve and blood vessels pass over the front of the pelvis into the thigh; in the male they are accompanied by the vessels and duct (vas deferens) of the testis. The sciatic nerve enters the back of the thigh through a gap between the sacrum and hip-bone, below the sacroiliac joint.

2. Disorders

Deformity of the pelvis, however slight, is important to women because it may cause difficulty with childbirth – even a normal pelvis leaves little room to spare. The so-called *contracted pelvis* is not deformed but simply the relatively small pelvis of a woman with small bones, which may cause trouble if she has a large baby. A more real and serious deformity is caused by rickets in childhood, or any other illness that interferes with the growth of bones. In all these cases, Caesarean section solves the problem.

If the sacrum and hip-bone were completely united like the vertebral elements of the sacrum, the sacroiliac joint would cause no trouble. But since the joint allows some slight movement it is prone to the ailments of joints in general, such as rheumatic diseases. Sacroiliac strain is a difficult diagnosis to prove, but what appears to be a strain of this joint is common, especially in women.

Fractures of the pelvis are a result of considerable violence, usually crushing injuries, associated with serious damage elsewhere. As a rule the fracture itself heals without difficulty, but there is a danger of injury to the underlying organs by fragments of bone. The bladder is especially vulnerable, and needs prompt surgical repair if it is damaged.

pemphigus. A name applied to several skin diseases, none of them common, characterized by blisters.

Acute (contagious) pemphigus is a sort of impetigo, caused by streptococci or staphylococci and treated with penicillin or sulphonamides. *Pemphigus neonatorum* is a similar condition in small babies.

Pemphigus vulgaris is a rare generalized disease in which the blisters are an incidental symptom; it appears to be one of the ◊ *collagen* diseases, and responds to treatment with corticosteroids.

Types of pemphigus related to many infections (diphtheria, syphilis, leprosy) have been described.

penetrance. The extent to which an inherited character or *gene* manifests itself. This concept is needed because one can inherit, for instance, a tendency to gout without ever having symptoms of the disease. An inherited tendency that only seldom reveals itself is said to be of low penetrance; one

that regularly does so is of high penetrance. This is a much more complex affair than the simple binary arithmetic of theoretical genetics. ◊ *genetics.*

penicillin. The first antibiotic to be used (1941), and still one of the most valuable. The discovery and action of penicillin are described under ◊ *antibiotic.*

Since the original discovery of *penicillin G* many closely related antibiotics have been isolated. They are all compounds of 6-aminopenicillanic acid. In addition to natural penicillins several useful derivatives of this acid have been synthesized; the acid itself being first extracted from moulds.

Penicillin G has to be injected, but penicillin V is active when taken by mouth.

Some of the newer penicillins such as ampicillin destroy not only bacteria sensitive to penicillin G but also several other types including intestinal bacteria.

The names of penicillins are distinguished by the suffix *-cillin.*

penis. Male copulatory organ. The penis is constructed of 3 columns of erectile tissue: the two *corpora cavernosa* placed side by side, and the *corpus spongiosum* below them. The end of the corpus spongiosum is enlarged to form the conical tip (*glans penis*). Erectile tissue consists mainly of a labyrinth of blood vessels. Erection is simply distension of the tissue with blood: the veins are compressed by reflex contraction of muscle fibres around them while the arteries are dilated.

The urethra, a tube for the passage of urine or semen, traverses the corpus spongiosum. The muscles that close the veins during erection also close the outlet from the urinary bladder.

The *prepuce* is a loose fold of skin partly covering the glans (◊ *circumcision*).

pentamidine. A synthetic drug for treating sleeping sickness and related diseases (◊ *trypanosomiasis*).

pentose. A sugar with 5 carbon atoms in its molecule, e.g. *ribose*, a component of nucleic acids.

pepsin. An enzyme formed in the stomach for the digestion of protein.

peptic ulcer. Erosion of a small patch in the lining of the stomach (gastric ulcer) or duodenum (duodenal ulcer), or occasionally of other parts of the digestive tract. It is easy enough to see that this might happen, and rather surprising that it does not happen all the time. People manage to digest tripe, and tripe is very like their own stomachs.

Several factors normally prevent the stomach from digesting its own lining.

The enzyme pepsin is secreted as *pepsinogen*, which is inactive until mixed with acid. The acid is formed in different cells from pepsinogen. The active mixture of the two is not formed until they are free in the cavity of the stomach.

The mucous membrane is protected from this destructive mixture by a layer of mucus.

Acid is not normally formed unless there is food in the stomach to absorb it.

As soon as the acid contents of the stomach flow into the duodenum the acid is neutralized by the alkaline secretion of the duodenum.

Even with these safeguards the mucous membrane suffers considerable injury, but damaged cells are very quickly replaced, probably within 24 hours. Small breaches are very common, but they seldom lead to ulcers.

If the regulation of movement and secretion of the stomach (◊ *stomach* (1)) is disturbed, a small breach of the surface may erode the deeper layers and form a definite ulcer. Excess of acid, and especially the secretion of acid when the stomach is empty, is an important factor in duodenal ulceration. Gastric ulceration may be related to delayed emptying and stagnation of digestive secretions in the stomach. Emotional stress can promote secretion of acid and is almost certainly a cause of peptic ulcers, and certain types of physical stress, e.g. extensive burns, can have the same effect. But for the most part the causes of this disease are unknown. Faulty diet is easy to accuse and hard to convict.

The symptoms always include stomachache. The pain may be anywhere in the upper part of the abdomen, but is usually in the mid-line. If the patient happens to vomit the pain generally goes, and it is nearly always relieved by food or antacid drugs such as magnesium trisilicate; these are all ways of dealing with excess acid, the immediate cause of the pain. Heartburn and nausea are other common symptoms. Most if not all peptic ulcers bleed from time to time and can cause anaemia.

Serious complications include sudden and severe bleeding, perforation of the stomach or duodenum with leakage into the abdominal cavity and peritonitis, and narrowing of the outlet of the stomach. These complications are, as a rule, treated surgically.

Nearly all peptic ulcers can be persuaded to heal by medical (i.e. non-surgical) treatment. The most important part of the treatment, and often the most difficult, is rest. The stomach itself is protected against both distension and complete emptying by small, frequent meals. Smokers can hasten their recovery by not smoking. The drug carbenoxylone (◊ *liquorice*) promotes the healing of gastric ulcers. The activity of the stomach (movement and secretion of acid) is damped down by drugs that suppress the parasympathetic (vagus) nerves – belladonna is the prototype, but newer compounds such as propantheline are pleasanter. Because physical and mental rest are so important, sedatives may be needed for a time. Antacids relieve symptoms, but they are not the first line of defence. Magnesium compounds are favoured because they are not absorbed from the stomach, and do not disturb the chemical balance of the blood as sodium bicarbonate may do (◊ *alkalosis*).

Various forms of surgical treatment are used when simpler treatment fails or when dangerous complications arise. They include removal of the lower part of the stomach where most acid is formed, and operations to by-pass the duodenum. The branches of the vagus nerves that stimulate the stomach can be cut.

There is no sound evidence that peptic ulcers turn to cancer. Duodenal ulcers certainly do not do so: cancer of the duodenum is practically unknown. Cancer of the stomach is so common that mere coincidence might account for an apparent association with gastric ulcer, but a likelier explanation is that some gastric cancer begins with the symptoms of an ulcer. This may be playing with words, and the practical conclusion is that anything that looks like a gastric ulcer needs investigation and treatment.

Some methods of investigation are discussed under ◊ *stomach* (2).

peptone. Partly digested protein.

percussion. A method of examining the chest and other parts of the body by tapping them and listening to the quality of sound, as an inn-keeper judges the amount of beer in a cask from its resonance; described by Auenbrugger in 1761.

Healthy lung tissue emits a clear resonant sound; a pocket of air, as in the stomach, sounds like a drum: solid tissue such as the heart or other muscle sounds dull. Thus the outlines of various organs can be roughly plotted by percussion. If part of a lung is not properly ventilated, or there is fluid between the lung and the chest wall, resonance is lost.

Tapping the skin with a bare finger does not give a very distinctive sound. Auenbrugger overcame this difficulty either by percussing through the patient's shirt or by wearing a glove. A better method is to lay a finger of the other hand on the chest and lightly tap that.

perforation. Piercing of an organ by disease, e.g. of the ear-drum by an abscess (otitis media) or the wall of the stomach by a peptic ulcer.

pericarditis. Inflammation of the pericardium, sometimes a complication of infectious diseases, rheumatic fever and other conditions; sometimes the cause is unknown. Many cases need no special attention beyond the treatment of the primary disease. If fluid collects (pericardial effusion) the heart may be embarrassed and the fluid has to be removed with a hollow needle. But the common causes of effusion are infection, particularly tuberculosis, which can be treated with antibiotics, and thyroid deficiency (myxoedema), treated with thyroid hormone. Another complication of tuberculous pericarditis is thickening and hardening of the pericardium (constrictive pericarditis) which may have to be treated by removing part of the pericardium to prevent mechanical interference with the heart.

pericardium. Fibrous sheath of the heart, enclosing a lubricated membrane like the lining of a joint and allowing the heart to beat almost without friction.

perilymph. Fluid surrounding the organs of hearing and balance in the inner ear.

perinatal. Of the period shortly before, during and shortly after birth. An international standard has not yet been laid down, but the period is roughly from the 28th week of pregnancy until the infant is a month old.

The perinatal mortality rate is the sum of stillbirths and neonatal deaths.

perineal. Of the perineum.

perineum. The external aspect of the outlet of the pelvis, i.e. the region enclosed by the thighs and the lower part of the buttocks, including the external genital organs and the anal canal (◊ *pelvis* (1)). The term is often – especially in midwifery – limited to the bridge of muscle and fibrous tissue between the genital organs and the anus, which is very liable to be injured during childbirth.

periosteum. Fibrous coating of a bone; it carries a network of nerves and blood vessels and is essential to the nutrition of the bone, and is also the sensitive part of the bone. When growth is complete, the periosteum is the one place where new bone can be formed. Fractures do not heal if the periosteum is destroyed. When this happens (it is fortunately a rare occurence) a graft has to be taken from another bone.

peripheral nerves. Cords of nerve fibres, radiating from the central nervous system (brain and spinal cord) and conducting impulses to and from all parts of the body – usually called simply *nerves*.

peristalsis. Rhythmic squeezing movements, flowing along tubular organs such as the intestine and propelling the contents. The rate and force of the contractions is regulated by autonomic (sympathetic and parasympathetic) nerves, but peristalsis itself is an intrinsic property of the muscles in the walls of these organs.

peritoneum. The lining membrane of the abdominal cavity; it forms a thin, transparent layer over the walls of the cavity and the abdominal organs. In effect it is a single closed bag, completely empty. The organs said to be within the cavity – stomach, intestine, liver, spleen etc. – are in fact *behind* it, but they grow forwards, pushing the peritoneum ahead of them. The intestine wanders so far forwards that the two layers of peritoneum join behind it to form the *mesentery*, in which the intestine hangs as if in a fold of a curtain.

The peritoneum is provided with blood vessels, which enable it to exude a thin film of fluid, so that the abdominal organs are lubricated in the same way as the moving parts of a joint. Its nerves convey a sensation of pain if it is stretched or inflamed. Sensation from the peritoneum over the organs is ◊ *referred* to various places, e.g. from any part of the stomach or intestine to the mid-line of the abdomen; but sensation from the peritoneal lining of the belly-wall is correctly localized. Hence with appendicitis the pain from the appendix itself is felt at the navel, but as the inflammation spreads to the neighbouring peritoneum the pain seems to move to the actual site of the appendix, below and well to the right of the navel.

With failure of the heart or kidneys, when fluid tends to leak away from the blood, large quantities may collect in the peritoneal cavity. This type of dropsy is known as *ascites*. Similarly, fluid collects if the peritoneum itself is inflamed.

The peritoneum has remarkable powers of healing. When a section of the intestine is surgically removed and the cut ends have been stitched together, the peritoneal coating forms a watertight seal within a few minutes. When the peritoneum is inflamed (*peritonitis*), for instance after perforation of a diseased appendix, the great danger is that the whole peritoneum will be involved – a most lethal condition. This danger is greatly lessened by the tendency of the inflamed surfaces to stick together – in other words to heal – and so wall off the trouble. This readiness to heal may be a nuisance. Any disturbance such as injury, operation, or infection, may cause two surfaces which should be separate to stick together. Adhesions formed in this way interfere with the normal movements of the intestine or even cause obstruction.

peritonitis. Inflammation of the peritoneum, the result of irritation within the abdominal cavity. The intestines and other organs are regarded as lying outside the true cavity, separated from it by their coating of peritoneum. As long as this coating remains intact it is almost impossible for peritonitis to develop. But if the peritoneum is punctured in any way it is extremely vulnerable. The cavity is a perfect incubator for bacteria, and infection spreads very rapidly from an abdominal wound or from the intestine if, for instance, the appendix is inflamed and

bursts. Until the discovery of antiseptics abdominal surgery was so dangerous as to be virtually impossible, because every attempt was bound to cause peritonitis, which at that time few survived.

Peritonitis can be severe even without bacteria. Acid leaking from a perforated gastric ulcer or bile from a duodenal ulcer irritate and inflame the peritoneum. Chemical inflammation of this kind is soon followed by bacterial infection.

The surface area of the peritoneum is very large. If much of it is inflamed the effect is similar to that of a very extensive burn with profound ◊ *shock*. The abdominal muscles tighten, as muscles over an inflamed area always do, but the intestine is paralysed while the inflammation lasts. The whole abdomen is painful. Fortunately, inflamed surfaces of peritoneum tend to adhere and so to restrict the spread of peritonitis. If this were not so, untreated peritonitis would almost always be fatal within a day or two. As it is, the condition is serious enough, but with the help of antibiotics and surgical operation to deal with the source of the trouble (e.g. repair of perforated intestine, removal of appendix) most cases can now be controlled.

The formation of an abscess – a localized collection of pus – is usually described as a complication of peritonitis. It is certainly a common sequel, but on the whole a desirable one because it is much less dangerous than diffuse inflammation throughout the peritoneum. The usual site is the pelvis, whence the pus can be released into the rectum. The patient with peritonitis is often nursed sitting rather than lying so that if pus should be formed it will gravitate to the pelvis. If infection is allowed to spread upwards a less accessible abscess may be formed between the liver and the diaphragm.

Women are more exposed to peritonitis than men because their Fallopian tubes open directly into the cavity, and infection in the female reproductive organs can spread by the tubes to the peritoneum. This type of peritonitis nearly always results in a pelvic abscess.

Occasionally tuberculosis causes chronic peritonitis. This is not a violent illness like the acute condition described above; it causes ill-defined abdominal symptoms of which the nature is often discovered only at operation. Tuberculous peritonitis is now much less common than it used to be.

peritonsillar abscess. Abscess around a tonsil; quinsy. ◊ *pharynx* (1).

pernicious anaemia (Addisonian anaemia). Defective formation of red blood cells through lack of vitamin B_{12}. ◊ *anaemia* (B.2).

pernio = ◊ *chilblain.*

peroneal. Of the ◊ *fibula*; of the outer side of the lower leg. The peroneal muscles, attached to the fibula, run to the outer side of the foot and are concerned with turning the foot outwards, an important movement when walking on rough or sloping ground and also in adjusting the balance.

perspiration. Since the two words are available, it seems worth while to keep a distinction between perspiration and sweating. Perspiration (insensible perspiration) is passive transudation of almost pure water from the surface of the body at a constant rate of 500–700 c.c. daily – a considerable loss to anyone deprived of water. Perspiration is 'insensible' because the water immediately evaporates.
(Cf. ◊ *sweat* – an active secretion of salt water for the regulation of body temperature.)

Perthes' disease. (Georg Perthes (1869–1927), German surgeon.) Osteochondrosis of the hip; a deformity of the head of the femur (the ball of the ball-and-socket hip-joint) in children, commoner in boys than girls. The cause is unknown, but may be interference with the blood supply by injury. Movement of the affected joint in certain directions, especially outwards, is limited and uncomfortable. The bone can usually be persuaded to grow normally by splinting.

pertussis = ◊ *whooping cough.*

pes cavus. Abnormally high arches of the foot, the opposite condition to flat foot.

pes planus. Flat foot. ◊ *foot.*

pessary. 1. Soluble gelatinous preparation for introducing antiseptic or other drugs into the vagina; vaginal suppository.
2. Appliance inserted into the vagina to support weak ligaments or as a contraceptive.

petechia. Minute fleck of blood in the skin from a bleeding capillary vessel, e.g. with the rashes of some fevers.

pethidine. A synthetic drug related to morphine, with similar pain-relieving properties but less tendency to depress respiration.

petit mal. A minor form of ◊ *epilepsy.*

petrous. Rock-like: the petrous temporal bone houses the inner ear.

phaeochromocytoma. A rare tumour of the medulla of the ◊ *adrenal* gland.

phagocyte. Cell able to engulf and digest bacteria, dead cells etc. The white cells of the blood and certain mobile cells at large in the tissues are phagocytes.

phalanx. A segment of a digit, or the bone of the segment. The thumbs and big toes have each 2 phalanges; the other fingers and toes have each 3. ◊ *hand; foot.*

phantom limb. The illusion that a limb is still present, and sometimes even painful, after it has been amputated. Nerves in the remaining part of the limb contain fibres that used to serve the amputated part, and if these fibres are stimulated the sensation is still ◊ *referred* there.

pharmaceutical. Concerning pharmacy.

pharmacology. Scientific study of drugs – their chemistry, effects on the body, useful and dangerous actions, dosage – including research into new drugs. It is distinct from pharmacy, though the two overlap. Pharmacology is a fairly young science. Until the 19th century it was generally enough to know that a drug was good for this or that disease. Critical studies were rare, and most drugs were given for no better reason than that they were traditional. Withering's study of digitalis (1785) and Jenner's of vaccination were among the very few scientific assessments of methods of treatment before experimental chemistry and biology had advanced far enough for pioneers like Magendie (1783–1855) in France and Buchheim (1820–79) in Germany to make a systematic study of drugs.

pharmacopoeia. List of approved drugs, with notes on their preparation, standards of purity, doses etc.

Between the beginning of the 16th century and the middle of the 19th many academic centres had their own pharmacopoeias for the guidance of local physicians and apothecaries. One of the most useful functions of these books was to ensure that a prescription meant the same thing to the man who wrote it and the man who dispensed it.

From the middle of the 19th century, official national publications began to replace local pharmacopoeias. The London Pharmacopoeia, first published in 1618, gave way in 1864 to the first British Pharmacopoeia, published under government authority by the new General Medical Council. The United States Pharmacopeia, first published in 1820, became official in 1907. The World Health Organization publishes an International Pharmacopoeia, which has no statutory authority but is a valuable guide to national compilers.

pharmacy. Preparation and care of drugs; it is an applied science, related to pharmacology in much the same way as building to architecture. ⟡ *apothecary.*

pharynx. Muscular back-wall of the nose, mouth, and throat, extending from the base of the skull to the entrance of the oesophagus (gullet) half-way down the neck. Its muscle fibres are attached to the underside of the skull, to the ⟡ *hyoid* bone, and to the sides of the *thyroid* and *cricoid* cartilages (⟡ *larynx*). The fibres curve back to meet in the mid-line in front of the backbone.

As regards function the pharynx is in three parts. Above the level of the palate it is the back of the nose, the *nasopharynx*, and concerned only with breathing. During swallowing this part is closed off by raising the soft palate. The lowest part, the *laryngeal pharynx*, behind the larynx, is only for swallowing. Between the two, from the palate to the opening of the larynx, the *oropharynx* is a passage for both air and food.

Swallowing begins as a voluntary action of the tongue and cheek muscles. When they have pushed food to the back of the tongue the action becomes reflex, though all the muscles involved are structurally voluntary muscles (⟡ *muscle*). The palate is raised to close the back of the nose, the epiglottis covers the entrance to the larynx, and the vocal cords close (⟡ *larynx*). Waves of contraction then push the food down to the oesophagus. Gravity plays little part.

The nasopharynx opens into the cavity of the middle ⟡ *ear* by the *Eustachian tube.* This is a narrow channel about 1½ ins. long. From the side of the nasopharynx above the soft palate it runs between walls of cartilage to enter the temporal bone of the skull. It serves to balance the air pressure at the two sides of the ear-drum. A slip of muscle joining the tube to the larynx contracts during swallowing; this pulls the entrance to the tube and allows air to pass if the pressure inside the ear-drum differs from that of the outside ear.

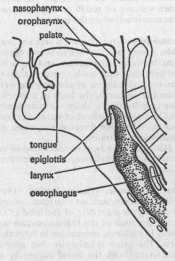

Pharynx (diagrammatic).

The pharynx is encircled with lymphoid tissue (⟡ *lymph*) of which two collections are large enough to deserve names. These are the *adenoids* at the back of the nasopharynx, and the *tonsils* between the pillars of the arch of the ⟡ *palate.* Similar clumps of lymphoid tissue are scattered through the length of the digestive tract. Like the spleen and lymph glands they set up resistance to infecting microbes (⟡ *immunity*). It has been said that the tonsils and adenoids sample the microbes in the inhaled air and form suitable antibodies. This they may well do, but there is little evidence that it is a very useful occupation. In fact, no special function can be ascribed to them.

1. Disorders

Pharyngitis or sore throat is among the commonest of all infections, and fortunately one which usually resolves itself. Bacteria, notably streptococci, tend to be more harmful than viruses in this area. *Scarlet fever* is infection of the pharynx with streptococci which happen also to cause a rash. In children, ◊ *rheumatic fever* is preceded by a streptococcal infection, usually of the pharynx. This type of pharyngitis responds quickly to penicillin and other antibiotics.

Tonsillitis, inflammation of the tonsils, is common in children but not in adults, because the tonsils usually shrivel and virtually disappear in late childhood. So far from combating streptococcal infection some tonsils seem to nurture it, perhaps because their defensive function has been destroyed by previous infection. Surgical removal of the tonsils and adenoids is done much less than it used to be, but it still has a place in the treatment of recurrent sore throat in childhood when the tonsils are obviously unhealthy. Between the two World Wars tonsils were removed wholesale. That the operation has since fallen from favour is partly due to penicillin, but also to the length of hospital waiting-lists. After several months' delay many children have been found not to need the operation after all, and the tendency now is to reserve it for selected cases.

Spread of infection from the pharynx to the surrounding tissues causes unpleasant and possibly dangerous abscesses. The usual site is around the tonsil: this is a *quinsy*. In addition to antibiotics to control the infection a minor operation is often needed to release the pus and prevent it from spreading.

Oedema of the glottis is distension by tissue fluid of the mucous membrane around the entrance to the larynx. It may follow infection but typically it is an allergic reaction like nettle-rash. Anywhere else it would be a minor nuisance, but here it is dangerous because the swelling may be enough to obstruct the airway. Prompt injection of adrenaline or of corticosteroids may reduce the swelling, but an artificial airway may be needed for a time.

phenacetin; phenazone. Two of the earliest synthetic drugs. ◊ *analgesic.*

phenindione. A drug used to prevent blood from clotting, similar to the derivatives of coumarin. ◊ *anticoagulant.*

phenobarbitone. A hypnotic and sedative drug, with a more sustained action than other barbiturates. To a great extent it superseded the bromides, and in the first half of the 20th century was the most popular drug for relieving anxiety. For this purpose the newer tranquillizers have a more selective action, causing less drowsiness. Phenobarbitone is one of the most effective drugs for controlling epilepsy.

phenol (carbolic acid). The prototype of antiseptics and disinfectants: with it, Lister revolutionized surgery. ◊ *infection; antiseptic.*

phenolphthalein. An irritant purgative. Part of a dose is absorbed from the intestine, concentrated in the liver, and returned to the intestine with the bile; the purgative action is then repeated.

phenothiazine. A compound with insecticidal properties. Derivatives of phenothiazine have several medicinal uses. Some are ◊ *antihistamine* drugs for the control of allergic symptoms; these also inhibit vomiting and can be used to treat sea-sickness etc. A drawback is that they sometimes cause drowsiness, but this property has been put to good use: phenothiazine derivatives such as *chlorpromazine* are among the most effective tranquillizers, especially with the more serious forms of mental disturbance.

phenylalanine ◊ *phenylketonuria.*

phenylbutazone. An analgesic drug, particularly effective against the inflammation of rheumatic disorders. ◊ *analgesic.*

phenylketonuria. A rare cause of mental deficiency. It is an inherited recessive character – i.e. both parents must carry the abnormal gene, with a 1:4 chance that a child of theirs will develop the disorder. The actual defect is absence of an enzyme for dealing with the amino-acid *phenylalanine*, which is a component of proteins. An excess of phenylalanine accumulates, and in some unknown way this affects the nervous system.

The condition can be detected soon after birth by chemical analysis of the urine. If the affected child is fed on protein foods from which phenylalanine has been removed, his brain develops normally.

phenytoin. A drug used to control epilepsy.

phimosis. Abnormally tight foreskin, sometimes requiring circumcision.

phlebitis. Inflammation of a vein, generally associated with blockage of the vein by a blood-clot (*thrombosis*). A healthy vein has a smooth, unwettable lining on which blood cannot clot. If the lining is damaged or irritated the surface is roughened and clots can form on it. In fact, one way of treating varicose veins is to inject an irritant, which sets up a mild phlebitis and closes the vein. But with spontaneous phlebitis, such as sometimes occurs in the legs after childbirth or surgical operations, the sequence is probably reversed: the first event is thrombosis, and phlebitis follows as an effect and not a cause. The term *thrombophlebitis* describes the condition and leaves open the question of which comes first.

After an injury such as an operation blood clots more readily than usual – a protective mechanism – but the main reason for thrombophlebitis as a complication of childbirth and operations is immobility, which allows blood to stagnate. The risk has been much less since surgeons gave up insisting on prolonged and complete rest in bed.

The readjustment of a woman's sex hormones in pregnancy causes blood to clot more readily. Oral contraceptives cause a similar readjustment, which may account for the slightly increased tendency to thrombophlebitis among women who take these drugs.

Circulation of blood is impaired only if a very large vein is involved. The part beyond the obstruction (nearly always a leg) then swells, and may remain swollen for weeks or months while new channels are established. A more serious risk is that a piece of clot may be dislodged and travel to the lungs and obstruct a branch of the pulmonary artery. This condition, *pulmonary embolism*, is a danger to life if the piece of clot is large enough to block a major branch of the pulmonary artery. Smaller clots cause a kind of pneumonia; very small ones probably pass unnoticed.

The use of anticoagulant drugs to discourage clotting has lessened the dangers of thrombophlebitis. Occasionally an affected vein has to be sealed with a ligature to prevent the clot from moving. The affected part may need complete rest during the attack, but on the other hand the most effective treatment has been prevention of the attack by precisely the opposite means – avoiding complete immobility – for the flow of blood in veins depends largely on the squeezing action of the neighbouring muscles.

Phlebotomus fever. ◊ *Sandfly* fever.

phlebotomy. Venesection; withdrawal of blood from a vein. ◊ *blood-letting*.

phlegm = ◊ *mucus*; one of the four humours of classical medical theory.

phobia. A kind of neurosis, in which symptoms of ◊ *anxiety* are aroused by a particular object or situation.

phocomelia. A grave congenital defect of the limbs: the hands and feet are fairly normal, but the arms and legs fail to grow. The hands and feet spring from the shoulders and hips like the flippers of a seal. This rare deformity suddenly became much commoner when the drug ◊ *thalidomide* was on the market.

phonocardiogram. Recording of heart sounds.

phosphorus. A non-metallic element, one of the components of living matter. Most of the phosphorus in the body is combined with calcium in bone, and the balance of assimilation and excretion of phosphorus is closely linked to that of calcium.

Certain phosphates, e.g. those of adenosine and creatine, are readily broken down, with release of energy, or re-formed with storage of energy. These reactions play an important part in body chemistry (◊ *energy*).

Most tissues incorporate small amounts of phosphorus. The presence of phosphorus compounds in the insulating sheaths of nerves led to the absurd belief that phosphates must be good for nerves, and to the prescription of 'tonics' containing wholly useless doses of phosphorus in various forms.

The pure element is a most dangerous poison. There are several forms or allotropes (as pure carbon can be charcoal or diamond), of which the white and yellow are dangerous and the red fairly safe.

Phosphorus poisoning has been rare since the prohibition of yellow phosphorus in match-heads.

photophobia. Intolerance of bright light, a common symptom of inflammation of the eyes, of dilatation of the pupils (e.g. by drugs), of migraine, and of meningitis.

photosensitivity. Increased sensitivity of the skin to light, usually of a particular wavelength; exposed areas become inflamed after a very brief spell of direct sunlight. This is an exaggeration of a reaction that anyone suffers with sufficient exposure. ◊ *sunburn.*

phrenic. Of the diaphragm. The *phrenic nerve*, the nerve of the diaphragm on which breathing largely depends, has to traverse the length of the neck and chest before reaching its destination (◊ *diaphragm*). Before the introduction of effective drugs for tuberculosis around 1950, surgical interference with this nerve was often used to paralyse one side of the diaphragm in order to prevent the affected lung from moving while it healed.

Many ancient Greek philosophers regarded the diaphragm as the seat of the mind, and *phren* meant either diaphragm or mind. The second meaning still appears in *schizophrenia.*

phrenitis (archaic). Delirium, frenzy (if the word were used now it would mean inflammation of the diaphragm as such and not of the supposed seat of the disordered mind).

phrenology. An attempt to study the brain from the outward shape of the skull. It was introduced by an able Viennese physician and anatomist, Franz Josef Gall (1758–1828). Phrenology has no basis in fact, but besides this lapse Gall made several valid observations on the anatomy of the brain.

phthisis. Consumption; pulmonary ◊ *tuberculosis.*

physic. The practice of medicine (in the limited sense, excluding surgery and obstetrics); also medicine in the sense of a remedy to be taken.

physician. Medical doctor; specialist in internal diseases. ◊ *doctor.*

physiology. Study of function of living organisms and their different parts. It is the companion of anatomy, which deals with structure. 'Function' is meant in the widest sense, including everything that happens in a living body and how it happens. Physiology is concerned with normal, healthy function, but the boundary between normality and abnormality – the concern of pathology – is not always clear. Similarly, function is so closely related to structure that physiology and anatomy are not as distinct from each other as one might suppose.

Ancient physiology was based largely on speculation, and while serious errors about anatomy persisted, speculation was almost bound to go astray. The early Greek philosophers evolved variations on the theory of ◊ *humours* as the basis of life and matter. None of these was related to fact.

Erasistratus (*c.* 300 B.C.) is generally regarded as the first man to have studied physiology as opposed to thinking about it. He was a junior colleague of Herophilus (◊ *anatomy*) in Alexandria. Erasistratus recognized the main functions of the nervous system and muscles, and came closer than anyone in the next 2000 years to understanding the action of the heart.

After Erasistratus, the next man who might have extended physiology was Galen (2nd century A.D.); but Galen was so wedded to his own mistakes that he made little progress. After Galen, all science came to a halt until the Renaissance.

Of necessity, all other medical sciences had to wait for anatomy to be revived. As the anatomists of Padua revealed structure, so their successors were enabled to make the first proper studies of function.

The earliest of the Paduan physiologists was Sanctorius (1561–1636), who introduced measurement to medical science. (It has been argued that science *is* measurement. By this definition, Sanctorius's studies of pulse rate, body temperature, and the diurnal variation of body weight would make him the originator of modern scientific medicine.) But the turning-point was the discovery by another graduate of Padua – Harvey – of the circulation of the blood, published in 1628. Without this knowledge one can make little sense of the human body: it is like trying to account for the electrical fittings in a modern home without having heard of electricity.

After a considerable pause for Harvey's discovery to sink in, physiology took shape in the hands of scientists such as Hales and Haller in the 18th century, Magendie and Müller in the early 19th century, and Magendie's illustrious pupil Bernard.

The subject is discussed further under the names mentioned in this article, and under such headings as ◊ *circulation; endocrine; nervous system; stomach; vitamins.*

physiotherapy. Treatment of illness by physical means such as massage, exercise, heat and electricity. Massage is a very ancient craft, but it has only recently had much recognition in orthodox medical practice. In Britain, it was not an officially recognized and chartered profession until 1920, and the Chartered Society of Physiotherapy replaced the Chartered Society of Massage and Medical Gymnastics in 1943.

The scope of physiotherapy is now very wide. Its traditional role – the palliative treatment of rheumatic aches and stiff joints – is only one of many, including maintenance or restoration of function after injury (there is not much point in setting a broken bone if the limb is allowed to become stiff and useless), attention to breathing with bed-ridden patients who would otherwise be liable to pneumonia, and training of joints and muscles to be of at least some use after nerve injuries, strokes etc. This last is perhaps the most rewarding part of physiotherapy. Even people with very severe physical disability can be educated to independence, including many with complete paralysis below the level of a spinal injury.

pia mater. Gossamer membrane over the brain and spinal cord, the innermost of the 3 *meninges.*

pica (= magpie). Eating earth or other unsuitable material; a habit of early childhood with obvious dangers. It is generally regarded as a sort of neurosis aroused by insecurity, but some cases have been attributed to iron deficiency.

picrotoxin. Drug extracted from a subtropical berry, used to stimulate respiration.

piles. An *external pile* is a blood-blister at the margin of the anus, which arises from bursting a small vessel while straining. It is harmless but very painful. The pain is promptly relieved by opening the blister, and releasing the clot of blood.

Internal piles: ◊ *haemorrhoids.*

(Other conditions such as *fistula* and *fissure* of the anus are sometimes misnamed piles.)

pilocarpine. Alkaloid extracted from a Central American shrub, with similar actions to *acetyl choline*, occasionally used to constrict the pupil of the eye in treating ◊ *glaucoma.*

pilonidal sinus. A trivial malformation, representing a minor degree of ◊ *spina bifida.* The sinus is a pit in the skin at the base of the spine containing a tuft of hair. As a rule it is harmless. If it becomes a nuisance by getting infected it is easily removed.

pineal body. A small protrusion from the centre of the brain. Its function in man is not known. The pineal body has evolved from a primitive central eye. In a few reptiles it still responds to light and may control the darkening of the skin when the animal is in a bright light. It may also be associated with sexual development. There is some evidence in mammals that chemicals concerned with transmitting impulses in the brain are formed in the pineal body.

Descartes insisted that the soul resided in the pineal body.

pink disease. A rare disease of infants, with redness of hands and feet, neuritis and other symptoms, probably due to mercury poisoning (e.g. from teething powders).

pink-eye = ◊ *conjunctivitis.*

pinna. The visible part of the ear; the auricle.

pinta. A skin disease of tropical America, due to infection with a spirochaete similar to those that cause syphilis and yaws.

piperazine. Synthetic drug for treating intestinal worm infestation.

pituitary body (pituitary gland; hypophysis). The most complex of the ◊ *endocrine* glands; consisting of two distinct organs, the anterior and posterior lobes.

The *anterior lobe* (adenohypophysis) develops in the embryo from the roof of the mouth. It is a typical endocrine gland, composed of hormone-secreting cells of several kinds. The *posterior lobe* is a downgrowth from the floor of the brain, and is a modified part of the nervous system, in effect, a protusion of the *hypothalmus*. The two lobes grow together and hang like a berry from the underside of the brain, occupying a small hollow in the floor of the skull.

The hormones of the anterior lobe regulate growth and the activity of several other endocrine glands. The following hormones have been identified:

1. ACTH (*adrenocorticotrophic* hormone; *corticotrophin*) stimulates the adrenal cortex to secrete cortisol (◊ *adrenal*; *corticosteroid*).

2. *Thyrotrophic* hormone stimulates the ◊ *thyroid gland*.

3. Two *gonadotrophic* hormones stimulate the gonads (ovaries or testes). One, the follicle-stimulating hormone, controls the formation of ova by the ovary or sperms by the testis. The other, the luteinizing hormone, controls the secretion of sex hormones by the gonads. The gonadotrophic hormones are the same for either sex.

4. *Growth hormone* is the principal factor for maintaining growth in childhood and adolescence. It promotes the synthesis of protein and other components of tissues. In adult life the pituitary still secretes small amounts of growth hormone, which influence the control of sugar in the body by the pancreas.

5. *Lactogenic hormone* (prolactin) regulates the secretion of milk.

6. *Melanophore-stimulating hormone* acts on melanophores (pigment cells) in the skin. Its significance in man, if any, is not known.

The hormones of the anterior pituitary are themselves regulated by the *hypothalamus*, a part of the brain immediately above the pituitary. The hypothalamus thus provides a link between the nervous system and the endocrine glands.

Growth hormone and lactogenic hormone act directly on the tissues. The 'trophic' hormones act through other glands, and are regulated by feed-back mechanisms. For instance, ACTH stimulates the adrenals to secrete cortisol. But as soon as there is enough cortisol in the blood, this suppresses the formation of ACTH, by its effect on the hypothalamus, and the stimulus to the adrenals is removed until the concentration of cortisol in the blood falls again. The amount of cortisol needed varies according to factors such as stress,

and the circuit pituitary/adrenal/hypothalamus/pituitary is adjusted in the hypothalamus, which in turn responds to other parts of the brain.

Glands that are regulated by trophic hormones cease to work if the pituitary fails. Conversely, if these glands fail, the pituitary pours out more and more trophic hormones to no purpose.

Complete failure of the anterior pituitary causes *Simmonds' disease*. The symptoms are those of simultaneous failure of thyroid, adrenal, and sex glands, which are very like those of extreme senility. This disease – fortunately rare – is fatal unless regular doses of the missing hormones are provided. Sometimes only one pituitary hormone is lacking, and the symptoms are those of deficiency of the associated gland. Lack of growth hormone in childhood causes *pituitary dwarfism*; these people generally develop normal intelligence but their bodily growth is arrested in childhood unless hormone supplements are given early. Growth hormone has no effect unless it is given early in life.

An excess of growth hormone from a pituitary tumour in childhood causes *gigantism*: the bodily proportions are normal but the dimensions are too big. A similar excess in adult life causes ◊ *acromegaly*.

Cushing's syndrome, an excess of adrenal hormones, can arise from over-activity of the pituitary, with too much stimulation of the adrenals by ACTH.

The *posterior lobe* (neurohypophysis) secretes two hormones:

1. *Oxytocin* stimulates contraction of the uterus at the end of pregnancy and initiates labour. It also promotes the secretion of milk. This seems to be partly a direct action on the breast and partly an indirect action by stimulating the anterior lobe to secrete lactogenic hormone.

2. *Antidiuretic hormone* (ADH) causes water to be retained by the kidneys and restored to the blood, preventing excessive loss of water in the urine. When the blood is slightly diluted after drinking water this hormone is suppressed and the control over the kidneys is relaxed until the surplus of water has been eliminated. A larger amount of ADH than the pituitary normally forms increases the blood pressure. and for this reason the hormone is also called *vasopressin*. Preparations of ADH or a synthetic substitute can be used to sustain

the blood pressure in states of collapse.

A deficiency of ADH causes excessive flow of urine with constant thirst, i.e. ◇ *diabetes insipidus.*

pityriasis. Any skin disease with which dandruff-like scales are shed. *Pityriasis rosea* is a common and harmless rash which clears up in a few weeks, possibly due to a mild infection of the skin surface. Generally a single oval spot, the 'herald patch', appears a week before the main crop of smaller spots.

placebo. A remedy without any direct action on a disease, given to keep the patient happy, or to persuade the prescriber that he is doing something positive and useful, or both. Many carefully conducted trials have shown that some three quarters of all patients feel better after taking placebos (provided that they believe the placebos to be active medicines), and objective tests show that many of them are in fact better. This makes the assessment of a new drug difficult: if the drug is completely inert it will still seem effective. To get a true picture one must compare the new drug either with an old one or with a placebo, given to a similar group of patients. Even toxic effects of new drugs have to be studied with the placebo effect in mind: many of the control subjects given only a placebo (e.g. coloured water) find that the 'medicine' causes drowsiness, insomnia, nausea etc.

placenta. Organ by which an unborn infant gets nourishment from its mother. The placenta develops from the layer of cells surrounding those destined to form the body itself (◇ *embryo*). It is a part of the growing infant's tissues, not the mother's, and its dense network of blood vessels communicates by way of the umbilical vein and arteries with the circulation of the infant. The placenta is firmly attached to the lining of the mother's uterus, but no blood passes between the two. Dissolved oxygen and nutrients diffuse from the mother's blood to the placenta, and carbon dioxide and other waste products diffuse in the opposite direction.

The placenta is released shortly after the birth of the infant, to whom it is still joined by the umbilical cord. At this stage it forms a thick disc, some 6 ins. across, weighing about a pound.

In addition to its main functions as an organ of respiration, nutrition, and excretion for the infant, the placenta acts as an endocrine gland for the mother, secreting hormones that diffuse into her circulation and maintain pregnancy.

placenta praevia. An unusual situation of the placenta, which lies across the opening of the uterus instead of high up and out of the way during birth. It is a cause of bleeding before or during labour, and may necessitate Caesarean section.

plague. A severe infectious fever, due to a bacterium *Pasteurella pestis* transmitted by rat-fleas. The disease is primarily one of rats and other rodents, but spreads to man in times and places where rats and men are in close contact. As rats die of the disease, so their parasites the fleas seek other hosts. The pneumonic form of plague can be transmitted from man to man by coughing.

Bubonic plague is the common form. In addition to the symptoms of any severe infection (fever etc.), buboes appear after a few days. A bubo is a swollen, acutely inflamed lymph node. These painful swellings occur in the armpits and groins and at the sides of the neck. Dark blotches from bleeding into the skin are one reason for the name *black death.*

Pneumonic plague is a fulminating pneumonia due to infection of the lungs with these bacteria. The slate-blue complexion of sufferers from this form of plague was a second reason for calling it the black death.

Without treatment, bubonic plague is fatal in well over 50 per cent of cases, and pneumonic plague in 100 per cent. But streptomycin and other antibiotics control the infection, and if they are given without delay the outlook is good.

At present plague is a rare disease, but it still smoulders in some hot countries, and rats and their fleas are ubiquitous. When sanitary services are disrupted, e.g. by warfare or natural disasters, major outbreaks are still possible. A specific vaccine, repeated yearly, gives good protection.

Some of the great epidemics of antiquity may have been plague, but they cannot be identified with certainty. About the Black Death of 1346–9, the eye-witness accounts of Guy de Chauliac (a physician who had the disease and recovered), Boccaccio (in the introduction to the *Decameron*) and others leave no reasonable doubt: this was wave upon wave of bubonic and pneumonic plague. It killed perhaps half the population of Europe. For the next 3 centuries, plague swept across Europe at intervals, then mysteriously receded. Since the Great Plague of 1665 there have only been local outbreaks.

plantar. Of the sole of the foot. *Plantar warts* are like any others, probably due to a virus infection, but they are more troublesome because of their position. They may disappear if pads are applied to take the weight off them, but a caustic of some kind is often needed to destroy them. Occasionally they have to be cut away.

plasma. The fluid component of blood. ◊ *blood* (1).

Plasmodium. A genus of protozoa, including the parasites of ◊ *malaria*.

plastic surgery. Plastic surgery includes the well-known cosmetic operations such as face-lifting and modifying unshapely noses, but it also deals with repair of lost or damaged tissue. Skin-grafting (◊ *graft*) after extensive burns or other injuries is not done merely to improve the final appearance. It provides the best possible dressing to protect exposed areas from infection and loss of body fluid; it prevents shrinkage of large scars, with deformity and loss of movement, and greatly hastens recovery. Nor is cosmetic surgery only a means of satisfying a patient's whims. It often relieves very real distress.

platelet (thrombocyte). The smallest of the solid particles suspended in the blood, formed by the fragmentation of large cells in the bone marrow and necessary to the clotting of shed blood and the sealing of injured blood vessels. ◊ *blood* (4).

platysma. A thin sheet of muscle fibres under the skin of the neck.

pleura. A double layer of thin membrane surrounding the lungs, analogous with the *pericardium* round the heart and the *peritoneum* in the abdomen, and resembling the *synovial membranes* of the joints. ◊ *lung* (3).

pleurisy. Inflammation of the pleura, practically always due to infection by bacteria or viruses. *Dry pleurisy* causes a characteristic

pain on coughing or taking a deep breath. *Pleurisy with effusion*, where fluid accumulates in the space between lung and chest wall, is painless because the fluid protects the inflamed membrane from friction. *Empyema* is pleurisy with effusion of heavily infected fluid, i.e. pus; it is a kind of abscess.

Bacterial pleurisy is a common accompaniment of underlying infection in the lung, especially of pneumonia. The lungs themselves are insensitive, and the typical pain of pneumonia is entirely due to pleurisy. Pleurisy without apparent cause, especially where there is a large effusion, is often due to unsuspected tuberculosis.

Epidemic pleurisy is a virus infection (◊ *Bornholm disease*).

Treatment of pleurisy itself is mainly palliative: analgesic drugs, warmth, restricting movement of the affected side to relieve pain; removal of fluid, etc. The bacterial types subside as the underlying infection is treated, and virus pleurisy subsides of its own accord. ◊ *empyema*.

pleurodynia. Pain such as that of pleurisy; epidemic pleurisy (◊ *Bornholm disease*).

plexus. Network of veins or nerves. Nerve plexuses include the *brachial* plexus, a system of communicating branches between nerves destined for the arm, at the root of the neck; the *lumbo-sacral* plexus, a similar arrangement for the leg; the *coeliac* (*solar*) plexus of sympathetic nerves in the upper part of the abdomen, and the *cardiac* plexus next to the heart.

Pliny the Elder (A.D. 23–79). Roman civil servant and writer; author of a massive compendium of scientific knowledge and superstition, which included several books on medical matters. Pliny had no personal knowledge of medicine, but because he wrote so much about it he was approved as an authority for many centuries.

plumbism. Chronic poisoning by ◊ *lead*.

pneumoconiosis. Disease of the lungs caused by inhaled dust of various kinds; a common industrial hazard.

At least three types of disease can be distinguished. Simple pneumoconiosis is merely a deposit of inert dust in the lungs, without apparent harm, e.g. the carbon that all city dwellers inhale (*anthracosis*). (City air is poisonous, but not because of carbon particles.) This fairly innocent dirt in the lungs hardly counts as a disease, but with some harmless dusts such as iron (*siderosis*) shadows appear in X-ray pictures of the lung that could be mistaken for more serious conditions.

Irritant dusts such as silica or asbestos inhaled over many years can cause chronic debilitating illness (*silicosis*, *asbestosis*), with formation of fibrous scar-tissue in the lungs. Silicosis is a disease of miners, sand-blasters and others. It is often complicated by tuberculosis. Since affected lungs are permanently impaired, prevention by suppression of dust and regular examination to allow a change of job at the first sign of trouble is more important than treatment.

Another type of pneumoconiosis is due to allergy to dusts such as cotton (*byssinosis*) or moulds (*farmer's lung*). These diseases behave like bronchitis with asthma.

pneumonia. Inflammation of the lungs from infection by viruses or bacteria. It is quite distinct from bronchitis, with which the lining of the main air-passages is inflamed and swollen; with pneumonia the trouble is further down, in the tiny pockets (*alveoli*; see *lung* (1)) at the ends of the air-passages. The walls of the alveoli have to be thin enough to allow oxygen to pass freely from the air to the blood, and they are also thin enough to allow inflammatory exudate – the fluid that leaks from blood vessels during any inflammation – to pass into the alveoli. The distinguishing feature of pneumonia is waterlogging of the alveoli in the affected part. Inflammatory exudate can form a solid clot, so that the part has the consistency of liver, as first described by Morgagni (1761).

Pneumonia can be classified by the distribution of the affected alveoli. In *lobar pneumonia* the whole of one lobe or segment is involved. *Broncho-pneumonia* affects groups of alveoli close to the larger air-passages, so that small patches of inflammation are scattered through the lungs. In a third type, *hypostatic pneumonia*, gravity determines the pattern. In this type of pneumonia the alveoli in the lowest parts of both lungs collect fluid because of poor circulation, just as the feet swell when blood does not circulate properly in the legs. Stagnant fluid in the lungs is a good breeding-ground for bacteria, and hypostatic pneumonia is bacterial infection of fluid already there, unlike other types of pneumonia where the fluid is the result of infection. It is seen only as a complication of other diseases, when an already sick person lies still in bed for a long time.

Since the discovery of antibiotic drugs for treating infection there has been less emphasis on the various patterns of pneumonia and more on the species of microbe, which determines the choice of drug. The commonest bacterial causes of pneumonia are streptococci (including the *pneumococcus* which is the usual cause of lobar pneumonia), staphylococci, and the 'influenza bacillus' (which does not cause influenza). Viruses can be the sole cause of pneumonia, or they can pave the way for bacterial infection, as when pneumococci take over from a common-cold virus.

A text-book case of lobar pneumonia starts either without warning or after a short minor illness with sudden fever, pain in the chest (from inflammation of the ◊ *pleura* or coating of the lung; there is no feeling in the lung itself), and a cough with blood-tinged sputum. (There is no pain if the trouble is in the centre of the lung far from the pleura, and for a time the pneumonia is almost unrecognizable.) After a few days any pain goes, because the inflamed pleura is cushioned by fluid, the cough becomes easier and more effective, but the fever persists. After a week or so the patient may undergo a *crisis* when the fever vanishes almost as suddenly as it appeared together with the other symptoms; or the fever goes by *lysis* (gradually); or the infection spreads outside the lung (◊ *empyema*); or the patient dies. But text-book cases are no longer the rule. With antibiotic drugs the symptoms of bacterial pneumonia usually begin to improve soon after the start of treatment. Whereas previously some 20 per cent of the patients died (in some series as many as 40 per cent) nearly everyone who is reasonably fit before the attack now recovers. Furthermore, bacterial pneumonia is less common than it was; it seems to be giving place to virus pneumonia, which is much less dangerous and runs an altogether less dramatic course.

Despite antibiotics, pneumonia is still a fairly common cause of death, but not among the young and middle-aged who used to be its principal victims. The people still apt to succumb are those who are already debilitated by chronic disease and put up no natural resistance – not even, in some cases, a raised temperature. In them, pneumonia is not so much the true cause of death as the mode of dying from some disease such as failure of the heart, liver, or kidneys.

Until recent years, pneumonia was a common and dangerous complication of major operations, especially operations on the abdomen. Anaesthetics certainly prepared the ground by irritating the lungs, but the main cause was prolonged and complete immobilization in bed, often with tight bandages (to support the wound – and impede breathing). Improved anaesthetics, breathing exercises, and above all a minimum of complete bed-rest have now made post-operative pneumonia a rarity.

pneumothorax. Air in the pleural cavity, between the lung and the chest wall, preventing normal expansion of the lung and so impairing respiration.

Pneumothorax is a complication of penetrating injuries of the chest and of disease of the lungs – in the latter case the air leaks out from the affected lung. Some cases arise without any apparent cause (spontaneous pneumothorax); these may be due to congenital weaknesses in the outer walls of the lungs.

As soon as the leak heals, the air is gradually absorbed until the lung can expand fully again.

Artificial pneumothorax is produced by letting a measured amount of air into the pleural cavity with a hollow needle. It has been much used for treating tuberculosis: the effect is to rest a severely affected lung by preventing its expansion, and allow the inflammation to subside. Since the discovery of streptomycin and other effective drugs this treatment has been used much less than formerly.

podagra = ◊ gout.

poison. Water, oxygen, and the ingredients of a good diet are all poisonous in excess, but the term has to be limited to substances that are harmful in small quantities. If the toxins of bacteria and the venoms of insects, snakes etc. are excluded the list of poisons is still very long. It includes practically all drugs and many minerals and synthetic substances. As a rule, poisons and drugs extracted from plants are dangerous in smaller doses than mineral poisons, but not in quite such minute doses as toxins and venoms.

Corrosive poisons such as acids, alkalis, and many disinfectants alter the chemical state of proteins and therefore indiscriminately damage all living matter. Other poisons interfere with particular chemical reactions in the body; for instance, cyanides prevent the transfer of oxygen in living cells and produce chemical suffocation. Vegetable poisons are often chemically related to substances in the body, which they displace in vital reactions. Their use as drugs depends on these effects, and poisoning is generally an exaggeration of the medicinal effect.

Some of the commoner poisons are described under their own headings. Only a few generalizations can be made here.

Irritants may help to eliminate themselves by causing vomiting or diarrhoea before all the poison has been absorbed from the stomach and intestine. Otherwise the stomach may have to be emptied by means of an emetic such as salt and water or, better, a stomach tube – but this needs expert handling. With corrosive poisons, recognized by staining or burning of the mouth, emetics and purgatives only make matters worse; and if a patient who is not fully conscious is given an emetic he may inhale vomited fluid and so die of the remedy rather than of the poison.

General antidotes include charcoal, which takes up many kinds of poison, and tannic acid (e.g. as strong cool tea), which neutralizes some vegetable poisons by making them insoluble. White of egg may protect the stomach from further damage by corrosive poisons. Milk is probably as good a household antidote as any.

Specific antidotes for some poisons are mentioned under the names of the poisons. Very few are completely effective. More than anything else it is skilled nursing that saves lives after severe poisoning, and all but the most trivial cases are safest in a hospital. The full effects of poisoning may not develop for some hours, and the victim may need continuous artificial respiration or even, with some poisons, the use of an artificial kidney in which the poison is washed from the blood.

policlinic. A clinic or health centre in a town, generally dealing only with out-patients (cf. ◊ *polyclinic*).

poliomyelitis (acute anterior poliomyelitis; infantile paralysis). A virus infection of grey matter in the front part of the spinal cord, affecting the nerve cells responsible for stimulating contraction of muscles. If some of these cells are damaged by the infection the corresponding muscles can no longer work.

The virus is fairly common. In the great majority of cases infection is confined to the throat and intestine, and the symptoms – if any – are those of a minor digestive upset. In a few cases, perhaps only 1 per cent, the spinal cord is involved and groups of muscles are weakened or paralysed. Sensation is not affected. There is little danger to life unless the muscles of the throat and of breathing are paralysed, but in about a quarter of all cases with involvement of the spinal cord there is some permanent loss of muscle power, sometimes confined to small groups of muscles, sometimes more widespread.

Since the virus can be carried by human excrement, good sanitation reduces the risk of infection. This has not been an advantage. Where sanitation is poor, most people are infected in infancy, when paralysis is unusual. In more hygienic surroundings there are enough children and adults who have never been infected, and therefore have no immunity, for epidemics to occur; and these older patients are more prone to serious effects of the disease. But even during an epidemic paralysis is rare in comparison with the numbers who either escape all symptoms or recover completely.

In view of good evidence that fatigued muscles are the most likely to suffer, children under the least suspicion of poliomyelitis are kept as quiet as possible. It is usual to close schools, swimming baths etc. during an epidemic, but since most cases are without symptoms and cannot be traced such measures have little effect; they may, however, help to prevent some of the children at risk from over-exertion. Much the most important method of prevention is the routine use of vaccines. With these, poliomyelitis can be virtually exterminated. Two kinds of vaccine are available, one given by mouth (◊ *Sabin*) and the other by injection (◊ *Salk*).

pollex = thumb.

polyarteritis nodosa. A rare disease, with inflammation of small arteries and impaired circulation in the tissues that they supply, which may be anywhere in the body; thus polyarteritis may show itself as a disease of skin, kidneys, joints, lungs etc. Cases associated with rheumatic fever or tuberculosis may be allergic reactions to some product of the primary disorder. Other cases show many signs of a protracted allergic reaction though no cause can be found. The most successful treatment is with corticosteroid drugs.

polyclinic. Hospital with various specialist departments (cf. ◊ *policlinic*).

polycythaemia. Excess of red blood cells. The number of these cells is normally about 5 million per cubic millimetre of blood (◊ *blood* (2)), with fairly wide variation among healthy people. A figure below 4 million is proof of ◊ *anaemia*, and above 6 million of *polycythaemia*.

Relative polycythaemia is seen with dehydration: the total number of red cells in the circulation is still normal, but they are suspended in a smaller volume of fluid. This state often follows severe injuries, especially burns where large amounts of fluid are lost into the damaged tissues.

Absolute polycythaemia – more cells than usual in the normal volume of fluid – is a natural response to prolonged shortage of oxygen. People who live at very high altitudes have it to compensate for the rarefied atmosphere, and it is also seen with chronic disease of the heart or lungs when oxygen is not delivered to the body at the normal rate.

Polycythaemia vera is a very rare disease in which for no known reason the patient has too many red cells, sometimes as many as 9 million per cubic millimetre. The blood can become so thick that it does not flow properly, and the patient has then to be treated either by blood-letting or by suppressing the formation of new cells with drugs or radiation.

polygraph. An apparatus for simultaneous recording of pulses, invented by ◊ *Mackenzie* for studying heart disease, and later reintroduced in a modified form as a 'lie-detector'.

polymorph (polymorphonuclear leukocyte). A white blood cell with a segmented nucleus. ◊ *blood* (3).

polymyalgia rheumatica. An uncommon but painful affliction, with stiffness and severe aching of muscles, usually worst around the shoulders but sometimes affecting much of the body. The patients are seldom younger than 65. The disease is associated with an obscure type of inflammation of arteries, commonly affecting the temporal artery at the side of the scalp, from which it may spread to the arteries of the eyes. The condition responds well to small doses of corticosteroids, and treatment not only relieves the muscles but prevents damage to the eyesight.

polymyxin. Several antibiotics from the bacterium *Bacillus polymyxa*, of which polymyxins B and E are used medicinally. They are rather toxic, but valuable against infection by the bacterium *Pseudomonas*, which withstands other antibiotics.

polyp (polypus). A tumour, usually harmless, attached to a mucous membrane by a stalk, like a berry. Polyps are common in the large intestine, where they need surgical attention because some intestinal polyps are precursors of cancer. Polyps of quite a different type are often found in the nose. These are not real tumours but simply swellings of the mucous membrane caused by infection or allergy (hay fever).

polypeptide. A compound of two or more amino-acids joined by peptide bonds. The amino (NH_2) group of one joins the acid (COOH) group of the next, with the loss of water. Thus alanine, $CH_3.CH(NH_2)COOH$ and glycine, $CH_2(NH_2)COOH$ (which may be written $HNH.CH_2COOH$), form alanylglycine:

$$CH_3.CH(NH_2)CO\overline{/OH} \; + \; \overline{H/NH}.CH_2COOH$$
alanine $\qquad\qquad\qquad$ glycine
$$\downarrow$$
$$CH_3.CH(NH_2)CO.NH.CH_2COOH \; + \; H_2O$$
alanylglycine $\qquad\qquad$ water

A ◊ *protein* is simply a polypeptide in which hundreds of amino-acids are joined in this way.

When proteins are digested they are broken down to individual amino-acids.

Several hormones are polypeptides. For instance, A D H and A C T H (◊ *pituitary body*) are respectively chains of 8 and 39 amino-acids; insulin, of 51.

polyposis. A hereditary tendency to form numerous polyps in the large intestine.

polysaccharide. A compound sugar, of which each molecule is made up of several molecules of simple sugars; e.g. *starch*, a long branching chain of glucose molecules. Polysaccharides are the principal carbohydrates and main source of energy in most normal diets.

polyuria. Formation of an excessive volume of urine. The word *diabetes* has much the same meaning.

pons (pons Varolii). Part of the brain-stem, above the *medulla oblongata* and below the *midbrain*; it appears to be a broad horizontal band of nerve fibres across the front of the brain-stem. The nerve cells of the 5th, 6th, and 7th cranial nerves are in the pons. Many of the transverse fibres enter the *cerebellum*, which protrudes from the back of the brain-stem at this level.

Bleeding in or around the pons upsets the regulation of the body temperature. Some of the highest fevers are from this cause; on the other hand the patient's temperature may fall to that of the surroundings. But the centre for regulating temperature is not in the pons. This strange effect may be due to compression of fibres passing through the pons from the real centre in the *hypothalamus*.

The name *pons Varolii* ascribes the discovery of the pons to Costanzo Varolio (1543–78) of Bologna. In fact it is clearly shown in earlier drawings of Eustachius, but Varolio was the first to name it.

popliteal. Of the back of the knee. The *popliteal fossa* is a lozenge-shaped space bounded by the tendons of the hamstring muscles above and the calf muscles below. It contains the *popliteal artery* and *vein*, which are the continuation of the femoral vessels into the calf, and the *popliteal nerves*, which are the two terminal branches of the sciatic nerve.

porphyria. A group of hereditary disorders of body chemistry, with excessive production of *porphyrins*, which appear in the urine either as red pigments or as colourless compounds that blacken on exposure to light. All types of porphyria are rare.

In the type with red urine the other important symptom is sensitivity of the skin, especially to sunlight. Disturbances of skin pigmentation and hair growth can also occur.

Other types of porphyria cause episodes

of abdominal pain, mental confusion, and skin disorders. Sometimes attacks are precipitated by other illnesses or by drugs.

porphyrin. A substance combined with iron and protein to form the oxygen-carrying blood-pigment *haemoglobin*. Similar porphyrins are found in most living organisms, e.g. in the green pigment of plants, chlorophyll.

portacaval shunt. Surgical operation to establish a short-circuit between the portal vein and the inferior vena cava, for treating obstruction of veins in the liver. ◊ *portal vein*.

portal vein. A large blood vessel formed from the veins of the stomach, intestine, and spleen. It enters the liver and distributes the materials assimilated from the diet (◊ *digestion*) to the cells of the liver to

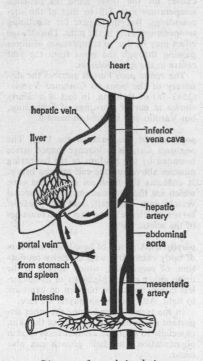

Diagram of portal circulation.

be stored or resynthesized. The blood is returned to the general circulation by the hepatic veins, which enter the inferior vena cava. The portal vein is an ordinary vein as far as the intestine is concerned, removing blood that has already circulated; but to the liver it behaves as an artery delivering blood.

Until birth an infant has no need of its own liver because it has nothing to digest, and the portal circulation is by-passed by the *ductus venosus*, a vessel passing straight from the portal vein to the inferior vena cava. At birth this vessel closes.

Disease of the liver, especially ◊ *cirrhosis*, may impede the flow of blood in the small branches of the portal vein and raise the pressure (*portal hypertension*). This causes leakage of fluid (◊ *oedema*), and large amounts of water may accumulate in the abdominal cavity. The small veins at the entrance to the stomach, where tributaries of the portal vein communicate with veins belonging to the general circulation, become overloaded and may bleed dangerously.

A rare form of portal hypertension arises in infancy from thrombosis (clotting) in the portal vein, probably caused by infection of the umbilical cord.

Portal hypertension can be successfully treated by surgery. Several operations have been devised for diverting some of the blood in the portal vein into the general circulation without its passing through the liver. This relieves the pressure and symptoms, and since the liver has a considerable reserve of function there is little impairment of nutrition.

postmaturity. Condition of an infant at birth after unduly prolonged pregnancy. If labour is delayed beyond a week or two after the normal time for pregnancy to end, the risk to the child may be almost as great as that of prematurity, because the placenta is no longer able to nourish the child sufficiently. The mother's difficulties may be increased if the child's bones begin to harden. Postmaturity is treated either by artificial ◊ *induction* of labour, or by Caesarean section.

posture. In physiological terms, posture is a complicated system of reflexes. The muscles used to maintain posture are the same as those used for voluntary movements – mainly those of the backbone and legs, but also many others – but their governing nerve cells receive unconscious as well as conscious stimuli. These are co-ordinated by the cerebellum and other unconscious parts of the brain, responding to unconscious sensation such as imminent loss of balance. Normally, the muscles of posture are so nicely balanced that they do practically no work. Some muscular pain ('fibrositis') is probably due to abnormal posture, e.g. the slumped posture of depression or the taut posture of anxiety,

potassium. Metallic element, similar to sodium. In test-tube chemistry these two elements are almost interchangeable, but in the body life itself depends on the correct balance between a high concentration of potassium inside the cells and a high concentration of sodium in the surrounding fluids. Nerve impulses are transmitted by electrical currents associated with a momentary exchange of sodium and potassium. A small excess or deficit of potassium interferes with the action of the heart, and larger changes are enough to stop it. When fluid is lost from the body, e.g. from diarrhoea or burns, or when the balance between intake and loss of potassium is disturbed by certain drugs, the correct amount of potassium may have to be maintained artificially. Most fruits provide a good supply, but sometimes potassium salts have to be given medicinally.

Pott, Percivall (1714–88). London surgeon; he gave the first description of the injury since known as *Pott's fracture*. With this serious injury of the ankle, the foot is twisted outwards (in the opposite direction to the common sprain). The fibula, at the outer side of the leg, is broken above the ankle joint, and at the inner side of the joint either the lowest part of the tibia breaks or the ligament binding it to the foot tears. The ankle joint is then unsupported and becomes dislocated. Pott is usually said to have suffered this fracture himself when crossing London Bridge, but it seems that his leg was broken higher up. He bought the front door of the nearest house for a stretcher and had himself carried to Guy's Hospital, saying that the only good surgeon at his own hospital, St Bartholomew's, had just broken his leg.

Pott's disease is paralysis of the legs through damage to the spinal cord by tuberculosis of the backbone.

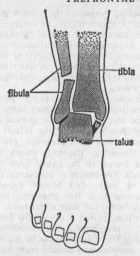

Pott's fracture-dislocation. The supporting bones at each side of the ankle are broken and the foot is displaced outwards.

Pott was the first man to identify a cause of cancer: chimney-sweep's cancer of the scrotum from repeated contamination with soot.

poultice. A kind of dressing applied hot to inflamed areas to relieve pain by *counter-irritation* and perhaps to increase resistance to infection by increasing the flow of blood. The objection to poultices is that they tend to make the skin soggy and liable to harbour further infection.

practolol. Drug with similar effects to ◊ *propranolol*.

prediabetes. A condition without symptoms thought to precede real diabetes mellitus, and to account for the fact that dietary indiscretion (and also certain drugs) can precipitate diabetes in some people but not in others.

prednisolone; prednisone. Synthetic derivatives of ◊ *corticosteroid* hormones.

prefrontal lobe. The foremost part of the brain; apparently concerned with intellect and personality. Some severe forms of mental disorder have been relieved by operations to isolate the prefrontal lobes (◊ *leukotomy*).

pregnancy. Pregnancy lasts from conception until labour. It lasts, on average, for 38 weeks. Because the date of conception is often uncertain, it is convenient to date pregnancy from the first day of the last menstrual period, which is likely to be a fortnight before conception, making a total of 40 weeks.

The many changes that occur – provision for nourishing the developing baby, cessation of menstrual periods, growth of the uterus, development of the breasts – are brought about by a hormone, progesterone, formed in the early stages by the *corpus luteum* in the ovary, later by the placenta. The ending of pregnancy, formation of milk, and labour depend on hormones from the pituitary, but the mechanism is not fully understood.

A missed period is usually the first indication of pregnancy, but it is not completely reliable. The diagnosis can be made with some confidence by clinical examination of the uterus a few weeks later, and it is absolutely proved when the heart beat of the foetus is heard half-way through pregnancy (much sooner with an electronic stethoscope) or movements are felt; the woman herself is aware of these movements some weeks before the examining doctor or midwife. The characteristic hormones in the urine can be detected about a month after conception by tests with animals: Aschheim-Zondek (mice), Friedman (rabbits), or Hogben test (xenopus toads).

Biologically it can be argued that childbearing is the normal condition of fertile women. This at least gets away from the idea of pregnancy as a sort of illness – a puritanical idea that accounts for some of the disagreeable symptoms associated with pregnancy. Symptoms such as nausea, fainting (commoner in fiction than fact), and emotional instability are due in the first place to incomplete adaptation to the altered output of hormones. They seldom last more than a few weeks, but they can be aggravated and prolonged by worrying about them.

A pregnant woman can easily eat more than she needs, either because she is anxious not to deprive the baby or simply because she feels hungry, and afterwards it may be difficult to lose the extra weight. In fact, the *quantity* of food she needs is not much increased, but the *quality* needs attention. In particular she may need supplementary iron and vitamins.

Although pregnancy is normally a healthy state, certain precautions are needed. With adequate ante-natal care the risks of pregnancy and labour can mostly be overcome, because the more dangerous complications can be anticipated and dealt with. Careful explanation is almost as important as the routine check of progress of the developing infant and health of the woman; her labour is much easier if she knows exactly what will be expected of her.

prematurity. An infant is said to be premature if its birth-weight is less than 2·5 kg. (5½ lb.). This is an unsatisfactory definition because it suggests that new-born babies should all be the same size. In fact, small parents can expect to have perfectly healthy babies that would be premature according to the definition, and other people may have babies of 'normal' weight that are underdeveloped at birth and need special care. What matters is the stage of the baby's development at birth. A baby that is born too soon is not yet able to maintain a normal body temperature, mainly because the protective fat develops only in the final weeks of pregnancy. The truly premature baby is also more vulnerable to temporary lack of oxygen than a full-term baby. A normal full-term baby can manage without oxygen for some minutes, presumably by converting glucose to lactic acid (◊ *muscle* (1)); but a premature baby cannot because he has no store of glucose.

The term 'small for dates' describes babies whose development is not as advanced as it should be at a given stage of pregnancy: thus at full term, i.e. after 9 months' pregnancy, the baby may have reached only the stage that it should have reached at 8 months. This is a kind of prenatal malnutrition due to a defective placenta. The remedy is not to try to prolong pregnancy, but on the contrary to get the baby born as soon as it is safe and then treat it as a premature infant. ◊ *postmaturity.*

premenstrual tension. Some women have emotional disturbances, headaches and other symptoms for a few days before menstruation, because the normal changes in the secretion of hormones at this time are exaggerated and cause salt and water to accumulate; this particularly affects the nervous system. The symptoms are relieved by ◊ *diuretic* drugs, which promote the excretion of salt and water by the kidneys.

Premenstrual tension affects judgement. Affected women are prone to accidents and abnormal behaviour. Many industrial accidents are avoided by transferring female workers to safer jobs during the premenstrual phase.

presbyacusis. Loss of hearing in old age – a gradual process that starts in adolescence. High-pitched sounds are most affected, so that consonants are not distinguished though vowel sounds can still be heard.

presbyopia. Loss of the ability to focus the eyes in old age.

prickly heat (miliaria). An itchy rash due to blockage of sweat glands, with the formation of minute blisters, commonest among newcomers to tropical climates. Various lotions are used and may help, but the only completely effective treatment is to keep cool. Light clothing – cotton for choice – is essential.

primaquine. A synthetic drug for treating malaria.

primidone. A drug used for controlling epilepsy.

probenecid. A drug that interferes with the passage of certain substances from the kidneys to the urine or vice versa. It prevents the excretion of penicillin into the urine, and so enhances the effect of a dose of penicillin. On the other hand it prevents the kidneys from reabsorbing uric acid into the blood-stream from the urine, and is therefore used to eliminate uric acid in the treatment of gout.

procaine. One of the most successful local anaesthetic drugs.

proctology. Study and treatment of disorders of the rectum.

progesterone. A hormone secreted by the *corpus luteum*, i.e. the small gland that develops in an ovary each month at the site from which an ovum or egg has been released. Progesterone stimulates development of the uterus to receive a fertilized ovum and nourish the embryo. If the ovum is fertilized and pregnancy occurs, the corpus luteum and later the placenta continue to form progesterone, which pre-

vents menstruation and the release of more ova. If pregnancy does not occur, the corpus luteum withers.

The action of progesterone in preventing ova from being shed is the basis of the contraceptive pill.

prognosis. Prediction of the course of an illness.

progressive muscular atrophy. A form of ◊ *motor neurone disease*

proguanil. A drug used for treating and preventing malaria.

prolactin. Lactogenic hormone, formed in the anterior lobe of the pituitary and stimulating the formation of milk.

prolapse. Displacement of an organ from its normal position, usually by gravity as a result of weakness of the supporting tissues. Prolapse of the rectum – extrusion of a segment of bowel through the anus – is not uncommon in children. Most cases respond to simple measures such as holding the buttocks together with adhesive plaster and education of the muscles, but a few need surgical reconstruction.

Prolapse of the uterus is common in women who have borne several children, especially if the supporting muscles and ligaments have been badly stretched or torn. A supporting ring (pessary) in the vagina often controls a slight prolapse but many patients find this unpleasant and unhygienic, and prefer a surgical operation. More severe prolapse can only be treated surgically, either by reconstructing the supporting tissue or, in extreme cases, by removing the uterus.

pronation. Turning the hand palm downwards; the opposite movement is *supination*.

prontosil. The precursor of the ◊ *sulphonamides*, and indirectly of penicillin and other antibiotics.

prophylaxis. Prevention of disease: anything from vaccination to a daily walk.

propranolol. A drug used to impede certain effects of adrenaline and of stimulation by sympathetic nerves. In particular, it prevents excessive stimulation of the heart, and is used to forestall attacks of angina when the capacity of the heart for work is limited by a poor blood supply.

proprioception. Sensation from muscles, joints etc., conveying information (not always consciously perceived) about their position in relation to the rest of the body so that posture is maintained by reflex movement.

prostaglandins. A group of substances derived from fatty acids, first identified in 1935 and thought to originate in the prostate gland, but now known to occur in most tissues. Under experimental conditions they have various biological actions, but it is not yet known whether in the living body they serve as hormones or are incidental by-products. They stimulate the pregnant uterus, and are used to procure abortion or induce labour. Reports from China suggest that they may promote the healing of gastric ulcers.

prostate gland (prostata). One of the male sex organs: it is a rounded mass of muscle fibres and small glands immediately below the urinary bladder, surrounding the outlet of the bladder (urethra). It secretes a part of the seminal fluid in which sperms from the testis are suspended.

Inflammation of the prostate is an occasional complication of infection elsewhere in the urinary system (tuberculosis, gonorrhoea etc.). The prostate can be injured by a blow between the buttocks, and it may be irritated by continuous pressure – e.g. in a long-distance lorry driver with a badly sprung seat. With all disorders of the prostate a firm seat is more comfortable than a soft one that can press upwards between the buttocks.

Much the commonest disorder of the prostate is overgrowth of its glandular elements in middle or old age. The ill effects are purely mechanical. Because the enlarged gland causes a sensation of pressure at the outlet of the bladder, the patient has a frequent urge to pass water (as a patient with large piles feels that he has to open his bowels). And the encroachment on the urethra tends to obstruct the flow of urine. In time, it may be impossible to empty the bladder completely, and the stagnant remainder of urine is liable to become infected with bacteria and damage the bladder and kidneys. If a large amount of urine is retained, the added pressure is a further embarrassment to the kidneys.

Removal of the enlarged part of the prostate is a fairly simple operation. Most surgeons advise early operation, because the risk is much increased if the kidneys are already damaged. If the operation is done when the symptoms first become a serious nuisance the results are extremely good.

Another reason for early attention is that a few cases of enlarged prostate are due to cancer, which become incurable if treatment is delayed. The best treatment of cancer of the prostate is to remove it, but if this is not possible or not advisable the cancer can be effectively discouraged by disturbing the hormones that regulate the prostate, by removing the testes or giving drugs such as stilboestrol.

prosthesis. Artificial substitute for a part of the body (e.g. false teeth, glass eye, wooden leg).

protamine. A protein derived from fish, used (1) as an antidote to the ◊ *anticoagulant* drug heparin, and (2) to form compounds with ◊ *insulin* with a prolonged effect.

protein. Proteins are essential ingredients of all living matter. They make up about 12 per cent of the weight of the human body (water is 70 per cent, fat 15 per cent). A molecule of protein is a chain of several hundred amino-acid molecules (◊ *polypeptide*). Amino-acids are composed of carbon, hydrogen, oxygen, nitrogen, and sometimes sulphur. Some 22 different kinds of amino-acid are involved. The biological properties of a protein depend on the exact sequence of different amino-acids in the chain (primary structure), their orientation (secondary structure), and the shape of the chain as a whole (tertiary structure). Small differences make for totally different proteins, and the possible permutations are almost unlimited. Other components of living matter vary little; it is in the arrangement of their proteins that species and individuals differ.

The proteins of the food (◊ *diet*) have to be broken down so that the amino-acids can be rearranged as specifically human proteins. A non-human protein introduced into the tissues provokes a defensive reaction (◊ *immunity; allergy*) and is rejected. Similarly a human protein that differs in any respect from the recipient's proteins is treated as non-human: this is the obstacle to transplantation of organs from one person to another.

Most of the protein dissolved in the blood (plasma protein) is assembled in the liver. The cells of the various tissues form their own proteins from amino-acids that diffuse from the blood into the tissue fluid. The exact structure of a protein is determined by the particular nucleic acid, in the cell nucleus, responsible for its synthesis. Nucleic acids for the synthesis of all the proteins of the body are determined at the time of conception, and hereditary characters depend on their precise nature. In essence, what parents pass to their children is the ability to form particular proteins. Many proteins are common to the whole race, but many show minor individual variations. Apart from identical twins, no two people are likely to have an exactly similar set of proteins.

Protein is mainly used in the structure of tissues. Any surplus can be used as fuel (◊ energy). The nitrogenous portion of amino-acids is converted to urea and excreted by the kidneys, and the residue is oxidized to carbon dioxide and water. If the diet does not contain enough ordinary fuel (carbohydrate and fat) the subject may be short of protein because he burns it instead of using it for growth and repair of tissue. Protein-energy malnutrition is thought to arise in this way. Two severe and superficially very different forms are ◊ kwashiorkor and ◊ marasmus. Treatment with a high-protein diet is not enough; the other ingredients of the diet also need attention, as do concurrent infections.

Proteus. A genus of bacteria: as a rule they are harmless but they can cause serious trouble when other bacteria have been eliminated from wounds, etc., with antibiotics.

prothrombin. A substance dissolved in blood, necessary to clotting. Prothrombin itself is inactive, but when blood is shed prothrombin is converted to thrombin, which together with several other factors causes blood to clot.

protoplasm. The characteristic material of most living tissue, based on a jelly-like suspension of protein in water.

protozoon. The protozoa are the smallest and simplest creatures that can be called animals. They form a diverse group with the common characteristic that their bodies are not divided into separate functional units or cells. They differ from simple plants such as algae in depending on other living creatures for their food; but the distinction between plants and animals at this low level is vague, and there are many borderline cases. The sizes of protozoa lie between 0·005 and 0·5 mm.

In general protozoa reproduce themselves by dividing into two equal parts, each of which grows to a replica of the original organism, able to divide again when it is large enough. In some species there is also a kind of sexual reproduction. At its simplest this is merely a fusion of two seemingly identical 'parents' which later split into 'offspring'. Some protozoa, such as the malaria parasite, have an elaborate life-cycle in which male and female forms appear.

A few species of protozoa are parasitic to man: ◊ dysentery; giardia; leishmania; malaria; toxoplasmosis; trichomonas; trypanosome.

proximal. Nearer to the centre of the body or to the trunk (as opposed to distal).

pruritus = ◊ itch.

pseudarthrosis. False joint, resulting from failure of a broken bone to heal: instead of joining, the broken ends become sealed with hard bone, and the fracture cannot then heal without a surgical operation. ◊ fracture.

pseudocyesis. False pregnancy, with symptoms of a real pregnancy. The basis is emotional, but emotion affects the formation of hormones by the pituitary gland, with physical effects like those of pregnancy. This is a rare neurosis in Western society, but much commoner where husbands may disown barren wives.

pseudomembrane. A skin of dried secretion at the back of the throat, as in diphtheria.

Pseudomonas. A genus of bacteria. One species, Ps. aeruginosa, can cause very troublesome infection, especially in hospital wards. It forms a characteristic blue pigment. This organism was formerly called *Ps. pyocyanea* with reference to the bluish pus.

psittacosis. Pneumonia due to a virus carried by birds of the parrot family; a kind of ◊ *ornithosis*.

psoas. A large muscle attached to the front of the lumbar vertebrae and passing in front of the hip-joint to the femur. It flexes the hip-joint, i.e. draws the thigh forwards and upwards.

psoriasis. A common disorder of the outer layer of the skin. The typical appearance is of thickened red blotches with a scaly surface, most often on the scalp, back, and arms. Fortunately the face is hardly ever affected, even when the blemishes are very wide-spread. In most cases the blemishes are the only symptom. Itching is unusual, and the general health is affected only in rare cases where the disease spreads rapidly and becomes dangerous unless treated. What distresses the patient is the disfigurement and the feeling – associated with any obvious skin disease – that he is somehow 'unclean'. In the past this feeling was wholly justified, because psoriasis was confused with leprosy and syphilis, both considered marks of divine disapproval.

Contagion plays no part in this disease. Only people with a hereditary predisposition ever suffer from it. Probably 1 per cent of people have psoriasis at some time in their lives; the true figure may be much higher because not every sufferer has it badly enough or for long enough to get medical advice. An actual attack can be precipitated by injury, acute illness, or, it seems, by emotional upsets.

Skin is adapted to wear and tear by continuous replacement of its surface. The tough protective outer layer consists of dead, flattened cells like scales. As these are shed the next layer of cells is adapted to take their place on the surface, to be replaced by fresh living cells from still deeper in the skin. New cells are formed in the deeper layer as fast as dead cells are shed from the surface, and the thickness of the skin remains constant. In psoriatic skin the whole process is accelerated; new cells are formed more quickly than dead cells are being shed, and the living undercoat of the skin becomes too thick. Various abnormalities of microscopical structure and tissue

chemistry have been described, but whether they are causes or effects of the visible changes is not known. The primary defect may be in the capillary blood vessels of the skin, which are abnormally tortuous and dilated in predisposed people whether or not psoriasis has developed.

Psoriasis may be accompanied by a peculiar form of arthritis resembling but distinct from rheumatoid arthritis.

Even without treatment psoriasis tends to come and go. With treatment it can nearly always be cleared up, at least for a time. But the predisposition remains, and more often than not the trouble returns and has to be treated again and again. The simplest remedy is sunlight or artificial ultraviolet radiation, and it improves all but a few psoriatics who cannot tolerate it and are made worse. Coal tar acts by sensitizing the skin to light. Many other applications have been used. Different patients respond differently and the best treatment has usually to be found by trial and error. Most forms of treatment work by hastening the shedding of dead skin to keep pace with the overproduction in the deeper layers. Recently, cytotoxic drugs which discourage the over-production have given promising results. But no lasting cure has yet been found, and the luckiest patients (apart from those whose psoriasis vanishes of its own accord) are those who can come to terms with it as an idiosyncrasy that is unlikely to endanger them and cannot possibly harm anyone else.

psychiatry. Study and treatment of mental and emotional disorders; it is related to *psychology* as surgery to anatomy. (For a general discussion and references to particular disorders, ◊ *mental deficiency; mental illness*.)

psychoanalysis. A method of treating mental illness, originated by Freud. The illness, expressed in the conscious mind, is seen as the result of conflicts between instinct and conscience, or of fears aroused by early memories that are too painful to be borne and are therefore pushed into oblivion – where they persist, beyond the reach of reason, to trouble the conscious mind. Psychoanalysis attempts to bring these suppressed conflicts and fears to the patient's consciousness. This precipitates an emotional crisis or release (*abreaction*) after which the patient is better able to understand and cope with his problem. Even very early memories can be revived, but it is a slow process. Under hypnosis it can be done much more quickly and easily, but without the same success, for then it is the hypnotist who uncovers suppressed memories. The point of psychoanalysis is that the patient must do this for himself. The analyst usually knows what the answer will be after only a few sessions, but he must wait until the patient is ready to overcome his own resistance to facing it.

Psychoanalysis has aroused a great deal of controversy. To the uninitiated it may seem more like a cult than a science; it even has its own semi-mystical vocabulary, and tends to dismiss its critics as merely ignorant. The schisms within psychoanalysis make it still harder for unbelievers: unless analysts can agree among themselves they are not likely to persuade the sceptics. Yet nobody doubts that psychoanalysis has theoretical and practical merits. Perhaps so much depends on the analyst himself that what is true for one may be untrue for another, and no general rules are valid.

An important objection to psychoanalysis is that it takes far too long: months or even years. Few patients can afford the treatment, and in any case there could never be enough trained analysts to go round. But if the number of people who have been directly helped is small, every part of psychology has been illuminated by Freud's work. Simpler forms of treatment that a purist might reject, but that work in practice, have been evolved. Many patients are helped by studying particular aspects of their suppressed conflicts rather than reconstructing their whole emotional life-history.

psychology. Study of the mind – of perception, thought, emotion, learning, behaviour. No simple definition is possible, because not all psychologists agree about what, precisely, they are studying. It is perhaps best to leave the word *mind* out, because it is itself such a vague concept. Modern psychology is mainly concerned with behaviour and the factors that determine it. *Behavioural psychology* is in one sense the part of psychology that deals with responses that can be observed and objectively recorded, but in another sense it is the whole of scientific psychology, because science is a matter of observations and the con-

clusions that can be logically drawn from them. Psychology approached from this direction claims ◊ *Pavlov* rather than ◊ *Freud* as its patron, and is a part of general physiology. *Experimental psychology* is of necessity based largely on behavioural studies, because the Freudian and other analytical schools of thought are concerned with abstract concepts that are not open to subjective experiment.

Psychiatry is a part of medical practice, the specialty that is concerned with mental abnormality exactly as cardiology is concerned with the heart. *Clinical psychology* is not quite the same thing as psychiatry. A clinical psychologist usually works with psychiatrists, but does not necessarily hold a medical qualification. He may be involved in psychiatric research, in specialized forms of diagnosis such as testing intelligence, or in treatment such as behavioural therapy or analysis (which is diagnosis and treatment combined).

psychoneurosis = ◊ *neurosis.*

psychopath. A term that embraces anyone whose behaviour is unacceptable to the society in which he lives; a psychopath might be defined as someone with a defective conscience – leaving conscience still to be defined.

The Mental Health Act of 1959 defines *psychopathic disorder* as 'a persistent disorder or disability of mind (whether or not including subnormality of intelligence) which results in abnormally aggressive or seriously irresponsible conduct on the part of the patient, and requires or is susceptible to medical treatment'.

Psychopaths include road-hogs, moral delinquents, and violent criminals. The common factor is lack of regard for others, of a social sense. They may require, but are not always susceptible to, medical treatment. Their trouble (or rather the trouble that they give to society) seems to arise from emotional isolation in childhood, a lack of warmth or affection. Better training in parenthood is the most hopeful remedy. But in some cases there may also be a constitutional defect. A significant number of habitual criminals have abnormal sex chromosomes (an additional X chromosome), and some show a characteristic anomaly in the electroencephalogram.

psychosis. Severe mental disorder involving

loss of touch with reality; insanity as ordinarily understood. ◊ *mental illness.*

psychosomatic disease. Any illness in which disturbance of the mind causes physical changes in the body.

Emotion is expressed in the conscious mind, and also at a completely unconscious level of the brain where it stimulates reflex action in the sympathetic and para-sympathetic nerves, which are distributed throughout the body and regulate functions such as rate of blood-flow and digestion. Emotion also affects the activity of the ◊ *pituitary* gland, which in turn regulates several other glands.

Few if any physical diseases are due entirely to emotional upset; what emotion does is to exaggerate the effects of physical causes. Individual cases of a disease differ widely in the relative importance of physical and emotional causes. For example, *asthma* is a narrowing of the air-passages in the lungs. Emotion may cause reflex spasm of the muscle fibres in the walls of these passages and so precipitate an attack of asthma – but it can do so only in some-one who is liable to asthma because of a physical anomaly. There is an emotional element in asthma, slight in some cases, predominant in others; but it is combined with allergy and other physical elements.

Diseases in which emotion can play a major part include various disorders of the skin, where blood vessels and sweat glands can both be affected; digestive disorders including overeating, duodenal ulcer, colitis with chronic diarrhoea; migraine; high blood pressure and perhaps other disorders of the heart and circulation. For many experts (if there can be experts in such an ill-defined branch of medicine) even this short list is too long; for others the list should be expanded to include dozens of diseases that might appear to have purely physical causes.

If conditions ascribed to ◊ *stress* are included, then psychosomatic diseases are a very large group. It is a commonplace that tuberculosis and other infections can light up under emotional strain. After severe injuries, the patient's anxiety contributes to the danger. It has been suggested that in these and similar situations emotional stress overworks the adrenal glands and lowers resistance, with serious, even lethal physical effects.

psychotherapy. Treatment of mental dis-orders, especially by teaching as opposed to drugs or physical interference. Examples of large-scale psychotherapy are ◊ *behaviour therapy* and ◊ *psychoanalysis.* But nearly all forms of treatment include an element of psychotherapy. A physician making brief notes of a patient's symptoms is establishing the facts from which he will infer a diagnosis, but at the same time he is allowing the patient to unload some of his worries. And even the most useless pre-scription (◊ *placebo*) conveys a measure of confidence.

ptomaine. A product of decomposition of protein by bacteria, i.e. of putrefaction. Ptomaines are poisonous and were once thought to be a main cause of ◊ *food poisoning.* In fact it is the bacteria, not the ptomaines, that cause the trouble.

ptosis. Sagging or drooping of an organ, especially of the upper eyelid from weak-ness of its muscle.

ptyalin. An enzyme in saliva, promoting the conversion of starch to sugar.

puberty. Onset of sexual maturity or fertility, brought about by stimulation of the gonads (ovaries or testicles) by hor-mones from the pituitary gland. The gonads begin to form fertile ova or sperms, and also to secrete hormones that promote adult sexual characters (body hair, female breasts, male voice etc.). The time of puberty is established in girls by the first menstrual period, following the first ovulation; in boys there is no such precise moment.

For a year or two after puberty the whole body seems to be adjusting itself to the altered system of hormones – not sur-prisingly, since the whole body chemistry is affected to some extent. The difficulties of puberty are mainly emotional. Physical readjustment is seldom a problem, except that a sudden burst of activity in the grease glands of the skin causes *acne* at precisely the time of life when a disfiguring skin complaint is hardest to bear.

The age of puberty varies widely among perfectly normal children; and even when it is several years away from the average there is generally no abnormality. Delayed puberty may sometimes be due to a relative deficiency of pituitary hormones; but the

363

causes of puberty – normal or abnormal – are not really known.

It is not true that puberty occurs at a younger age in the tropics or in dark-skinned people. It is, however, true that the average age of puberty in Western Europe has decreased considerably in the past century – from over 15 to about 13 in girls, and a year or two later in boys. The reason is not known. It may simply be that the average child of a century ago was under-fed and therefore underdeveloped; this would also explain why the average English boy now grows an inch or two taller than the average boy of 100 years ago.

pubis. A bone forming part of the ◊ *pelvis*.

puerperal. Related to childbirth; affecting a woman who has recently given birth.

Puerperal fever (puerperal pyrexia) can mean any high temperature following child-birth, but is generally taken to mean infec-tion of the birth-passage as a result of childbirth.

No child is born without some injury to the mother. The soft linings of the uterus and vagina are at least bruised by the head and shoulders of the child, and the placenta, having been firmly stuck to the inside of the uterus, leaves a raw area when it is expelled. If labour is difficult, more extensive injury is likely; but these tissues heal quickly, and as a rule are repaired within a couple of weeks. But until healing is complete the birth-passage is vulnerable to infection. What was an ideal incubator for the baby becomes an ideal incubator for bacteria. Streptococci cause some of the worst cases, but in such an environment most kinds of bacteria can set up rapidly spreading and dangerous infection.

Until the mid 19th century death from puerperal fever was appallingly common, and the growth of hospitals was making matters worse because infection was carried from patient to patient. Estimates run as high as one death among every 4 nursing mothers in some hospitals. ◊ *Semmelweis* in Vienna wrote that until he insisted on routine disinfection of the attendants' hands, patients whose labour was pro-longed nearly all died of puerperal fever. But by that one simple precaution, Semmel-weis brought the mortality below one in 100. By the turn of the century the figure had fallen to one or two per thousand, where it remained until effective drugs were found – sulphonamides in 1935, penicillin in 1941. In recent years, mortality from puerperal fever has fallen almost to vanish-ing point: it has been of the order of one in 100,000 births in England.

In the United Kingdom and some other countries puerperal pyrexia (high tempera-ture after childbirth, regardless of cause) is a ◊ *notifiable disease*.

pulmonary. 1. Of the lung (e.g. pulmonary tuberculosis). **2.** Of the pulmonary arteries (e.g. pulmonary embolism, stenosis).
Pulmonary artery. The right ventricle of the heart pumps blood from the veins into the right and left pulmonary arteries, to be circulated through the lungs and replen-ished with oxygen. Because these vessels carry dark blood, depleted of oxygen, un-like the bright red oxygenated blood of other arteries, Galen called them the *venous arteries*.
Pulmonary embolism. A clot of blood in a vein has a clear passage through the right side of the heart to the pulmonary arteries, if it is dislodged. The original site of such a clot is usually a vein of the pelvis or lower limb. A clot large enough to rest at the division of the pulmonary trunk can be rapidly fatal unless it is surgically removed within a few minutes; this is among the most urgent of all surgical operations. Pul-monary embolism has never been a com-mon disaster. It used sometimes to follow surgical operations, but with the practice of getting patients out of bed as soon as poss-ible, so that blood does not stagnate in the veins, it is now very rare.
Pulmonary oedema. The pulmonary veins open into the left side of the heart. With left-sided ◊ *heart failure* the pulmonary veins become congested with blood that a healthy heart would pump away; the pres-sure in them rises, and fluid is forced out of the capillaries into the lungs, which become waterlogged (◊ *oedema*). Any other cause of oedema can affect the lungs, but pul-monary oedema is typically due to heart failure.
Pulmonary stenosis. Abnormally narrow pulmonary artery. ◊ *heart* (4).
Pulmonary veins. Two large veins leave each lung and enter the left atrium of the heart. These veins carry arterial (oxygenated) blood; Galen called them the *arterial veins*.

pulmonic. Pulmonary (US more than UK).

pulse. Pressure-wave in an artery, corresponding with the heart beat. Arteries are elastic and therefore expand with each wave; it is this rhythmic expansion that is felt. The main beat is followed by a rebound wave, which is easily recorded mechanically but scarcely possible to feel.

The pulse in an artery surrounded by soft tissues (muscle, fat) can seldom be detected, but a pulse can be felt wherever an artery can be lightly compressed against a bone. These are the pressure points, familiar to first-aiders, where arteries can be compressed to stem heavy bleeding.

In most people the resting pulse rate is between 60 and 70 beats per minute, but in individual cases rates as slow as 50 or as fast as 100 may be normal. Changes in pulse rate are much more significant than the precise rate at a given moment. For instance, when a patient is first seen after an injury a pulse rate of 90 means very little, but an increase from 80 to 90 may be the only clue to internal bleeding. The force of the pulse is even more significant than the rate as an index of the state of the circulation.
◊ *arrhythmia*.

pupil. Circular hole in the centre of the iris, by which light reaches the back of the eye. The iris consists largely of muscle fibres. They are controlled by *sympathetic* nerves, which cause the pupil to enlarge, and *parasympathetic* nerves, which cause it to contract. The pupil is reflexly contracted in bright light and also when the eye is focused on close objects. Excitement and fear increase the flow of adrenaline into the blood-stream, which dilates the pupils in the same way as stimulation of their sympathetic nerves. Drugs such as belladonna dilate the pupils by abolishing the action of the parasympathetic nerves, leaving the sympathetic unopposed.

purgative; purge. Any drug given to induce opening of the bowels (defaecation). Until modern times, purges were by far the most widely used medicines. To clear the system must be good, the doctors argued. They did not stop to wonder what they meant by the system, or of what they wished to clear it. In the present century, there has been talk of eliminating poisons that might be absorbed from the intestine into the blood-stream; but this is almost certainly a myth (◊ *constipation*).

The terms aperient, laxative, purgative, and cathartic have been used in ascending order of severity, but they are not very useful because the classification of a particular drug may depend on the dose as much as the nature of the drug. Purges are better classified by the way in which they act.

Some of the most effective purges act solely by their bulk. The intestine will usually empty itself regularly if its muscles have something to grip. A good mixed diet contains enough undigested residue (roughage), mainly vegetable fibres, to provide this. A diet of milk and eggs is constipating because it is wholly digested. Bulk purges include methyl-cellulose and agar-agar, and also salts such as magnesium sulphate, which draw an excess of water into the large intestine by *osmosis*.

Indigestible oily fluids such as liquid paraffin act partly by their bulk but mainly by simple lubrication.

Most other purges stimulate the intestine by irritating its lining. The vegetable laxatives such as senna, cascara, and rhubarb all contain irritant compounds of anthracene. Jalap and colocynth contain more violent irritants; they act partly by direct stimulation and partly by causing inflammation with exudation of fluid from the lining of the intestine. They are unpleasant and seldom used. Castor oil is itself bland, but the acid of the stomach decomposes the oil and releases the irritant ricinoleic acid. All irritant purges cause griping if the dose is at all excessive, and the right dose for an individual has often to be guessed. The synthetic irritant bisacodyl is less troublesome in this respect than the older drugs.

purpura. Spontaneous bruising of the skin. ◊ *bleeding disorders*.

purulent. Containing pus.

pus. A by-product of ◊ *inflammation*, especially local inflammation due to certain bacteria. It is commonly a thick yellow fluid, but may be watery or almost solid. The physical properties – consistency, colour, smell – depend on the kinds of bacteria.

During inflammation, fluid and white blood cells leak from the blood vessels. These are the main components of pus. To them are added living and dead bacteria and the remnants of tissue damaged by infection.

pustule. Small abscess in the surface layer of the skin; a small pus-blister.

Malignant pustule = ◊ *anthrax* of the skin.

putrefaction. Decomposition of animal or vegetable remains by bacteria.

pyaemia. Spread of bacterial infection by the blood-stream, usually from an abscess, with the formation of new abscesses.

pyelitis (pyelonephritis). Inflammation of the renal pelvis, i.e. of the receptacle at the outlet of the ◊ *kidney*. The pelvis is a hollow cone into which urine formed in the kidney flows. From the apex of the cone a slender pipe, the *ureter*, conveys the urine to the *bladder*.

Pyelitis is due to bacterial infection, often by bacteria which occur in great profusion in the healthy large intestine and cause trouble only if they stray from their natural habitat. It is possible for them to be carried straight to the renal pelvis in the blood, but usually the infection spreads up the ureter from the bladder. The female bladder with its short outlet (*urethra*) is not nearly as well protected from extraneous contamination as the male bladder, and pyelitis is much commoner in women than in men.

Stagnant urine is very liable to infection. Any impediment to the flow of urine predisposes to pyelitis, which often complicates pregnancy, stone in the kidney or bladder, enlargement of the prostate gland, and narrowing of the ureter or urethra. (A stone may be the result of infection.)

A valve where the ureter enters the bladder normally prevents urine from flowing in the wrong direction when the bladder is full, and is a fairly effective barrier against the spread of infection in the bladder (cystitis) to the ureters and pelvis. In children with pyelitis this valve is often defective. Infection might well injure the valve, but it seems likelier that the defective valve precedes the infection. Operations for repairing these valves have been devised.

Acute pyelitis need not cause much in the way of symptoms. In children particularly it can be a very vague illness, recognized only when the urine is found to harbour large numbers of bacteria. More often, however, there is a high temperature with pain over the affected kidney(s) or in the lower part of the abdomen (right-sided pyelitis can mimic appendicitis). The accompanying cystitis causes frequent and painful passage of urine.

Chronic pyelitis is the same disease continuing for months or years, with attacks of acute pyelitis at intervals and few if any symptoms between attacks. It accounts for a good deal of vague ill health, especially in middle-aged women.

Pyelonephritis (inflammation of renal pelvis *and* kidney) describes the condition better than the older term, *pyelitis*, because the kidney substance is also affected to a greater or lesser extent. The distinction is worth making because it draws attention to the potential danger of the disease. Pyelitis pure and simple would be unpleasant but fairly harmless, and until recently few doctors took it very seriously. It is now clear that if chronic pyelonephritis is not treated the kidneys may gradually approach a condition very like advanced ◊ *Bright's disease* and ultimately fail. In most cases the infection is eradicated by sulphonamide drugs. If these fail, antibiotics such as tetracyclines are used. Predisposing factors such as obstruction to the flow of urine may need surgical correction.

pyelography. X-ray examination of the kidneys (1) by injecting into a vein a substance opaque to X-rays that is concentrated by the kidneys and passed into the urine (intravenous pyelography), or (2) by injecting a similar substance into the ureters towards the kidneys by way of a cystoscope passed into the bladder (retrograde pyelography). Method (1) works only if the kidney is functioning and able to concentrate the substance. It is therefore a test of function as well as of structural defects. Method (2) shows the outlet of the kidney regardless of function.

pyelonephritis = ◊ *pyelitis*.

pyknolepsy. An uncommon form of epilepsy in childhood, with repetitive fleeting loss of consciousness. The distinction from *petit mal* is not clear.

pyloric stenosis. Narrowing of the outlet from the stomach. In adults this may be due to scarring from a duodenal ulcer, but the term is usually reserved for a disorder of infancy, congenital hypertrophic pyloric stenosis. This condition afflicts boys more than girls (3 or 4:1), and is said to be commonest in first-born children. The condition is simply over-development of the muscle in the wall of the pylorus. It is a genetic disorder, but nothing more is known of the cause.

A few weeks after birth the baby begins to vomit. The vomiting, described as 'projectile', is quite different from the spilling-over of feeds that most babies show from time to time: the milk is really ejected. The baby loses weight and dies if not treated. The standard treatment is Ramstedt's operation, by which the constricting muscle fibres are split longitudinally. This operation is safe and completely effective.

Some babies appear to recover without operation if given drugs which act like atropine to suppress stimulation of the stomach muscle by the vagus nerves. Many surgeons would insist that these are not true cases of pyloric stenosis. It is difficult to argue the point without arguing in a circle, but since pyloric stenosis is a definite structural fault it may well be that every true case needs operation.

pylorus. Outlet from the stomach; narrow muscular tube joining the stomach to the beginning of the intestine (duodenum).

pyo-. Prefix = 'pus'.

pyorrhoea. 1. Any discharge of pus. **2.** *Pyorrhoea alveolaris*, infection of the gums. ◊ *gingiva; teeth.*

pyrexia = ◊ *fever.*

pyridoxine = ◊ *vitamin B₆.*

PZI. Protamine-zinc insulin, a compound of insulin with a more delayed action than ordinary insulin. It enables some diabetics to manage with one injection instead of two or three in a day.

Q

Q-fever. An infectious disease very like a virus pneumonia, due to a similar microbe (*Rickettsia*) to that of typhus. It is carried by sheep and other livestock, which themselves suffer no ill effects. Like other rickettsial diseases, Q-fever responds well to treatment with antibiotics.

quadriceps (quadriceps femoris). The large (four-headed) muscle of the front of the thigh: its 4 heads are *vastus lateralis, vastus intermedius,* and *vastus medialis,* all arising from the shaft of the femur, and *rectus femoris,* arising from the pelvis above the hip-joint. The whole mass is attached to the front of the tibia by a broad tendon. A bone set in this tendon, the knee-cap (*patella*), acts to some extent as a fulcrum, but the muscle works well after loss of the patella.

The muscle serves to extend or straighten the knee, and is perhaps the most important of the various supports of the knee joint. A healthy quadriceps is essential to recovery from injuries of the knee.

The kind of sudden jerk that in a younger person might fracture the patella sometimes tears the quadriceps in middle-aged or elderly people.

quarantine. Originally an attempt to prevent plague from spreading: at Mediterranean seaports (Ragusa, Rhodes, Venice) incoming ships were isolated, and their crews forbidden to disembark, for 40 days. The system started in the 14th century and had been adopted in most European ports by the 16th. There was no sort of agreement between countries until the advent of cholera in the 19th century brought governments together. Even then, discussions lasted from 1851 till 1903 when the first international regulations were drawn up. By that time it was clear that control was needed only when there was good reason to suspect cholera or plague on board. Later,

yellow fever, smallpox, and louse-borne relapsing fever and typhus were added to the list of diseases subject to international regulations.

Quarantine is now seldom rigidly enforced, and the period of 40 days has been shortened to a time corresponding with the known incubation period of each disease. It is nearly always enough to keep people who have been in contact with infection under medical supervision, without strict isolation unless symptoms develop; but with several types of infection contacts may have to be kept away from places such as schools, cinemas, and public transport.

quartan fever. ◊ *Malaria,* with a bout of fever every 4th day by the old notation (1st, 4th, 7th . . .) or every 3rd day as one would now say.

quassia. A bitter appetizer, with some reputation as a cure for worms.

quinacrine. A synthetic drug for treating malaria.

quinidine. An alkaloid from cinchona bark, chemically similar to quinine, but used only for treating certain irregularities of the heart beat (◊ *arrhythmia*). Quinidine impairs the conduction of impulses in the heart. In some cases of total irregularity (auricular fibrillation), the drug cuts out aimless, conflicting impulses and leaves a steady rhythm.

quinine. The principle alkaloid of ◊ *cinchona.* It was the first effective drug against malaria, and perhaps the first drug to tackle the cause of any disease.

quinsy. Abscess round the tonsil; an occasional complication of a sore throat. ◊ *pharynx* (1).

R

rabbit fever = ◊ *tularaemia*.

rabies (hydrophobia). A virus infection, unusual in its severity and in the number of different kinds of animal that it can affect. Human rabies is fortunately rare even in countries where the virus is common among wild animals. When it does occur it is nearly always the result of a bite from an infected dog. The virus enters the skin and slowly travels along nerves to the spinal cord and brain. The incubation period between infection and first symptoms lasts between 10 days and several months. The actual illness, with fever, delirium, muscle spasm and paralysis is fatal within a few days. The patient may be unable to drink because of painful spasm of the throat muscles: hence the alternative name *hydrophobia*.

Although there is no effective treatment for rabies, it can be prevented. It has been eliminated from the British Isles by strict quarantine for imported dogs and cats, but this method is possible only in an island. Elsewhere these animals are usually vaccinated against rabies so that an occasional case is unlikely to spread. People who have been exposed to the risk of infection can be protected by the vaccine invented by Pasteur (1885).

rachis. Spine; backbone. (The word is seldom used except as an element of compound words such as the following.)

rachischisis. A congenital defect of the backbone; ◊ *spina bifida*.

rachitis = ◊ *rickets*. Literally, rachitis means inflammation of the backbone (*spondylitis*), which rickets is not. The word appeared in one of the first scientific accounts of the disease, by Francis Glisson (1650), who adopted it as a Latin name for 'the disease of children commonly known as the rickets'. A few years later, John Aubrey insisted that the disease was named after a Dr Ricketts of Newbury, who specialized in its treatment, adding 'and now 'tis good sport to see how they vex their Lexicons, and fetch from it the Greek *rachis*, the backbone' (*Aubrey's Brief Lives*,

ed. O. L. Dick, Secker & Warburg, 1960, p. xlvi). Or the word may be much older and related to 'wrick' (twist, sprain).

radial. Of the radius, the outer of the two bones of the forearm.
Radial artery. In front of the elbow the brachial artery divides into two branches, *radial* and *ulnar*. The radial artery runs down the forearm to the thumb side of the wrist, where it can easily be felt for examining the pulse. It curls round the base of the thumb, and rejoins the ulnar artery in the palm.
Radial nerve. A branch of the brachial plexus, supplying branches to the muscles and skin of the back of the upper limb. It winds round the back of the shaft of the humerus, where it is liable to injury if the bone is broken.

radiation. Exposure to ionizing rays. All living creatures receive constant radiation from outer space (cosmic radiation) and radioactive deposits in the soil, but the dose is too small to have any obvious effect. It is possible, however, that natural radiation may play a part in evolution by causing mutation (◊ *genetics* (4)).

With the discovery of X-rays in 1895 and radium in 1898 two potentially dangerous sources of ionizing rays were uncovered, and the new uses of atomic energy in war and peace have added greatly to the dangers.

All forms of life are destroyed by large enough doses of radiation. The main effect is on cell division, the process by which tissues reproduce themselves or grow. Therefore a growing child is more susceptible than an adult, and an embryo even more than a child. The most susceptible parts of the body are those that grow or replace themselves most rapidly: blood-forming tissues and sex glands, followed by lining membranes and skin. The constantly multiplying cells of a cancer are more susceptible than healthy tissue – hence the treatment of cancer with radium, X-rays etc.

People far enough from an atomic explosion or a major accident in a nuclear reactor to escape immediate death from burning can still get a rapidly lethal dose of radiation. The brain is among the least susceptible organs; if the dose is enough to damage brain cells the victim dies within a few hours. People a little further from the disaster die in a few days from damage to the lining of the intestine, and those in the next zone die in a few weeks from failure of the blood-forming tissues. Some in this third group may be saved by a graft of healthy bone marrow.

A far commoner hazard is lasting damage to a single tissue. This can happen not only to the remoter victims of atomic explosions, but to people over-exposed to X-rays or radioactive matter used in medicine and industry. Irradiation of the sex glands causes sterility; but a rather smaller dose may disturb the sex cells without destroying them and so cause deformity in the next generation. Disturbance of other tissues can make them liable to cancer, especially of the skin and of the blood cells (leukaemia). Before suitable precautions were enforced many X-ray workers developed cancer of the skin.

Whether radiation arrests or causes cancer depends on whether the dose is enough to destroy or merely disturb the parts of a cell concerned in growth. Some of the drugs for treating cancer have a similar effect.

radioactive isotopes ◊ *isotope.*

radiography. Examination by X-rays.

radiology. Study of radiation, especially its medical uses for diagnosis and treatment of disease ◊ *X-rays.*

radiotherapy. Treatment of disease with ionizing radiation from radioactive substances or X-rays. The earliest form of radiotherapy was the treatment of cancer with radium, which has given place to substances such as radioactive cobalt (^{60}Co) which are easier to get and to handle. An alternative is exposure of the cancer to high-voltage X-rays. Useful as these measures are, they have the disadvantage that sufficient radiation to suppress a cancer often has ill effects on the body as a whole; but some surface cancers are cured by radiotherapy without upsetting the patient at all.

Other uses of radiotherapy include the treatment of *polycythaemia vera,* an ab-normal proliferation of red blood cells' with radioactive phosphorus (^{32}P), and that of toxic *goitre* with radioactive iodine (^{131}I). Ankylosing ◊ *spondylitis* can be treated with X-rays. Skin diseases characterized by proliferation of the surface layer of the skin used often to be treated with small doses of X-rays, but this technique is now thought too drastic for all but a few cases.

radium. Radioactive element, discovered by Marie and Pierre Curie in 1898; used for destroying cancer cells near the surface of the body.

radius. One of the two bones of the forearm; the other is the ulna.

With the palm of the hand facing forwards the two bones are parallel, the radius lying on the outer or thumb side. At the elbow the ulna takes most of the strain, but at the wrist the strain falls on the radius. The ulna is the longer of the two because it extends beyond the elbow joint to form the *olecranon,* the point of the elbow. The two bones form joints with each other at each end.

At the upper joint the head of the radius turns in a notch on the side of the ulna. At the lower joint the arrangement is reversed: a notch at the lower end of the radius fits the rounded lower end of the ulna. Rotation of the forearm is a movement of the radius around the ulna. In *supination* the bones are parallel, the palm faces forwards or upwards. In *pronation* the bones are crossed; the head of the radius is still in its notch at the outer side of the ulna, but the lower end has rolled over the ulna to lie on its inner side, and the palm faces backwards or downwards.

Because supination brings the powerful biceps muscle into play it is a stronger movement than pronation. If the right hand is turned clockwise as in driving a screw the biceps can be felt to contract.

1. INJURIES

It is difficult to break one bone of the forearm without disturbing the other. Often both are fractured. With fracture of the radius alone the ulna is likely to be dislocated at the wrist and with fracture of the ulna, the radius may be dislocated at the elbow. Such injuries are unstable and difficult to manipulate. They often need surgical operation and internal fixation (◊ *fracture*).

The commonest fracture of the forearm is ◊ Colles' fracture, in which the lower end of the radius is displaced backwards by a fall on the palm of the hand. In Smith's fracture the broken end is displaced forwards; this is also called chauffeur's fracture because it can be caused by a blow on the back of the wrist from a starting handle.

With all these injuries, unless the alignment of the bones is restored rotation of the forearm is disturbed. This can be a serious disability.

râle. Abnormal sound from the lungs, fainter and higher pitched than a wheeze (rhonchus), generally indicating moisture in the lungs.

Ramazzini, Bernardino (1633–1714). Italian physician; professor of medicine at Modena, Padua, and finally Venice. Famous in his own time as an authority on epidemics, he is now remembered mainly for the first systematic account of the relation between diseases and trades (◊ occupational disease).

rat. Rats live as close to man as they can safely get, and share several of his nastier diseases. These include a common type of bacterial food poisoning, and Weil's disease, rat-bite fever, flea-borne typhus, flea-borne relapsing fever, and plague.

rat-bite fever. Fever with swollen lymph nodes, from infection either with the spiral bacterium Spirillum minus or the mould Streptobacillus moniliformis, both of which are common in rats. Human infections are rare only because rat-bites are rare. Neither form is very dangerous. Both respond to penicillin.

rauwolfia. Kinds of tropical plant. The root of R. serpentina is a very ancient Indian remedy for insomnia and certain types of insanity. It was first used outside India in 1953 after laboratory investigation in India, Switzerland, and the United States. Several alkaloids have been isolated from rauwolfia, of which the most important is reserpine. The drugs induce mental calm and also lower the blood pressure. Although they are traditionally supposed to induce sleep they do so only by relieving the anxieties that kept the patient awake. Reserpine was the first drug that could be called a ◊ tranquillizer. It is still used for

certain types of mental agitation, but its greatest value is in the treatment of high blood pressure (◊ blood pressure (1)).

Rauwolfia probably acts by reducing the stores of adrenaline and similar substances in parts of the brain concerned with the emotions.

Raynaud's disease. (M. Raynaud (1834–81), French physician.) A disorder of small arteries, especially in the hands and feet, with sudden attacks of pallor and coldness of the fingers or toes, lasting from a few minutes to an hour or more. The attacks are due to reduction of the flow of blood by spasm of the arteries.

Contraction of arteries near the surface of the body is a natural reponse to cold. By restricting the flow of blood through the skin it prevents loss of heat. These arteries also contract when blood is diverted to the muscles to prepare for physical exertion, e.g. in response to fear or anger. In people with Raynaud's disease the natural response of the small arteries is grossly exaggerated. Attacks may be brought on by slight cold, emotion or stimuli such as vibration. Sometimes Raynaud's disease is a symptom of a disorder of the nerves or endocrine glands; in these cases it clears up when the primary disorder is treated. But more often the defect seems to be in the arteries themselves. Drugs that dilate blood vessels may help, and in severe cases cutting the sympathetic nerves to the affected limb, to prevent reflex contraction of the arteries, alleviates the symptoms. The most effective treatment is to identify the factors that precipitate attacks and avoid them.

receptor. 1. Nerve-ending adapted to a particular kind of sensation.
2. Chemical component of a living cell (a part of a much larger molecule), with which a foreign substance combines to alter the functioning of the cell. The idea of chemical receptors was first suggested by Ehrlich to explain the interaction of antigens and antibodies to neutralize the effects of bacteria in the body (◊ immunity), but it can be extended to explain the effects of many hormones and drugs.

rectum. The last few inches of the large ◊ intestine, terminating in the anal canal.

The rectum is likely to be involved in diseases of the large intestine such as dysentery or ulcerative colitis. It is the commonest site of cancer in the intestine. The early symptoms – passage of blood or mucus, or a change in the usual bowel habit such as unaccustomed constipation or diarrhoea – often bring the patient to a surgeon in time for this type of cancer to be cured.

Haemorrhoids (piles) are swollen veins at the junction of the rectum with the anal canal.

rectus. Straight (muscle), e.g. *rectus abdominis*, a strap-like muscle at each side of the mid-line at the front of the abdomen; *rectus femoris*, a vertical muscle at the front of the thigh, forming part of the quadriceps muscle.

recurrent laryngeal nerve. Branch of the ◊ *vagus nerve* to the muscle of the vocal cords. Its fibres run with the vagus nerve down the neck and into the thorax, then leave the vagus and return to the neck, to pass behind the thyroid gland into the larynx. These nerves are exposed to injury by disease of the thyroid gland or operations on the gland, with impairment of the voice.

reduction. Restoration of the natural position of a displaced organ, e.g. setting a broken bone, or replacing an organ that has protruded into a hernia.

referred pain. Pain felt in a different part of the body from the site of injury. A blow on the inner side of the elbow causes pain in the little finger, which has not been touched. This is because the pain is neither in the finger nor the elbow; it is awareness that a nervous impulse has reached the brain by a particular pathway. In this case the pathway is by certain fibres of the ulnar nerve, which run from the little finger up the inner side of the arm and ultimately via the spinal cord to the brain. The brain 'knows' only that it has received a signal from somewhere on the pathway, and it always interprets the signal as an insult to the little finger. It would still do so if the finger had been amputated.

Some pathways from different organs converge in the spinal cord and brain. Many of the internal organs first appear in one part of the embryo and later migrate to another part, trailing their original nerves with them. Pain signals in these migrant nerves are interpreted as coming from the original site of the organ. For instance, the diaphragm, separating the heart and lungs from the stomach and liver, first grows in the same part of the embryo as the shoulders. Irritation of the diaphragm by pleurisy, or inflammation of the liver, causes pain to be felt in the shoulder – it is 'referred' to the shoulder.

reflex (adj., or n. = reflex *action*). Involuntary response to a stimulus, determined by impulses in nerves. There are three components: the *receptor* reacting to the stimulus, the *effector* responding, and the *reflex arc*, the pathway of the nervous impulse. A familiar example is the *knee-jerk*. The quadriceps muscle of the thigh is slightly stretched by a tap with a rubber hammer on its tendon. The receptors are the muscle-spindles, sensory organs in the muscle which set off a nervous impulse in response to stretching. The impulse passes up the femoral nerve to the spinal cord. Here it is transmitted to motor nerve cells and down their fibres to the effector organ, the muscle itself, which contracts.

The knee-jerk is an instance of the general principle that muscles automatically resist any tendency to stretch them. This is how balance is maintained: any disturbance of position is resisted unless a movement is actually needed. Even voluntary movements include a reflex element. The will determines what movement is to be made, but the choice of which muscles are to contract, and the inhibition of the opposing muscles that have to be stretched in the process, are reflex.

Many reflexes, including the knee-jerk, are *inborn*. They have evolved just as ears and fingers and kidneys have evolved, and are part of everyone's hereditary constitution. Most bodily functions are controlled mainly by inborn reflexes. The effectors are either muscles or glands; receptors are more diverse. Dilatation of blood vessels in the skin and sweating are responses to heat; constriction of the vessels and shivering, to cold; deep breathing, to acidity of the blood; slowing of the heart beat, to increased blood pressure; passage of urine, to distension of the bladder; constriction of the pupils, to bright light; salivation, to eating. Some reflexes, such as breathing and passing urine, can be modified for a time by nerves under voluntary control, but in the end reflex action is stronger than will. Nobody can hold his breath or his water for ever. Reflex actions effected by ◊ *sympathetic* or ◊ *parasympathetic* nerves may be greatly modified by emotion; this is the basis of most ◊ *psychosomatic* illness.

Only two nerve fibres are involved in the knee-jerk. Most reflex arcs are more complicated, several nerve cells intervening between receptor and effector; and a number of reflexes may combine to produce a single effect. A man keeps his balance by adjusting the tension of muscles in his trunk and legs, a reflex action determined by sensations from muscles, joints, eyes, and the balance organs of the ears. The transmission of the impulse is discussed under ◊ *nervous system*.

Not all reflexes are inborn. *Conditioned* reflexes are either modifications of inborn reflexes or completely new automatic responses, developed as a result of the individual's experience. Such reflexes were first demonstrated by Pavlov at the end of the 19th century. By an inborn reflex a dog's mouth waters when it eats. But the sight of food also stimulates a flow of saliva, before eating begins. This, Pavlov argued, cannot be a predetermined inborn reflex, because the dog must learn to recognize food before the stimulus can work. Next, Pavlov taught a dog to associate the ringing of a bell with food. In time the bell alone, without food, made the dog's mouth water. This is still a pure reflex – there is no question of the dog's deliberately producing saliva – but it has to be learnt. Actions as varied as fainting at the sight of blood and stopping a car at a red traffic light may be reflexes of the same type: an involuntary response to a learned stimulus.

A different type of conditioned reflex is acquired by learning that some action has a particular consequence. A rat in a cage seems to move aimlessly, but learns to repeat a movement that releases food into the cage. Here there is no external stimulus as there is in the first type, unless hunger or merely enjoying food is regarded as a stimulus. The response has no counterpart among inborn reflexes.

Conditioned reflexes do not override the principle that a reflex arc is invariable; they are new reflexes added to existing ones. Pavlov's bell did not replace food as a stimulus. The inborn reflex worked as before, and the bell was a new stimulus operating a new reflex. Indeed, the response differed slightly: saliva after the bell

had not quite the same chemical composition as saliva when eating.

Inborn reflexes, then, are standard equipment which everyone inherits and transmits to his offspring. Conditioned reflexes are optional extras to be acquired by each generation in response to the environment. The extent to which learning is merely the acquisition of conditioned reflexes is still open to speculation.

refraction. Deflection of light by the surfaces of glass, water etc., which accounts for the action of lenses. In medical usage, refraction refers to the focusing mechanism of the eye, or to the testing of this mechanism before prescribing spectacles.

refractionist. A person who tests the refraction of the eye.

regime; regimen. In French, the word *régime* must do duty for both, and many writers make it do so in English. Since English has the two words it is worth preserving the distinction: *regime* in the political sense; *regimen* in the medical sense of a set of rules prescribed for treating illness or preserving health.

regional enteritis. Regional ileitis; Crohn's disease. ◊ *enteritis.*

registrar. In British hospitals, a junior specialist, the first assistant to a consultant physician or surgeon.

Reiter's disease. A feverish illness, characterized by inflammation of the urethra, sore eyes, and painful joints resembling those of rheumatoid arthritis. The pattern of the illness strongly suggests an infection, and in the past cases of Reiter's disease have been ascribed to gonorrhoea, which can cause the same symptoms. But although from circumstantial evidence Reiter's disease appears to be a venereal infection this has not been proved, and no infecting organism or germ has been definitely identified.

relapsing fever. Intermittent fever caused by a spiral bacterium, *Borrelia*. One type is carried by lice, the other by ticks.

About a week after infection, the patient has a severe attack of fever, which completely subsides after a few days, to return a week or ten days later. There may be as many as 10 of these relapses if the infection is not treated. It is believed that several strains of bacteria infect the patient together, or that fresh strains evolve from those originally injected by the insect, and that the patient has to acquire immunity to each strain in turn before he finally shakes the disease off. Though very debilitating, relapsing fever is seldom fatal even without treatment, and the infection responds well to penicillin.

Louse-borne relapsing fever (famine fever), like louse-borne typhus and plague, typically follows a breakdown of hygienic services, e.g. in wartime or after natural disasters. All three of these diseases are internationally ◊ notifiable.

Tick-borne relapsing fever is common in some tropical countries. The ticks live in crevices in the walls of mud huts. The disease can be controlled by spraying houses with insecticides.

relaxant. Drug used for relieving spasm of muscles, or for preventing muscles from contracting. The prototype is *curare*, which prevents the transmission of impulses from nerves to muscles. These drugs are used during surgical operations. By keeping the patient's muscles loose they make it easier for the surgeon to get at the diseased organ and to see what he is doing, and they also make it possible to use smaller doses of anaesthetics. In both ways they reduce the risks of surgery.

Relaxants are also used to control dangerous muscle spasm, e.g. in the treatment of tetanus.

Since these drugs temporarily paralyse all muscles, including those of breathing, some form of artificial respiration is needed while they are being used.

Some of the drugs used as ◊ *tranquillizers* have a slight relaxant effect.

relaxin. A hormone that loosens the ligaments of the pelvis at the end of pregnancy and facilitates birth. It is known to be important in some animals, but whether relaxin plays any part in human labour is uncertain. The laxity of the baby's ligaments associated with congenital dislocation of the ◊ *hip* is possibly an effect of this hormone.

remission. Temporary freedom from symptoms in the course of a disease.

renal. Of the kidney. The *renal arteries*, one

for each kidney, are very large branches of the aorta; between them, they receive about a quarter of the output of the heart. Congenital anomalies of these arteries are occasionally troublesome. An abnormally narrow renal artery is a rare cause of high blood pressure; and an abnormally situated branch of the artery may pinch the ureter and impede the flow of urine from the kidney, a condition needing surgery.

Renal hypertension: high ◊ *blood pressure* caused by disease of the kidneys.

Renal rickets: ◊ *rickets*.

renin. A hormone formed by the kidneys, concerned with the regulation of blood pressure. ◊ *circulation* (1).

rennin. An enzyme that clots the protein *casein* as the first step in the digestion of milk, found in the stomachs of most young mammals, including human babies.

research. Medical science, which is applied human biology, is a branch of natural science in general, and research in any branch of science is apt to affect any other branch. Basic medical research is research in the theoretical sciences on which medical practice is based: ◊ *anatomy,* ◊*physiology,* ◊ *pathology,* ◊ *pharmacology* and others. This entry is concerned with clinical research, or the application of the results of basic research to sick people, and in particular with the problems of trying out new drugs.

In principle, basic research is the concern of universities, and investigation of new drugs is that of the chemical and pharmaceutical industries. The two fields overlap considerably, and all research is becoming so expensive that few universities can manage without some financial help from industry or elsewhere. Basic research indicates the kind of substance that is likely to turn into a useful drug, and, coupled with clinical observation, the actions that should be sought in new drugs. A manufacturer often has to start from the other end. His plant is adapted to the synthesis of certain classes of compound. It is no mere chance that most of the early synthetic drugs were related to dyestuffs: the modern chemical industry began in the second half of the 19th century with dyes and other substances needed by the textile industry. As chemists began to see the possibility of synthesizing new drugs, with the advantages over the old herbal remedies that they could be exactly standardized, modified, and produced in the required amounts, they naturally turned first to the substances on hand or to compounds easily derived from these. There is no theoretical limit to the number of different substances that might be synthesized, but even the largest chemical plant cannot attempt more than a few of them without heavy capital expenditure. Therefore a manufacturer, whether capitalist or state-controlled, has to be fairly sure of his ground before starting work on a new type of chemical compound.

Often the starting point is a known drug, and many new drugs are simple modifications of old ones, in which a change of chemical structure has enhanced the desired effect or decreased the toxicity. Or a chemist may synthesize a new substance and pass it to the biologists to see whether it has any potential as a drug. This all sounds like a hit-or-miss research, but there is no alternative while so little is known about how drugs work. Two closely related compounds may have similar, or opposite effects. Thus isoprenaline and methyl-dopa are both related to adrenaline. One is a useful alternative to adrenaline in the treatment of asthma, whereas the other is a direct antidote, used for lowering high blood pressure.

The first step in testing a possible new drug is to give it to small animals such as frogs and mice, and test its effect on each of the organs in turn, to see whether the compound shows any promise or whether it is too toxic to be worth further study. Most compounds are rejected at this stage. Sometimes there are wholly unexpected rewards. In the late 1950s, when a series of compounds was being studied in the hope of finding a new treatment for worms, one of them (guanethidine) did not cure the rats of their worms but caused an alarming fall in their blood pressure. The research changed course, and later guanethidine emerged as one of the most valuable remedies for high blood pressure.

If the new compound promises to be useful, it is tested with higher animals (e.g. dogs, monkeys) including – since the disaster with thalidomide – pregnant animals, with particular attention to the margin between effective doses and dangerous doses, the *therapeutic index*. Unless the index is reasonably high the research is discontinued. Otherwise, the compound can be tested for untoward effects on healthy human volunteers, usually members of the research team.

From this point, in many countries further research comes under official scrutiny: in Britain by the Committee on Safety of Drugs, and in the United States by the Food and Drugs Administration. The clinical trials, i.e. tests on actual patients, are conducted under an agreed code of ethics, with these government agencies to arbitrate. The manufacturer must satisfy the agency that his drug is likely to be useful and reasonably safe, and he must then find a physician with facilities for clinical research who is willing to conduct the first trials, usually one working in a large hospital attached to a university, for only a large medical unit has the laboratories and other elaborate diagnostic aids for recognizing ill-effects before serious harm is done. And, apart from safeguards, the manufacturer's claims will have to be supported by unimpeachable authority when he comes to market his new product.

Only rarely can a new drug be assessed from its effect on a handful of patients. An example was the first treatment of tuberculous meningitis with streptomycin in 1944. The mortality from this disease had been 100 per cent; no patient had ever recovered. A single patient cured was virtual proof that the new drug worked. But this is quite exceptional. With most other diseases, the patient might have recovered without the drug. This problem can be overcome by comparing the new drug with the results of giving no active treatment. A valid comparison needs a large enough series of cases to exclude, within reason, the workings of pure chance – another reason for choosing a large hospital: ◊ *statistics*.

Two groups of patients are studied together. They are matched as nearly as possible for age, sex, severity of illness, race, social background and other factors that might affect the outcome. Ideally, the only difference between the groups would be the drug itself.

To give one group the new treatment and the other no treatment at all would not serve, because the patients who knew that they were being treated would inevitably do better than the others. So the control (untreated) group must be given medication that looks like the real thing, a ◊ *placebo*, and none of the patients is told until later to which group he belongs. Neither should the physician be told, because knowing which patients are getting the drug can affect both his manner with them (and therefore their response) and his judgement of the results. The trial is then *double-blind*, with neither the doctor nor the patients knowing how the two groups are allocated. The hospital pharmacist does know, and breaks silence if there is any sign of trouble.

In a *cross-over* trial, the two groups, still without knowing, change sides at half-time, so that all the patients at one stage or the other receive the drug. With chronic disorders needing prolonged treatment, the patients thus serve as their own controls.

The ethical questions include these. The physician must be sure that the trial is justified. In 1865 Claude Bernard summed this up by saying that a trial likely to make the patient worse was forbidden, one likely at least to do no harm was permissible, and one likely to make the patient better was obligatory. This does not go quite far enough. To justify a clinical trial, a new drug should offer some prospect not merely of working, but of being better than existing and tried remedies. 'Better' need not mean more efficient: it can also mean safer, or more convenient. For example, many drugs derived from adrenaline are offered for the relief of asthma. Probably none of them stops an asthmatic attack more efficiently than adrenaline itself. The first of them, ephedrine, is much less efficient, but it is safer and has the great advantage that it can be taken by mouth instead of by injection. Because its action is slow, ephedrine is better for preventing attacks than for treating them. A later development, isoprenaline, is taken under the tongue or inhaled and works quickly enough to stop an attack. But all these drugs irritate the heart. The latest ones, such as salbutamol, are much safer in this respect. Thus all these drugs justify themselves, though none is more efficient than the prototype. Often, though, a new drug offers no advantage other than circumventing a rival's patent; this is a common source of discord between doctors and manufacturers. On the other hand, a drug that is neither better nor

worse than another, but cheaper, would be justified.

Next, the patients have to be told exactly what is happening. Unless they fully understand the nature of the trial and agree to take part, it is unethical to include them. With children, the parents' consent is needed, and with mentally deranged patients, that of the relatives. In both cases the doctor has to some extent to accept the responsibility of acting *in loco parentis*, which poses its own ethical problems.

There is then the question of treating dangerous illness. If, for example, a new treatment for typhoid fever is proposed, to give half the patients a placebo would be grossly improper because their lives would be in danger. In such cases, the new drug is compared not with a placebo but with an established remedy such as chloramphenicol. In this instance, the new drug could be only marginally more effective since chloramphenicol is highly active against typhoid bacilli, and a large series of cases would have to be studied to show a statistically significant advantage. But a slightly less active drug might be acceptable if it proved to be safer. Hundreds of cases might have to be studied before one could be sure.

If the first trials are successful, the drug is tested at other centres before the Committee on Safety of Drugs makes its recommendations to the medical profession in general.

It should be mentioned that only about one compound in every 200 studied ever reaches the stage of being given to patients. So that the cost of the research leading to one new drug is enormous. Even among the few that find their way into clinical practice there are many disappointments. New drugs often seem better than they really are. It may be months or years before their drawbacks come to light, and despite all the precautions doctors have to be constantly on guard when handling new remedies. Alexander Pope was no pharmacologist, but in one couplet he summed up this problem:

'Be not the first by whom the new are tried
Nor yet the last to lay the old aside.'

reserpine. Active principle of ◊ *rauwolfia*.

respiration. Exchange of gases between an

organism and its environment. All living tissues need a constant source of energy, which is supplied by burning fuel (carbohydrate, fat, or protein) – i.e. combining fuel with oxygen. Fat in the fire or fat in the body produces exactly the same amount of heat when it is oxidized; only the rate of oxidation differs. An average man at complete rest needs about 1·2 Calories per minute, and to generate this amount of heat he uses 250 c.c. of oxygen.

A man at rest breathes in about 3·75 litres of air per minute. This air contains 750 c.c. of oxygen of which he uses a third, or 250 c.c.

With deep and rapid breathing he takes in about 15 times as much air, and during exertion he takes up more oxygen from it. Thus the *oxygen* uptake can be increased about 30 times.

The end-products of oxidation in the body are energy, water, and *carbon dioxide*. Oxygen is carried by the blood to the tissues, where it is exchanged for carbon dioxide, which the blood carries to the lungs. This exchange of gases in the body is called *internal respiration*. The opposite exchange in the lungs, where oxygen is taken in and carbon dioxide is breathed out, is *external respiration*. A third term, *tissue respiration*, is applied to the actual process of oxidation inside the living cells.

1. MECHANICS OF BREATHING

The lungs are elastic bags, together holding about 6 litres of air when fully expanded and about half this amount at rest. During quiet breathing the air in the two lungs fluctuates between, say, 3 and 3·4 litres. The extremes, during forced breathing, are 1·5 and 6 litres.

Air is inhaled when the diaphragm and intercostal muscles enlarge the cavity of the chest, and atmospheric pressure forces air into the empty space provided.

The diaphragm is a sheet of muscle attached to the lower ribs and the lumbar vertebrae and rising in the centre to form a dome. As the muscle contracts the centre is pulled down, and the thorax is enlarged at the expense of the abdomen. The belly bulges to make room for the displaced abdominal organs.

The intercostal muscles span the gaps between the ribs. By contracting they make the chest deeper from front to back by raising the front of the ribs, and also wider by splaying the ribs. This enlargement of the rib-cage makes more room for the abdominal organs and so draws the belly *in*. During quiet breathing the opposed actions of the diaphragm and the intercostals on the abdomen about cancel each other. When breathing is distressed the muscles of the neck and shoulders reinforce the usual respiratory muscles.

Expiration, on the other hand, is mainly passive. The lungs and chest wall are elastic. When the pull of the muscles is relaxed, the recoil is enough to expel the air. But during forced breathing the abdominal muscles are used to compress the belly and push the diaphragm up.

A *cough* works like an air-gun: the chest is 'loaded' with compressed air by contracting the abdominal muscles while the outlet – the ◊ *larynx* – is held firmly shut. The gun is fired by sudden relaxation of the larynx.

Singing makes very special demands on breathing. The singer breathes as much as possible with his diaphragm, which contracts more rapidly than the intercostals, and is thus a better means of snatching a quick breath. But a more important part of singing is controlled breathing *out*, and again the diaphragm is a better mechanism than the intercostals. If a singer tries to breathe with his intercostals – i.e. from the ribs – he has to control the out-flow by constricting the throat (as in 'loading' the lungs for a cough), and this produces the strangled tone of a bad singer. But if he breathes in with his diaphragm he distends the abdominal muscles, which he can then balance against his diaphragm to regulate the out-flow. The stream can be a torrent or a trickle, and the larynx plays no part in its regulation; its muscles need be used only to determine the pitch of the note. The same principles apply to public speaking. The medical significance is that people who have trouble with breathing, such as asthmatics, or people who run a risk of infection of the lungs, such as patients recovering from major operations, can be taught better breathing. This is an important branch of physiotherapy.

2. REGULATION OF BREATHING

Breathing appears to be a deliberate action, and the muscles are voluntary muscles under conscious control. But free will in this respect is largely an illusion. Only a particular breath or short series of breaths can be adjusted at will; breathing as a whole is a reflex action. A given demand for oxygen may be satisfied by 20 moderate breaths in a minute. A sobbing child may take twice as many shallow breaths, or a singer half a dozen deep ones, but neither changes the volume of air exchanged in the given time. This balance can be deliberately upset by holding the breath or over-breathing, but only for a very short time; the subject's will is soon overruled by mechanisms outside his consciousness.

The process is co-ordinated by the *respiratory centre*, a group of nerve cells in the lowest part of the brain. Lack of oxygen in the blood is at best only a weak stimulus to the respiratory centre, and severe short-age of oxygen *suppresses* the centre. The really important factor is the acidity of the blood. This depends on the ratio of circu-lating bicarbonate (alkaline) to carbon dioxide (acidic). An excess of carbon diox-ide makes the blood less alkaline, and stimulates the respiratory centre. Breathing becomes deeper and faster, and more car-bon dioxide is expired. Any acid in the blood (e.g. lactic acid formed in the muscles during exercise) has the same effect. The more acidic the blood, the greater the stimu-lation.

There is an important difference be-tween *anoxia* (lack of oxygen) and *asphyxia* (*suffocation*). With asphyxia, the blood is short of oxygen and at the same time car-bon dioxide formed in the tissues is not eliminated. This carbon dioxide stimulates breathing and so tends to correct both faults. With anoxia, for example at very high altitudes, there may be just enough oxygen in the air to keep a man alive if he breathes rapidly and deeply, but he has no stimulus to do so. At first, the shortage of oxygen may provide a weak stimulus. But deep breathing eliminates carbon dioxide – and with it the most effective stimulus to the respiratory centre. The centre is then in-hibited both by lack of carbon dioxide in the blood and *severe* lack of oxygen, and breathing stops. Lack of oxygen also de-presses the brain, so that even if an oxygen mask is to hand the man quickly becomes too dazed to use it.

respiratory syncytial virus (RSV). A virus first identified in 1954 but not recognized as a cause of human illness until 10 years later. When RSV is grown in tissue culture there is a tendency for the cells of the cul-ture to merge with each other and form a conglomerate or *syncytium*. RSV infection is common in the first two years of life. Older children and adults are generally immune.

Most RSV infection is mild and con-fined to the nose and throat, and the illness is exactly like a common cold. In some cases it is more like influenza.

Less commonly, RSV infection causes *bronchiolitis*. This is a severe illness of early childhood, with symptoms suggesting both pneumonia and asthma. The importance of bronchiolitis was not recognized until the mid-1960s, and before then it was surely the cause of some mysterious 'cot-deaths', apparently from suffocation. Antibiotics that would cure pneumonia can do no more than prevent secondary bacterial in-fection, and drugs that relieve the spasm of asthma have no effect because the bronchi-oles are blocked not by spasm but by in-flammation. In severe cases the child needs oxygen and artificial respiration, and also constant supervision of the fluid intake to avoid dehydration. In practice this means that he has to be treated in hospital.

rest. Until recently, rest was regarded as a sort of panacea, or at least as a necessary supplement to all other medical treatment. Its most famous champion was a London surgeon, John Hilton (1804–78), whose *Rest and Pain* was among the most influ-ential medical books of the 19th century. Hilton did more than anyone else of his time to teach surgeons to let well alone. His doctrine that diseased parts need rest – for many years a medical axiom – is still accepted, but only with some reservations. Where there is definite inflammation, or where damaged tissues are healing, move-ment delays or prevents healing, and also encourages the spread of infection to neighbouring tissues if bacteria are the cause of the trouble. To some extent, rest is automatic, because loss of function is one of the effects of inflammation. With pneu-monia, for instance, the chest fails to ex-pand on the affected side and breathing is one-sided. One cannot use a septic finger or a badly sprained ankle. Nobody with a fever wishes to exert himself.

Sometimes it is necessary to help. A broken bone does not heal unless the ends are held in place. Before effective drugs were found, prolonged rest was the most hopeful treatment of an organ affected with tuberculosis, and surgical methods were used to prevent a severely affected lung from being used. An inflamed joint may need a splint not only to prevent the pain of movement but to allow the inflammation to subside. In these and many other cases there are definite reasons for encouraging rest, and nobody doubts its value.

But rest for its own sake is no longer accepted as good medicine. A generation ago, candidates for medical degrees could safely begin an answer to almost any question by saying that they would order a bland diet, a laxative, and complete rest. Today, they would be expected to say why, and also what they meant by rest.

The surgeons were perhaps the first to recognize that rest could be overdone, when they discovered that many of the complications that arose while their patients spent a mandatory fortnight in bed after operations arose precisely because the patients *were* in bed, and could be avoided by getting the patients up as soon as possible. In fact, many patients are able to walk around a few hours after major surgery, without ill effects. And loss of function after injuries can often be blamed on failure to get the injured part moving as soon as possible.

Much the same is true of other branches of medicine. If there is no definite reason for patients to rest, they are no longer forced to do so. Even those who do not feel well enough to get up are, with few exceptions, at least encouraged to move around in bed. In defiance of all that was taught until quite recently, exercise is prescribed in certain cases of serious heart disease. It has to be closely supervised, because overexertion would be dangerous, but the heart specialists who advocate this treatment claim to reduce the risks of angina by cautious physical training.

Rest does not necessarily mean physical rest. Much illness is largely due to mental stress. This calls for rest, but of a kind that may be better taken behind a lawn-mower than in bed.

resuscitation. Revival of patients who appear to be dead, e.g. from drowning, electrocution or heart attacks. By any definition, death is irreversible, and anyone who can be resuscitated is still alive, however desperate his condition. But to decide whether a person is dead and beyond resuscitation or still alive may be very difficult

indeed; and the decision has become much harder in recent years. When resuscitation meant only artificial respiration it was hard enough to decide when further attempts would be useless. Now that a heart can be kept beating with an electrical impulse, while the lungs are ventilated mechanically, or the whole work of heart and lungs can be done by a machine, it may be almost impossible to say whether someone is alive or dead. One can remove an animal's heart and keep it beating almost indefinitely with a supply of oxygen and other essentials: in a sense the heart still lives while the animal is undoubtedly dead. Similarly it may be possible to keep most of a patient's organs 'alive' long after he has ceased to be a living person in any complete sense.

reticular formation. A tangle of nerve cells and fibres in the brain-stem in which impulses between the brain and the periphery are switched into appropriate pathways (◊ *midbrain*).

reticulocyte. A newly formed red blood cell, distinguished from mature cells by a fine network revealed by staining. An unduly large proportion of these cells is evidence that red cells have been rapidly replaced, e.g. after bleeding.

reticuloendothelial (RE) system. A community of cells scattered around the body. They are *phagocytes*, i.e. they can engulf and destroy foreign matter, such as bacteria, or worn-out tissue due to be replaced, such as blood cells that have served their useful term. Stationary RE cells line bloodspaces in the bone marrow, spleen and lymph nodes, and are also found in the liver and other tissues. Some authorities limit the RE system to these cells, but others include cells wandering at large in the blood and connective tissues. RE cells are closely related to blood cells.

The RE system seems to play an essential though ill-defined part in immunity to infection.

◊ *spleen; lymph.*

reticulosis. Any disorder mainly affecting the reticuloendothelial system, including infections such as typhoid and malaria with a predilection for RE cells, and conditions such as Hodgkin's disease.

retina. Light-sensitive membrane lining the back of the ◊ eye.

retinaculum. Retaining band of connective tissue, such as the *flexor retinaculum* at the front of the wrist (◊ *carpal tunnel*).

retinitis. Inflammation of the retina. ◊ *eye* (3); *retinopathy*.

retinoblastoma. A tumour of the retina; one of the rare cancers of infancy.

retinol = ◊ *vitamin A*.

retinopathy. Any disease of the retina. It is a better word than the widely used 'retinit- is' for conditions without inflammation, such as the damage to the retina by severe diabetes or high blood pressure arising from degeneration of small arteries in the retina.

retroflexion ◊ *retroversion*.

retrolental fibroplasia. Proliferation of connective tissue behind the lens of the eye, impeding the passage of light and ultimate- ly causing blindness. It appeared as a new disease of infancy in the 1940s, and dis- appeared when the cause was found to be over-use of oxygen in the first few days of life. Asphyxiated babies need oxygen, and it had not occurred to anyone that they could be given too much. When new-born babies are given oxygen it is now either diluted with air or given intermittently.

retroversion. Backward displacement of an organ, especially the uterus. A normal uterus slopes downwards and backwards; a retroverted one may lie vertically or slope downwards and forwards. *Retroflexion* is a somewhat different condition: the uterus is arched backwards. Both conditions are so common among healthy women that one may doubt whether they should be regard- ed as abnormalities. Nevertheless, symp- toms such as backache and menstrual dis- turbances are sometimes relieved by cor- recting the position of the uterus.

rhesus factor (Rh factor). A factor in blood determining one of the systems of blood groups (◊ *blood* (5); *transfusion*).

An independent system of blood groups discovered in 1940 in experiments with rhesus monkeys has been named the

rhesus system. It involves half a dozen factors, of which one ('D') is especially important. In 85 per cent of people the red blood cells carry factor D; these people are rhesus (Rh) positive. The 15 per cent with- out D are Rh negative.

If Rh-positive red cells find their way in- to a Rh-negative person's blood-stream, their D factor excites a defensive reaction: it is a 'foreign' substance, and an *antibody* is formed to neutralize it, exactly as though it were a harmful bacterium. The effect of this reaction is to destroy the foreign red cells. If a Rh-negative person is given a transfusion of Rh-positive blood, antibod- ies are formed too slowly to cause much trouble. But the person is then *immune* to D, and remains so. If he ever has another transfusion of Rh-positive blood, his anti- bodies will promptly destroy the foreign cells, just as antibodies first formed during an attack of measles will ever afterwards destroy the virus of measles and prevent a second attack (◊ *immunity*).

Like all blood groups, the Rh group is inherited. If a Rh-negative woman marries a Rh-positive man, there is a fair chance that her children will be Rh-positive. Since blood cells are too large to pass from the baby to the mother during pregnancy, his Rh-positive red cells have no chance of making her form antibodies, and unless she has previously had a Rh-positive blood transfusion all is well. But at the time of birth the mother bleeds from the uterus and the baby bleeds through the placenta. If some of the baby's cells get into the moth- er's veins, she forms antibodies against them. She is then immune to D, and if she has another Rh-positive baby her anti- bodies filter across the placenta and dam- age the baby's red blood cells.

Although 15 per cent of women are Rh- negative, and 85 per cent of their husbands are Rh-positive, only about one baby in 200 is affected by Rh-incompatibility. Firstly, not all babies of these mixed marriages are Rh-positive, and the negative ones run no risk. Secondly, most women do not actually form the antibodies, or they do so only after two or three successful pregnancies. Thirdly, even when there are antibodies the damage to the baby's red cells may not be enough to give serious trouble. But in a few babies this is a fatal disease. Some are stillborn, some are born with heart failure due to profound anaemia, and some devel- op severe jaundice soon after birth, because broken-down blood-pigment forms bile-pigment, and jaundice is simply an excess of bile-pigment. The babies with heart failure seldom live more than a few hours, but after the first day the jaundice becomes more lethal than the anaemia. Bile-pigment is highly poisonous to the new-born baby's nervous system, much more so than in older children or adults. The *untreated* babies who survive may have permanent damage to the brain (◊ *spastic paralysis*).

The standard treatment is *exchange transfusion*. An ordinary transfusion might help the anaemia but would do nothing to lessen the destruction of the baby's own red cells and the resulting jaundice. Exchange transfusion is done with a large hypodermic syringe and a three-way valve with leads to (1) the baby, (2) a supply of Rh-*negative* blood, (3) waste. Blood is drawn from the baby a syringeful at a time and replaced with the fresh blood which, being Rh-negative, cannot be harmed by the mother's antibodies still in the baby's blood. By the time half a litre of blood (twice the volume of the baby's blood) has been withdrawn both antibodies and bile-pigment are usually reduced to safe levels. By this means some 95 per cent of affected babies can be saved. Methods of getting fresh blood into the baby before birth are now being studied, and there is promising research on ways of suppressing the mother's antibodies before they can do any harm. An antibody against the D factor is used to prevent Rh-negative women from developing antibodies of their own that would be a danger to a subsequent baby. The immunization is carried out immediately after the first confinement. If any Rh-positive cells have entered the mother's blood, they are neutralized by the injected antibody before they have time to do any harm. The patient develops no lasting immunity to Rh-positive cells.

rheumatic fever. An acute illness, commonest among children and adolescents, with raised temperature, and centres of inflammation arising and subsiding unpredictably in connective tissues. The tissues most affected are those of the larger joints and the lining and valves of the heart. Characteristically, one joint after another becomes swollen and painful for a few days.

Sometimes the disease seems to run a very mild course with little or no fever, and only fleeting pains in the limbs. Many such cases have been lightly dismissed as 'growing pains', but growing pains are a myth.

Many children develop curious involuntary movements during an attack of rheumatic fever, a condition known as Sydenham's ◊ *chorea*.

The joints always recover completely, and chorea always subsides. But the heart may be permanently affected. Inflammation of the heart valves may leave scars that deform the valves. The *mitral valve*, which allows blood to flow from the left atrium to the left ventricle but prevents flow in the opposite direction, is most often damaged. There may be narrowing of the valve (mitral stenosis) and also leakage (mitral incompetence). Both defects increase the work to be done by the heart, sometimes to a point where the heart muscle (which may itself have been weakened by rheumatic fever) can no longer meet all normal demands (◊ *heart failure*).

The cause of rheumatic fever is still not known. It is always preceded by infection with the same species of bacterium, the haemolytic streptococcus (severe sore throat, scarlet fever etc.), the rheumatic attack coming on a week or two after recovery from the infection.

In some ways, rheumatic fever resembles an allergic reaction. It does not seem to arise from allergy to streptococci, but the trouble might be caused by the antibodies that the patient himself forms to destroy the streptococci. If the precise nature of the disease remains a mystery, it is at least clear that rheumatic fever is prevented by prompt and adequate treatment of streptococcal infection. This has been possible since the discovery of sulphonamides, and since 1936 the disease has become less and less common.

Salicylates such as aspirin control the symptoms of rheumatic fever. Corticosteroid hormones are equally effective, but they have numerous drawbacks and have not replaced salicylates as the routine treatment.

The treatment of late complications – rheumatic heart disease – has been greatly improved by operations for restoring the efficiency of damaged valves.

rheumatism. Any painful disorder of joints or muscles not directly due to infection or injury. This rather ill-defined group includes rheumatic fever (acute rheumatism), rheumatoid arthritis, osteoarthritis, gout, and 'fibrositis' – itself an ill-defined group of disorders in which pain felt in muscles is the common factor.

rheumatoid arthritis. A chronic disease of connective tissue, commoner in women than men. In Britain at least one person in 20 has it at some time; the figure may be much higher because mild cases are not reported.

The characteristic feature is a small knot or nodule of inflamed fibrous tissue; these tender nodules are often just under the skin. Any organ may on occasion be affected, but most of the symptoms arise from inflammation of the fibrous connective tissue around the joints. Any joint may be affected but the knuckle-joints and wrists tend to suffer most.

The course of the disease varies widely. In most cases the inflammation subsides without doing much damage, though further attacks are possible. Less often a sort of grumbling inflammation persists and the affected joints are stiffened by damage to their linings of smooth cartilage. In severe cases joints may become crippled. This is partly due to direct damage to the joint linings, and partly to the action of muscles around the joint. The muscles over any seat of inflammation tighten as a defensive reaction, and when this happens around a damaged joint the joint may in time be deformed or even dislocated.

In rare cases, rheumatoid arthritis takes the form of a generalized feverish illness like a protracted attack of rheumatic fever.

The cause of rheumatoid arthritis is not known. There is evidence that it may be an instance of ◊ *autoimmunity*, i.e. of a sustained allergic reaction to some component of the patient's own tissues. Physical and emotional stresses play some part in setting off attacks, and there may also be hereditary factors. The immediate damage to joints is probably due to the release of destructive enzymes from inflamed cells, and some research is directed at the source of these.

Rheumatoid arthritis is not likely to be completely curable until more is known of its causes, but much can be done to alleviate it. Pain and inflammation can be controlled with various drugs such as aspirin, phenylbutazone, and indomethacin (◊

analgesic), and in most cases this is enough.

Compounds of gold are sometimes given to suppress the underlying process rather than the symptoms of rheumatoid arthritis. The results are often good, but the dose is not easy to regulate, and the treatment is suitable only for selected cases. The antimalarial drug chloroquine is also sometimes effective. How these drugs work is unknown.

Steroid hormones (◊ *corticosteroid*) give quite dramatic relief in severe cases. This disease was the first for which these drugs were used, and for a short time it seemed as though a cure had been discovered. But it soon became clear that the disadvantages of the treatment outweighed the benefits except in severe, progressive disease; in such cases these hormones are invaluable.

Acutely inflamed joints can be protected from harmful wear and tear and from deformity by splinting, but as inflammation subsides controlled exercises are used to preserve function. Patients who have lost the use of one joint are taught to make the best use of unaffected joints, and many ingenious gadgets have been devised to assist severely handicapped patients. Devices as simple as a higher toilet seat or a knife and fork with handles large enough to be grasped by stiff fingers may be enough to restore a patient's independence.

Some joints can be treated surgically. Surgery can be used to correct deformity, to immobilize a badly damaged joint and prevent painful and useless movement, or to construct an artificial joint.

rhinitis. Inflammation of the lining of the nose, e.g. by common cold or hay fever.

rhodopsin. Light-sensitive pigment in the retina. ◊ *eye* (2).

rhonchus. Wheeze; an abnormal breath sound with bronchitis, asthma etc.

rhythm method. Safe-period method of birth control. ◊ *conception.*

rib. The rudiments of a pair of ribs project from the sides of every ◊ *vertebra*. As a rule only those of the 12 thoracic vertebrae form separate bones, but an additional pair may be attached to the 7th cervical or 1st lumbar vertebra. These are unimportant unless a cervical rib compresses one of the nerves to the arm.

The ribs have rounded heads to fit shallow sockets on the vertebrae, and each makes a second joint with the transverse process of the vertebra. The front part of each rib is of cartilage, not bone. The cartilages of the upper seven ribs are directly attached to the sternum, and the next three each join the cartilage above. The last two ('floating ribs') end blindly in the muscles of the back.

A rib is easily broken and easily mended. The fracture is effectively splinted by the adjacent ribs. The object of strapping fractured ribs is not so much to promote healing as to relieve the pain of breathing. If the ribs are held firmly respiration is carried on by the diaphragm. The danger of a fractured rib is injury to the underlying organs – lungs, liver, spleen – with internal bleeding. But apart from small punctures of the lung (◊ *pneumothorax*) which usually heal well, these complications are rare except in cases of severe multiple injuries. Some of the worst are caused by the impact of the steering wheel in motor accidents, with fractures of the ribs or costal cartilages on both sides and depression of the sternum against the heart.

riboflavin = ◊ *vitamin B₂*.

ricinus. Plant of which the seeds yield castor oil.

rickets. Defective growth of bone due to lack of vitamin D. The vitamin is formed in human skin exposed to sunlight. Children deprived of sunlight need vitamin D in their diet (fish, milk, eggs). Rickets affects those who lack either source. It was therefore rife among poor children in English towns during the Industrial Revolution. In many countries it is known as the English disease.

Without vitamin D, not enough calcium salts are deposited in bone to make it rigid. The cartilage at the growing ends of long bones is enlarged, e.g. at the front ends of the ribs and at the knees; and weight-bearing bones are twisted out of shape.

A rare condition, *renal rickets*, is due to incompetence of the kidneys, which allow phosphates to escape in the urine in such amounts that not enough calcium phosphate can be deposited in the bones.

Neither sunlight nor a normal diet provides enough vitamin D to cure rickets; a concentrated supply such as halibut-liver oil or synthetic vitamin D is needed.

For the origin of the word, ◊ *rachitis*.

Rickettsia. A genus of small bacteria, responsible for typhus and several other fevers transmitted by insects.

Rift Valley fever. An influenza-like illness, due to a virus found in East Africa. It is transmitted from animal to man by mosquitoes.

rigor. Violent attack of shivering at the start of a fever, indicating a rapid rise of body temperature.

ringworm. One of the commonest skin diseases; it is an infection of the outer layer of the skin with a microscopical fungus or mould. With certain types the infection tends to spread outwards as a disc; the centre heals while the circumference is still active, forming a ring.

Common sites are the scalp (true 'ringworm'), the groin ('dhobie itch'), and between the toes ('athlete's foot').

Itching is common to all forms. With ringworm of the scalp, small patches of hair are temporarily lost. The nails of the fingers or toes may harbour the fungus and become deformed, often in association with athlete's foot.

Sometimes small itchy blisters appear at some distance from the site of infection, e.g. on the fingers with athlete's foot. This *id reaction* is not a spread of the infection, but an allergic reaction to it.

Many ointments and lotions can be applied to the affected skin, including preparations of salicylic acid, antiseptic dyes, aluminium acetate, and undecylenic acid. There are many species of fungi among the causes of ringworm and they respond to different remedies, but even when the fungus has been identified the best treatment may have to be found by trial and error.

The antibiotic griseofulvin, taken by mouth, cures cases of ringworm that resist all local treatment. It is most often needed with infection of the hair and nails, and renders unnecessary the older, drastic remedies which involved removing large areas of hair or infected finger-nails.

RNA. Ribonucleic acid. ◊ *genetics* (1).

rodent ulcer. A kind of cancer of the skin, practically confined to the face and scalp. It starts as a small, round, painless hard lump in the skin. As the lump grows its centre tends to break down, forming an open sore (ulcer) with a raised circumference. Like any cancer, a rodent ulcer destroys any healthy tissue in its path. Unlike most other cancers it is nearly always restricted to the area in which it is seen. If, therefore, it is removed surgically or destroyed with drugs or radiation it is almost certainly cured. This property, together with the fact that the disease occurs where it is easily noticed, makes rodent ulcer the least dangerous of cancers.

Roentgen, Wilhelm Conrad (1845–1923). German physicist, awarded the first Nobel Prize for physics in 1901 for his discovery of X-rays. When studying the behaviour of electricity in a vacuum in 1895, Roentgen found that a covered photographic plate had been exposed. He made a rapid yet thorough investigation of the event, and within a few weeks was able to publish an account of the physical properties of the new rays, the use of photographic plates or fluorescent screens to observe them, and the degree of transparency to them of different substances including human tissues.

Roentgenography. Radiography; the use of X-rays to reveal internal structure.

Rokitansky, Carl von (1804–78). Viennese pathologist; the most indefatigable observer of the processes and physical effects of disease. He personally made and described more than 30,000 postmortem examinations, and directed twice that number. This mass of reports is a foundation-stone of modern pathology. Rokitansky was no experimental scientist, and he was an unlucky theorist ($\Diamond$ *pathology*), but it was on his observation of fact that scientists like Virchow were to build.

rosacea. Abnormal redness of the skin of the nose and sometimes of large areas of the face. It is popularly attributed to heavy drinking, but in fact there are many other causes. In sensitive people – the tendency is at least in part hereditary – anything that causes temporary flushing of the face, such as strong tea, very hot or cold or spicy food, or emotion, can lead to permanent flushing in time. Sometimes a kind of acne accompanies rosacea, and the affected skin may become thickened. The treatment is mainly to find and eliminate causes. The lotions and ointments used for acne sometimes help.

roseola. Any pink rash, but especially that of measles (rubeola).

Ross, Sir Ronald (1857–1932). British physician, in the Indian Medical Service; he proved that malaria was transmitted by mosquito bites. Ross was awarded a Nobel Prize in 1902.

roundworm. A common parasite of the intestine. $\Diamond$ *worms.*

RSV = $\Diamond$ *respiratory syncytial virus.*

rubefacient. Medication applied to the skin to increase its flow of blood and redden it. $\Diamond$ *counter-irritation.*

rubella = $\Diamond$ *German measles.*

rubeola = $\Diamond$ *measles.*

rubor. Reddening (of the skin) as a sign of inflammation.

rugae. Wrinkles or folds, e.g. those of the lining of the intestine and some other mucous membranes.

rupture. 1. Bursting of a hollow organ such as an inflamed appendix. **2.** = $\Diamond$ *Hernia.*

rutin. A substance obtained from buckwheat, said to strengthen capillary blood vessels and sometimes used as a vitamin. Its value is doubtful.

S

Sabin vaccine. A vaccine against polio-myelitis, prepared by growing the virus under artificial conditions until it loses its ability to cause the disease. When this attenuated virus is taken by mouth it confers immunity in the same way as an attack of poliomyelitis, but without causing symptoms.

sac. A pocket or bag of tissue, e.g. *amniotic sac*, the fluid-filled membrane surrounding an unborn baby; *hernial sac*, a protrusion of peritoneum (lining membrane of the abdomen) through a gap in the muscles (◊ *hernia*).

saccharose. Ordinary sugar; sucrose.

sacral. Of the sacrum.

sacroiliac joint. Joint at the base of the spine between the sacrum and hip-bone (◊ *pelvis*).

The sacroiliac joints carry the weight of the body to the legs; the sacrum belongs to the backbone and the ilium to the lower limb. The joint surfaces do not interlock, and since the plane of the joint is almost vertical there is a considerable shearing strain. Unlike most joints, the sacroiliac joint gets little support from muscles. This is one of the few joints supported almost entirely by ligaments, and since there is virtually no movement between the bones the ligaments are all taut the whole time. Yet there is a real joint-space, lined with cartilage, as though this were a movable joint. Towards the end of pregnancy the ligaments of the sacroiliac joint may loosen, allowing the baby's head to push the sacrum back a little and so enlarge the birth-passage. The strain on the slackened ligaments would explain the dull ache at the base of the spine so often felt in the last weeks of pregnancy.

sacrum. The continuation of the backbone below the lumbar vertebrae; it consists of 5 vertebrae joined together. The sacrum is the central bone of the ◊ *pelvis*.

safe period ◊ *conception*.

St Anthony's fire. 1. = ◊ *Erisypelas*. **2.** Ergot poisoning.

St Louis encephalitis. A virus disease, affecting the brain, occasionally carried from animals to man by mosquitoes.

St Vitus's dance. Sydenham's ◊ *chorea*, a complication of rheumatic fever.

salicylate. A salt of salicylic acid; the term generally includes derivatives such as acetylsalicylic acid (aspirin). ◊ *analgesic*.

saline. A common abbreviation of 'normal (or isotonic) saline solution', a solution of sodium chloride in water in a concentration, about 0·9 per cent, which balances the osmotic action (◊ *osmosis*) of the body fluids, so that it can be injected without disturbing the amount of water inside the cells of the body. A stronger (hypertonic) solution would draw water out of the cells, and a weaker (hypotonic) would waterlog them. In this context, 'normal' means physiological; it has nothing to do with the normal solution of chemistry, which is nearly 7 times stronger.

Normal saline solution is used in large quantities to replace fluid in cases of dehydration, and in small quantities as a vehicle for drugs to be injected. There are several more elaborate variations in which a part of the sodium chloride is replaced by other salts of which the body has been depleted, or by glucose. In addition to their clinical uses, these are used in the laboratory for keeping alive fragments of tissue to be studied.

saliva. Watery fluid secreted by the salivary glands into the mouth. The flow of moisture keeps the mouth clean, facilitates speech, and makes it possible to ◊ *taste* solids (the nerve-endings for taste respond only to dissolved substances). One phase of ◊ *digestion* begins in the mouth: saliva contains an ◊ *enzyme, ptyalin*, which splits starch into smaller molecules to be broken down in the intestine to simple sugars.

There are 3 pairs of *salivary glands*: parotid, submandibular, and sublingual. The *parotid* gland extends from the root of the cheek bone in front of the ear down to the angle of the jaw which it overlaps. The external carotid artery and the facial nerve are embedded in the gland. The duct runs forwards to open inside the cheek. The *submandibular* gland lies under the jaw, below the back teeth, and the *sublingual* in the floor of the mouth behind the chin. The ducts of both open at either side of the *frenulum* of the tongue.

Salivation is a ◊ *reflex* carried by ◊ *parasympathetic* nerves. The stimulus may be food in the mouth (inborn reflex) or mere anticipation of food (conditioned reflex). The very opposite of appetite – nausea – can also cause salivation, but this is only a part of widespread over-activity of reflexes.

By far the commonest disorder of the salivary glands is ◊ *mumps*, a virus infection which may involve other glands.

Like all glands the salivary glands can be affected by cancer, but most salivary tumours are not cancerous and are easily cured by surgical removal.

The duct of a salivary gland may become blocked by a *calculus*, a deposit of insoluble chalky matter. Small calculi are easily removed; with large ones the whole gland may have to be removed – no great loss since it has probably ceased to work, and the remaining 5 are more than enough.

Salk vaccine. A vaccine against poliomyelitis, prepared by killing the virus with formaldehyde and adding a small amount of penicillin. When the dead virus is injected it cannot cause the disease but confers immunity to infection by a live virus.

Salmonella. A genus of bacteria, including the causes of typhoid and paratyphoid fevers and some common types of food poisoning.

salpingitis. Inflammation of the Fallopian tubes from infection with gonococci, streptococci or other bacteria. The infection may be carried to the tubes in the bloodstream, but more often reaches them by direct spread from the vagina and uterus. An acute attack causes severe pain in the lower abdomen like that of appendicitis, and like appendicitis it can lead to widespread and serious infection of the peritoneum.

Probably most cases subside if they are treated promptly with antibiotics, but quite often the affected tube has to be removed, because the trouble is not reported until an abscess has formed. If both tubes are seriously inflamed they may remain blocked by scar tissue; the patient cannot then conceive.

salt. 1. Any compound formed by replacing the hydrogen of an acid with ammonium or a metal, i.e. neutralizing an acid with an alkali.

2. Sodium chloride; common salt. Salt is an essential component of all living matter. The idea that all living cells are bathed in dilute sea-water is considered under ◊ *kidneys*.

The concentration of salt in the body fluids is kept steady by the kidneys. If the concentration rises the salt passed in the urine can reach 2 per cent; if it falls no salt is allowed to escape in the urine. But some salt is inevitably lost in sweat, and this must be replaced in the diet.

If too much salt is retained, e.g. because of deficient flow of blood through the kidneys with heart disease, or with deficiency of the kidneys themselves, the correct dilution of the body fluids is maintained by keeping an equivalent excess of water (◊ *oedema* (2)). It is only in conditions such as these that the intake of salt may have to be restricted. A healthy person can deal with any amount of salt that he is likely to eat. But the gross excess taken by drinking sea-water is poisonous, because sea-water is 3 per cent salt and the most concentrated possible urine only 2 per cent. To get rid of the salt in a pint of sea-water the kidneys must pass a pint and a half of water, and if this goes on the body becomes dehydrated.

If too much salt is lost, e.g. by heavy sweating, vomiting, or leakage of body fluids as a result of burns or other injuries, the correct concentration could be maintained only by reducing the amount of water in the body. What in fact happens is that the concentration is allowed to fall. Salt depletion is quite common after exertion in hot surroundings. The victim feels unduly weary and incompetent, and he is apt to suffer painful muscular cramps, or even prostration. The condition is often mistaken for heat-stroke. The remedy is salt. Anyone who is short of salt can drink a solution of salt in water that would make him vomit in ordinary circumstances.

sal volatile. Ammonium carbonate, used as smelling salts. The pungent smell of ammonia is supposed to revive people who faint, but lowering the patient's head is more effective.

Sanctorius (Santorio) (1561–1636). Italian physician; professor of medicine at Padua; one of the first men to apply science, in the modern sense of drawing inferences from exact observation and measurement, to the study of the human body. He used a cumbersome thermometer to measure the temperature of the body (a practicable instrument was not devised until the 19th century), compared the pulse rate with a pendulum of variable length, and spent many hours of his life suspended from a balance, estimating the fluctuations of his body weight. This was a completely new approach to physiology: it marked the transition from believing in what ought to happen to observing what does happen in the healthy body.

sandfly. A small insect, *Phlebotomus*, of which different species carry the two forms of Leishmaniasis (◊ *kala-azar*, ◊ *oriental sore*) and sandfly fever.

Sandfly fever (three-day fever, Pappataci fever), transmitted by the bite of *Phlebotomus paptasi*, occurs in the countries around the Persian Gulf and the eastern Mediterranean. The patient has aches all over the body and sore eyes, but the disease is not dangerous and does not last long. It is due to a virus.

saphenous veins. Superficial veins of the lower limb; they include the *long* or *great saphenous vein*, which runs from the base of the big toe up the inner side of the limb to the groin, where it joins the femoral vein, and the *short* or *small saphenous vein*, which runs up the back of the calf to enter the popliteal vein behind the knee. There are communicating branches between the two, and between them and the deep veins. The usual one-way valves ensure that the flow is upwards, and valves in the deep branches open inwards so that the flow is from the saphenous to the deep veins under the muscles. If any of these valves fail the saphenous veins become engorged: ◊ *varicose veins*.

sarcoid; sarcoidosis. A sarcoid is a small focus of chronic inflammation without evidence of infection; the name implies a similarity to sarcoma (a kind of cancer) but the two are quite unrelated. *Sarcoidosis* is

the disease in which sarcoids occur. They may be scattered throughout the body. Often they cause no trouble, but when they happen to be concentrated in particular organs or tissues they can imitate many diseases, including disorders of the skin or the lymph nodes, bronchitis, and rheumatism. The liver, nervous system, and blood-forming tissues may also be involved.

This rather uncommon disease is much less dangerous than the diversity of its symptoms would suggest. The sarcoids tend to disappear as mysteriously as they arrived, though sometimes only after a long time. The cause is unknown. This is neither a tumour nor an infection, but it is so often associated with tuberculosis that it may be an abnormal reaction to tuberculous infection (rather as rheumatic fever is an abnormal reaction to streptococcal infection).

Many kinds of treatment appear to succeed, usually because the disease was going to clear up in any case. If symptoms become a serious nuisance, corticosteroid hormones can be given to suppress them.

sarcoma. Cancer arising in bone, connective tissue or muscle, i.e. the tissues mainly derived in the embryo from mesoderm (as opposed to *carcinoma*, arising in covering or lining membranes). Sarcoma is much less common than carcinoma. ◊ *cancer*.

sarcoptes. Acarus, a mite, of which one species causes ◊ *scabies*.

sartorius. A very long strap of muscle at the front of the thigh, attached to the pelvis above the hip-joint and the upper part of the shin. Its action is to flex both hip and knee, as when sitting cross-legged, tailor-fashion.

scabies (the itch). A minor but distressing skin disease caused by a tiny insect, the itch-mite (*Sarcoptes scabei*), of which the female burrows just under the surface of the skin to lay her eggs. The usual sites are soft moist skin, as in front of the elbows or in the groins. The main symptom is itching, which may be complicated by infection of scratch marks with bacteria. Benzyl benzoate emulsion, applied all over from the neck down after a bath, is a rapid cure.

scalp. The skin over the vault of the skull; it is peculiar in several respects. It is extremely tough and inelastic, and it is firmly attached to an underlying muscle, the *epicranius*. This muscle extends as a thin sheet (*frontalis*) from the eyebrows over the forehead and (*occipitalis*) from the nape of the neck over the back of the skull; the central portion is a broad, flat tendon joining the two sheets of muscle. The connective tissue between the epicranius and the skull is very loose and flimsy.

Because the scalp is unyielding, a blow with an instrument as blunt as a rubber truncheon or a boxing glove splits it as cleanly as a knife. The pull of the attached muscle causes the wound to gape, and the blood vessels, of which there are many, are held open. The arteries of the scalp intercommunicate freely, so that there may be arterial bleeding from both sides of the wound. The bleeding can be stopped either by firm pressure over the whole injured area or by stitching the wound.

The loose tissue under the muscle allows bleeding to seep under the whole scalp (whence the black eye from a blow on the forehead). Similarly, pus spreads easily, and abscesses under the scalp are especially dangerous. The flimsiness of this tissue makes it possible for large areas of the scalp to be torn off, e.g. if the hair is caught in machinery.

scaphoid. A small bone in the wrist, at the base of the thumb. It is the most easily broken of the carpal bones (the 8 small bones in the ball of the hand), and the fracture is often difficult to recognize in an X-ray picture. As a rule, a fractured scaphoid heals if the wrist is kept in plaster for a few weeks, but in some cases a surgical operation is needed.

scapula. A triangle of bone about the size of a hand. It lies over the upper ribs and so is slightly concave to fit their curvature. Most of the bone is very thin, but the outer border, running from the lower angle of the scapula to the *glenoid fossa*, is rounded and strong. The glenoid fossa is the socket of the shoulder-joint. Unlike the socket of the hip, it is too shallow to contribute much to the stability of the joint. The *spine* of the scapula is a triangular projection from the back of the bone. Its base runs horizontally from the inner border almost to the glenoid fossa. Its crest, easily felt through the skin, is carried above and beyond the shoulder-joint, to end in a flat plate of bone, the

acromion process. Here the outer end of the clavicle is attached, forming the *acromio-clavicular* joint. From just above and medial to the glenoid fossa a stout projection arises, the *coracoid process*. This points forwards below the clavicle, which is bound to it by strong ligaments.

The scapula is embedded in powerful muscles. Their actions, and the movements of the scapula, are discussed under ◊ *shoulder*.

Because it is well padded and very mobile the scapula is not often broken. If a fracture does occur it is supported by the muscles. Since only a direct and heavy blow is likely to damage the scapula there are usually other injuries in more urgent need of attention.

The scapula is the sole representative in man of the primitive *pectoral girdle* (◊ *skeleton* (2)). Each limb girdle is derived from three elements, seen in the lower limb as *ilium*, *ischium*, and *pubis*. The scapula corresponds with the ilium. The other two elements have dwindled to the coracoid process; they grow separately but are completely integrated into the adult bone. The clavicle is an evolutionary afterthought and not part of the primitive girdle.

scapular (adj.). Of the scapula. (The noun 'scapular' has no anatomical meaning: it is a garment.)

scarlatina = ◊ *scarlet fever.*

scarlet fever (scarlatina). An infectious fever, mainly of childhood, caused by the bacterium *Streptococcus pyogenes*. It is a streptococcal sore throat with the addition of a scarlet rash.

Scarlet fever is spread from case to case by coughing, but many healthy people carry the bacterium and can infect others at any time. The infection can also be spread by contaminated milk or other food.

The symptoms begin about 4 days after infection with fever, sickness, and sore throat. The face is very flushed except that the skin round the mouth remains pale. A day or two later a rash of tiny raised spots, redder than the surrounding skin, spreads over the body.

Apart from the rash, which is unimportant, scarlet fever is no different from any other streptococcal infection. It responds to the same treatment – usually penicillin – and unless treated threatens the same complications (◊ *streptococcus*).

Schick test. A test of susceptibility to diphtheria: a minute dose of diphtheria toxin is injected into the skin, where an inflamed spot appears if the person is susceptible. The test can be used to show whether people exposed to diphtheria need to be immunized.

Schistosoma = ◊ *bilharzia*.

schistosomiasis. Bilharzial disease.

schizoid personality. A term applied to people who avoid emotional involvement with others and tend to be aloof, withdrawn, over-sensitive, and sometimes decidedly eccentric. Although 'schizoid' implies 'like schizophrenia', and schizophrenia is a sort of caricature of a schizoid personality, the two conditions are quite distinct. The most that can be said is that if a schizoid person should ever become mentally deranged he would be more likely to develop schizophrenia than any other psychosis.

Schizomycetes. A class of microbes to which bacteria belong.

schizophrenia. A kind of psychosis or mental derangement; it is probably a pattern of symptoms with various causes rather than a single disease, and some psychiatrists therefore prefer the term 'schizophrenic reaction'.

If one symptom can be said to typify schizophrenia it is the impossibility of making any emotional impact on the patient. The term schizophrenia (split mind) does not mean dual personality, but dissociation of the patient's thoughts from the physical reality of his own body and surroundings – it is no mere slip of the tongue when a schizophrenic refers to himself as 'he' and not 'I'.

When once thought is divorced from reality all kinds of mental symptoms can arise. A healthy mind seems to filter a mass of impressions, and pass to full awareness only those that appear to make sense. To a schizophrenic, sense and nonsense may be all one. The jumbled fantasies, the absurd patterns of words and half-formed ideas that most people have when falling asleep give some hint of what may go on in a schizophrenic's mind. His delusions (e.g. of his own importance, or of persecution by others) and hallucinations (e.g. 'hearing voices') are as real to him as anything else,

for he accepts everything that comes into his mind as valid. His intellect is not impaired, but he fails to apply it.

The causes of schizophrenia are largely unknown. To call it an abnormal response to intellectual or emotional conflict only pushes the question one step backwards: why should a few unfortunate people respond in this way? Heredity certainly plays some part but not, it seems, the leading part; it is hard to distinguish hereditary from environmental factors because families tend to share the same environment. Several chemical abnormalities in the brain have been identified. They relate to *adrenaline* (and drugs such as amphetamine that mimic adrenaline can cause an illness like schizophrenia), *serotonin* (and hallucinogenic drugs such as LSD cause symptoms like those of schizophrenia, and they interfere with serotonin), the copper-containing protein *ceruloplasmin*, and many others. But these changes could as easily be effects of the disease as causes. At least some of them are sure to be effects, for the mental turmoil of schizophrenia must be reflected in chemical changes. The idea of schizophrenia as a chemical anomaly like diabetes or gout is attractive, and would hold out better hopes of cure than any other explanation, but much more evidence is needed – especially about the detailed chemistry of the healthy brain.

Until recently, most schizophrenics were certified insane and confined to mental hospitals until they recovered. Many did not recover, or if they improved enough to be released they had been in hospital so long that they were unable to cope with the outside world and soon relapsed. It is now known that apart from a minority of severe progressive cases there is no need to keep schizophrenics in hospital for long periods, and that the atmosphere of an institution can easily make them worse by depriving them of their remaining shreds of identity. All schools of psychiatry agree that these patients should and can be integrated with the general public like any others with non-infectious illnesses. Since progress in treatment has made this policy possible it has been found that most patients are soon able to live and work with other people – a normal job of work is itself a useful form of treatment. Some patients relapse, but can be expected to recover after further treatment. A few remain ill, but even these seldom need special hospitals. While the illness is at its height, schizophrenics can be difficult to live with, but they are seldom dangerous.

Psychological treatment such as psycho-analysis has its advocates among those who regard schizophrenia as the patient's attempt to adapt himself to conflicts that he cannot resolve. Freud, the founder of psychoanalysis, said that it would be an error in schizophrenia. There is even a possibility that analysis may make things worse, and most psychiatrists feel that the place for psychotherapy is in helping the patient to readjust himself when the worst of his symptoms have been allayed by other means.

◊ *Electroconvulsive therapy* is some-times used. It is not as dramatically help-ful with schizophrenia as with severe de-pression, but it is effective in some cases.

Much the most important advance in the drug treatment of schizophrenia was the introduction in 1954 of the potent tranquil-lizer, chlorpromazine. This drug, or newer ones of the same type, has made it possible to return severely disturbed patients to their homes in a few weeks instead of years, and with this form of treatment many patients lead normal working lives instead of being restrained in institutions.

Schwann, Theodor (1810–82). German anatomist, a pupil of Müller in Berlin; later professor of anatomy at Louvain. He was the first to recognize that animal tissues were composed of ◊ *cells*, and so paved the way for his colleague Virchow to establish the modern science of pathology.

The *sheath of Schwann* is a membrane around a nerve fibre.

sciatic. Of the *ischium* (rump), one of the bones of the pelvis. The *sciatic nerve* is the principal nerve of the lower limb, the larg-est nerve in the body. It is formed in the pelvis from branches of several of the lum-bar and sacral spinal nerves, passes below the sacroiliac joint to the buttock, then be-hind the hip-joint to the back of the thigh. It is deeply buried in muscles throughout its course. Above the knee it divides into tibial and peroneal branches, which be-tween them supply all the structures below the knee. Above this division, small branches of the sciatic nerve go to the muscles and skin of the back of the thigh.

sciatica. Persistent pain in the area of the sciatic nerve, i.e. the back of the thigh, calf, and foot; the whole area is not necessarily or even usually involved.

Sciatica is a symptom and not a disease, and in each case it is the cause that has to be identified and treated, and not the scia-tica itself. The commonest cause is pressure on a spinal nerve destined for the sciatic nerve, usually by an intervertebral disc ('slipped disc'; ◊ *vertebra* (1)). Less often sciatica is due to pressure on the nerve in the thigh from a bad sitting posture or a badly designed seat. Any disease that causes irri-tation of nerves, e.g. diabetes, alcoholism, may involve the sciatic nerve and cause a kind of sciatica.

scintigram. Record of the distribution of radioactivity in an organ after introduction of a small dose of a radioactive substance. The pattern may represent the flow of blood in the organ, or a particular function such as storage of iodine in the thyroid gland. The method is used to define and localize disease processes within the substance of an organ.

sclera (sclerotica). The white shell of the eye.

sclerosis. Thickening or hardening of tissue; e.g. *arteriosclerosis*, hardening of the arteries; *multiple (disseminated) sclerosis*, deposits of abnormal connective tissue in the central nervous system.

scoliosis. Sideways curvature of the spine (cf. *lordosis*, forward curvature; *kyphosis*, backward curvature).

Scoliosis may be due to weakness of the muscles of one side of the back, e.g. as a result of poliomyelitis; to disease of the vertebrae such as rickets; to chronic disease of one lung, when the muscles on the affected side are held taut; to sciatica or disease of a hip-joint, when the pelvis is tilted to relieve strain on the painful side and the spine is bent in the opposite direc-tion to compensate; or to no apparent cause.

scorbutic. Affected with scurvy (lack of vitamin C).

scorpion. Scorpions are found in most hot countries. They are related to spiders, but whereas a spider injects poison by biting, a scorpion has a poisonous sting in its tail.

Scorpion venom is a nerve poison as strong as cobra venom, but the quantity is much less.

A scorpion sting is painful and may be followed by transient weakness of the muscles in its vicinity, but there is little danger except to small children; a child stung by a scorpion is a case for hospital. An antivenene can be given in serious cases. Local anaesthetics are sometimes injected to relieve pain. A dressing soaked in a cold solution of epsom salt or even cold water may help, and the injured part (usually a leg) needs to be kept still. Pain-killing drugs and alcohol do more harm than good.

scotoma. A blind spot in the eye.

scrofula. Tuberculosis of lymph nodes at the side of neck with ulceration of the overlying skin; the King's evil, supposed until the time of the Stuarts to be cured by the Royal Touch.

scrotum. A loose bag of skin containing the testes, which function at a few degrees below the temperature of the rest of the body.

scurvy. A defect of the substance that binds cells together, especially in connective tissue and capillary blood vessels, due to lack of vitamin C. The usual cause is lack of fresh vegetables or fruit; but healing of severe injuries or inflammation makes heavy demands on the supply of vitamin C and may cause a relative deficiency even with an average diet. The symptoms include bleeding into the skin, around bones, into joints, and from the gums. The teeth become loose and misshapen. Resistance to infection is lowered. ◊ *vitamin*; *vitamin C*.

sea sickness ◊ *travel sickness*.

sebaceous. Of *sebum*, a greasy substance formed by the sebaceous glands of the skin. A *sebaceous cyst* or *wen* is a lump in the skin, often at the back of the neck or on the forehead, filled with sebum because of blockage of one of these glands. If the cyst is unsightly or in any other way a nuisance it is easily removed.

seborrhoea. Excessive activity of the sebaceous glands, often associated with acne or dandruff. A kind of eczema, *seborrhoeic dermatitis*, sometimes develops in greasy skin, especially on the scalp. It consists of small, inflamed, itchy spots, with a tendency to form loose scales. Seborrhoeic dermatitis usually responds to simple lotions and dusting powders, but the spots are prone to bacterial infection, and affected skin has to be kept very clean.

sebum. A greasy substance formed by the sebaceous glands around the roots of hairs. It keeps the skin supple.

secretion. The formation by an organ (a gland) of a substance that is needed by some other organ or by the body as a whole. The secretions of *exocrine* glands are carried away in tubes (ducts), or poured straight into the place where they are to be used; e.g. the secretions of the digestive glands and the glands of the skin. The secretions of *endocrine* glands – hormones – are released into the blood.

sedative. A medicine for soothing a patient or making him drowsy. The older sedatives are simply small doses of hypnotics, i.e. of drugs that would send the patient to sleep in larger doses. A newer class of drugs, the tranquillizers, allay anxiety without much dulling the patient's general awareness.

semen. Seed; the secretion of the testes, consisting largely of sperms, to which is added fluid from the prostate and other smaller glands opening into the urethra.

seminoma. A cancer of the testis.

Semmelweis, Ignaz Philipp (1818–65). Hungarian obstetrician, a pioneer in the prevention of ◊ *puerperal* fever, then a very common cause of death after childbirth, due to bacterial infection of the birth-passage.

Before Semmelweis, Charles White (Manchester, 1773) and Alexander Gordon (Aberdeen, 1795) had written of puerperal fever as a form of contagion; Gordon actually recognized that doctors and midwives could carry the infection on their hands and clothes. Next, Oliver Wendell Holmes (Harvard, 1843) wrote a paper in which he stated: 'The disease known as puerperal fever is so far contagious as to be frequently carried from patient to patient by physicians and nurses'. He warned against the possibility of carrying infection from postmortem room to labour ward. Nobody paid him the least attention.

In about 1847 Semmelweis, an assistant

in the university department of obstetrics in Vienna, noticed firstly that puerperal fever was commoner in his wards (where 10 per cent of the women admitted died of it) than in the wards where the midwives were taught; and secondly that a colleague who died of blood-poisoning after doing a postmortem examination had the same symptoms as the women. He then realized that his students were in the habit of going straight from the postmortem room to attend confinements, and he inferred that they carried the infection.

The role of microbes in causing infection was not yet known; nevertheless Semmelweis insisted that everyone attending a confinement should first wash in chlorine water, an efficient antiseptic. The death rate fell at once. Only 1 per cent of the patients still died. Semmelweis published an account of his work in 1861. His views were not only not accepted; he was so abused by his colleagues that he left Vienna and went back to Hungary. He fared better overseas. As early as 1855, Holmes heard of his success and wrote a second paper, to which American doctors did begin to pay attention. A few years later Pasteur and then Lister set the control of infection on a scientific basis and the doctrine of Semmelweis became generally accepted as one of the most important advances in the whole history of medicine.

senility. Although it could mean the sum of all the changes due to old age, senility is generally taken to mean the changes in the brain. All the cells of the body have a limited span of life, but most types of cell can regenerate by dividing to form two new cells. Nerve cells cannot do this, and throughout adult life the number of active cells in the brain gradually decreases. An old brain therefore has less potential than a young one. But a much more important factor is the condition of the arteries of the brain. If they degenerate the brain does not get enough blood and is deprived of oxygen. The amount of arterial degeneration varies greatly, and some people have lively minds at 100 while others begin to deteriorate at 60.

These gradual processes are not the only causes of mental change in old age, for the chances of having a minor stroke or other illness affecting the nervous system inevitably become greater as the years pass.
    ⟡ *ageing.*

sensation. There are several kinds of *receptor*, each responding to a particular kind of stimulus by starting an electrical impulse in an adjacent nerve fibre. The receptors include the rods and cones in the retina of the eye, responding only to light, the organ of Corti in the ear, responding to sound, the taste-buds, the olfactory nerve-endings responding to smells, structures in the skin responding to touch, pressure, and temperature, and receptors for unconscious sensations such as balance and blood pressure. The nerve impulses for all these sensations are identical. They are carried to the brain, where impulses in particular fibres are identified with their sources and translated into information about the environment. Unconscious sensation is conveyed to outgoing (motor) nerve fibres to evoke reflex actions that adjust the body to meet change. Some conscious sensation is also diverted to reflex action, e.g. a bright light is consciously perceived but also causes the pupil to constrict so that the eye is not over-stimulated.

Sensations are essentially events in the brain. If an impulse reaches the brain by a particular sensory nerve then the sensation associated with that nerve is evoked. Dreams and hallucinations must represent spontaneous activity without the usual stimulus to the appropriate receptors, but as far as the brain is concerned the sensations are real.
    ⟡ *referred pain.*

sepsis. Destructive infection of tissue by bacteria such as streptococci or staphylococci.

septicaemia. Spread of sepsis by carriage of bacteria in the blood; blood-poisoning.

septum. A partition such as the sheet of bone and cartilage between the nostrils.

sequestrum. A loose fragment of dead bone, formed as a result of infection of bone (osteomyelitis) and then providing a safe shelter for bacteria so that the infection persists until the sequestrum is removed.

serology. The study of serum, especially of the reactions of serum with microbes. If serum from a person's blood contains antibodies that react with a particular species of microbe, that is good evidence that the person is or has been infected with the same kind of microbe – a useful aid to diagnosis of infectious diseases. Conversely, microbes can be identified from their reactions with sera containing known antibodies.

serotonin. 5-Hydroxytryptamine (5-HT); a substance found in many tissues; it is released from blood platelets at a site of bleeding and helps to control the bleeding by causing constriction of small blood vessels. It seems to play an important part in the working of the brain; it may transmit impulses between nerve cells. Some hallucinogenic drugs interfere with the action of serotonin.

serratus anterior. A large muscle arising from the sides of the ribs and drawing the shoulder-blade forwards, as when punching. If the arms are fixed, the muscle lifts the ribs and helps breathing. A person out of breath will therefore clutch a fixed object.

serum. Clear yellow fluid that separates from clotted blood. ◊ *blood* (1; 4).

Servetus (Miguel Servet y Reves) (1511–53). A Spanish theologian sometimes credited with the discovery of the circulation of blood through the lungs.

Galen's doctrine that blood passed from the left to the right side of the heart through holes in the dividing wall had been accepted for 13 centuries. Servetus said that the blood passed not through the middle wall of the heart but 'by a very ingenious arrangement' through the lungs. He proposed a similar arrangement between the arteries and nerves in the brain. The first theory is correct; the second is nonsense. Neither is based on observation, but the first may have been inspired by a similar suggestion in the 13th century by Ibn an-Nafis.

Servetus's fellow-student Vesalius, a scientific observer, merely said that he could find no holes and that he did not see how Galen's theory could work. Servetus, a dreamer, proposed the right theory without evidence. The real discovery, i.e. demonstration, of the pulmonary circulation was by Vesalius's pupil Colombo. Servetus was concerned not with the flow of blood but with how the Divine Breath reached the remoter parts of the body. Another passage in the same book, *Christianismi Restitutio*, questioned the doctrine of the Holy Trinity. Servetus fled from the wrath of the Spanish Inquisition to the protection of Calvin in Geneva, but Calvin also thought him a heretic and had him burnt at the stake.

sesamoid. A bone formed in a tendon at a point of great friction, e.g. the patella (knee-cap) in the tendon of the quadriceps muscle in front of the knee.

sex. Most bodily functions are concerned with the survival of the individual. Sex ensures the survival of the species. The central event is the *fertilization* of an *ovum* by a *sperm*, and the primary sex organs are the *ovary* and the *testis* in which these germ cells are formed. The accessory sex organs facilitate fertilization and the development of the fertilized ovum. The principal ones are the *Fallopian tubes, uterus* and *vagina* in the female, and the *vas deferens, prostate* and *penis* in the male. These organs are described under their own headings, and the physiology is further considered under *puberty, pregnancy, labour, menopause, sex hormones, genetics.*

Sexual intercourse, or coitus, the process by which fertilization occurs, is based on a simple reflex action: continued stimulation of the penis causes waves of contraction in the involuntary muscles along the urethra, and the ejaculation of a few c.c. of semen containing some hundreds of millions of sperms, swimming in all directions. One of these may find its way into the uterus, and along a Fallopian tube to penetrate the waiting ovum. This reflex is determined at a very primitive level of the nervous system: the nerves involved go no further than the spinal cord. But, like many other reflex actions, it is influenced and modified by many conscious and unconscious factors, and it is preceded and accompanied by many other inborn and conditioned reflexes. These are concerned mainly with the arousal of sexual desire, which prepares the accessory organs for coitus. Unless the male is aroused coitus is not possible, and if the female is not aroused it may be possible but it gives her no pleasure and may be painful. The essential physical changes are erection of the penis by distension with blood, and a similar swelling of tissues at the entrance to the vagina together with secretion of a lubricant fluid. These effects are reflex actions governed by ◊ *parasympathetic* nerves, but they are affected by all the senses, and by memory, fantasy, the mood of the moment, moral and aesthetic feelings, and idiosyncrasy. Only a few of these responses appear to be instinctive, e.g. those to certain smells or to contact with lips, breasts or genitalia, and even these few are profoundly affected at higher levels of consciousness: thus intimate contact that by instinct should excite may embarrass or repel if the other person is unattractive or the circumstances are inappropriate.

Most sexual stimuli are learnt and become conditioned reflexes. When skirts reached the ground the sight of a woman's ankles was exciting. In modern western society, breasts have usurped ankles – but in societies where breasts are normally bare the men are not disturbed by them. Kissing is an expression of love, but only among people who are brought up to this idea. And, within a society, individuals differ very widely in their acquired tastes, which may have their origins in infancy or early childhood.

Sexual arousal, if it is continued, culminates in *orgasm*, a sudden burst of activity in the ◊ *sympathetic* nervous system, of which the effects in the male include ejaculation of semen, and in both sexes a kind of pleasurable convulsion followed by a profound sense of release and satisfaction. Thus one half of the involuntary (autonomic) nervous system, the parasympathetic, prepares for the climax, and the other half, the sympathetic, achieves it. But the division is not so clear; the two systems work together throughout, and their activity is influenced by hormones and by the conscious elements of the nervous system.

Before considering one or two of the more common medical aspects of the sexual act it may be worth noting the analogy between sexual appetite and the much less complicated appetite for food. At its most primitive, the desire to eat arises from having an empty stomach. The desire is reinforced by the taste or smell of food. That is about all that is inborn or instinctive. The rest has to be learnt, as Pavlov's dogs learnt to associate a bell with food until the bell alone stimulated appetite and they had acquired a conditioned ◊ *reflex*. We learn to respond with appetite to the sight of food, talk of food, the trimmings of a well served meal, or merely knowing that it is dinner time. Appetite is enhanced by pleasant surroundings, con-genial company and a relaxed mood. Unattractive looking food, wholesome as it may be, worry, or illness suppress appetite. A delicacy in one society may disgust another. Religions lay down dietary rules that other religions think absurd. Unhappy associations can create dislikes and fads, and within a social group individual tastes differ greatly for no apparent reason.

Sexual feelings develop in the same way and under similar influences, but they are subject to far more public and private censure than tastes in food. A man who eats peanut butter with smoked salmon may seem eccentric, but nobody fetches a psychiatrist or a policeman to him. Even in sexual matters, what matters most is not what society really thinks, but what the individual supposes that society thinks. One of the commonest sources of unhappiness in sex is the fear of falling below a required standard. The conflict between instinctive sexual desire and indoctrinated moral standards is, according to Freud and his disciples, a common source of anxiety and neurosis in general. This may or may not be true, but the conflict is undoubtedly a source of trouble with sex itself. Even in these days of open discussion, people still marry believing, consciously or not, that sex is dirty and wrong. But prudery is not the only tyrant. Permissiveness also has its tyrannies, and girls whose great-grandmothers worried themselves into a decline over losing their virtue are now apt to worry if they remain virgins, or are less promiscuous, or more conventional, than seems right to them. The leaders of subcultures sometimes forget that there are people who prefer simple home cooking to the exotic fare that they advocate.

Inadequacy, real or supposed, is the commonest reason for people to consult their doctors about sex. *Frigidity* is lack of sexual desire, sometimes amounting to positive aversion. The term is nearly always applied to women rather than men, perhaps because the medical vocabulary has been coined by men, and frigid men prefer to call themselves continent. *Impotence* is inability to perform coitus. A woman can be impotent if physical obstruction at the entrance to the vagina makes coitus impossible: ◊ *dyspareunia*. But impotence is primarily a male disorder, usually a failure of the penis to erect, but it can also take the form of *ejaculatio praecox*, when orgasm occurs and erection subsides either before or at the moment of entry.

These conditions can have physical causes. Sexual activity, like other physical functions, is depressed by general ill health, and by various drugs. Heavy drinking is a common cause of impotence; on the other hand a reasonable drink at bedtime (which in this context does not have to be any fixed hour) can allay the anxiety that is causing the trouble. Hence the reputation of alcohol as an aphrodisiac. Most impotence and most frigidity are emotional states or frames of mind. It is relevant that a few men are impotent with their wives yet potent with prostitutes. This has been rather pompously ascribed to an incest-taboo, the man unconsciously identifying his wife with his mother. A simpler explanation might be that he loves his wife and is afraid of hurting her, physically or mentally. Clear thinking would tell him that his going with prostitutes would hurt her more, but logic has no place in sexual behaviour. Similarly, frigidity has been ascribed to anxieties arising from psychological trauma in childhood, but often it would be simpler and clearer to blame shyness, from which either sex can suffer. And pretended frigidity is natural in women, as in females of other species. A woman is seldom aroused as quickly as a man, and her apparent disinclination is sometimes an invitation to woo her. Unless both partners are prepared for it, coitus is not as satisfying as it should be to either, and may be positively distasteful to the woman.

Most people do not discuss the details of their sex-life, even with their best friends, and those who do are not always truthful. (This casts doubt on some surveys of sexual behaviour.) Young couples disappointed by their first attempts would do well to ignore the glowing accounts that other people offer them. They can take it that most honeymoons are something of a fiasco. A few couples achieve sexual harmony at once, but many more need months or even years. It requires patience and above all consideration. This may sound sanctimonious, but it is true. Instinctive sex is a selfish urge, but civilization is largely a process of modifying and subduing instinct, and civilized sex is a partnership. Professional help is needed if neurosis or physical illness interferes with sex, but in the countless cases where the trouble is ignorance, thoughtlessness or shyness the remedy is largely, perhaps literally, in the partner's hands. It is silly to pretend that sex is not important to a stable marriage. It is supremely important, but not so important that it can never be ridiculed. Laughing at it, and at ourselves for taking it too seriously, often brings it comfortably to earth.

Some other medical aspects of sex are briefly discussed under ◊ *contraception*; *fetishism, homosexuality, masturbation*.

sex chromosomes ◊ *genetics* (3).

sex hormones. A person's sex is determined by the sex chromosome from the father at conception. With an X chromosome the gonads become ovaries; with a Y chromosome they become testes. All the other distinguishing marks of sex (sex characters) are determined by hormones formed by the gonads. These hormones are all closely related *steroids*. There are three groups: *androgens, oestrogens,* and *progestogens*. Both sexes have all three, but the proportions differ.

If androgens predominate, male characters (broken voice, facial hair, muscular physique etc.) develop. These characters can be induced in females by giving the hormones artificially, or with certain disorders of the adrenal glands where an excess is produced. In the absence of androgens, female characters develop. Androgens promote the synthesis of protein and the growth of muscle and bone. After puberty the increase of sex hormones causes the ends of the bones, where most growth occurs, to harden, and growth ceases. Because they lack hormones with this effect, eunuchs tend to grow unusually tall.

Oestrogens are the primary female hormones. They influence bodily character less than androgens, because female characters seem to represent the basic human form; it is the male who is a modification. But without these hormones a female remains immature. Their action is more concerned with function than structure; they determine the female sexual cycle, on which fertility depends.

Progestogens are much more specialized hormones, concerned with the preparation and maintenance of pregnancy.

In the body the androgens are represented mainly by *testosterone*, the oestrogens by *oestradiol*, and the progestogens by *progesterone*. The actions of oestradiol and

progesterone are considered further under
◊ *menstruation* and ◊ *ovary*.

Many related hormones have been synthesized for medicinal use. Most are derived from the natural hormones, but synthetic oestrogens such as stilboestrol are not steroids. They are used to make up deficiencies, e.g. of oestrogens after the menopause or of progesterone in some women who tend to miscarry. Some cancers of the reproductive organs can be held in check by altering the balance of sex hormones. Some of the modified androgens promote growth of muscle and bone without stimulating the sex characters.

The sex hormones formed by the gonads are supplemented by varying amounts formed in the cortex of the adrenal glands, which accounts for abnormal sexual development in some disorders of these glands.

The formation and release of sex hormones by the gonads is governed by other hormones from the pituitary gland. If the pituitary is defective there is no stimulus to the gonads and therefore a deficiency of sex hormones.

shaking palsy = ◊ *parkinsonism*.

shell shock. A very severe form of anxiety neurosis among soldiers exposed to trench warfare in the First World War. The term was dropped because the blast of shells was no more than a contributory cause; but at least it was better than the term thrown up by the Second World War – *lack of moral fibre* – with its implication that the patient and not the war was to be blamed.

shingles. ◊ *Herpes* zoster.

shock. Failure of the circulation of blood when the blood pressure is too low to maintain an adequate flow through the tissues and back to the heart; often the immediate cause of death from injury or acute illness. The lethal factor is a reduced flow of blood through the brain. Other organs can manage for a while with a reduced supply, but the brain cannot.

In health, the calibre of the blood vessels is such that they offer a steady resistance to flow. As a result, an even pressure is maintained, enough to ensure that sufficient blood is pumped through the vessels of the

brain to keep up a supply of oxygen and glucose and to remove waste.

Unless some compensating mechanism operates, the pressure must fall if (1) the volume of blood is decreased, or (2) the capacity of the vessels is increased, or (3) the heart pumps less vigorously. All three can contribute to shock. A fourth but less likely cause of a fall in blood pressure would be decreased viscosity of the blood.

1. When someone donates a pint of blood his vessels contract so that the remaining 7 pints still fill them at the original pressure. Later, the volume is restored from the tissue fluid, and the lost protein and cells are replaced more gradually. But after more serious bleeding, with the addition of damage to tissue, the vessels cannot contract enough, and the pressure falls. The bleeding need not be apparent. Enough blood can be lost into the muscles of the thigh around a fractured femur to cause shock. A very large amount of fluid, much of it derived from the blood, can accumulate in a burn, with similar effects on the circulation to severe bleeding. Diarrhoea or vomiting can be so profuse that all the tissues, including the blood, are short of water; for instance if people die of cholera they are in effect killed by shock.

2. An ordinary faint is due to reflex activity including sudden widening of blood vessels to internal organs. The simultaneous constriction of vessels in the skin, causing pallor, does not nearly compensate, and for a moment – until he lies down – the patient is in a state of shock. A similar reflex may operate after injury, and increase the effect of bleeding. Pain and anxiety make it worse. Anything done to relieve pain or calm fear is more than mere kindness – it may be life-saving. With some very severe infections and some types of chemical poisoning the control of blood vessels by the nervous system may become so disorganized that shock develops. It is in this type of shock that the corticosteroid drugs are sometimes very helpful.

3. The efficiency of the heart may suddenly fall off after damage to the heart muscle, e.g. by coronary thrombosis, causing the blood pressure to fall to a dangerous level.

Any of these three types of shock can occur together. If the circulation is impaired for any reason the heart and blood vessels are deprived of oxygen like any other organs, and this causes the blood vessels to dilate and the heart to beat less effectively. A very dangerous vicious circle is then established, and without prompt treatment the patient is unlikely to live.

The treatment of shock obviously depends on the cause. With injuries the first step is to ensure that no further injury is done. Many people who might have survived their original injury are killed by unskilful attempts to move them. Bleeding has to be stopped if replacing lost blood is to do much good. Quite light pressure over an artery or around the edges of wound is enough, or a well applied bandage. When bleeding has stopped, interference with the wound may start it again.

Movement of broken limbs increases the damage and the pain; both contribute to shock.

In the past great stress was laid on the value of warmth, but in fact warmth can do harm by dilating the blood vessels of the skin. It is enough to keep the patient comfortable and prevent him from shivering; cooking him does no good.

Morphine or some such drug may help by relieving pain and calming the patient. Alcohol, on the other hand, promptly lowers the blood pressure and is dangerous. Anything at all given by mouth has to be avoided until it is certain that none of the digestive organs is damaged.

With most types of shock the definitive treatment is to replace lost fluid, with blood transfusion if possible, though other kinds of fluid are also valuable. Drugs to raise the blood pressure, such as noradrenaline and angiotensin, are occasionally helpful but their usefulness is limited.

shock therapy. Treatment of severe mental disorder by abrupt stimulation of the brain cells sufficient to cause a kind of epileptic seizure. Nobody knows how this works, but in practice it often gives quick and lasting relief from severe depression and some other disorders. Various drugs have been used for the purpose, but their effects are difficult to control, and at present the standard method is by applying a small electric current to the scalp (◊ *electro-convulsive therapy*).

shoulder.

1. STRUCTURE

The shoulder is a ball-and-socket joint between the rounded head of the ◊ *humerus*

and the glenoid fossa of the ◊ *scapula*.

The shape of the bones lends little stability to the joint, for the glenoid fossa is small and shallow. While in the hip the head of the femur sits like an egg in an egg-cup, in the shoulder the head of the humerus is more like a golf ball on a tee. Like all movable joints, the shoulder is enclosed in a fibrous capsule, but the capsule is slack and gives little support. Nor is there much support from accessory ligaments. The stability of the shoulder depends almost entirely on muscles.

Fan-shaped muscles from both surfaces of the scapula converge on the upper end of the humerus, to which they are attached behind, above, and in front of the joint. Their tendons merge with the joint capsule, and serve as adjustable ligaments, of which the tension can be maintained in any position.

The deltoid muscle covers the joint and its scapular muscles. Below the joint the nerves and vessels of the arm are close enough to be involved occasionally in fractures or dislocations.

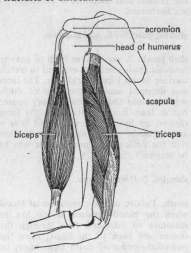

Dissection of left shoulder.

2. MOVEMENTS

The shoulder has a wide range of movement in all directions.

In all but slight movements of the shoulder the scapula moves with the arm. A straight punch is ineffective if the shoulders are braced back. But if the scapula is swung round so that the glenoid fossa looks forwards, the humerus has a firm backing.

When the arms are raised above the head through 180°, about 90° of the movement takes place at the shoulder-joint itself, and 90° comes from rotation of the scapula. If for any reason the shoulder-joint should become immobilized there may still be a good deal of useful movement from the scapula.

3. DISORDERS

The shoulder is more readily *dislocated* than any other joint in the body. This is the price of mobility. It is embraced by muscles on three sides, but below there is little to keep it in place. Dislocation of the head of the humerus is nearly always downwards and forwards. Hippocrates rightly said that dislocation in other directions seemed possible, but he added that he had not seen a case. Simple manipulation is usually all that is needed, but occasionally there are complications. The nerves and vessels below the joint may be involved. The tendons that merge with the capsule may be torn, in which case the dislocation will be liable to recur. There may be an associated fracture, especially since the tendons may be more resilient than the bone to which they are attached. But a fracture is less troublesome than a torn tendon, because bone heals better than fibrous tissue.

These tendons lie in a narrow gap between the joint and an overhang of the scapula, the acromion process. Injury or inflammation of the tendons, or of the subacromial bursa, leads to painful friction when the shoulder is abducted, and sometimes to the painful stiffness known as ◊ *frozen shoulder.*

shoulder-blade = ◊ *scapula.*

sickle-cell anaemia. A hereditary defect of red blood cells. ◊ *haemoglobin; genetics.*

side-effect. Unwanted action of a drug, e.g. drowsiness from an antihistamine given to relieve allergic symptoms, or acceleration of the heart by a drug given for asthma. The term is not usually applied to the toxic effects of an overdose, but to an effect of a standard therapeutic dose. ◊*drug.*

sidero–. Prefix = 'iron', e.g. *sideropenia*, iron deficiency; *siderosis*, deposition of excess iron in the tissues.

sigmoid. S-shaped. The sigmoid colon is the last part of the large intestine before the rectum, lying in the left side of the pelvis.

sigmoidoscopy. Direct examination of the rectum and sigmoid colon with a lighted tube.

sign. Objective indication of disease, i.e. one found by examining a patient, as opposed to a ◊ *symptom*, reported by the patient himself.

silicosis. Deposition of silica dust in the lungs, an occupational disease of miners. ◊ *pneumoconiosis.*

silver nitrate. Dilute solutions of silver nitrate or colloidal suspensions of silver salts were formerly much used as antiseptics in the treatment of infected mucous membranes, and for preventing infection in the eyes of new-born babies. Penicillin generally superseded them.

Simmonds' disease. (Morris Simmonds (1855–1925), German physician.) Failure of the ◊ *pituitary* gland.

Simpson, Sir James Young (1811–70). Scottish gynaecologist; a pioneer of anaesthesia. ◊ *anaesthetics* (2).

sinew. Tendon or ligament.

sinus. 1 (path.). Burrowing ulcer in the form of a blind tube, usually a track by which pus formed at the blind end reaches a body surface. A *fistula* is similar but open to body surfaces at both ends (a body surface may be the skin or the lining of a hollow organ).

2 (anat.). (a) Recess or cavity opening off a hollow structure, e.g. the *air sinuses* around the nose; (b) natural bulge in a tube, e.g. the *carotid sinus*, a dilated segment of the internal carotid artery, sensitive to pressure changes; (c) blood-space with inelastic walls, e.g. the *venous sinuses* around the inside of the skull carrying blood from the brain to the jugular veins; (d) any cavity not otherwise classified.

The *paranasal air sinuses*, or simply 'the sinuses', are extensions of the cavity of the nose into the surrounding bones. The largest is the maxillary sinus or antrum, which occupies most of the bone between the floor of the orbit and the roots of the upper teeth. The maxilla looks solid but is only a shell of bone, lined with an extension of the mucous membrane of the nose. There are similar sinuses over the eyebrows (frontal), in the roof of the nose (ethmoid), and at the back of the nose (sphenoid). All open by narrow channels into the side of the nose, and all are in effect extensions of the nose. The middle ear and ◊ mastoid antrum communicate with the nose by the Eustachian tube and are part of the same system.

The sinuses act as resonators for the voice; otherwise they have no known function, except to reduce the weight of the skull.

The mucous membrane of the nose swells quickly when it is inflamed with a common cold or hay fever, and may block the openings of the sinuses. A sudden change of air pressure, e.g. with change of altitude, is then painful because the air trapped in the sinuses is still at the original pressure. The discomfort is usually worst in the ears because the ear-drums are very sensitive to differences of pressure inside and out, but the maxillary and frontal sinuses can also be painful. Even at ground level air is slowly absorbed from the sinuses into the blood, and cannot be replaced if the openings are blocked. The partial vacuum is as uncomfortable as raised pressure.

Inflammation of the sinuses (◊ sinusitis) is discussed below.

sinusitis. Inflammation of the mucous membranes lining one or more sinuses of the nose due to spread of infection from the nose, often a complication of allergy (hay fever). Since the sinuses are merely a continuation of the cavity of the nose some degree of sinusitis accompanies every cold. The condition becomes troublesome when the infection is trapped and persists. The passages from the nose to the sinuses are narrow at the best of times, and when the mucous membranes are congested and swollen these passages are easily blocked by quite small quantities of mucus. Any deformity of the cartilages of the nose increases the chance of blockage.

Sinusitis causes moderate to severe headache or faceache with an unpleasant sense of stuffiness in the nose. In an acute attack the patient may be ill and feverish for some days. With chronic sinusitis the nose always feels blocked, and acute attacks may be precipitated by colds, hay fever, damp foggy weather or even emotional upsets.

Acute sinusitis needs thorough treatment, not only because it is disagreeable, but to avoid the remote danger that the infection might spread inwards and cause meningitis. Antibiotics are used to clear up infection in the sinuses and have largely overcome the need for surgical treatment. Nasal drops to shrink the mucous membrane give prompt but temporary relief. After their brief effect has worn off the condition may be worse than it was beforehand, especially if they are used habitually. Bland solutions, e.g. of sodium bicarbonate, are used to rinse out infected sinuses.

skeleton.

1. ORIGIN

The highest status reached by animals without some sort of rigid framework is that of the earthworm and the octopus.

Skeletons are of two kinds: a shell of hard, inert material exuded by the skin (exoskeleton), and an inner framework of living tissue (endoskeleton). An exoskeleton is a good passive defence, but leaves little scope for initiative. It is a dead thing that has to be cast off to allow growth, leaving the animal helpless until another is formed. If a shell is heavy enough to protect, it is also cumbersome.

All creatures that can be called higher animals have an internal framework. The simplest endoskeleton is the notochord, a crude, unjointed forerunner of a backbone. This is an improvement on the condition of the spineless worm, for it enables muscles to work without contracting the whole body – a worm trying to advance on a smooth surface only manages to squirm.

On its own, a notochord is by no means better than a shell. The defenceless owners of these primitive skeletons, such as the lancelet, bury themselves in tidal sand, with only their mouths protruding to gather such food as comes their way; they seldom risk a nocturnal swim. In comparison, the swift and voracious lobster seems a very lord of creation. But the humble lancelet, or a similar creature some 500 million years ago, was the ancestor of all vertebrates – fish, flesh, fowl. The notochord has all but disappeared in these more complex animals, but even in man it is important to the embryo, where it precedes the vertebral column. Traces of it persist into adult life in the intervertebral discs.

From the forward end of the notochord a living skull, able to grow with the brain, has been evolved. The addition to the skull of a mobile lower jaw is among the most important steps in evolution, for more than anything else it marks the transition from passive to active existence.

Limbs within shells can be serviceable, as the claws of a lobster or the hind legs of a grasshopper, but they are not as versatile as limbs built round a central core – wings, fins, hooves, hands.

Even a vertebrate may have a supplementary exoskeleton. Tortoises have an obvious one, and the skin of a shark is like a flexible shell. A man's hair, finger-nails, and dental enamel are derived from his skin.

2. THE VERTEBRATE SKELETON

The skeletons of all land-dwelling vertebrates (and of a few whose terrestrial ancestors returned to the water) are modifications of a single basic plan, conveniently divided into an *axial* and an *appendicular* skeleton.

The *axial skeleton* consists of a skull, a backbone, and a tail, with a set of ribs encircling the forward part of the trunk.

The skull is a mosaic of tightly jointed bones, surrounding the brain and housing the special sense organs. Its underside serves as a fulcrum for a mobile jaw, and also as a fixed upper jaw for the lower to bite against.

The backbone is made up of rigid units (vertebrae) jointed to make a flexible rod. It serves principally as a firm anchorage for muscles, allowing movement while maintaining the general shape of the body (thus preventing internal organs from being crushed), and it also encloses the tailward continuation of the brain: the spinal cord.

The tail is an extension of the backbone beyond the end of the trunk; it is found (if only as a vestige) in all vertebrates.

All the ribs are attached at one end to vertebrae, and at least some at the other end to a sort of keel, the sternum. The sternal end of a rib is often of cartilage instead of bone.

The *appendicular skeleton* consists of two limb girdles (pectoral and pelvic), each with a pair of limbs attached.

Each girdle forms a more or less complete ring of flattened bones, but the pectoral girdle, carrying the forelimbs and making with them the shoulder-joints, is much lighter than the pelvic girdle, to which the hindlimbs are joined at the hips. These girdles have grown *towards* the vertebral column, and only the pelvic girdle is actually joined to it. (In more primitive creatures such as fish, neither girdle reaches the axial skeleton.)

In any limb, fore or hind, the segment attached to the girdle has a single bone (humerus or femur). The next segment, from elbow to wrist or from knee to ankle, has a parallel pair (radius and ulna or tibia and fibula). Next comes a cluster of small bones (carpus or tarsus) from which radiate 5 jointed digits.

With very little modification this account – or indeed a much more detailed one – describes the skeleton of a brontosaurus, a sparrow, or a man. The differences between them are not so much of kind as of size and proportion. Among the more obvious ones are the relative size of the brain-box or cranium, the form of the jaws and teeth, and the adaptation of the limbs to widely different functions. But limbs, whether used for flying, swimming, running, or grasping, are all built to the same pattern. A horse's hooves correspond with the nails of our middle fingers and toes; a cow's, with the nails of our 3rd and 4th digits. Only vestiges of the other digits remain, but the evolution of these highly adapted limbs from the primitive 5-digit pattern can be traced. Similarly the feathers of a bird's wing are suspended from an enormous index finger; the other fingers have vanished.

3. THE PRIMATE SKELETON

The order of mammals to which man belongs, the *primates*, includes lemurs, bushbabies, monkeys, and apes. The primates are essentially tree-dwellers. They have depended for survival on agility rather than strength or speed, and on being able to treat on its merits each new situation in their ever-changing habitat, rather than on automatic responses to the repetitive demands of life on the ground, in the air, or under water. In terms of structure this means that their limbs are *unspecialized* and so able to serve various functions. The

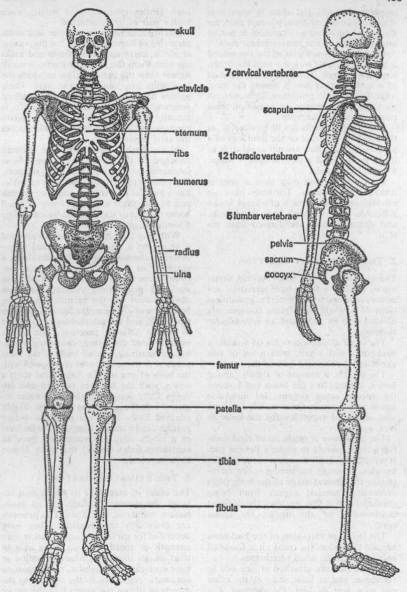

skull

7 cervical vertebrae

clavicle

scapula

sternum

ribs

12 thoracic vertebrae

humerus

5 lumbar vertebrae

radius

pelvis

ulna

sacrum

coccyx

femur

patella

tibia

fibula

highly developed limbs of a bird or a horse can do one job supremely well, and no other; whereas those of the primates, with little change from the most primitive pattern, can be used for running, climbing, grasping and above all for exploring. The skull is dominated by a very large brain-

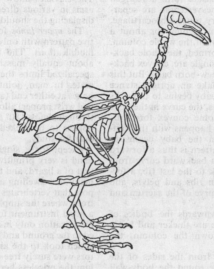

skeleton of bird

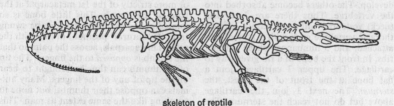

skeleton of reptile

box, which has grown at the expense of the face. These animals rely more on sight and hearing than on smell; thus the nose has receded. The eyes point straight forwards, allowing stereoscopic vision, and are set in deep, well protected sockets. A very mobile neck compensates for the resulting loss of mobility of the eyes themselves.

4. THE HUMAN SKELETON

Some human characteristics are related to man's unique upright stance; others, to the use of the forelimbs for feeding, for defence, and above all for learning.

Axial skeleton. The *skull* has to house a relatively enormous brain, and the cranium is accordingly much larger than the face. With the great development of the frontal lobes of the brain, the large forehead forms a shelf above the eyes. As in other primates, but not in lower orders, the deep eye-sockets are walled off from the temples by bone. The nose is prominent not because it is important, but because the teeth below it have receded. For the same reason man (alone among animals) has a chin.

The *backbone* is composed of 33 vertebrae. The first 24 make a flexible column from the nape of the neck to the small of the back; the next 5 are fused to form the sacrum, to which the pelvic girdle is attached; and the last 4 form a vestigial tail, the coccyx. The vertebrae are separated by discs of very tough fibrocartilage, which between them account for about a quarter of the height of the whole column.

When it is first formed, the whole backbone is curved in a single arc, convex backwards. It is so in a new-born baby. But this curvature would make an upright stance impossible. As the baby begins to move its head and use its eyes, the curve in the neck is reversed, to become convex forwards, and the same thing happens with the lumbar vertebrae when the baby begins to stand. The adult pattern is thus a forward curve in the neck, a backward curve from the root of the neck to the last rib, a forward curve between ribs and pelvis, and lastly a backward curve of the sacrum and coccyx.

From above downwards the bodies of successive vertebrae are thicker and heavier: the further down the column, the greater the load.

The *ribs* project from the sides of the vertebrae and curve round the body-wall to enclose the heart and lungs, sloping downwards at about 45°. Every vertebra includes a rudimentary pair of ribs, but only 12 pairs, from the 8th vertebra down, develop. The others become absorbed into the vertebrae. Thus there are 7 cervical (neck) vertebrae without separate ribs, 12 thoracic vertebrae each with a pair of ribs attached, and 5 lumbar vertebrae without ribs. In front the bone of a rib gives way to cartilage. The upper 7 cartilages join a flat bone at the front of the chest, the *sternum*. The next 3 join the cartilage above but do not reach the sternum. The last two are unattached.

Ribs 1–7 are sometimes called 'true' ribs, 8–10 'false' ribs, and 11–12 'floating' ribs.

Appendicular skeleton. The elements of the primitive pectoral girdle are fused to form the *scapula* or shoulder-blade, which with its attached muscles is free to slide over the upper ribs, carrying the arm with it. A ridge of bone projects from the back of the scapula above and beyond the shoulder-joint. To it is attached the outer end of the *clavicle* or collar-bone. This is a simple strut, joined at its inner end to the sternum. Animals which use their forelimbs only for running, and so need only a pendulum movement at the shoulder, have a rudimentary clavicle or none (e.g. dog, horse). The clavicles allow muscles to move the arms in various directions without simply displacing the shoulders.

The *upper limbs* follow the most primitive pattern with only slight, but important modifications. The radius and ulna are about equally massive, whereas in more specialized limbs the ulna tends to degenerate. In man, joints between these two bones at either end (additional to the elbow and wrist proper) allow the forearm to twist through almost 180° (⧓ *radius*). This allows objects to be picked up and then turned over for study.

Except for a single feature the human hand is very primitive. It looks much like that of a lizard, and the type is common to many tree-dwelling animals. We may suppose that vertebrates took very early to the trees, where the simple 5-fingered hand was a good instrument for climbing. It needed modification only in animals which returned to the ground and had to run, or in those which took to the air. Man's latest ancestors were surely tree-dwellers, and they left him the priceless heritage of an unevolved carpus with 5 intact digits: priceless, because unspecialized and therefore adaptable. The one special feature of the human hand is the extreme mobility of the thumb, or more strictly of the 1st metacarpal at the base of the thumb. This little bone is so jointed at the carpus that it can be swung from its 'natural' position, in line with the other 4 metacarpals, across the palm so that the thumb is *opposed* to the fingers. The tip of the thumb can thus be brought to bear on the tip of any of the fingers. Many animals can oppose their thumbs, but none to anything like the same extent as man. This movement accounts more than any other for man's dexterity, and so, to a great extent, for his general pre-eminence among animals.

The pelvic girdle is a rigid structure, firmly attached to the backbone. The last 5 vertebrae (excluding the rudimentary tail) are fused to form the sacrum. To either side of this massive bone is attached a hip-bone which curves round to meet its fellow in front. On the outer side of each hip-bone is a deep socket (contrasting with the very shallow cup on the scapula) into which the head of the femur fits to make the hip-joint. Since the hips are widely separated by the pelvis, whereas the knees are together, the two femora are set at a V-shaped angle.

called *ligaments*, but the stability of the system depends much more on the inter-action of the muscles, which serve not only to move the joints but also maintain their posture.

◊ *bone*; *joints*; and the bones and joints named above.

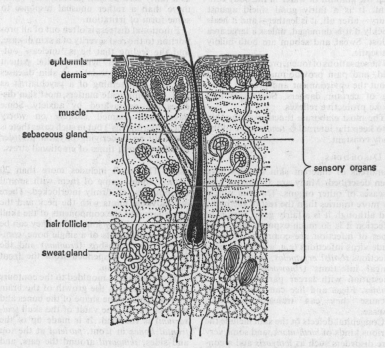

Section of skin, magnified.

Throughout the lower limb, mobility is sacrificed to stability. It is much more specialized than the upper limb. The hip, as a ball-and-socket joint, has some move-ment in all directions, but movement at the knee and ankle is limited to one plane. The fibula is no more than an appendage of the tibia, and no movement between the two is possible. The bones of the foot are jointed to allow twisting movements. They are arranged to form flexible arches along and across the foot; man thus walks on springs. No other creature has arched feet, just as no other creature walks quite upright.

The 206 bony elements of the skeleton are held in place by tough fibrous bands

skin. The two principal layers of the skin are the *dermis*, composed of tough, elastic connective tissue with a rich network of blood vessels and nerves, and the *epidermis*, a protective outer layer without blood vessels. The epidermis has a deep layer of growing cells and a covering of dried dead cells that are constantly shed and replaced from the growing layer.

The sweat glands are curled tubes of epi-dermis that grow down into the dermis. The nails and hair are also derived from epi-dermis. Like sweat glands, hair follicles (roots) grow down into the dermis. Each follicle gives rise to a few sebaceous or grease glands.

The skin is more than a waterproof jacket for the body. It is an active and versatile organ of sensation and of adaptation to a changing environment.

Since it is almost waterproof, the skin prevents rapid absorption or evaporation at the surface of the body and so helps to keep the amount of water in the body constant. It is a fairly good shield against injury – after all, it is leather – and it heals quickly if it is damaged, unless a large area is lost. Sweat and sebum are both mildly antiseptic.

The sensations of touch, pressure, warmth, cold, and pain provide much information about the environment and provide warning of certain dangers. Sometimes they evoke protective reflexes.

The most elaborate function of the skin is to keep the internal ◊ *temperature* of the body constant.

1. Disorders

Hundreds of different skin diseases have been described. Many are analogous with diseases of other organs. The skin suffers far more injuries than the rest of the body, and although it is a fairly good barrier to infection it is so much exposed that many types of infection are common. They include virus infections (e.g. *warts*), bacterial infections (*boils; erysipelas; impetigo*), and fungal infections (*ringworm*), and also infestation with larger parasites such as *scabies*. Fleas and lice can be dangerous because they can transmit infectious disease.

Congenital defects of the skin include the various kinds of *birth-mark*, and some very rare disorders such as *icthyosis* and a congenital lack of sweat glands (which makes it impossible to live in a hot climate).

Cancer of the skin is generally safer than most forms of cancer, partly because it is noticed while it is likely to be curable, and partly because one form, the rodent ulcer, does not migrate to other parts of the body.

Allergy and irritation by noxious substances cause many kinds of *dermatitis* (eczema). These are the commonest of all occupational diseases.

Because it is open to inspection, the skin often shows signs of illness of the body as a whole; e.g. the rashes of many fevers or the skin changes of vitamin deficiencies.

The skin has more unexplained diseases than other organs, perhaps because disorders that would be too slight to arouse comment in any other organ are enough to irritate the skin and – which is much more important – arouse a sense of disgust. *Acne*, for instance, brings great distress to adolescents, yet in purely physical terms it is hardly worth calling a disease. Even *psoriasis*, which most people would regard as a fairly serious skin disease, may be no more than a rather unusual response to some form of irritation.

Emotional distress is often out of all proportion to the real severity of a skin disease, and the feeling that he is 'unclean' outweighs any other symptoms the patient may have. The specialist in skin diseases has to be something of a psychiatrist as well. To complicate matters, most skin diseases are aggravated by anxiety. Some have been blamed entirely on worry ('neurodermatitis') but in such cases there is probably an underlying physical disorder that flares up at times of emotional stress.

skull. The skull includes more than 20 named bones, some of them with several components, all firmly interlocked. There are movable joints with the neck and the lower jaw, but the components of the skull itself are so tightly joined that they can be considered as parts of a single bone, comprising the brain-box (*cranium*) and the face, which is suspended from the front half of the cranium.

The cranium is moulded to the contours of the brain; it is the growth of the brain that determines the shape of the bones and not vice versa. The vault of the skull (*calvarium*) is rounded. It is made up of the *frontal bones* in front, *parietal* at the top and sides, *temporal* around the ears, and *occipital* at the back. These consist of two thin sheets of ivory-like bone separated by a spongy layer, the diploë. Although the structure appears flimsy, the round form gives it considerable strength.

The floor or base of the cranium includes parts of the frontal, temporal, and occipital bones joined to a bridge, the *sphenoid bone*, which spans the skull behind the eyes. It is arranged in descending tiers or *fossae*. The foremost and highest is the anterior *fossa*, supporting the frontal lobes of the brain and roofing the orbits and nose. Next, the middle fossa behind the eyes supports the temporal lobes, and below and behind is the posterior fossa containing the cerebellum. On the underside, the front part of the floor of the cranium forms the roof of the

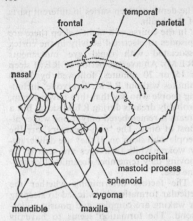

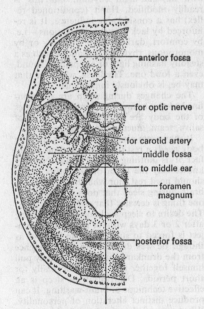

Skull: left side, and floor from above.

face, and the back part is the anchorage of the muscles of the neck.

A large hole in the centre of the floor, the *foramen magnum*, allows the stem of the brain to enter the spinal canal where it is continued as the spinal cord. There are numerous smaller holes for the passage of nerves and blood vessels.

The bones of the face are arranged round the openings for the eyes, nose, and mouth. The centre-piece on either side is the maxilla, which provides the floor of the orbit, the side of the internal part of the nose, the base of the cheek, and the upper jaw. It appears to be massive, but it consists mainly of a thin-walled cavity, the maxillary sinus (antrum). Several of the other bones are hollowed out by sinuses, all opening into the nose. The cheek bone (zygoma) forms an arch, fastened like the handle of a jug to the maxilla in front and the temporal behind.

1. DISORDERS

Various congenital malformations are occasionally seen. Because the development of the skull follows that of the brain, a deformity of the skull does not affect the brain. One type of mental defect, microcephaly, is associated with an abnormally small head, but the primary defect is in the brain; and because the brain fails to grow properly the skull remains small. With hydrocephaly, when an excess of fluid accumulates around the brain, the skull enlarges to accommodate the excess; this is no problem because the bones of the calvarium are separate in early life, and the fibrous bridges between them can expand. With the hereditary type of dwarfism, achondroplasia, the bones of the limbs and face are underdeveloped but the cranium grows to the normal size, and the brain is not affected.

Fractures of the skull are common and important injuries. Those that are confined to the face are managed according to the same principles as fractures of the limbs, with the object of restoring the position of the broken bone and keeping it still while it heals. There are special problems because it is difficult to find anywhere to apply a splint, and these fractures provide a good example of modern surgical teamwork. They may need the combined efforts of dental, plastic, and nose-and-throat surgeons. A common method of temporary fixation is to insert pins into the bone on either side of the fracture and join these with a metal bridge when the fragments have been set in place. With fractures of the jaws a method described by the ancient Egyptians is still in use: that of joining the teeth with wires so that the intact jaw splints the broken one.

With fractures of the cranium, the fracture itself is of little importance. The complications are all that matters. The underlying vessels are likely to be damaged, and the bleeding is extremely dangerous to the brain. There is no room for expansion in the skull, and quite a small amount of blood can cause fatal pressure on the brain. If the signs are recognized at once it is usually possible to operate and stop the bleeding. If the fracture is associated with an open wound there is a danger of infection inside the skull, which again can be dealt with if it is recognized in time. Hence when there is the least suspicion of a fractured skull the patient needs to be under close supervision.

A depressed fracture – a dent in the bone – is treated by replacing the fragment, which may otherwise cause localized pressure. The method was described by Hippocrates (5th century B.C.).

⟨⟩ *head injury*.

sleep. Although we spend about a third of our lives asleep, and it is apparently necessary to health that we should do so, we know little of the nature of sleep and almost nothing of its purpose.

The activity of the brain, as shown by the electroencephalogram, is altered but not suppressed. The cerebral cortex, where most of the conscious activity of the brain seems to take place, is still electrically active during sleep, but the activity is unconscious because the impulses from the reticular formation of the midbrain are cut off. The reticular formation acts as a switching station between the highest levels of the brain and the rest of the nervous system, and it seems to have the power of determining whether one is awake or asleep. When the reticular formation is switched to sleep, nervous impulses continue to circulate in the cortex and the rest of the brain, but they are no longer dependent on incoming impulses from the sense organs.

The electrical waves from the waking brain are rapid and irregular, averaging about 10 per second. In very light sleep the waves become smaller and rather slower. In deep sleep the waves are slow and regular, about 1 per second, and much larger than the waking waves, from large numbers of nerve cells acting synchronously.

The depth of sleep varies in different parts of the brain.

In the course of a night's sleep there are episodes of electrical activity in the cortex associated with rapid eye movements (REM). An average period of REM sleep is 15 or 20 minutes, followed by 70–90 minutes without REM. Everyone, including people who say that they never dream, probably dreams during REM sleep. But a dream is remembered only if one wakes almost at once. The 'non-dreamers' are the people who sleep on. If they are deliberately woken while their eyes are seen to be moving they remember dreaming like anyone else.

The factors determining whether the reticular formation is switched to sleeping or waking are complex and poorly understood. The formation seems to have its own day-and-night rhythm, but this is readily modified. Habit (conditioned reflex) has a considerable influence. It is reinforced by lack of strong sensations – i.e. by comfort, darkness and silence – or by monotonous, rhythmic sensations such as a steadily flashing light or a repetitive sound, even a loud one. Tiredness, whatever that may be, is obviously important.

The changes during sleep are not confined to the brain. The chemical processes of the body are slowed, and the flow of saliva, tears, mucus, and urine decreases.

It may seem almost self-evident that the body needs a rest from time to time, but in fact it is nothing of the kind. Nobody knows why the brain or any other organ should need rest, nor what happens to the brain during sleep that does it good. Only one thing is certain: that sleep is necessary. The desire to sleep is almost overwhelming after 2 or 3 days without sleep. If the subject is forced to stay awake he behaves as though he was drunk, with the difference from the drunkard that he can usually pull himself together and behave normally for short periods. Deprivation of sleep is an effective technique of brain-washing. It can produce distinct alteration of personality. When normal sleep is restored, the subject sleeps longer and deeper than usual for some nights, with frequent long periods of REM sleep.

The subject can be selectively deprived of REM sleep by waking him as soon as his eyes begin to move, and although he is allowed his usual hours of sleep the loss of REM sleep has similar effects to depriving him of all sleep. This rather suggests that dreaming is a necessary function.

Insomnia is a very common symptom. It can be a direct result of physical symptoms such as pain, itching, or indigestion. Anxiety makes it difficult to go to sleep, and depression causes early waking, but here one may confuse cause with effect. A person who thinks that he does not sleep enough develops anxiety about it. Many people feel tired because they cannot cope with their affairs, and persuade themselves that they cannot cope because they are tired. They theretore take sleeping pills that make them still less able to cope. There is a clear analogy between insomnia and constipation, where worry about a supposed disorder becomes a real disorder.

None of the time-honoured rules about hours of sleep is valid, except that everyone needs what is enough for him. Most children sleep a good deal longer than adults, but there are healthy children who sleep much less than most. A child in good physical health is unlikely to go short of the sleep that he, individually, needs. Old people tend to sleep less, but they are apt to get too little sleep because of depression arising from loneliness or physical ailments.

sleeping sickness. An infectious disease confined to tropical Africa, transmitted by tsetse flies. ◊ *trypanosomiasis.*

sleepy sickness. ◊ *Encephalitis* lethargica, an epidemic virus infection.

slough. A fragment of dead tissue cast off from living tissue, e.g. the core of a boil.

smallpox (variola). A highly infectious virus disease. Smallpox is unrelated to climate and was once a common pestilence everywhere. It is now mainly a tropical disease only because in many tropical countries routine vaccination is still not usual.

About 12 days after infection the patient develops a fever like a severe attack of influenza. The only clues to the diagnosis in the next 2 days are a history of exposure and a worse backache than with most other fevers. On the third day the rash appears. It may be difficult to distinguish from chickenpox, especially when there is no reason to suspect that the patient may have been in contact with smallpox. There are a few distinguishing features: the spots of small-

pox begin together, and at any one time are all more or less at the same stage of development; the spots are all the same size; they lie more deeply in the skin than those of chickenpox; they are more profuse on the face than the body; some occur on the palms and soles and inside the mouth. The evolution of the spots over two or three days is similar in both diseases: flat spots (macules) – raised spots (papules) – watery blisters (vesicles) – pus-filled blisters (pustules).

This description is of a typical case. The diagnosis is difficult because many cases are not typical. Sometimes the virus itself has to be examined in a specially equipped laboratory before smallpox can be certainly identified.

Most patients recover in the course of a week or two, though it may be longer before all the spots completely heal, and there is usually some permanent scarring. Two types of case can be fatal. A few patients succumb to an overwhelming virus infection with bleeding into the rash, the spots so numerous that they almost overlap, and extension of the rash into the air-passages. Some of these can be saved by creating an artificial airway (tracheostomy), but the outlook in such cases is poor. Another group survive the initial infection, but their resistance to other infection is so lowered that they die from invasion of the rash by the common bacteria of the skin, or from pneumonia. These lethal complications are forestalled with pencillin.

Until lately there has been no effective treatment of the primary virus infection, but the new thiosemicarbazone drugs seem to reduce the severity of the attack if they are given soon after exposure, before symptoms develop.

Alastrim (variola minor) is a variant of smallpox with milder symptoms and few if any deaths. An individual case cannot be distinguished from a mild case of ordinary smallpox (variola major), but epidemics of alastrim breed true – none of the contacts develops variola major.

Smallpox can be controlled by vaccination, which is infection with a virus that confers the same immunity as an attack of smallpox without producing the disease. A few vaccinated people may still develop a mild form of smallpox, but most are completely immune for at least 3 years.

Children with eczema are liable to very dangerous reactions and cannot be vaccinated, and vaccination is not advised during pregnancy or illness. People who should not be vaccinated can be given temporary protection with an immune serum or with a thiosemicarbazone drug.

New cases of smallpox in nearly all countries are immediately notified to the World Health Organization, which in turn notifies all the other countries so that returning travellers can be supervised. In Britain, possible contacts are vaccinated on arrival, and those suspected of already having the disease are isolated. Medical Officers of Health, usually assisted by smallpox consultants with tropical experience, keep a daily watch on contacts. While a risk of smallpox lasts, chickenpox is generally made notifiable to lessen the danger that a mild case of smallpox may be overlooked.

smoking ◊ *tobacco*.

snake bite. Most snakes are not poisonous, though it is wise to regard them all as dangerous until proved safe. Poisonous snakes carry venom in modified salivary glands. When they bite, the venom flows into the wound along grooved or hollow fangs.

Snake venoms are of two principal types: nerve poisons which paralyse the victim, and tissue poisons which destroy cells and interfere with the clotting of blood.

The only poisonous snake in Britain and most of Europe is the common adder. Its bite is unpleasant but seldom deadly. All the other continents have numerous species of highly poisonous snakes, mostly in tropical regions. As a rule they are timid creatures and bite man only as a last resort in self-defence, though a few seem to be aggressive, e.g. mamba (Africa), fer-de-lance (tropical America), hamadryad (Asia). Puff adders are dangerous because they are too sluggish to get out of the way, and kraits because they are too small to be noticed. More people die from snake bite in India than in the rest of the world together.

With dangerous snakes the best treatment is the appropriate antivenene as soon as possible. Hospitals in tropical countries keep a *polyvalent serum*, effective against all the local snakes, and people exposed to the risk of snake bite far from medical help carry a supply in a snake-bite kit. As symptoms may be delayed for a day or more,

anyone bitten by a tropical snake is best taken to hospital even if he does not appear to be in trouble.

There is some controversy over first aid. A splint is needed to keep the limb still (it is nearly always a limb); and a tourniquet or bandage above the bite only tight enough to grip the limb *lightly* may help, but it has to be released for a full minute every half-hour and reapplied higher up.

Some people cut the punctures open and rub in potassium permanganate crystals; others inject a solution of epsom salt. Unless they are done with some skill these more heroic measures (including the tourniquet) can do more harm than good, and they are useless after a few hours when the poison has spread. An important part of first aid is to give no alcohol.

Snow, John (1813–58). London physician, the first to specialize in anaesthesia. Even more celebrated than his many contributions to the technique of anaesthesia was Snow's investigation of an outbreak of cholera, worthy of the best detective fiction, which he traced to an infected water supply when nothing was yet known of infection by microbes, and everyone else thought that cholera was due to noxious vapours in the air.

sodium. A metallic element distributed throughout the body, most abundant in the body fluids outside the cells; within the cells it is largely replaced by potassium. It is taken into the body mainly as sodium chloride (common ◊ *salt*). Most diets contain slightly more than is needed, and the excess is passed by the kidneys into the urine. If there is a shortage the kidneys pass none, but some salt is inevitably lost in sweat and this has to be replaced in the diet.

soft sore ◊ *chancroid*.

solar plexus ◊ *coeliac plexus*.

soldier's heart = ◊ *effort syndrome*.

somatic. Of the body as opposed to the mind, or of the body with the exception of the reproductive cells (which are in a sense immortal).

Soranus of Ephesus (*c*. A.D. 100). Roman physician; by repute a prolific writer on many medical topics, but most of his work is either lost or survives only in much later translations. He is regarded as the best gynaecologist of antiquity, and the leading authority on mental illness.

spasm. Sustained involuntary contraction of muscle, often caused by inflammation in a neighbouring structure, for instance the stiffness of the jaw muscles with an infected tooth socket. Spasm can also be caused by interference with the nervous control of muscles, e.g. with ◊ *tetanus.* ◊ *spastic paralysis.*

spastic paralysis. Loss of voluntary movement together with spasm of the affected muscles.

A muscle is activated by nerve cells in the spinal cord which communicate directly with the muscle by their nerve fibres. If these fibres are cut (e.g. by a penetrating wound of a limb), or if the nerve cells themselves are damaged (e.g. by poliomyelitis) the muscle ceases to act at all; it is limp and the paralysis is said to be *flaccid.*

These nerve cells are themselves activated by various other cells in the brain and spinal cord, some concerned with voluntary movement and others with reflex action, some with stimulating and some with suppressing muscular activity. If parts of the brain concerned with movement are damaged, reflex pathways in the spinal cord are left intact with nothing to oppose them or co-ordinate their effects; the muscle is kept permanently taut, and the paralysis is said to be *spastic.*

Congenital spastic paralysis (*cerebral palsy*; *Little's disease*) in its various forms is among the commoner physical handicaps of childhood. It has come into prominence in recent years not because it is on the increase – if anything, it is becoming rarer – but because many other kinds of physical handicap that used to be common are no longer so (e.g. those resulting from poliomyelitis, tuberculosis of bone, rheumatic fever, and rickets), and because the needs of spastic children are better understood.

The paralysis is due to failure of groups of nerve cells in the brain. There are three main types. Spasm predominates if the affected cells are in the cerebral cortex, lack of co-ordination if they are in the cerebellum, and uncontrolled purposeless movements (athetosis) if they are in the basal ganglia, the grey matter in the centre of the brain. Common to all types is weakness of groups of muscles with persistent spasm that interferes with useful movement. The trouble is often confined to the legs, but in the worst cases it may be very much more wide-spread, even involving the muscles of speech.

Paralysis in this condition is relative. It does not mean that an affected limb cannot be deliberately moved at all, but that voluntary movement is impaired. A totally paralysed baby would be stillborn or die soon after birth. The disability varies between trivial defects that do not affect the patient's life in the mildest cases and life-long dependence on other people's help in the severest cases.

Mental development is often but by no means always retarded. It is difficult to assess because the physical handicap can make an intelligent child seem backward.

The cause cannot always be found, but very often it can be traced to a particular type of injury to brain cells. These include severe jaundice (◊ *rhesus factor*), physical injury during birth (less common than one would expect), temporary shortage of oxygen to the brain during the transition between the baby's getting oxygen from the mother's blood and breathing for himself, and lack of glucose as a result of immaturity at birth. In theory these are all largely preventable conditions.

A spastic baby cannot always be recognized at birth. All new-born babies work by reflex action, and the damage may not show itself until purposive movements should begin. This creates a false impression that the disorder is progressive, but in fact all the damage is done at or shortly after birth. From then on there is no further loss of brain cells, and the condition can only remain stationary or improve. Unlike other tissues, nerve cells cannot regenerate; but much can be done to make the most of all the unaffected areas of the brain. Healthy muscles can be taught to take on at least some of the work of paralysed muscles, occasionally with the help of surgery. Severely affected children may need special education for a time at least, and some need speech training before they can communicate and make the most of their intelligence. All this kind of work is still at an early stage, but it has been advancing rapidly in recent years.

species. Although the classification of

animals and plants is based on the concept of species there is no exact definition. When reproduction is sexual it can be said that members of the same species can breed and produce fertile offspring, but with simple creatures such as bacteria the only criterion is very close similarity.

Related species are grouped together as a *genus*. Within a species there may be distinct races or breeds. Bacteria that are apparently of the same species may differ in such respects as the severity of the disease that they cause and may be classed as strains, varieties etc.; but the classification of bacteria and viruses is unsatisfactory and subject to frequent change.

spectacles ◊ *vision.*

speculum. Lighted tube or other instrument for enabling openings or cavities of the body to be inspected.

speech. Words are formulated in the speech centre of the cerebral cortex, at the side of the brain. This centre lies next to the zone of cerebral cortex that controls the dominant hand. Since the main nervous pathways cross the mid-line, the speech centre is on the left side of the brain in right-handed people. The centre is closely co-ordinated with centres for hearing (comprehension), vision (reading), and hand movement (writing).

Vowel sounds are produced by the ◊ *larynx* and shaped by the mouth, and consonants are formed by the tongue and lips.

A defect anywhere in a long and complicated chain can impair speech. To begin, a certain level of general intelligence is needed. But delayed or defective speech in childhood need not mean that the child is stupid; children of equal ability do not all develop at the same rate. Sometimes a first child does not speak as early as subsequent children because he does not hear speech going on around him all day – children learn more easily from each other than from their parents. Defective hearing, easily overlooked, is an obstacle to learning and is a common cause of backwardness in speech. Emotional disturbances and mental illness can affect speech in various ways. Their symptoms range from occasional stammering to complete failure to communicate.

The speech centre can be affected by injury or disease such as a stroke; in these cases paralysis of the right hand is often accompanied by loss of speech. Any disease of the neck or throat can affect the larynx or its nerves. Defects of the mouth affect the quality of speech.

Any illness that affects the co-ordination of movements, e.g. parkinsonism, may cause difficulty with speaking.

Speech therapy, a young and highly skilled profession, teaches patients to overcome defects that would have been thought incurable a generation ago. It embraces not only the training of children who have never learnt to speak distinctly but also the re-education of adults such as those whose speech has been impaired by injury or disease.

sperm. Male germ cell. A human sperm consists of an oval *head* about 0·005 by 0·003 mm. and a slender whip-like tail about 0·05 mm. (1/500 in.) long. The testes produce sperms in vast numbers; some two hundred million are released in an orgasm.

spermatic cord. A bundle containing the duct of the testis (vas deferens) and blood vessels, wrapped in fibrous tissue and a rudimentary muscle (cremaster), suspending the testis. The passage of the cord through the groin creates a weak point where a ◊ *hernia* may develop.

spermatozoon (spermatozoön) (pl. *spermatozoa*). Sperm.

sphenoid. A large bone spanning the base of the skull behind the eyes.

sphincter. Ring of muscle fibres around the entrance or exit of a hollow organ.

sphygmomanometer. Pressure gauge for measuring the blood pressure. When extreme accuracy is needed, as in some experimental work, the pressure is measured directly with a tube in an artery, but an ordinary sphygmomanometer records the pressure of air needed to stop the flow of blood into a limb.

spica. Bandage applied with successive turns crossing each other; figure-of-eight bandage.

spider. Spiders bite their prey and inject poison. Only a few are dangerous to man.

The worst are members of the genus *Latrodectus,* small black creatures with red markings found in most warm countries. They include the *black widow* (America), the *button spider* (S. Africa), the *karakut spider* (Russia and near East), and the *night stinger* (Australasia). The poison stimulates nerve cells and causes trembling, sweating, vomiting, and severe pain. If these general symptoms overshadow the pain of the bite itself the condition suggests some acute abdominal disorder, and patients unaware that they had been bitten have been subjected to abdominal operations. Severe bites from these spiders can be lethal, especially to children.

A few other kinds of spider, e.g. the funnel-web spider of Australia, are also dangerous. The tarantula and the still more alarming tropical bird-eating spiders are comparatively harmless; their bites may be painful but that is all.

Tarantism or dancing mania, a strange medieval affliction, appears to have been some kind of mass hysteria not due, as people thought, to the bite of the tarantula.

spina bifida. A congenital defect of one or more vertebrae, generally in the lowest part of the backbone. Each vertebra in the backbone should have a weight-bearing portion (body) in front and an arch of bone to protect the spinal cord behind. The series of arches forms a strong flexible tube, the spinal canal. This canal is a downward extension of the cavity of the skull, and the spinal cord that it encloses is a downward continuation of the brain. With spina bifida one or more of the arches fails to develop, leaving a gap into which the delicate spinal cord bulges.

With a minor degree of spina bifida there are no troubles: it is an insignificant anomaly. But with a larger defect the spinal cord becomes involved before birth, and there is some amount of paralysis, varying in different cases between a small patch of numbness and complete lack of control from the waist down.

Spina bifida is commonly associated with defective drainage of cerebrospinal fluid from the cavities of the brain, causing pressure on the brain and abnormal enlargement of the skull (hydrocephalus).

Both defects can be repaired – spina bifida by plastic surgery, and hydrocephalus by fitting a one-way valve to drain the excess fluid into a vein. By these means further damage to the spinal cord or brain can be prevented, though nerve tissue already destroyed by pressure cannot be replaced. The sooner the operations are done, the less the established damage and the greater the chance of success. The surgeons who specialize in this work generally operate within 24 hours of birth if possible. As a result, many of the affected children develop almost or quite normally, and others who would not have survived long are able to lead useful lives. Some of the worst affected cannot be altogether independent, but with early operation on the defect and orthopaedic treatment later on most of them learn to walk. Management of a paralysed urinary bladder is generally the greatest difficulty.

spinal cord. The continuation of the brain below the skull; it is a column of nervous tissue enclosed in the *spinal canal,* a tunnel in the backbone. The spinal cord is not a distinct organ from the brain. Both are parts of a single unit, made up of nerve cells (grey matter) and conducting fibres (white matter). The spinal cord is a conductor between the brain and the rest of the body, but that is not all. It deals with many reflex actions without reference to the brain: for instance, the familiar knee-jerk depends only on the spinal cord (◊ *reflex*). Passing urine is also a spinal reflex, though its timing is controlled by the brain.

The ◊ *spinal nerves* carry impulses between the cord and the trunk and limbs. They leave the backbone by the gaps between the vertebrae. Originally a pair of nerves emerges from the cord opposite to each gap, but the backbone grows more than the cord. In adult life the cord ends at the first lumbar vertebra, just below the 12th ribs, and the spinal nerves for the lower vertebrae are carried down the rest of the spinal canal as a leash, the *cauda equina.*

The *meninges,* the surrounding membranes of the brain, are continued down the whole length of the spinal canal to form a waterproof sheath for the spinal cord, filled with *cerebrospinal fluid.*

1. Injuries

The spinal cord is well protected by bones and muscles, and considerable violence is needed to damage it. The danger is from a fracture of a vertebra with displacement of the fragments. Not all injuries of the spinal cord occur at the time of the accident.

Unskilful handling of the patient can displace a fracture that did not at first involve the cord to a position where a fragment of bone can do permanent damage. If there is the least suspicion of an injury to the back it is a safe policy for only people trained in this kind of first aid to move the victim.

A severe jolt may cause temporary interference with the working of the spinal cord. But nerve fibres that are cut or torn do not regenerate in the cord or brain as they can in peripheral nerves. This means that communication between the brain and the parts of the body below the injury is interrupted, with loss of sensation and voluntary movement. Below the injury the spinal cord can still maintain reflex actions.

The treatment of spinal injuries is largely a matter of making the best of the remaining function, and of preventing complications such as deformity produced by uncontrolled muscle reflexes and damage to skin that has lost its sensation. Before the Second World War cases of severe damage to the spinal cord were generally regarded as hopeless because the cord itself could not be repaired, and most of the patients died of infection within a year or two of the injury. The outlook was completely changed by surgeons such as Guttmann, who recognized that the spinal cord was only a part of the whole patient, and that with skilled training and perseverance people with spinal injuries could acquire new skills and pleasures. From the start the patient is set the objective of leading an independent life.

2. OTHER DISORDERS

Compression of a nerve fibre interferes with the conduction of impulses, and pressure on the spinal cord can cause anything from minor disturbances of sensation to complete paralysis. If the pressure is relieved without delay, normal conduction is likely to return. Sources of pressure include results of injury such as blood-clots, and abscesses and tumours. All these are amenable to surgery.

A congenital defect of the vertebrae, ◊ *spina bifida*, causes the spinal cord to be pinched in a gap in the backbone. With the uncommon condition ◊ *syringomyelia* a cyst in the centre of the cord causes pressure from within; this also is probably a congenital defect.

Infections that cause inflammation of the brain (encephalitis) may also involve the spinal cord. Many of the common viruses can do this, but in fact such infection is rare, with the exception of *poliomyelitis*. Even poliomyelitis, which has a special affinity for the motor nerve cells of the spinal cord, causes serious trouble in only a small minority of cases. *Tabes dorsalis* is involvement of the cord at a late stage of syphilis, affecting mainly the sensory fibres.

Several diseases cause degeneration of the insulating (myelin) sheaths of nerve fibres in the cord. These include deficiency of vitamin B_{12} (pernicious anaemia), and *multiple sclerosis*, of which the cause is still unknown.

spinal nerves. Branches of the spinal cord from which the nerves of the trunk and limbs are derived. There are 31 pairs, each pair corresponding with a vertebra, and emerging from the sides of the backbone through a gap between two vertebrae. In principle the nerves encircle the body, each pair supplying a segment, but this simple arrangement is modified for the limbs. The nerves from the upper and lower ends of the spinal cord form networks, the brachial and lumbosacral plexuses, from which branches supply the upper and lower limbs; thus each limb nerve contains elements of several spinal nerves.

At their origin from the spinal cord the motor and sensory fibres are in separate bundles or roots, motor in front of sensory. The two roots merge as the nerves pass out of the backbone.

There is little room to spare in the gaps between the vertebrae, and with many disorders of the backbone the emerging nerves may be compressed, causing mainly disturbances of sensation such as numbness, tingling, or pain. The commonest source of pressure is a 'slipped disc' (◊ *vertebra* (1)), and the commonest sites are the lumbar and sacral vertebrae where the pressure causes lumbago or sciatica.

spine. 1. Any sharp projection from a bone, such as the spinous process (neural spine) projecting from the back of each of the vertebrae that make up the backbone. **2.** The backbone (spinal column) as a whole. ◊ *skeleton* (4); *vertebra*.

spirochaete. A spiral bacterium. Most spirochaetes are harmless, but the group includes Vincent's spirochaete (*Borrelia vincenti*), associated with Vincent's angina, and the causes of syphilis, yaws, relapsing fever, Weil's disease, and a kind of rat-bite fever.

splanchnic. Of the viscera (internal organs of the abdomen and thorax).

spleen. Large purple, rubbery abdominal organ. It is the size of the whole hand, rather larger than a kidney, under the ribs on the left side between the stomach and the left kidney. The spleen is a fibrous sponge full of blood and lymphoid tissue. It is an offshoot of the supporting tissue of the stomach, and is supplied by large blood vessels branching off those of the stomach. It is an important element of the *reticulo-endothelial system*, which is a collective term for scavenger cells scattered throughout the body.

In classical and medieval medicine the spleen was the seat of one of the four humours, the black bile (melancholy). The blood in the spleen is rather tarry because the lymphoid tissue acts as a filter bed, tending to concentrate the solid blood cells and let the fluid plasma pass.

An unborn infant's bone marrow does not start forming blood cells until the 5th month of pregnancy. Until this time the blood cells are all formed in the spleen, thymus, and liver, but by the time the child is born the only blood cells still being formed there are lymphocytes. In many animals the spleen continues to make red blood cells throughout life, and even in adult man it can do so if there is a sudden demand, e.g. during recovery from severe anaemia.

The spleen is also concerned with the destruction of spent red blood cells. The useful life of a red cell is 4 months. It is then broken down in the reticuloendothelial system and replaced by a new cell from the bone marrow. The spleen also appears to carry out a quality control: faulty or misshapen red cells are removed from the circulation and destroyed.

In carnivorous animals the spleen is a reservoir of blood cells for emergencies. When the animal has to go into action the spleen contracts under the influence of adrenaline, forcing additional cells into the circulation. In man, this function is only rudimentary.

Like other lymphoid tissues (lymph nodes, thymus) the spleen forms antibodies, on which ◊ *immunity* largely depends.

Apart, perhaps, from the quality control of red cells, all the function of the spleen can be carried on by other organs, though children without spleens are said to develop less immunity to infection than they should. In adults, surgical removal of the spleen has no ill effects.

1. DISORDERS

The ribs and diaphragm generally protect the spleen from injury, but it can be torn by a really heavy blow on the left side, or punctured by a broken rib. It then bleeds freely into the abdominal cavity. The spleen is too spongy to be easily repaired, and the usual treatment of a ruptured spleen is to seal off its blood vessels and remove it. The operation is not difficult, because the spleen is on a sort of stalk. A ligature tied round the stalk cuts off the whole blood supply.

The spleen has few if any diseases of its own, but it is involved in various widespread disorders of the lymphoid and blood-forming tissues, e.g. ◊ *leukaemia*, ◊ *Hodgkin's disease*. In some types of anaemia due to excessive destruction of blood cells (◊ *anaemia* (A.2)) the spleen is enlarged, and removing it may help the patient.

Almost any kind of infection can cause the spleen to enlarge, and with some tropical diseases the spleen becomes enormous (◊ *malaria*, ◊ *bilharzia*). A diseased spleen protruding beyond the margin of the ribs is vulnerable, and ruptured spleen is a very common accident in the tropics. The large malarial spleen is packed with red blood cells damaged by malaria parasites and therefore removed from the circulation to be broken down (the spleen is carrying out its function of 'quality control'). With bilharzial disease the main reason for the large spleen is damage to the liver by the parasites.

Many chronic diseases of the liver affect the spleen, because the splenic vein is a tributary of the ◊ *portal vein*; therefore blood from the spleen has to pass through the liver to get back to the heart. Any obstruction in the liver causes back-pressure and congestion in the spleen.

splenic anaemia = ◊ *Banti's disease*.

splenomegaly. Abnormal enlargement of the spleen. *Egyptian splenomegaly* is due to infection with ◊ *bilharzia*; it arises partly from direct involvement of the spleen and partly from interference in the liver with blood vessels that should drain the spleen. In this latter respect it is a variant of Banti's disease. In most cases the effect of malaria is added to that of bilharzia.

spondylitis. Inflammation of vertebrae. *Ankylosing spondylitis* is a rheumatic affection of the vertebrae (bamboo spine) related to rheumatoid arthritis. There is gradual loss of mobility in the joints between the vertebrae. In severe cases the normally flexible ligaments supporting these joints acquire almost the consistency of bone, and the affected part of the spine resembles a bamboo rod. The patient is liable to episodes of backache, and in severe cases breathing may be hindered. The treatment is similar to that of rheumatoid arthritis. X-rays have been used to slow the process, but may damage the bone marrow of the vertebrae, an important blood-forming tissue, and cause anaemia.

spondylolisthesis. A partial dislocation of one of the joints of the spine; it is commonly the 5th lumbar vertebra (carrying the rest of the backbone with it) that slips forward on the top of the sacrum. The condition is associated with a congenital defect of a vertebra. The affected joint may need surgical fixation.

spondylosis. A degenerative process or ◊ *osteoarthritis* of vertebrae and the joints between them, usually diagnosed from X-ray pictures which show narrowing of the joint spaces and small irregular protuberances of bone around the joints. Spondylosis may cause stiffness or aching in the affected segment of the spine, and spondylosis in the neck, causing pressure on the nerve roots which emerge between vertebrae, is often blamed for ◊ *fibrositis* in the back and shoulders, perhaps for want of a more convincing cause. Though spondylosis can cause symptoms, most people over the age of 30 show signs of it without suffering any discomfort.

spore. Seed of a fungus; some bacteria (e.g. that of tetanus) form spores as a kind of hibernating or dormant phase in which they are remarkably resistant to antiseptics. Bacterial spores may survive even in boiling water for half an hour or more, but they are readily killed by compressed steam in an autoclave.

spotted fever. 1. Epidemic meningitis. **2.** A kind of typhus.

sprain. An injury to a joint without fracture or separation (dislocation) of bones but with torn fibres of the supporting tissue. The pain is usually enough to prevent movement that would interfere with healing. Cold compresses, or merely raising the limb, may help to reduce swelling. A skilfully applied bandage supports the joint and takes strains off the damaged ligament while it heals. The ankle is much more often sprained than any other joint. Sprains elsewhere have to be treated with suspicion because they are apt to disguise small fractures.

sprue. Chronic diarrhoea, loss of weight, and anaemia from failure to assimilate fat and vitamins from the intestine. The diarrhoea is due to unabsorbed fat, and the anaemia to lack of folic acid, which has much the same effect as the vitamin B_{12} deficiency of pernicious anaemia (◊ *anaemia* (B.2)).

Tropical sprue occurs in parts of Asia and America. It is not clear whether lack of folic acid causes defective function of the intestine or vice versa, but treatment with folic acid generally cures the diarrhoea as well as the anaemia.

Non-tropical sprue is like the coeliac disease of infants, and is treated by excluding gluten (wheat-protein) from the diet.

sputum. Mucus (phlegm), often with pus, coughed from the air-passages. Sputum, as opposed to saliva or spittle formed in the mouth, is proof of inflammation. Even a very small amount, which most smokers consider normal ('clearing the chest'), is a definite sign of bronchitis. Microscopic examination of bacteria, cells etc. in the sputum is helpful in the diagnosis of many diseases of the lungs.

squill. A vegetable drug with similar properties to digitalis.

squint. Faulty alignment of the axis of an eye. A squint may be *convergent* (inward), *divergent* (outward), or, rarely, vertical. The obvious cause, paralysis of one of the muscles of the eye, is rather uncommon, but a squint that first appears in adult life is likely to be paralytic. A paralytic squint arises from damage to one of the nerves of the eye muscles, and generally causes double vision. These squints call for prompt investigation because they are symptoms of irritation or compression of the nerve.

Congenital squint is by far the commonest type. The muscles and their nerves are healthy, but the two eyes are wrongly coordinated. The squint is said to be *concomitant* because the eyes move together, with the same degree of squint in all positions (whereas the degree of a paralytic squint varies with the direction of gaze). A concomitant squint may not be obvious until the child begins to use his two eyes as a unit, and not always then, for some squints remain latent for years.

Concomitant squint is often due to faulty accommodation (focusing). If the child is long-sighted, nothing is in focus with the eyes at rest. To see a distant object clearly, he has to focus the lenses as a normal child would do to see a near object. But the reflex for focusing is linked to reflexes controlling the eye muscles, so that the eyes automatically turn inwards when they are focused for near vision, like a coupled range-finder on a camera. In a long-sighted child, the two reflexes are thrown out of step. As he focuses on the horizon his eyes turn inwards as though he were looking at a near object, and he squints and sees double. But his young brain is still learning to translate nerve impulses from the eyes into pictures, and to overcome the nuisance of double vision it ignores the impulses from one eye. Unless the squint is treated, the habit of ignoring one eye becomes fixed; when the squint is finally corrected it is too late for the brain to learn and the eye remains useless. Squints have therefore to be recognized and treated early.

The treatment includes correction of focus by glasses, exercises for the eye muscles (orthoptics), and in some cases surgical adjustment of the muscles.

stapedectomy. Surgical treatment of deafness due to *otosclerosis*, an abnormal deposition of bone in the cavity of the middle ◊ *ear* that interferes with sound conduction from the drum to the organ of Corti by the chain of small bones. The disease prevents the innermost of the 3 bones, the stapes, from vibrating. The operation, done with a binocular microscope, consists of removing the stapes and replacing it with a tiny plastic piston. It is both safer and more reliable

than the former treatment, fenestration, which involved making a new opening to the inner ear.

stapes. One of the small articulated bones of the middle ear.

staphylococcus. A spherical ◊ *bacterium*, diameter 0·001 mm. (1/25,000 in.); a single staphylococcus looks exactly like a ◊ *streptococcus*, but a family forms a cluster instead of a chain. Two kinds of staphylococcus are important:

1. *Staph. albus* inhabits healthy skin, seldom causing trouble. It may be the only microbe in cases of trivial infection such as pimples, but more often it merely joins in when some more virulent microbe has already started an infection. Like the bacteria of the intestine, it can become dangerous if it strays from its natural environment, e.g. into the urine.

2. *Staph. aureus* (*Staph. pyogenes*) is much more harmful. It is called *aureus* because of its yellow pigment, and *pyogenes* because it provokes the formation of pus. About half the population harbours it either in the nose or on the skin. It is the usual cause of infection in wounds and of abscesses, boils, and impetigo. Staphylococcal infection tends to be localized, but even a small abscess can cause fever and other general symptoms because staphylococci form various toxins (poisons) which circulate in the blood. If, as rarely happens, the staphylococci themselves invade the blood-stream they can cause a most lethal ◊ *septicaemia*.

Natural resistance to staphylococci is fairly good, considering that everyone has a boil or an abscess at one time or another and serious complications are rare. The natural tendency for these microbes to become walled off in abscesses helps to prevent spread but hinders destruction of the microbes by white cells and antibodies in the blood. (With *streptococci*, which tend to spread, the opposite holds.) Even with drugs to assist the natural defences, a surgical operation is often needed to provide an outlet for the pus (◊ *abscess*).

Antiseptics readily kill staphylococci, but no drug was both safe and effective against staphylococci in the body until the discovery of ◊ *sulphonamides*. All sulphonamides inhibit staphylococci, but embarrassingly large doses of the earlier ones were needed. Suitable sulphonamides were overshadowed by the introduction of penicillin in 1941, since when many other effective antibiotics have been discovered. It is as well that there are many, because staphylococci are prone to become resistant to a particular drug in time, and another must be used against them. This danger is greatest in hospitals, where only the 'fittest' microbes are likely to survive.

Food poisoning by staphylococci is different from infection: it is due to chemical poisons formed by staphylococci which contaminate the food before it is eaten.

starch. A carbohydrate found in many plants; it is the basis of most diets. A molecule of starch is a long branched chain of molecules of *glucose*, to which it is converted by digestion. Starch is very similar to cellulose, but the human digestive system has no enzymes for separating the glucose molecules of cellulose and cannot therefore use foods such as grass.

Starch has no special fattening properties. Reducing the amount of starch in the diet (potatoes, bread) is merely the most convenient way of reducing the total intake of food without impoverishing the diet.

Starling's law. (Ernest H. Starling (1866–1927), professor of physiology at University College, London.) The force with which the heart contracts is proportional to the rate at which it is filled from the veins and the resistance against which it has to pump; in other words the heart adapts itself to the needs of the moment. Heart failure means that the heart cannot comply with this law. It is only a matter of degree. No heart can obey Starling's law beyond a certain level of work, but with heart failure this level is lower than it should be.

starvation. Even when the body is at rest it needs a continuous supply of energy for chemical processes and for the work of its vital organs; and the materials of many tissues need constant replacement.

When no food is taken, the carbohydrate stored in liver and muscle as glycogen can be converted to glucose and used as fuel, but even a well-fed body has only a few hours' supply. After this, the fat deposited under the skin and elsewhere can be consumed. Complete starvation for several days – under the closest supervision – is an effective method of losing weight. Other fat, an integral part of most tissues, is not available as fuel.

If the available store of fat is depleted, other sources of fuel are brought in. The most important is protein; but as soon as the body begins to consume its own protein its health begins to suffer.

The heart and nervous system are spared to the end, but the rest of the body can lose up to half its weight before the victim dies of starvation. This may take a month or more, but in the meantime resistance has become so low that the least infection may be fatal. With severe starvation the digestive organs may be so injured by lack of vitamins and other necessities that they can no longer take up ordinary foods if they are provided. People in this state may need food that requires little digestion for some time.

A severely starved person may not, at first sight, look thin, because lack of protein in the blood allows water to collect in the tissues and produce a kind of ◊ oedema.

statistics. There are two meanings, both of medical interest. The original meaning is the compiling of numerical data about populations for official use: a statist was a statesman or politician. The basic form is the census, used since the earliest historical times for taxation. Census data together with statistics such as birth-rate, death-rate, and ages and causes of dying are obviously very important in studying the health of the community, in identifying the problems to be tackled or the success with which they are being tackled, and in studying the natural history of epidemics. Causes of lung cancer and arterial disease, two of the leading causes of death, have been identified in this way. A population under study is simply all the people, or as many as can be traced, within a defined group. For example, the World Health Organization collates statistics from all over the world for studying the control of major pestilences such as malaria and tuberculosis, whilst a municipal health department may be concerned with the population of a single school.

Medical historians usually credit John Graunt of London with being the first to apply statistics ('political arithmetic') to the study of public health. He began to publish his *Natural and Political Observations made upon the Bills of Mortality* in

1662. But 50 years before this Felix Platter wrote his observations on 7 outbreaks of plague that he had lived through in Basle, including a house-to-house census of the town with notes on everyone who had caught the plague in the outbreak of 1609–1611. The M S is still in the University Library; it has not been published in full.

The second meaning of statistics is the analysis of representative samples. Clinical research usually has to deal with fairly small groups of patients, i.e. samples of the whole population. The sample is compared with a *control*, which may be a second sample differing only in respect of the factor to be studied (e.g. a new drug not given to the control group). Or the control may be the same group studied at a different time, or it may be a known standard such as an average for the population as a whole. The results are expressed in figures and analysed to show whether differences between the study group and the control are *significant*, i.e. unlikely to have arisen by pure chance. Statistical analysis never proves anything in the absolute sense of proving a theorem in geometry. It aims at the same kind of proof as a court of law. In abstract theory, the man with the jewels in his knapsack and his fingerprints on the latch could be the victim of a series of misunderstandings, but his guilt is established beyond *reasonable* doubt. In most clinical work, 'significant' means 95 per cent sure, i.e. a 5 per cent chance that the result was a fluke. With a new drug, this could justify further trials provided that no serious drawbacks had arisen, always bearing in mind the 5 per cent chance that the new will finally turn out to be no better than the old. 'Highly significant' is 99 per cent sure, and 'very highly significant' is 99·9 per cent. The greater the difference between sample and control, and the larger the sample (number of patients studied), the higher the significance is likely to be. A crude example will show the effect of the two factors.

Suppose that a man is taking bets on a 50–50 chance such as whether a card drawn from a pack will be black or red. The 'sample' is a series of consecutive draws. The 'control' is the theoretical distribution of an infinite number of draws governed by chance. The man should win twice in a row once in 4 attempts if he bets on 2 reds (R R), since the possible results are R R, R B, B R, B B. He should win 3 in

a row once in 8 attempts, 4 in 16 attempts, and 5 in 32 attempts, i.e. the odds against 5 reds in a row are 31 to 1, so we are about 97 per cent sure that this result will not arise by chance. This is more than the limit of significance, and we may suspect the man of cheating. After 7 consecutive wins, due to arise by chance only once in 128 attempts, we are more than 99 per cent sure: 'highly significant'. After 10 consecutive wins (1 in 1024 by chance) we are more than 99·9 per cent sure and may well feel that it is time to call a policeman. Thus a very small sample, only 10 draws, can give a very highly significant result if the difference from the expected result is great enough: here, it is the maximum. In medical research, this kind of thing happens only rarely, e.g. when an effective drug is discovered for a previously incurable disease. As a rule, the differences to be studied are more subtle. If our card-sharper is wise he will cheat only half the time, to win 3 draws in 4. Then his 6 wins in 8 draws will arouse no suspicion, because this would occur by chance once in about 7 attempts, whereas 8 wins would be well past the limit of 'highly significant'. Even 18 wins in 24 draws would occur by chance once in about 80 attempts, which is 'significant' but a little short of 'highly significant'. The odds against his winning all 24 would have been over 16 million to one. At this rate we should need a sample of more than 40 draws before the man's 3 wins out of 4 became 'very highly significant'.

When the results of a clinical experiment have been analysed, then, a statistician can say with mathematical precision how likely or unlikely it is that the results are due to pure chance, but he cannot say what, other than chance, has affected the result. A trial may appear to show that a new drug is significantly better than an old one, or that a rich diet increases the risk of heart disease, but it shows nothing of the kind unless all other differences between sample and control are considered and their effects excluded. The effect on the patients of knowing that they are getting a new and promising drug is enough to invalidate a trial (◊ *placebo*; *research*). People with an over-rich diet might get heart disease because as a group they are also people who tend to go by car when a walk would do them good. It happens that both these factors, overeating and lack of exercise, endanger the heart, but this could be established only by considering each independently of the other. The commonest fallacy in research involving statistics is to mistake association for cause and overlook the essential factor. From the figures alone one might think that hot climates encourage typhoid fever and smallpox. Certainly they are associated, but only because so many of the countries that cannot afford an expensive public health service to prevent these infections happen to be hot countries.

Most people consider statistical evidence untrustworthy. This is not so. It is as precise as any other kind of evidence, but easier to misinterpret than most.

status asthmaticus. A severe and prolonged attack of asthma, persisting for 24 hours or more despite the usual remedies such as injections of adrenaline. ♢ *asthma*.

status epilepticus. A succession of epileptic attacks, or one very prolonged attack. Although status epilepticus is usually controlled by the drugs used for ordinary epilepsy, a prolonged fit needs hospital treatment because the muscle spasms may have to be controlled with drugs such as curare; breathing has then to be maintained artificially while the effects of the drug last.

status lymphaticus (status thymolymphaticus). A mythical disease until recently thought to be a cause of sudden death in childhood, in cases where the only apparent abnormality was enlargement of the thymus gland. The mistake arose because the normal weight of the thymus had been grossly underestimated. During severe illness or stress the thymus shrinks rapidly, and its average weight after death, on which the estimates were based, is much less than its average weight in life. But if death is very sudden the thymus has no time to shrink, and therefore appears to be abnormal. Most of the deaths ascribed to this 'enlargement' were really due to sudden suppression of breathing by anaesthetics.

steatorrhoea. Diarrhoea due to undigested fat in the intestine, e.g. with ♢ *coeliac disease* and ♢ *sprue*.

stegomyia. A kind of mosquito, *Aëdes*, able to transmit certain viruses.

stenosis. Narrowing of a tubular organ such as a segment of a blood vessel or of the intestine.

stereotactic surgery. A method of direction-finding that has much increased the scope of brain surgery, enabling the surgeon to work on areas of the brain that would otherwise be inaccessible. The exact location of the area, which may be a cluster of cells the size of a pinhead, can be inferred from the structure and dimensions of the inside of the patient's skull as shown by X-rays. These data are used to set an apparatus consisting of two arcs at right angles to each other, like the gimbals of a ship's compass, by which the point of a needle can be guided to the area within 0·1 mm. The calculations can be done by a computer, which also indicates the point at which the needle can be inserted without damaging the intervening brain tissue. A minute electric current passed down the needle then inactivates the tissue around its point. The method is mainly used for suppressing uncontrollable muscular activity such as the tremor of *parkinsonism*. It has also been used for destroying small tumours, for locating foreign bodies, and even for the treatment of serious behavioural disorders: this last is still at an experimental stage.

sterile. 1. Free from living microbes.
2. Unable to have children: not the same as *impotent* (unable to copulate). For instance, a eunuch is sterile but not necessarily impotent, and some people are impotent for psychological reasons although they are fertile if the emotional problem can be overcome. ♢ *fertility*.

sterilization. 1. ♢ *antiseptic*; *bacterium* (5).
2. Surgical operation to render the patient sterile. The most certain method would be removal of the gonads (castration), but this causes hormonal disturbance, because the gonads form important hormones as well as germ cells. In practice, males are sterilized by obliterating the vas deferens on each side (a simple procedure, because the vas lies just below the skin of the groin), and females by obliterating the Fallopian tubes. Either operation blocks the passage of germ cells (sperm or ovum). Although fertility can sometimes be restored by a second operation sterilization is

best regarded as irrevocable. In some countries it is illegal. On the other hand, the governments of some overpopulated and undernourished countries are doing all they can to encourage men to be sterilized while their families are still small.

sternomastoid. Large muscle at the side of the neck, extending from the top of the sternum and clavicle, to the skull behind the ear.

The sternomastoids acting together flex the neck. Either acting alone turns the head. They balance the vertebral muscles at the back of the neck, acting as guy-ropes to maintain the posture of the head.

Contracture of a sternomastoid causes a deformity, *torticollis* (wry-neck), by which the head is twisted to one side. In infants this is usually the result of injury during birth. It needs surgical correction to prevent further compensatory deformity such as uneven growth of the face.

sternum (breast-bone). A flat bone at the front of the chest to which the upper ribs are attached by their cartilages. The upper part or *manubrium* slopes downwards and forwards, making an angle (angle of Louis) with the more nearly vertical *body*. A joint between manubrium and body allows the sternum to straighten when the ribs rise during inspiration.

Fractures of the sternum generally heal without trouble, but since the heart lies just behind the bone they can be dangerous. They are the result of considerable violence and usually associated with other serious injuries.

steroid. A group of chemical compounds, widely distributed in nature, all with the same pattern of 17 carbon atoms arranged in 4 linked rings. Steroids with significant effects on the human body include substances as different as *vitamin D*, the drugs extracted from *digitalis*, male and female *sex hormones*, and the hormones of the *adrenal cortex*. The term is often confined to this last group, as an abbreviation of *corticosteroid*.

stethoscope. Instrument for examining the sounds in the chest (*stethos*) or other parts of the body, invented by Laënnec in 1816 and first described in his book *De l'auscult-*

ation médiate (Paris, 1819). 'Mediate auscultation' meant listening through an instrument, as opposed to 'immediate auscultation' with an ear on the patient's chest, the method of Hippocrates. The old method had been inefficient and undignified and little attention had been paid to the sounds of the heart and lungs. The new instrument, coupled with its inventor's clinical genius, transformed the diagnosis of disorders of the heart and lungs from a guessing-game to a science.

At first Laënnec used a roll of paper. Later, after much trial and error, he devised a straight wooden tube, widened at the patient's end for picking up the soft breath sounds. An adapter screwed into this end converted the stethoscope into a tube of uniform diameter for listening to the heart. The modern binaural stethoscope, with a flexible tube to each ear, often has interchangeable wide and narrow chest-pieces for the same purpose. A flexible diaphragm may improve the acoustic properties. Some sounds, e.g. an unborn baby's heart, are heard better with the original straight stethoscope.

Electrical instruments can be used for demonstrating sounds to a class, and for recording them (phonocardiography).

A kind of electronic stethoscope, depending on the deflection of high-frequency echoes, is used for studying the flow in arteries and for detecting the foetal heart in early pregnancy.

The sounds heard in a healthy chest are the soft rustling of air entering and leaving the lungs, and the heart sounds, two to each beat. The first heart sound is a dull thud as the ventricles, having filled, begin to contract, their inlet valves close, and blood begins to flow into the arteries. The second sound is sharper; it is heard when the ventricles have emptied themselves and the outlet valves close. Recorded tracings show third and fourth sounds, but these are faint or inaudible with an ordinary stethoscope.

If the texture of the lungs is altered by disease the conduction of sound may be enhanced or restricted and the air-stream is distorted. Different types of disease produce characteristic changes in the breath sounds, and various added sounds may be heard, such as the squeaky wheeze (*rhonchus*) of air being forced through narrowed tubes in asthma, or the crackling and bubbling sounds (*râles*) of fluid in the air-passages. Friction between inflamed membranes in pleurisy produces a sound 'like the creaking of leather', described by Hippocrates.

Disorders of the heart muscle affect the quality and timing of the heart sounds, and disorders of the valves cause added sounds (murmurs, *bruits*). The quality of an abnormal sound usually indicates the type of disorder, and the area where it is loudest indicates the site, but some sounds are almost impossible to interpret without further investigations. The murmurs that are sometimes heard from perfectly healthy hearts cause anxiety to both doctors and patients. A doctor hears a murmur that might indicate a defective valve. He cannot simply ignore it, because the heart needs attention if it is in fact abnormal. But as soon as the suspicion is mentioned the patient has something to worry about, and may go on worrying long after the heart has been proved innocent. Children are especially prone to harmless murmurs, and many healthy children have had to live like invalids because a suspicion once raised would not be stilled.

stilboestrol. A synthetic drug with similar actions to the oestrogens formed by the ovaries. ◊ *sex hormones.*

Still's disease. A rare form of ◊ *rheumatoid arthritis,* affecting children, with the important difference from the usual adult form of the disease that most patients recover completely.

stimulant. Drugs either increase (stimulate) or decrease (depress) the normal activity of organs. Depression is much commoner than true stimulation. This is to be expected, because healthy tissues generally perform as well as they can be made to, and unhealthy tissues can be improved only by removing the cause of ill health. Many apparent stimulants in fact depress. For instance, digitalis improves the performance of a *diseased* heart by suppressing useless activity; it does no good to a normal heart.

Alcohol needs special mention, because it is still often called a stimulant. Its sole effect is to depress all tissues, especially the nervous system; if it appears to stimulate, that is only because it suppresses inhibitions and worries.

Numerous drugs enhance the action of adrenaline and related substances that transmit impulses at relay stations in the brain. They include adrenaline substitutes such as ephedrine and amphetamine, and drugs used to relieve depression. Since they increase the activity (though not necessarily the efficiency) of the brain, any of these might be described as a stimulant. ◊ *analeptic.*

stimulus. Any event outside a living cell that causes change within the cell. In general, a particular kind of cell responds only to a particular stimulus. Cells at the back of the eye respond to light, cells in taste-buds to certain chemicals, muscle fibres to acetyl choline released from nerve-endings. An electric current serves as a stimulus to most cells that are capable of being stimulated, but it may act not directly on the cell but on its controlling nerve.

Stokes-Adams attack. (William Stokes (1804–78) and Robert Adams (1791–1875), Dublin physicians.) Sudden unconsciousness caused by heart-block. ◊ *arrhythmia.*

stomach. The part of the digestive tube between the lower end of the oesophagus and the beginning of the intestine, shaped like the bag of a bagpipe.

The first part of the stomach, the *fundus*, rises to the left of the oesophagus and forms a dome under the left side of the diaphragm. The second part, the *body* of the stomach, is a broad tube running down from the fundus. The third part, the *antrum*, is funnel-shaped. It runs upwards and to the right, and ends in the midline of the body at the *pylorus*, which is a muscular tube acting as a valve between the stomach and the *duodenum* or beginning of the intestine.

In very stocky people the stomach is almost entirely hidden by the left ribs, but in some thin people it hangs down in a loop like the letter J. The spleen lies to the left of the fundus, the left kidney behind the body, and the pancreas behind the antrum and pylorus.

The stomach is very muscular. Like the rest of the digestive tube it may contract in waves (peristalsis) to push its contents along but for some time after a meal the food is churned to and fro and thoroughly mixed with the digestive fluid (gastric juice) secreted by the stomach lining. The muscle is thickest at the pylorus, where it prevents food from passing too rapidly to the duodenum.

The lining membrane secretes large quantities of mucus, an effective barrier to prevent digestion of the stomach by its own enzymes. Three other important substances are formed by cells of this membrane: *hydrochloric acid*, *pepsin*, and *intrinsic factor*. The acid-forming cells are nearly all in the body of the stomach.

The *acid* is remarkably strong – gastric juice is about 0·4 per cent HCl, rather stronger than the decinormal solution commonly used in chemical laboratories. The synthesis is not fully understood; it is certainly complex. In brief, the cells take up acidic carbon dioxide from the blood, and return it to the blood converted to alkaline bicarbonate (the blood is slightly more alkaline after a meal). This active extrusion of alkali into the blood leaves the cell with a relative excess of acid to be secreted into the stomach.

Pepsin is an enzyme concerned in the digestion of protein.

Intrinsic factor is a protein without which vitamin B_{12} is not adequately absorbed.

The stomach has a good supply of blood from branches of the *coeliac* artery, which is a branch of the aorta. The blood is returned by way of the *splenic* vein to the *portal* vein and so to the liver.

1. REGULATION

The behaviour of the stomach has been directly observed in several classic studies. From 1823 to 1833 the American surgeon William Beaumont observed his patient Alexis St Martin, who had a permanent opening between his stomach and his abdominal wall after a gunshot wound. Through the opening Beaumont was able to study the secretions and movements of the stomach.

Pavlov 50 years later isolated a small pocket of a dog's stomach (Pavlov pouch) from which he could collect pure gastric juice, uncontaminated by food, and study the composition and rate of formation of gastric juice under various conditions. More recently S. Wolf and H. G. Wolff, in New York, have made detailed studies of their patient Tom. In this case an opening similar to that of Alexis St Martin had to be made surgically to relieve an obstruction.

These and other experiments have shown that:

1. Impulses in the vagus nerves stimulate movement of the stomach, dilate its blood vessels, and promote secretion.

2. The sympathetic nerves inhibit movement and constrict the blood vessels. They diminish secretion only indirectly, by reducing the blood supply of the mucous membrane. Adrenaline and similar drugs have the same effect.

3. The vagus nerves begin to stimulate the stomach at the sight and smell or even the prospect of food. The activity is greatly increased by eating. ۞ *reflex*.

4. The effects of emotional disturbances are varied, but on the whole they inhibit rather than stimulate the stomach. Symptoms with an emotional background are thus more likely to be due to stagnation than to excessive secretion.

5. Mechanical stimulation of the stomach by the pressure of food causes secretion independently of the vagus nerves. The action is indirect: *gastrin* (a polypeptide) is released from the lining of the antrum and stimulates the secreting cells higher in the stomach via the blood-stream. The gastric juice so formed is less acid than that promoted by nervous action.

6. Secretion is diminished by a high concentration of acid (a typical feed-back mechanism) and also by fatty food.

2. EXAMINATION OF THE STOMACH

A patient's symptoms may be a good guide to the state of his stomach, but more often symptoms such as loss of appetite, nausea, or stomach-ache do no more than point vaguely in the direction of the upper abdomen. Ordinary clinical examination seldom establishes the diagnosis: a gastric ulcer (which is most likely to be in the part of the stomach not covered by the ribs) may be tender, but that is about all.

The stomach can be examined by X-rays. The patient takes a draught of a fluid opaque to X-rays (e.g. barium sulphate suspension). This makes it possible to study movements, shape and size of the stomach, deformities, and the pattern of the mucous membrane.

A fractional test meal is a means of studying the secretion of gastric juice. The patient swallows one end of a long rubber tube, and a syringe is attached to the other end. A sample of gastric juice is first drawn off for analysis, and further samples are taken at intervals after various stimuli. The test meal itself usually consists of gruel, and secretion can also be stimulated by drugs.

The inside of the stomach can be examined with a gastroscope, which is simply a lighted tube passed down the oesophagus, with a system of lenses at each end. This instrument can also be used to take a small piece of mucous membrane for microscopical inspection.

3. DISORDERS

Only a few diseases of the stomach are common, but these few include some of the commonest of all ailments. Those mentioned here are discussed in more detail under their own headings.

Congenital ◊ *pyloric stenosis* is a hereditary affliction of babies, usually boys. The exit from the stomach is blocked by overgrowth of the muscle. It is treated surgically.

Inflammation of the stomach (◊ *gastritis*), unlike inflammation elsewhere in the body, is not often caused by infection, because the acid kills bacteria. It is more often due to irritation by swallowed poisons. The poison may have been produced by bacteria growing in food before it was eaten; the harm was then done before the acid had a chance to act (◊ *food poisoning*). The two commonest chemical irritants causing gastritis are alcohol and aspirin. Chronic, insidious gastritis has been attributed to every sort of dietary indiscretion. Some cases are certainly due to alcohol – all heavy drinkers are liable to chronic gastritis – but often the cause cannot be defined.

Gastric ulcer is discussed together with duodenal and other similar ulcers under ◊ *peptic ulcer*.

Cancer of the stomach is one of the commonest of cancers, second only to cancer of the lung in men and of the breast in women. In principle it should be easy to treat. The stomach is surgically accessible, and it can be removed without great danger. If, then, a cancer is recognized while it is still strictly confined to the stomach the chance of cure is good. The trouble is that these cancers are, more often than not, recognized only when surgical cure is already difficult or impossible. This is because the early symptoms are no more than those of some minor upset, and the diagnosis can be made only by one or more of the investigations described in section 2 above.

The surgical treatment of stomach cancer is not likely to be much improved, and no form of medical cure has yet been found. The high death rate from this cause can be reduced only by *early* investigation of trifling symptoms such as loss of appetite, abdominal discomfort, or 'indigestion'.

Achlorhydria is absence of hydrochloric acid from the stomach. The amount of acid is well below average in some 3 per cent of healthy people, and also in patients with chronic gastritis or cancer of the stomach. It is often reduced with gastric (not duodenal) ulcer. Complete failure to secrete acid, associated with inability to assimilate vitamin B_{12}, causes the usual type of pernicious anaemia; ◊ *anaemia* (B.2).

For surgery of the stomach, ◊ *gastrectomy*.

stomatitis. Inflammation of the mucous membrane of the mouth, often from invasion by types of bacteria that as a rule live harmlessly in healthy mouths. The mouth is generally resistant to infection – it needs to be, for it teems with microbes and is often injured. But stomatitis is a common complication of conditions that lower resistance, such as anaemia and vitamin deficiency. It can also follow treatment with antibiotics, which eliminate the normal bacteria of the mouth and so expose it to alien species. ◊ *noma; Vincent's disease.*

stone = ◊ *calculus.*

strabismus = ◊ *squint.*

stramonium. Datura, a poisonous plant with similar properties to belladonna. The active principle, *hyoscyamine,* is also found in belladonna (deadly nightshade) and hyoscyamus (henbane).

strangulation. Cutting off the blood supply to a part of the body, e.g. to a loop of intestine pinched in the opening of a *hernia.*

strangury. Difficult and painful passage of urine, e.g. with narrowing (stricture) of the urethra (the passage from the bladder), or a stone in the bladder, or spasm of the bladder muscle due to inflammation (cystitis).

strawberry mark ◊ *birth-mark.*

streptococcus. A spherical ◊ *bacterium,* diameter 0·001 mm. (1/25,000 in.). Unlike

staphylococci, which form clusters, streptococci grow in lines like beads on a string.
Three types are important in human disease:

1. *Str. viridans* is normally a harmless
inhabitant of the mouth and throat, which
can enter the blood stream when the lining
of the mouth is damaged, e.g. when a tooth
is extracted. This bacterium has little resistance to the natural defences and is
quickly destroyed in the blood. But a heart
valve with a congenital defect, or damaged
by rheumatic fever, sometimes offers a
sheltered anchorage where *Str. viridans* can
multiply. The resulting *bacterial endocarditis* is a serious condition; until the discovery of antibiotics it was always fatal, but
treatment with penicillin is effective.
Penicillin is also used to prevent the disease
by giving it to people with defective heart
valves before operations on the mouth.

2. *Str. faecalis* is equally harmless in its
natural habitat, the large intestine, but if it
contaminates the urine it can cause ◊ *pyelitis*.

3. *Str. pyogenes* is among the most
troublesome of all microbes. About one
person in 10 carries it in the mouth and
throat (whereas everyone carries *Str.
viridans* in the mouth and *Str. faecalis* in
the intestine).

It is one of the two main causes of infection and pus formation in wounds, the
other being *Staphylococcus pyogenes* (pyo-
genic = engendering pus). Streptococci are
much less prone than staphylococci to form
localized abscesses; streptococcal pus is
watery and tends to spread widely through
the tissues, and streptococci form a *toxin*
that breaks down fibrous barriers. The
lymphatic system, which serves to remove
foreign matter from the tissue fluid, becomes infected, and inflamed lymphatic
vessels may show as red lines joining a
wound to the nearest lymph nodes.
Streptococci may also enter the blood
stream and cause septicaemia.

Streptococci produce numerous other
toxins, which circulate and cause a severe
feverish illness in addition to damage at the
site of infection. Some strains of *Str. pyogenes* form a toxin responsible for the rash
of scarlet fever.

Because of their greater tendency to
spread, streptococci typically cause a more
fulminating type of infection than staphylococci, but for the same reason they are
more exposed to natural defences and to the
action of antibacterial drugs. In the great

majority of cases streptococcal infection can
be rapidly overcome, especially since nearly
all the usual drugs (sulphonamides, antibiotics) are effective.

The commonest streptococcal disease is a
sore throat, usually more severe than the
still commoner type due to viruses. Scarlet
fever is simply a streptococcal sore throat
due to a strain which also produces a rash.

At least two important diseases – rheumatic fever and acute nephritis – appear to
be after-effects of streptococcal infection,
though neither is directly due to infection.
They do not respond to antibiotics, but
they may be prevented by prompt treatment
of streptococcal disease. The mechanism is
not known, but a plausible theory is that
when the patient forms antibodies to combat streptococci some of the antibodies are
harmful to his own tissues.

streptomycin. An ◊ *antibiotic*, from the soil
fungus *Streptomyces griseus*, discovered by
Waksman in 1944. It is lethal to many types
of bacteria, including several against which
penicillin is ineffective. By far its greatest
value is in the treatment of tuberculosis.
After a time the tubercle bacilli develop resistance to streptomycin, but this trouble is
largely overcome by simultaneous treatment with drugs such as PAS and isoniazid
which attack the bacilli in other ways.

The principal drawback of streptomycin
is that it sometimes damages the auditory
nerve (◊ *ear* (4)) which conveys the senses
of hearing and balance from the ear.
Poisoning by streptomycin itself causes
giddiness; the closely related dihydro-
streptomycin causes deafness.

stress. Any influence that disturbs the
natural equilibrium of the living body. A
fundamental rule of physiology is that the
cells of the body need a constant environment, and that the primary function of any
organ is to maintain this internal environment despite changes in the surroundings
(◊ *Bernard, Claude*). Stresses in this sense
include physical injury, exposure, deprivation, all kinds of disease, and emotional
disturbance, any of which can disturb the
normal regulation of the internal environment.

According to the Canadian physician
Hans Selye and many others, prolonged
stress provokes first an immediate reaction,
then a more or less balanced state in which
the stress is resisted, and finally a break-

down of resistance. Many organs are involved, but most of all stress affects the adrenal glands: ◊ *adrenal* (2). If the resistance to change is depleted by any one kind of stress, there is less chance of resisting other stresses. Thus a serious injury increases susceptibility to infection, and worry aggravates physical illness.

◊ *psychosomatic disease*.

stricture. Narrowing of a tubular organ, e.g. by scarring.

stroke (apoplexy). More or less sudden interference with the circulation of blood in a part of the brain, generally with some permanent damage. Nerve cells can survive only a very short time without fresh supplies of oxygen and glucose, certainly not long enough for new paths for the circulation to be established, and lost nerve cells are not replaced.

Serious strokes are of three kinds: (1) *cerebral haemorrhage*, bleeding from a weakened artery into the brain; (2) *embolism*, sudden blockage of an artery by a flake of material that has come adrift from a diseased artery or from the heart; (3) *thrombosis*, a more gradual blockage by clot-formation within a diseased artery of the brain.

Sometimes a congenitally weak spot in an artery predisposes to haemorrhage. With or without such a weak spot, high blood pressure greatly increases the risk, and one of the main reasons for treating high blood pressure is that the risk of a stroke can be greatly diminished.

The disease of the arteries that predisposes to all three types is *atherosclerosis*. High blood pressure is again a contributory factor. A few strokes are due to embolism by fragments of clot formed in an unhealthy heart. A clot can find its way from a lung, through the heart to the brain. Sometimes a clot elsewhere, e.g. a vein in a leg, causes a stroke. It must reach the brain either via the lungs or through an abnormal opening between the right and left sides of the heart.

The effect of a stroke depends entirely on the size and situation of the affected area of brain. Some strokes cause no symptoms at all, and others are rapidly fatal. Between these extremes there are many degrees of impaired function, depending on the site and extent of the damage. If the patient survives the first week or two the final outcome is nearly always better than one

would expect. This is partly because of a zone of temporary loss of function around the permanently damaged area, and partly because the patient can often adapt intact muscles to take over the work of muscles that he can no longer control. A physiotherapist can do a great deal to help in this way; similarly speech therapists can sometimes teach people to speak again despite serious damage to the speech centre of the brain.

Strokes due to haemorrhage can sometimes be treated surgically, by removing blood-clot or by sealing a weak vessel. If an embolus can be traced to clotting in an accessible site such as an artery in the neck it may be possible to clear the artery surgically and prevent further attacks. Anticoagulant drugs to impede clotting are used after some types of stroke – not, of course, those due to bleeding.

Transient ischaemic episodes – 'little strokes' – have only recently been recognized. The patient has the symptoms of a stroke for a few minutes and then recovers completely. They may be due to temporary spasm of blood vessel in the brain, or sometimes to compression of an artery in the neck by an awkward posture. Sometimes they are due to a defect in an artery that could later cause a major stroke, unless it is corrected surgically.

stroma. The fibrous framework of a tissue (cf. *parenchyma*, its characteristic working cells).

strophanthus. An East African plant with similar actions on the heart to *digitalis*.

struma = ◊ *goitre*.

strychnine ◊ *nux vomica*.

stye (hordeolum). A boil in one of the skin glands of an eyelid.

subacute. Between acute and chronic.

subarachnoid. In the fluid-filled space between the coverings of the brain and spinal cord. ◊ *meninges*.

subclavian. Below the collar-bone (clavicle). The *subclavian artery* is a very large vessel arising on the left side directly from the aorta, and on the right from the innominate artery, a short vessel that divides into subclavian and right carotid arteries. After passing below the clavicle, the subclavian is continued as the axillary artery into the armpit.

The branches include the *vertebral artery*, which runs up the side of the backbone into the skull, and arteries to parts of the neck and chest.

The subclavian is accompanied by a *subclavian vein*, which joins the corresponding jugular to form an *innominate vein*.

subcutaneous. Under the skin.

sublimation. According to Freud, an unconscious process of diverting unseemly instincts into respectable channels.

subliminal. Term applied to sensations too slight or fleeting to be consciously perceived, though they may be unconsciously remembered; or stimuli too small to arouse a response in a nerve.

subluxation. Partial dislocation; displacement of bones in a joint without complete separation.

subphrenic. Below the diaphragm. A *subphrenic abscess*, in the space between the diaphragm and the top of the liver, sometimes arises from infection in the abdomen. It can be difficult to recognize because although the patient is obviously suffering from severe infection there is no indication of where the trouble lies. Sometimes a gas-bubble below the diaphragm is shown by X-rays, and sometimes the diagnosis is made by excluding all other possibilities.

substrate. The substance on which an *enzyme* acts; i.e. the raw material of a chemical process in a living organism.

Substrate competition is a common way for drugs to act. The drug so closely resembles a natural substrate that the enzyme reacts with it instead. For instance, *sulphonamide* drugs closely resemble a foodstuff of bacteria. The bacterial enzymes involve themselves with the useless drug and so deprive the bacteria of an essential food.

succus entericus. The digestive juice of the small intestine. ◊ *digestion*; *intestine*.

sudamen (pl. *sudamina*). Sweat blister; prickly heat.

sudor. Sweat.

sugar ◊ *carbohydrate*.

suicide. About 100 people are known to commit suicide in Britain every week. The rate is higher among the well-to-do than among the poor. Comparisons between countries, indicating for instance that suicide is much commoner in northern than southern Europe, may not be valid because in some countries doctors may be reluctant to upset relatives with the stigma of a mortal sin in the family. The formula of British juries 'suicide while the balance of the mind was disturbed' is a compromise between stating the fact and saving the family's face.

But the juries have been nearer the truth than they knew. Completely rational suicides are the exceptions. As a rule, something has gone wrong with the patient's thinking – and he really is a patient. Until 1961, he was officially a criminal in English law. Most people felt that the law was absurd, but it had the merit that anyone who attempted suicide could be legally detained, while someone investigated the case and found out why the prisoner (who was in fact kept under supervision in hospital) had tried to kill himself. The great drawback of this law was that it encouraged everyone concerned to conceal the 'crime', so that nothing was done to avert a second, possibly successful, attempt.

Suicide must now be regarded as the final symptom of a common illness, or group of illnesses. If the disease has a distinguishing feature it is the patient's feeling – perhaps unfounded – that he is cut off from the society or background he regards as his. In general, the patient also has some kind of mental instability, though there are circumstances in which a mentally stable person is so isolated from society that he kills himself. In these cases the society may be at fault. In the past an officer who behaved dishonourably, like a well-born Japanese who lost face, was expected to kill himself. Such suicides, dictated by public opinion, were little different from lynchings. But in most cases the sense of isolation is coupled with (and not the direct cause of) mental depression. If the depression is severe it may be the only real factor, though the patient imagines reasons for killing himself. These are often in the form of self-condemnation ('I have sinned – I am unfit to live').

The medical significance of suicide is that many cases could be prevented if the symptoms were recognized in time; and suicides are almost as numerous and quite as futile as deaths on the roads.

Several widespread and dangerous fallacies stand in the way of a rational view of suicide:

1. 'Attempted suicide is only moral blackmail'. Attempted suicide may well be moral blackmail (whether the patient knows it or not), but it is not *only* moral blackmail. The attempt may be a cry for help, but it is a desperate cry. The patient cannot be sure of surviving. He may hope to recover after giving everyone else a fright ('look what you made me do'). But he cannot tell how many pills will make him unconscious without killing him (nor, in the individual case, can a pharmacologist); he does not know how far he can fall without breaking his neck (nor does a surgeon). He may well hope to recover and find that things are better, but he does not much care about the risk of killing himself. Anyone in this frame of mind needs expert attention.

2. 'If one attempt fails, so will the next'. The patient is all too likely to try harder next time, because nobody was sufficiently impressed by the first attempt. This time he may try it with a motor car or a fire, and kill someone else by mistake.

3. 'The ones who talk about it never do it'. This is the most dangerous medical fallacy since surgeons gave up believing that pus was a good thing. *Most* people who commit suicide have dropped a hint to someone. It is a symptom to be taken as seriously as coughing up blood.

There are social services, official and voluntary, for dealing with the purely material reasons for suicide. The mental depression that underlies practically every case is a treatable illness.

sulphonamide. 1. The chemical group —SO_2NH_2.

2. Any compound that includes this group, especially one used to treat bacterial infection ('sulpha-drug'). Some diuretics and drugs used for treating diabetes are also sulphonamides.

In 1932 ◊ *Domagk* showed that the red dye *prontosil* controlled certain types of infection. The active principle of prontosil is sulphanilamide (*para*-aminobenzene sulphonamide), which was discovered in 1908 by Gelmo in Vienna and used in dyeing.

The anti-bacterial effect of sulphonamides depends on their similarity to *para*-aminobenzoic acid, which bacteria need as a vitamin. The bacteria mistake the drug for the vitamin and poison themselves.

Sulphonamides are effective against many kinds of infection, including common types of pneumonia, meningitis and cystitis, bacillary dysentery, gonorrhoea, trachoma, and streptococcal infection. Since their introduction in 1935, some of the most lethal diseases have been curable. There are now scores of drugs, of which the official names all have the prefix '*sulpha*-', derived from sulphanilamide but with fewer toxic effects, a wider range of activity, or smaller dosage. *Co-trimoxazole* is a mixture of a sulphonamide, *sulphamethoxazole*, with *trimethoprim*, which interferes with the synthesis of folic acid. This mixture thus disturbs the metabolism of bacteria at two points, and sometimes controls an infection against which neither ingredient would work on its own.

For a time after 1941 the sulphonamides were overshadowed by penicillin, but they still hold a place in the treatment of common infections.

sulphone. A kind of drug related to the sulphonamides; the sulphones were investigated during a search for a sulphonamide that would cure tuberculosis, and found to be an effective long-term treatment of leprosy. *Dapsone* is the usual form.

sunburn. Anyone with a fair skin is burnt by sufficient exposure to bright sunlight, especially when reflection from snow or water is added. In the tropics, enough ultraviolet rays find their way through even an overcast sky to cause some burning.

Several common drugs (e.g. sulphonamides) and a few uncommon diseases (porphyria; lupus erythematosus) sensitize the skin to sunlight. The antimalarial drug chloroquin sometimes suppresses an abnormal sensitivity.

The best treatment is to keep out of direct sunlight or protect the skin with long sleeves and a broad hat. Various creams and lotions filter off the harmful rays. They are selective, and it may be necessary to discover the wave-length of light to which a particular skin is sensitive, or try several preparations until a suitable one is found.

sunstroke ◊ *heatstroke.*

superego. Freud's term for a part of the unconscious mind that acts as a censor – the conscience.

super-female. A female with 3 instead of 2 X chromosomes to a cell. Such women are often sterile but are otherwise normal.

superinfection. During the course of one infection, a second infection by a different kind of microbe. The term is generally limited to a second infection by a microbe that is resistant to drugs being used against the first; the second microbe is sometimes a resistant variant of the first, and sometimes one of a type that is harmless until other types have been eliminated by drugs.

supination. Turning the forearm and hand palm upwards (cf. *pronation,* palm downwards).

suppository. A form of medication for insertion into the rectum, solid at ordinary room temperature but liquefying at body temperature, used either for a local effect such as relief of constipation or as a means of getting a drug into the circulation. (Chemical pessaries for vaginal use are also sometimes called suppositories.)

suppuration. Formation of pus.

suprarenal = ◊ *adrenal.*

surgery. The craft of surgery (*chirurgia* – hand-work, treatment of disease with the hands) is much older than recorded history. The Edwin Smith Papyrus, one of the earliest medical texts (*c.* 1600 B.C.), describes the splinting of fractures, the replacement of dislocated joints, the care of wounds – as today, contaminated wounds are left open but clean ones are stitched – and the drainage of abscesses.

Hippocrates (*c.* 400 B.C.) devotes one book to the treatment of head injuries and another to the surgery of piles. In a general treatise on surgery he insists on careful preparation and technical skill – his surgeons had to be professionals in any sense – and the Hippocratic Oath makes it clear that there were specialists.

After the Graeco-Roman era surgical practice deteriorated. The pious and scholarly physicians of the Middle Ages did not soil their hands on their patients, excepting

a very few great men such as Guy de Chauliac. For the most part, surgery was left to itinerant tradesmen with little if any training. But one group – the barbers – took this additional work seriously and in the end achieved something like professional status. In England, they received a charter in 1540. Three years later, Vesalius published the *Fabrica* and brought anatomy and surgery back into the realm of medical science. (◊ *Paré.*)

But another 2 centuries had to pass before surgery was wholly accepted as a part of medicine, and a surgeon had to be first and foremost a doctor. John Hunter (1728–93) put his chosen profession in its true perspective when he taught his students that a surgical operation was a last resort, an admission that other methods had failed: 'It is like an armed savage who attempts to get that by force which a civilized man would get by stratagem'. There must always be a place for surgery in the repair of damage or deformity, but for the rest the surgeon's ultimate goal is to work himself out of a job. Until recently, many forms of tuberculosis could be cured only by drastic surgery; now, streptomycin and other drugs offer a safer and surer remedy for all but a few cases.

By the middle of the 19th century surgeons had acquired almost unbelievable skill in the few operations that were possible. But the body cavities – abdomen, chest, skull – were forbidden territory except for desperate attempts to repair wounds, because any operation was almost bound to introduce fatal infection. Operations involving bones were almost equally dangerous. And since the patient was conscious, any operation lasting more than a few minutes was unthinkable. These two obstacles, infection and pain, kept surgery more or less within the bounds that the Greek doctors of the Roman Empire had known.

Then both obstacles were overcome at almost the same time. ◊ *Anaesthetics* were introduced in the 1840s, and 20 years later the principle of surgery without ◊ *infection* was discovered. All the old operations became safer, and for the first time, surgeons could reasonably treat diseases of the abdomen and of the bones and joints. With time no longer the first consideration, surgeons could work more like watchmakers than inspired butchers, and even the brain came within their scope.

Between the two World Wars the technique of anaesthesia improved rapidly. All surgery became safer, and with methods of maintaining respiration while the chest wall was open it was possible to operate on the lungs and the outside of the heart. The inside of the heart remained inaccessible until the introduction of heart-lung machines to take over the work of the heart during the operation.

suture. Surgical stitching, or the material used for it. Cotton or linen threads have been used for centuries. They are strong and easy to work with, but if the wound is infected these materials provide a safe refuge for bacteria. Catgut, popularized by Lister, is broken down in the tissues and disappears, and is particularly suited to stitches that have to be buried. The disappearance of the suture does not weaken the repair, because no suture is more than a splint to facilitate healing by living tissue. Occasionally even catgut provokes an adverse reaction. The ideal suture is a strip of the patient's own fibrous tissue, but the method is not often feasible.

Synthetic fibres are now used more often than natural ones because they are stronger and easier to sterilize, and various types of wire can also be used; all these remain in the tissues except where they are used in the skin and can be removed as the wound heals. Removable metal clips are a satisfactory alternative.

swallowing. The initial stage of swallowing is a voluntary act, though it is so well learnt as to be almost automatic. As soon as the food passes the back of the tongue a series of reflexes comes into play: the epiglottis closes the larynx and the food is pushed into the oesophagus by the muscles of the larynx.

sweat. A weak solution of salt, secreted by glands in the skin. Sweating is an active process, distinct from insensible ◊ *perspiration*, which is simply evaporation of almost pure water from the surface of the skin. The evaporation of sweat takes up a great deal of heat, and sweating is one of the principal means of regulating the temperature of the body. Unless the sweat can evaporate, no heat is lost. The air can take up only a limited amount of water vapour; therefore if the surrounding air is already saturated sweat merely accumulates on the

skin; an atmosphere that is both hot and humid is intolerable.

In cool surroundings no sweat at all is secreted. In very hot surroundings the sweat glands may pour out as much as 10 litres (2 gallons) in a day, together with 30 grammes (1 oz.) of salt. ◊ *heatstroke.*

Newly formed sweat has little smell. The unpleasant smell of stale sweat is due to the action of bacteria. Deodorants act mainly by destroying bacteria on the skin.

sycosis barbae = ◊ *barber's itch.*

Sydenham, Thomas (1624–89). 'The English Hippocrates'; next to Harvey the most celebrated of English physicians. Harvey in the laboratory and Sydenham at the bedside symbolize the two poles of the world of medicine. Sydenham was not concerned with scientific discovery for its own sake. Like Hippocrates, he was content to observe the course of illnesses, record neither more nor less than what he observed, and interfere as little as possible with the natural process of healing. Nobody has excelled Sydenham's accounts of symptoms nor his precise distinctions between various diseases.

Good remedies were few. Sydenham made the best use of those that he had, and established sound principles for treating malaria (then a common disease in England) with cinchona, syphilis with mercury, anaemia with iron, and severe pain or restlessness with opium.

His purely clinical study of disease led Sydenham to the conclusion that symptoms represent Nature's attempt to shake off disease. Although this is by no means the universal truth that Sydenham thought it to be, it remains one of the most important and most neglected principles of medical practice. Patients consult doctors to have their symptoms relieved, and every generation needs a Sydenham to point out that treating symptoms without first considering their causes may be the worst of disservices.

sympathectomy. Surgical operation to disconnect sympathetic nerves, with the object of preventing spasm of blood vessels or other effects of these nerves. Chemical sympathectomy is inhibition of sympathetic nerves with drugs; it has the advantage over surgery that it does no permanent damage and can be stopped at any time, but a drug affects the whole sympathetic system whereas surgery is confined to the particular branch that is to be put out of action.

Although sympathectomy would increase the flow of blood through healthy arteries it does not always improve diseased arteries, which may already be as wide as they can be. As a rule the operation is done only if a trial of blocking the nerve with a local anaesthetic improves the circulation.

sympathetic. One of the two divisions (cf. *parasympathetic*) of the autonomic or vegetative nervous system, which are responsible for the automatic, unconscious regulation of bodily function. Most parts of the body receive twigs from both of these divisions, generally with opposite actions.

The sympathetic nerves originate from cells in the spinal cord. These cells send fibres to relay stations (*ganglia*) which form a chain lying in front of the muscles at either side of the backbone. From the sympathetic nerves branches spread throughout the body, most of them accompanying the main arteries.

Sympathetic nerves have the following actions:

The sweat glands and the tiny muscles at the roots of the hairs (*arrectores pilorum*) are stimulated.

The upper eyelids are raised, and the pupils are dilated – the upper lids can, of course, also be controlled by voluntary nerves.

Arteries to muscles, including the coronary arteries of the heart muscle, are dilated, but other arteries (skin, abdominal organs etc.) are constricted.

The rate and force of the heart beat are increased, and more air is allowed into the lungs.

The activity of the digestive organs is suppressed.

With one exception, the sympathetic nerves act by releasing *adrenaline* and *noradrenaline*, and an injection of one of these substances has similar effects to direct stimulation of the nerves. The exception is the nerves of the sweat glands, which like parasympathetic nerves release *acetyl choline*.

Sympathomimetic or *adrenergic* drugs imitate the effects of the sympathetic nerves. Adrenaline itself is given for asthma and other severe symptoms associated with allergy. It works only if it is injected, and its action is rapid but short-lived. Many drugs have rather similar actions. *Ephedrine* can be given by mouth. It works fairly well against asthma, and is less likely than adrenaline to raise the blood pressure. But it causes unwanted mental excitement. This last effect is the principal one of *amphetamine* and related compounds, and accounts for their use by drug addicts. *Isoprenaline*, a derivative of noradrenaline, is especially suited to asthma because it relaxes the bronchi without constricting any blood vessels.

Sympatholytic drugs inhibit sympathetic nerves. The drugs used to treat high ◊ *blood pressure* are mostly of this type. They inhibit all the effects of adrenaline. Some others, e.g. *tolazoline*, selectively inhibit only the characteristic effects of noradrenaline (*alpha* effects) such as constriction of blood vessels, and can be used to treat spasm of blood vessels without disturbing the rest of the sympathetic system. *Practolol* and *propanolol* inhibit the other actions of the sympathetic nerves (*beta* effects) and can be used to prevent the nerves from over-stimulating the heart in conditions such as angina, again without disturbing the rest of the system.

symptom. In ordinary English a symptom is any indication that something may be wrong: a manifestation of disease. Symptoms in this sense may be subjective, i.e. observed by the patient, or objective, i.e. observed by his attendants. Medical usage restricts the term to what the patient himself reports. Abnormalities found by examining the patient are *signs*.

A *presenting symptom* is one which prompts a patient to seek medical advice – not necessarily the first he notices; he may ignore a cough and some loss of weight but consult a doctor when he finds blood on his handkerchief. Bleeding is then the presenting symptom, cough and weight loss are other symptoms, and the signs might include a slightly raised temperature and abnormal shadows in an X-ray picture of the lungs.

synapse. A junction or relay station between nerve cells. When an impulse travels down the conducting fibre (axon) of a nerve cell a chemical substance (usually acetyl choline) is released from the end of the fibre and sets off a new impulse in the next nerve cell of the chain of communication.

syncope = ◊ *faint*.

syndrome. A fixed pattern of symptoms, not necessarily with the same cause in all cases.

synovium. Smooth moist membrane lining a ◊ *joint*.

syphilis. An infectious disease caused by a spiral bacterium (spirochaete), *Treponema pallidum*. Since the spirochaete cannot withstand exposure in the open air the disease is transmitted only by close contact, nearly always sexual (but ◊ *yaws*). The infection enters through either a mucous membrane (vagina or male urethra) or a scratch in the skin; thus apart from frankly venereal infection there are rare cases from kissing and from touching an infectious patient with an unnoticed scratch on the hand – a risk to doctors and nurses. A greater danger is infection of an unborn infant, for *T. pallidum* is one of the very few microbes that can pass through the placenta to infect the infant.

There are no recognizable accounts of syphilis earlier than about A.D. 1500, but after the return of Columbus from the New World the disease spread as a plague from the Mediterranean across Europe. Nobody can prove that Columbus and his men imported syphilis, but it seems likely. There is, however, a considerable weight of contrary opinion, some of it well informed (◊ *yaws*). One need not take very seriously the scholars who have insisted that the leprosy of the Bible must have been syphilis because it is an apt punishment for sin, and congenital syphilis visits the sins of the fathers upon the children.

Syphilis was first named in 1530 by Fracastorius in a poem *Syphilis sive Morbus Gallicus*, where he describes the disease as hitherto unknown and gives an unmistakable account of its natural history. He then tells how an unfortunate shepherd named Syphilus cursed the Sun during a heat-wave and was promptly stricken with the new disease as a punishment.

All the protean effects of syphilis are due to localized, subdued and chronic inflammation wherever the spirochaetes take hold. The small blood vessels are more affected than any other structures, and many of the symptoms are from impaired circulation of blood in affected areas.

The first sign is a *chancre*, a hard small lump that may break down to form an ulcer at the site of entry. The nearest lymph nodes – in the groins if, as is usual, the chancre is on the genitalia – swell. The chancre appears at any time between a week and 3 months after infection, and gradually disappears even without treatment. In a few cases there is no chancre and the disease passes straight to the second stage.

In the second stage, beginning several weeks or even months after infection, the spirochaetes have been disseminated in the blood-stream and cause general mild illness and a skin rash with swollen lymph nodes. The rash may be localized or widespread, and can take so many forms that cases of secondary syphilis have been mistaken for most of the common skin diseases. This stage also subsides even without treatment, but the infection still lurks.

The third stage of syphilis does permanent damage. The spirochaetes form established colonies in various parts of the body and start a persistent grumbling inflammation followed by obstruction of small arteries and loss of normal tissue. Any tissue or organ in the body can be affected and almost any chronic disease can be simulated. Physicians of the 19th century, when advanced syphilis was rife, taught that any student who knew syphilis knew medicine. A sort of chronic abscess (*gumma*), consisting mainly of dead tissue and overgrown scar tissue, may appear anywhere in the body and cause symptoms by compressing healthy neighbouring tissue. Mucous membranes, skin, and bones are common sites of tertiary syphilis. Syphilis of the heart can be fatal. The initial attack is on small arteries that nourish the main artery – the aorta – which loses its resilience and becomes permanently stretched by the pressure of blood (◊ *aneurysm*). Later the valve that prevents blood pumped into the aorta from returning to the heart leaks, so that the heart is no longer an efficient pump.

The nervous system may be severely damaged at a late stage of the disease. Again the various types of syphilis can be confused with many other diseases, but there are two characteristic types. These are *tabes dorsalis* (locomotor ataxia), with loss of reflexes that co-ordinate voluntary movement and posture; and *general paresis* (GPI, dementia paralytica), with deterioration of personality, delusions (often of grandeur or self-importance), and at last total insanity.

As early as 1530 Fracastorius described the treatment of syphilis with mercury. It was unreliable and dangerous but much better than nothing, and for 4 centuries offered the only hope of a cure. In 1910, Ehrlich discovered arsphenamine (◊ *arsenic*), and for the first time it became possible to kill microbes in the body without great risk to the patient. Arsenic has now given way to penicillin as the standard treatment of syphilis. In the first and second stages syphilis can usually be cured because there has been no permanent damage. In the later stages it can only be arrested, for tissues already destroyed are not restored.

Prevention would be the best answer, but this is still no more than a dream (◊ *venereal disease*).

In the early stages, the spirochaete can usually be identified. Later it becomes difficult to isolate, but its presence can be inferred from blood tests such as the ◊ *Wassermann* reaction.

syringomyelia. An uncommon defect of the spinal cord. Small cavities filled with watery fluid appear in the centre of the cord and disturb conduction in adjacent nerve fibres. The fibres conducting the sensations of pain and temperature are the first to suffer, but other function may be impaired later (sometimes after decades). The cause is unknown, but there may be a congenital fault in the spinal cord. There is no reliable treatment. Surgical operations to relieve pressure within the cord sometimes help.

system. (1) A group of more or less distinct organs with a common function, e.g. the cardiovascular system (heart and blood vessels), the digestive or alimentary system (oesophagus, stomach, intestine, liver, pancreas and other digestive glands). (2) A school of medical or pseudo-medical opinion based on a few fixed axioms, e.g. homoeopathy. (3) The whole body regarded as a functional unit, now obsolescent as a noun but still alive as an adjective: see next entry.

systemic. Applying to or affecting the body as a whole, often opposed to *local* or *topical*. Thus the local symptoms of an abscess include swelling and pain, while the systemic symptoms include fever and proliferation of white blood cells. A drug may be given systemically, e.g. by mouth or by injection into a vein, to be taken into the circulation and distributed through out the body, or topically, e.g. in an ointment, to act only at the site of trouble.

systole. Contraction of the heart muscle, the active phase of its cycle when blood is pumped into the arteries (cf. *diastole*, the passive phase when the heart relaxes and blood flows into it from the veins).

T

TAB. Combined vaccine against typhoid, paratyphoid A and paratyphoid B fevers.

tabes (archaic). Any wasting disease. *Tabes dorsalis* = syphilis of the spinal cord. *Tabes mesenterica* = abdominal tuberculosis.

tachycardia. Unduly rapid heart beat.

tachyphylaxis. Decreasing effectiveness of a drug after repeated use; it occurs most often with drugs acting on the nervous system. ◊ *tobacco.*

taenia. Tapeworm. ◊ *worms.*

talipes = ◊ *club-foot.*

talus (astragalus). A bone of the foot. It fits into a mortise formed by the lower ends of the tibia and fibula to form the ankle joint.

tannic acid (tannin). Plant extract used for converting hide to leather. It is a powerful astringent, and it used to be a standard dressing for ◊ *burns* (in an emergency, in the form of cold tea). Tannin forms a crust, which was thought to protect the burn. But the crust is as likely to keep infection in as out, and if it encircles a part of the body such as a hand it may obstruct the circulation.

Tannin precipitates some alkaloid (vegetable) poisons, and is used as an antidote.

tapeworm ◊ *worms.*

tarsus. Base of the ◊ *foot.* Of the 7 tarsal bones, only one, the talus, articulates with the leg to form the ankle-joint.

taste. The mucous membranes of the tongue and palate contain numerous minute sensory organs, the taste-buds. Each bud is a round cluster of spindle-shaped cells, from which nerve fibres lead to the facial and glossopharyngeal nerves. Four types of sensation are received from the taste-buds: salt, sweet, sour (acid), and bitter. Of these, only sour is obviously linked to the chemical structure of the substance tasted. The buds all look alike, but four sensations suggest four types of bud. Furthermore some areas of the tongue are more sensitive than others to particular tastes: the tip to sweet and salt, the edges to sour and salt, and the back to bitter. There is, however, evidence that all taste-buds are able to respond to all four tastes, and that the long-accepted principle that one nerve fibre can do only one job may need modification. It may be that different tastes are transmitted by different patterns of impulses, decoded in the brain. The same applies to the different types of sensation from the skin.

This crude sensation promotes a reflex flow of saliva. But awareness of flavours depends more on smell (◊ *nose* (2)) and on information about consistency, texture, and even appearance.

teeth.

1. STRUCTURE

The exposed part of a tooth is the *crown.* the concealed part is the *root.* The slight constriction where the two meet is the *neck,* to which in health the mucous membrane of the gum is attached.

A tooth is a stout shell of *dentine* (ivory), which is like compact bone except that it has no blood vessels. The dentine of the root is coated with a thin layer of a similar but softer material, *cement.* The crown has a thick covering of *enamel,* which is much denser and harder than dentine or than any other animal matter. The cavity of the tooth is filled with the *pulp,* soft connective tissue rich in blood vessels and nerve fibres.

The arrangement of the teeth is the same in upper and lower jaws. On each side, counting from the midline, there are 2 incisors, 1 canine, 2 premolars, and 3 molars – 8 teeth in each quadrant or 32 in all. The *incisors* are chisel-edged. The upper ones close in front of the lower; together they act as scissors. The *canines* are conical, grasping teeth, especially well developed in carnivores, which use them for seizing their prey and wrenching off lumps of meat. Premolars and molars are adapted for grinding food between knobs (*cusps*) on their surfaces. The premolars, each with 2 cusps, are also called *bicuspid* teeth. The upper molars have each 4 cusps; the lower molars have 5.

Each upper molar has 3 roots. Lower molars have 2, and the other teeth usually have single roots. The roots are deeply embedded in sockets in the jaws, to which they are fastened by ligaments (*periodontal membrane*).

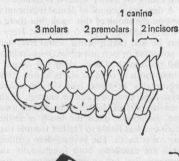

3 molars   2 premolars   2 incisors

1 canine

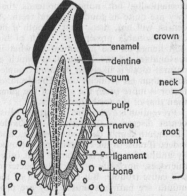

crown

enamel
dentine
gum   neck
pulp
nerve
cement   root
ligament
bone

(Above) *Arrangement of adult teeth.* (Below) *Section of tooth (diagrammatic).*

2. DEVELOPMENT

The elements of the teeth are formed before birth. The lining membrane of the mouth grows into the tissue from which the jaws are to develop, and forms the enamel. The rest of the tooth is modified connective tissue. Each tooth bud is enclosed in a little capsule or *dental follicle*. At birth the jaws are filled with these follicles.

The deciduous or milk teeth begin to erupt about half-way through the first year of life – the time varies and is unimportant. Only 20 milk teeth appear: in each quadrant 2 incisors, 1 canine, and 2 molars. The set is usually complete at about 2 years.

The first permanent teeth to erupt are the 1st molars at about 6 years. They are behind the deciduous molars, so no teeth are shed when they appear. Later the deciduous teeth are replaced by permanent teeth – deciduous molars by permanent premolars. The last milk teeth, the canines, are usually replaced in the 12th year. After that the 2nd permanent molars erupt. The 3rd molar (wisdom) teeth are delayed for a few more years and may not erupt at all.

Healthy development of the teeth obviously depends to some extent on the general health: the teeth are as susceptible as any other organ to malnutrition. Vitamin deficiencies, especially scurvy and rickets, impair the growth of the teeth. Dentine and enamel both need a supply of *fluorine*, and minute quantities of certain other elements appear to be needed – probably molybdenum and manganese, possibly vanadium and selenium.

Drugs given to pregnant women, notably tetracycline antibiotics, may affect the baby's teeth; the enamel is discoloured and sometimes defective.

3. DISORDERS

Human jaws have receded in the course of evolution, and there is now barely room for the full set of permanent teeth. But quite apart from overcrowding, teeth are apt to grow unevenly. Some of the effects are obvious: the teeth are unsightly, useless because they do not meet their opposite numbers (malocclusion), and hard to clean. The second and third effects make them liable to decay. These are more than enough reasons for energetic treatment. *Orthodontics* is the branch of dentistry which deals with misplaced teeth. It has become a very refined craft, and even quite gross deformities can be corrected if they are treated early. Some of the remote effects which have been ascribed to malocclusion, such as disorders of breathing, are open to doubt.

Tartar (calculus) is a chalky precipitate from the saliva. If it is not regularly removed it injures the gums and provides a shelter for bacteria.

Considering that the mouth teems with microbes the gums remain remarkably free from infection, but they can become infected and inflamed, especially if they are not kept clear of tartar and food residues. The inflammation – *gingivitis* – is disagreeable in itself because the gums are tender and the mouth tastes and smells unpleasant; in time the bone of the jaws recedes, the teeth become loose, and dentures may be difficult to fit. The condition of the gums deteriorates rapidly with anaemia, malnutrition, and many chronic infectious diseases.

Much the most important disease of the teeth is decay or *dental caries*. The enamel and then the dentine are dissolved from part of the tooth until the pulp is exposed and ultimately the tooth dies. The process is still not fully understood, but the usual sequence appears to be as follows. Bacteria in the mouth, perhaps lactobacilli, ferment sugar to form acids. The acids dissolve the calcium salts of the enamel and dentine to form a crevice in which the process can proceed more quickly. The bacteria are most active away from air. At first they are protected from air by particles of food between the teeth, but later the crevice that they have made protects them. Once a hole is established other types of bacteria can attack the pulp.

Enamel which lacks fluorine is especially vulnerable. Some people, perhaps 10 per cent of the population, are highly resistant to caries for no known reason. Clean teeth are safer than dirty teeth because on them bacteria are exposed to the air. The protective value of chewing is not clear. Chewing may do more for the supporting tissues than for the teeth themselves. Sugar is a better medium for the bacteria – i.e. more harmful to the teeth – than any other food, and sugar between meals is much worse than sugar with meals because saliva flows freely during a meal. Saliva itself is essential to the health of the teeth. If the saliva is deficient the teeth decay rapidly.

Next to caries the commonest cause of severe toothache is an *abscess* around a root. Such abscesses may be associated with caries or with inflamed gums, but they can also arise at the roots of healthy teeth. The tooth socket is of bone and therefore rigid, and the abscess cavity is plugged by the tooth. Since there is no room for expansion the abscess is painful even at the earliest stage, and the pus is liable to invade neighbouring tissue. The path of least resistance is usually into the mouth, but an abscess at the root of a lower back tooth may point below the angle of the jaw. The obvious treatment is to draw the tooth, which releases the pus and alleviates both pain and risk. This used to be the only way to manage an established abscess, but with antibiotics it is now possible to abort the process, at least in the early stages. Even when pus has formed it can sometimes be drained by drilling the length of the tooth and filling the cavity when it is clean.

A detailed account of dental treatment is beyond the scope of this book, but there is a historical note under ◊ *dentistry*. Here it may be said that modern dental treatment is governed by two principles: conservation and prevention. Caries does not attack a whole tooth at once. It starts at one point, presumably at some fault in the microcrystalline structure of the enamel. If the decayed part of the tooth is cleared away and the hole is filled the tooth is neither more nor less liable to further trouble than any other tooth. The best modern artificial teeth are excellent, both functionally and cosmetically, but nobody pretends that they are quite as good as natural teeth. A dentist will not, then, draw a tooth if he can reasonably preserve it. Much of his skill hangs on the judgement of what is reasonable, of the moment at which a natural tooth is likely to be more troublesome than an artificial one. The deciding factor is more often the state of the gums than that of the teeth themselves.

Prevention is even more important. Most dental disease is theoretically avoidable. The mouth cannot be freed of bacteria, and indeed if most of the bacteria are destroyed by antibiotics there is a danger that other microbes, normally opposed by bacteria, will cause trouble. But the bacteria of the mouth are harmless unless they are protected by particles of food between the teeth, or by tartar; if neither is allowed to collect the teeth and gums are safe. If no food, especially no sugar, ever remains between the teeth there is nothing for the bacteria to ferment. Perfect cleaning of the teeth immediately after eating and regular scaling of tartar by a dentist ought to protect the teeth for a lifetime. Whether it would in fact do so is not known, for nobody can be sure of removing every food particle with every brushing, and a few hours are enough to establish the first crevice that is the start of caries.

Diet is important in two ways. Firstly, it

must contain the factors necessary for the healthy growth of teeth, at least until growth is complete. Vitamin deficiencies are rare in prosperous communities but all too common elsewhere. ⟡ *Fluorine* deficiency is a result of living in an area where the drinking water contains too little. Secondly, the food should need chewing. It is difficult to prove the importance of this, but most authorities agree that the soft food of an over-civilized diet is a factor in dental ill health.

Finally, the actual treatment of diseased teeth and gums is also a means of prevention, for if lost tissue cannot be restored the processes of decay can at least be arrested or greatly slowed.

teething. Children may be fretful and even feverish when they are cutting teeth, but it does not follow that these symptoms are due to teething. The first teeth erupt at an age when children are meeting infections to which they have not yet developed any immunity. The child may be teething or ill or teething *and* ill. Each case needs to be investigated before the trouble can be dismissed as unimportant (⟡ *paediatrics*).

teleology. The doctrine of final causes: the assumption that events are ultimately due to the ends which they serve. In other words, things happen because it is necessary that they should happen. This is very nearly the same as saying that they happen because it is God's will.

In essence, the doctrine must be almost as old as abstract thought. Materialism can never wholly displace it, because man's finite intelligence cannot deal with infinite problems. Science is largely a matter of determining causes and effects. Progress means advancing the frontiers of what we can rationally define, but the frontiers remain, and discussion of anything beyond them is almost bound to be teleological. Aristotle thought in terms of a planned universe in which everything had its place. To say that events are caused by the need for them is no more than to say that they must suit the plan – or the purpose of the planner. The doctrine led to error only when later and lesser thinkers than Aristotle, such as Galen, presumed to know what this purpose was. The early Christians all but canonized Galen. If they had thought more deeply they would have disowned him for supposing he was party to

God's design. He was the greatest physician of ancient Rome, and a fine observer. But since he was determined that everything he observed should take its place in the grand design *as he saw it*, he was not always a reliable witness. For example, although his account of the muscles was detailed and reasonably accurate, he flouted the evidence of his own eyes by describing hollow nerves, in order to suit his theory of how muscles worked. He also described, as though he had seen them, channels between the chambers of the heart and an elaborate system of communication between the arteries and nerves at the base of the brain, because he thought that they should be there to convey the 'vital spirit'. Some of the most tenacious fallacies in medicine have arisen, and will continue to arise, in this way.

The belief that pus was necessary to the healing of wounds bedevilled surgery throughout the Middle Ages and almost into our own times. Observing that wounds usually formed pus, the surgeons argued that pus must have a useful purpose, so they irritated and infected wounds to encourage more pus to be formed. Thus they caused as much suffering as ever they relieved. Inflammation, the process by which pus arises, gives a more modern instance of the same kind of fallacy. John Hunter, who could use teleology without letting it blind him, correctly described inflammation as a means of defence and healing. From this it is all too easy to conclude that inflammation is *always* desirable, and therefore to be encouraged. It has only recently been shown that certain types of inflammation are harmful. ⟡ *allergy.*

Teleology, then, has no place in a 'pure' science such as physics, except as the last refuge of the man who knows that he has reached the limit of his ability to see or reason. The same is true of basic research in medicine, which has to seek out causes and not take them for granted. But in medical practice decisions have to be made which cannot be based on complete knowledge or mathematical proof. What the doctor cannot explain he must take for granted; beyond the frontiers of scientific knowledge he is inevitably a teleologist. This is the difference between the science and the art of medicine.

In speaking or writing about medicine, teleology can hardly be avoided. The critical reader will find instances on almost any page of this book. The heart *pumps* blood; the kidneys *filter* it; muscles *pull*, or *resist* gravity; white blood cells *attack* germs. All these verbs imply purpose. To a purist, each begs the question. Yet anyone who tried to avoid them would write so pedantically as to be unreadable even by a specialist. If one is to discuss these things at all one must discuss them in a language that can be understood, and as often as not this is the language of teleology. Even the experimental physiologist, running to catch his train, can be allowed to breathe fast in order to bring more oxygen to his overworked muscles. He will have time when he reaches his laboratory to reflect that he breathed fast, not *in order to* do anything, but *because* acid formed in his muscles stimulated the nerve centre controlling respiratory rate.

temperament. The four temperaments of ancient medicine were supposedly related to the four ◊ *humours*: *sanguine* to blood, *melancholy* to 'black bile' (the dark, viscous blood of the spleen), *choleric* to yellow (real) bile, and *phlegmatic* to phlegm or mucus.

temperature. The temperature of the body is not strictly constant, nor is it the same in all parts of the body. 'Normal' temperature, taken in the mouth, is close to the temperature of arterial blood. In the armpit the temperature is a little lower and in the rectum, higher. Most people have an average temperature in the mouth between 36° and 37·2° C. (97–99° F.), but the value fluctuates during the day (lowest in the early morning, highest in the evening), and, in women, during the month (lowest at menstruation, highest at ovulation).

The reflex control of temperature is modified by clothing. Tropical heatwaves apart, the body constantly loses heat to the environment by conduction and radiation and above all by evaporation of water from the skin. It gains heat from the combustion of fuel derived from food. Small variations are dealt with by adjusting the flow of blood through the skin. To conserve heat, the blood vessels of the skin contract and the skin pales; to lose heat they dilate and the skin flushes. Heat is gained rapidly when the muscles are made to work, for like all engines they dissipate some of the energy provided as heat. If no positive exercise is taken to work the muscles, they can work automatically to produce shivering. Heat is lost when the sweat glands pour water on to the skin to be evaporated. If the surrounding air is moving, sweat evaporates faster. Movement of the air also increases the conduction of heat away from the body. The warmth of clothing depends on the layer of enclosed, still air.

Raised body temperature is discussed under ◊ *fever*, and lowered body temperature under ◊ *cold*.

temper tantrums. Most small children have occasional episodes of uncontrolled rage, but frequent tantrums may need investigation. Often a child's feelings develop faster than his ability to express them; he is like an adult who finds foreigners intolerably stupid because he cannot communicate with them. Temper tantrums may of course be straightforward blackmail, but they may also be a desperate attempt to convey some real problem such as illness or emotional starvation.

temporal. Of the side of the cranium (temple). The *temporal bone* is the part of the skull around the ear. Its outer surface gives attachment to the *temporalis* muscle.

The (superficial) *temporal artery* runs in front of the ear, where its pulse can be felt, and over the scalp. This artery is occasionally the site of painful chronic inflammation (◊ *arteritis*).

The *temporal lobe* is a part of the brain under cover of the temporal bone. It records hearing, and appears to play an important part in the storage of memory.

temporalis. Large muscle at the side of the head for closing the jaw. In many animals these muscles are so large in relation to the head that there is a crest on top of the skull to accommodate them, much as the huge pectoral muscles of a bird raise a crest on the sternum.

tendon (leader; sinew). Fibrous cord joining a muscle to a bone. A tendon is a bundle of tough fibres of *collagen*, which are so strong that a violent jerk of the muscle is as likely to break off a piece of the bone as to snap the tendon.

An *aponeurosis* is a flat sheet of fibres representing the tendon of a flat muscle, as in the abdominal wall or scalp.

The sensory nerves in tendons transmit the unconscious sensation of stretch, setting off reflex contraction of the muscle to oppose the movement and maintain a given posture. This reflex is exemplified by the familiar knee-jerk: a tap of the examiner's hammer stretches the tendon in front of the knee and the muscle promptly responds. A tendon can also register pain if it is squeezed.

Tendons have their own blood vessels, and can heal if they are stitched together after an injury. The result is apt to be spoiled because in the process of healing the tendon sticks to neighbouring structures, and loses its mobility.

At the wrist and ankle the tendons are enclosed in slippery fibrous sheaths, which may be inflamed (*tenosynovitis*) by bacterial infection or rheumatism.

tennis elbow. Pain and stiffness in the muscles below and to the outer side of the elbow joint, commonly associated with a strain on the muscles such as a hard game of tennis when out of training, or unaccustomed effort with a screwdriver. The pain is variously ascribed to a partial tear of the muscle fibres, to pinching of the radial nerve as it passes through the muscle at this point, and to bursitis. It can be relieved by an injection of hydrocortisone into the painful spot, or by manipulation. Whether treated or not the symptoms disappear in time, but they may linger for many months.

tension ◊ *premenstrual tension*.

teratoma. 1. A grossly deformed foetus.
2. A kind of tumour of which the cells may develop into a semblance of almost any tissue; originating either from several different kinds of cell or from persistent embryonic cells that have kept their ability to develop in various ways.

tertian fever ◊ *malaria*.

testis (testicle). The primary organ of sex in the male. Like its counterpart the ovary, the testis has two distinct functions. It forms the male germ cells – sperms – and it is also an endocrine gland, secreting sex hormones into the blood-stream.

Within its tough fibrous shell, the *tunica albuginea*, the testis contains fine coiled tubes, the *seminiferous tubules*, lined with cells that from puberty until old age can develop into sperms. The seminiferous

tubules lead to the *epididymis*, a tangle of tubes in which newly formed sperms mature. The epididymis opens into the *vas deferens*, which carries the sperms through the groin, behind the urinary bladder, and through the prostate gland to the urethra.

Between the seminiferous tubules are collections of *interstitial cells* where hormones, mainly *androgens*, are formed (◊ *sex hormones*).

Both components of the testis are regulated by hormones of the ◊ *pituitary*.

The testes originate in the abdomen immediately below the kidneys. In fish (soft roes) and birds they remain there, but in man and most other mammals they migrate through the groins to the surface of the body where they are carried in a bag of skin, the *scrotum*. They work at a lower temperature than other organs. A testis that fails to descend to the scrotum generally fails to produce live sperms, but its output of hormones is not impaired. The testes usually descend before birth, but about 10 per cent of boys are born with one or both still on the way. In most of them the undescended testis arrives within a few weeks, but the condition has to be treated if it persists. Pituitary hormones may complete the process; otherwise the testis must be brought down surgically.

In its descent from the abdomen the testis brings with it its duct, the *vas deferens*, and its blood vessels, which arise next to those of the kidneys. All these form a leash, the *spermatic cord*. Occasionally the cord becomes twisted, causing severe pain in the testis and obstructing its supply of blood. This condition, torsion of the testis, needs prompt surgical treatment.

The passage of the cord through the muscles of the abdomen creates a weakness through which a *hernia* can protrude.

The commonest disorder in this region is a *hydrocoele*. This is a collection of fluid in the membrane surrounding the testis. The fluid can be drawn off with a hollow needle but it is likely to reappear; the condition is permanently cured by a small operation to remove a part of the membrane.

Inflammation of the testis (orchitis) is an occasional complication of mumps, gonorrhoea, tuberculosis and some other infections.

testosterone. A male sex hormone (androgen); the principal hormone of the testis.

tetanus. Spasm of voluntary muscles with convulsions, caused by infection with the tetanus bacillus, *Clostridium tetani*. This bacillus lives harmlessly in the intestines of various animals, especially horses and occasionally man. It can multiply only in the absence of air, but when conditions are unfavourable it forms spores, a sort of hibernating phase, from which active bacilli can develop after years of inactivity. Tetanus spores are often found in soil. Many wounds must be contaminated with tetanus spores, but nothing untoward happens unless the conditions exactly suit them. For this, the spores must be embedded in tissue that has been killed, e.g. by other bacteria, injury, or chemical poisons, so that it has no oxygen supply.

Even active tetanus bacilli do not harm the tissues in which they multiply; but they produce a *toxin* that is one of the most poisonous substances known. It has a similar action to strychnine, but the lethal dose is about 100,000 times less.

The toxin released by tetanus bacilli follows the path of the nearest nerve to the spinal cord. There, it blocks the automatic impulses that restrain motor nerve cells and so allow the selective stimulation that is the basis of controlled movement. When the motor cells are freed from this restraint they bombard the muscles with impulses, and the muscles respond either with convulsive twitching or sustained contraction. Co-ordinated movement is impossible because opposed muscles pull against each other.

Trismus – a spasm of the jaw muscles – gives tetanus its alternative name, *lockjaw*. It may be the first symptom, but any group of muscles can be affected first. Later, other groups follow; the patient is severely ill and may die from inability to control breathing or from sheer physical exhaustion. Symptoms may begin at any time from a few days to a month or more after the original wound – the later, the less the danger.

Tetanus can be prevented by vaccination, which has to be repeated every 5 years and immediately after a suspect injury. People who have not been vaccinated against tetanus can be given temporary immunity after a wound with an injection of anti-toxin.

The antitoxin is also used for treating an actual case of tetanus, but it neutralizes only toxin that has not yet invaded nerve cells – it prevents the disease from getting worse but does not cure symptoms that have already begun. Opening up the wound surgically exposes the bacilli to air, which they cannot tolerate. Oxygen can be used to reinforce this effect.

Since any sensation may trigger convulsions, patients with tetanus have to be nursed in quiet and shade, with sedative drugs. In severe cases a drug such as curare may be needed to prevent muscular action; this treatment paralyses the muscles of breathing along with the rest and therefore mechanical respiration is needed. In fact, the patient is treated in much the same way as one undergoing a major operation.

Untreated tetanus is often fatal, but with present-day treatment most patients recover, and suffer no lasting effects.

tetany. Twitching and spasm of muscles from any cause, e.g. disturbance of the calcium in the tissue fluid with disease of the parathyroid glands, vitamin D deficiency, or alkalosis.

tetracycline. An antibiotic prepared from chlortetracycline, which is extracted from the fungus *Streptomyces aureofaciens*. These and other related compounds are broad-spectrum antibiotics, i.e. they kill many different types of microbe. This versatility is useful with mixed infections, and when the infecting microbe cannot be identified. The disadvantage is that useful bacteria are also destroyed.

thalamus. Two masses of nerve cells, sometimes joined in the mid-line, at the headward end of the brain-stem, between the cerebral hemispheres. Sensations of all kinds are carried to the thalamus to be relayed to the cerebral cortex, where they are consciously perceived, or to lower centres where appropriate reflex actions are set in train. At least one sensation – pain – appears to be perceived in the thalamus itself, without having to be referred to the cortex. If the thalamus is damaged, pain is not so easily induced, but such pain as can be felt seems unnaturally severe.

thalassaemia. Cooley's anaemia, a hereditary anomaly of ◊ *haemoglobin*.

thalidomide. Sedative drug first used in Germany in 1958, and withdrawn in 1961 because of serious deformities among babies born to women who had taken the drug during pregnancy. Thalidomide is related chemically to drugs that have been used for many years. Its advantage was that overdoses were unlikely to be fatal. A few patients taking it developed a kind of neuritis, which was mistaken for a minor side-effect.

A well known but very rare congenital defect of the limbs, *phocomelia*, suddenly became commoner, and the increase was associated with thalidomide. At that time the routine investigation of new drugs did not include tests during pregnancy, because the risk to the embryo was unsuspected. Looking back, it seems that the action of thalidomide on adult nerve cells, which can cause neuritis, is far more injurious to the growing nerve cells of an embryo. The nerves are the first part of a limb to develop, and if their growth is impaired the bones and muscles also fail to develop.

Since 1961, drugs have been tested on pregnant animals before being considered for human use.

theine. Caffeine extracted from tea.

thenar. Of the ball of the thumb. ♢ *hand* (1).

theophylline. An alkaloid resembling theine, extracted from tea. ♢ *aminophylline.*

therapeutics; therapy. Therapeutics is the science of treating disease; therapy is the treatment itself.

thermometer. Sanctorius measured the body temperature before 1612 with a cumbersome modification of Galileo's thermometer, but for two and a half centuries no further progress was made for want of a convenient instrument. The 19th-century German physicians Carl Wunderlich and Ludwig Traube were the first to make any systematic study of the temperature in health and sickness. The modern clinical thermometer was designed by Sir Clifford Allbutt (1836–1925) in 1867.

A half-minute thermometer registers in half a minute under laboratory conditions but takes rather longer in the mouth and much longer under the arm. If the reading is going to be wrong, it will be too low – unless the thermometer has been rinsed in warm water or not shaken down.

The arrow indicating 'normal' (37° C.; 98·4° F.) is no more than a guide to an average temperature. A single reading, is not usually as important as the progress of the temperature. As with a barometer, the rise or fall is more significant than the exact level.

thiamine = ♢ *vitamin B₁*.

Thiersch graft. (Karl Thiersch (1822–95), German surgeon.) ♢ *graft.*

thigh. Region from hip to knee; functionally it includes the buttock.

The skeleton of the thigh is the ♢ *femur*, which for most of its length is surrounded by large muscles. These muscles are in four main groups: those of the buttock (♢ *gluteus*), the ♢ *quadriceps* at the front of the thigh and the ♢ *hamstrings* at the back, and the adductor muscles of the inner side of the thigh.

The *gluteal* nerves and arteries arise within the pelvis and pass under the hip-bone to supply the buttock. The *sciatic* nerve takes the same route, and then runs down the back of the thigh, giving branches to the hamstring muscles. The *femoral* nerve enters the thigh in the middle of the groin and supplies the quadriceps and adductor muscles. It accompanies the femoral artery, which is the main source of blood for the whole limb.

thiopentone. A short-acting barbiturate drug, injected into a vein as a general anaesthetic.

thiouracil. A drug that suppresses overactivity of the thyroid gland, used for treating toxic goitre.

thoracoplasty. A major operation on the chest wall in which several ribs are removed to allow the wall to collapse and close the cavity of a large abscess. With effective antibiotics against tuberculosis and other lung infections this drastic operation is now seldom used, but in the past it saved many lives.

thoracotomy. Any surgical operation that involves opening the thorax.

thorax. Compartment of the body enclosed by the ribs, extending from the first rib above to the diaphragm below. The word 'chest' generally means the same, but it has no clear anatomical definition.

The thorax is smaller than it appears to be. The shoulders fill out the contour of the living body, but the thorax itself is conical, and at the top it is no wider than the neck. Its floor is higher than the limit of the ribs, because the diaphragm is a dome, and the upper part of the abdomen is also enclosed by the ribs.

The thorax is divided by fibrous partitions into three compartments. The central compartment, the *mediastinum*, contains the *heart*, with the *oesophagus* behind it, and in its upper part the *trachea*, with the *thymus* gland in front of it. In addition, the mediastinum contains the blood vessels entering and leaving the heart, and several important nerves.

The two lateral compartments are the *pleural cavities*, which contain the *lungs*.

All three cavities are lined with slippery membranes to prevent friction: the mediastinum with the *pericardium*, and the pleural cavities with the *pleura*.

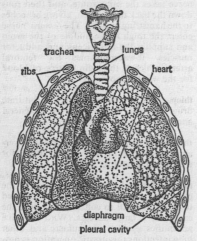

Principal thoracic organs, with part of the right lung removed.

1. THORACIC SURGERY

Penetrating wounds of the thorax always need attention, for two reasons. Firstly, if air can get between the chest wall and the lung, the lung may collapse like a balloon (◊ *pneumothorax*). Secondly, there is little to prevent infection from spreading throughout the pleural cavity. To prevent

air from getting in, the wound needs to be tightly covered, e.g. with a strip of sticking plaster, until it can be stitched; and anything lodged in the wound is best left until the patient reaches an operating theatre.

Apart from the repair of wounds, only one operation on the thorax was feasible until modern times. This was the drainage of pus from an abscess of the pleural cavity (◊ *empyema*). There was no danger that the lung would collapse, because the tissues round the abscess were stuck together by inflammation.

Now that infection can be controlled, and adequate breathing artificially maintained, the lungs are as accessible to the surgeon as any other organ, and with the invention of a heart-lung machine to act for the heart as well, the surgery of the heart has also advanced.

◊ *heart*; *lungs*.

throat. The word has no precise anatomical meaning: 'cut throat' refers to the front of the ◊ *neck*, and especially the carotid and jugular blood vessels; to throttle someone is to squeeze his windpipe (◊ *trachea*); a sore throat is inflammation mainly of the middle part of the ◊ *pharynx*, at the back of the mouth, spreading downwards to the voice-box or ◊ *larynx*.

Food passes through the mouth, pharynx, and oesophagus to the stomach; air passes through the nose (or mouth), pharynx, larynx, and trachea to the lungs. The pharynx thus serves both swallowing and breathing. Its continuation behind the larynx is a flat tube, of which the back wall (in contact with the backbone) and the front wall (which is the back of the larynx) are held together except during actual swallowing. The larynx, on the other hand, has a shell of cartilage which ensures that the airway is held open. Various reflexes ensure that food shall not be inhaled. The swallowing reflex is coupled to reflexes which stop breathing, draw the vocal cords together as a shutter across the larynx, and drop the epiglottis as a lid over the vocal cords. If a particle of food passes these barriers it stimulates nerve-endings in the larynx or trachea and sets off the cough reflex which expels it.

If an object such as a fish-bone sticks in the throat instead of being swallowed it may sustain the reflexes which prevent breathing: the subject chokes. As soon as the object is dislodged and returned to the mouth or swallowed, or at least moved to a less sensitive area, breathing is resumed. The usual first-aid methods – thumping the patient's back, holding him head down, hooking a finger behind the tongue – are attempts to move the object into a safer place. The rare cases in which choking persists are serious emergencies, because it may be impossible for the patient to breathe properly until the airway is cleared by means of surgical instruments, a simple procedure in an operating theatre but difficult elsewhere. There is less immediate danger from inhaling an object down the larynx and trachea into a lung. It is likely to be coughed up. If it is not it has to be removed through a bronchoscope – a lighted tube passed down the trachea – to prevent an abscess from forming beyond it.

thromboangiitis obliterans = ◊ *Buerger's disease.*

thrombocyte. Blood platelet. ◊ *blood* (4).

thromboendarterectomy. Surgical treatment of thrombosis in an artery by stripping the diseased lining of the artery together with the clot, leaving a free passage for the blood.

thrombophlebitis. Inflammation of a vein with obstruction by clotted blood. ◊ *phlebitis.*

thrombosis. Clotting of blood in an artery or vein, with partial or complete blockage of the circulation in the area. Although blood clots almost at once if it is shed, it cannot normally do so inside an intact blood vessel. But if the lining of the vessel is unhealthy and loses its water-repellent sheen a fibrous clot may form on it and increase until the vessel is obstructed. Thrombosis in veins is generally associated with inflammation (◊ *phlebitis*), and thrombosis of arteries with ◊ *atheroma.*

Thrombosis causes little trouble if there are adequate alternative (collateral) vessels to maintain the circulation in the area; if there are not, some tissue is inevitably damaged. Death of a segment of a tissue from blockage of its artery (e.g. of a segment of heart muscle after a coronary thrombosis) is *infarction.*

A second danger of thrombosis, whether or not there is any local damage, is *embol-*

ism, when a fragment of the clot (embolus) breaks off and blocks a vessel further along. Some strokes are due to thrombosis in the heart or in a carotid artery, when there is no significant blockage but a small embolus lodges in one of the arteries of the brain.

The enzyme *streptokinase,* injected into the affected vessel, may dissolve a recently formed thrombus. *Anticoagulant* drugs help to prevent thrombi from forming. An obstructed artery can sometimes be cleared by a surgical operation, *thromboendarterectomy,* or even replaced with a graft. Treatment and prevention are discussed further under ◊ *atheroma.*

thrombus. A clot formed on the lining of a blood vessel.

thrush. Infection of a mucous membrane, usually in the mouth, with the fungus *Candida albicans.* ◊ *Candida.*

thymus. A kind of gland in the root of the neck, mostly under cover of the upper part of the sternum. It consists largely of developing lymphocytes, the white blood cells concerned with immunity to infection. In relation to the size of the body, the thymus is largest around birth. Between birth and puberty it only doubles its size, and after puberty it very gradually shrinks. The residue of the thymus can be removed in adult life without ill effects.

The functions of the thymus in infancy are still little understood. It is concerned with the development of immunity to infectious microbes and of the similar process that causes the body to reject proteins other than its own, accounting for both allergic diseases and the rejection of transplanted organs. Conversely, the thymus before birth seems to be responsible for the selection that prevents the body's own proteins from being rejected. An important group of diseases is due to a partial failure of this last mechanism (◊ *autoimmunity*), and at least one of these diseases (*myasthenia gravis*) is sometimes cured by removing the thymus.

◊ *status lymphaticus.*

thyroid cartilage. The shell of the ◊ *larynx;* its protusion in the front of the neck is the Adam's apple.

thyroid gland. Endocrine gland in the front of the neck. It consists of two lobes, one at either side of the Adam's apple, joined at their lower ends by a bridge of glandular tissue across the upper part of the trachea. Although it lies near the surface the normal gland is small and soft and can scarcely be felt through the skin.

1. FUNCTIONS

The thyroid produces a hormone, *thyroxine*. This is a compound of iodine with the amino-acid tyrosine. Most of the iodine in the body is stored in the thyroid. A feedback mechanism controls the release of thyroxine into the blood-stream: if the concentration of thyroxine falls, *thyroid-stimulating hormone* (TSH) is released from the ◊ *pituitary*, whereas increased concentration of thyroxine inhibits the release of TSH. Therefore, if the pituitary fails, the thyroid, deprived of its stimulus, also fails. If the pituitary is over-active, so is the thyroid.

Thyroxine accelerates the release of energy in the tissues from combustion of glucose. How it does so is not known. It does not itself take part in the chemical reactions which produce energy. The enzymes which do so are stored in small compartments of the body-cells, the *mitochondria*, and thyroxine may facilitate the passage of reagents into the mitochondria.

With this accelerated combustion, breathing and the circulation of blood are increased to meet the added demand for oxygen; bodily and mental activity are stimulated; the body temperature is raised.

A second thyroid hormone, *calcitonin*, lowers the concentration of calcium in the blood, in opposition to the hormone of the ◊ *parathyroid* glands.

2. DISORDERS

In the embryo the thyroid grows downwards to the neck from the back of the tongue. Occasionally a fragment is left behind and forms a cyst. But the most important congenital disorder of the thyroid is *cretinism*, failure of the gland to develop. The new-born cretin is usually a normal baby, presumably because he has been able to use thyroxine from his mother's thyroid. After birth his physical and mental development are retarded. The child's appearance is characteristic: coarse hair and skin, protruding tongue, and pot belly. The untreated cretin remains undersized and below the mental level at which formal education is possible. If he is given thyrox-

ine from an early age he develops normally. Unfortunately cretinism is difficult to recognize in the first few months, and if treatment is delayed the patient may not quite catch up with normal children.

Thyroid deficiency starting in adult life causes *myxoedema*. The patient, often a middle-aged woman, loses energy and appetite; the body temperature is low; the skin is dry and puffy; the mind is dulled. All these changes are completely reversed by giving thyroxine. Some cases of myxoedema are due to ◊ *autoimmunity*, whereby a defence mechanism for rejecting invasion by parasites is directed against one of the body's own tissues. Rejection of an essential protein of the thyroid (Hashimoto's disease) was the first proven instance of autoimmunity.

Goitre is any enlargement of the thyroid gland. *Simple goitre* arises from lack of iodine in the diet. Deprived of its most important raw material, the thyroid is constantly stimulated to produce more thyroxine. It responds by overgrowing, and may become enormous. Only about 0·2 mg. of iodine is needed daily. In most parts of the world this is provided by sea-food, vegetables, or drinking water. Where the soil lacks iodine – usually in mountainous regions – goitre is endemic. This happens in the central parts of all the continents, and even in England a 'goitre belt' stretches from Derbyshire to Somerset. In many countries the prevalence of goitre has been much reduced by adding traces of iodine to table salt. Large goitres may have to be removed because neighbouring structures (trachea, veins, nerves) are compressed or because they are unsightly. Kocher was the pioneer in this branch of surgery.

Toxic goitre (thyrotoxicosis, Graves' disease, Basedow's disease) is over-activity of the thyroid. The goitre itself may be hardly noticeable; what matters is the increased fuel consumption. The patient becomes irritable and restless. She loses weight. The heart is over-active; its rhythm may be disturbed and it may fail. Most cases are due not to any fault in the thyroid itself but to abnormal stimulation of the thyroid. The stimulus is either an excess of the normal thyroid-stimulating hormone from the pituitary, or an abnormal hormone (*long-acting thyroid stimulator*) arising, perhaps, from the hypothalamus. This abnormal hormone, or a substance associated with it, causes the eyes to protrude (exophthalmos). When this symptom is added to the others the disorder is known as *exophthalmic goitre*.

Complete rest relieves many of the symptoms of toxic goitre, but cannot be prescribed indefinitely. The surest form of treatment is surgical removal of most of the thyroid. The operation would be dangerous, especially to the overworked heart, unless the activity of the thyroid were first damped down. Moderate doses of iodine are very effective (for no known reason), but since the good effects of iodine wear off in a few weeks iodine is only a preparation, not a substitute, for surgery.

Several newer drugs, most of them derived from thiourea, prevent the thyroid cells from forming thyroxine. They can be used instead of iodine to prepare the patient for operation. Some patients are apparently cured by taking them over a period of months or years, but more than half still need operation.

A radioactive isotope of iodine (^{131}I) can be used to suppress the over-active thyroid, which takes up the isotope as avidly as it takes up ordinary iodine (^{127}I) and thereby poisons itself. Very small, harmless doses of ^{131}I are used to study thyroid function; they provide a record of the rate at which the gland assimilates iodine. Some cancers of the thyroid have been successfully treated with ^{131}I, but the method works only with the few cancers which keep the affinity for iodine of healthy thyroid tissue.

thyroiditis. Inflammation of the thyroid gland. Bacterial infection, the usual cause of inflammation in most organs, is rare in the thyroid. Thyroiditis is more often due to ◊ *autoimmunity*.

thyrotoxicosis. Abnormal and excessive activity of the thyroid gland; toxic goitre. ◊ *thyroid gland* (2).

thyrotrophic hormone. The thyroid-stimulating hormone (TSH) of the pituitary gland.

thyroxine. Hormone formed in the thyroid gland.

tibia. The shin-bone, one of the two parallel bones in the lower leg, corresponding with the ◊ *radius* in the forearm (the fibula

corresponds with the ulna). The two forearm bones are equally important, but in the leg the tibia carries all the weight and is much more heavily built than its companion.

A flat surface of the tibia, from the front of the knee to the inner side of the ankle, lies immediately under the skin. The large muscles of the foot and ankle are attached to the other surfaces.

The commonest fracture involving the tibia is ◊ *Pott's* fracture-dislocation of the ankle.

Because the tibia is covered only by skin, fractures of the middle of the bone are more often compound than fractures of any other bone – a broken end is forced through the skin and the fracture is contaminated with bacteria from outside.

An intact fibula is a good splint for a fractured tibia, and fractures of the tibia alone are usually easy to manage. But an injury severe enough to break the tibia is unlikely to spare the fibula, and fractures of both bones together can be very unstable. If they are broken straight across, as by a direct blow, a plaster cast may hold them in place; but if the fracture is oblique or spiral the broken ends are liable to slip inside a cast, and a continuous pull against the muscles has to be maintained. This can be done by weights suspended from a wire passed through the heel. Otherwise, the fracture can be splinted internally with a metal pin down the centre of the shaft.

The blood supply of the tibia is not very good, and healing of fractures may be slow.

tic. Habit spasm; a purposeless stereotyped movement such as screwing up the eyes, shrugging the shoulders, or a 'nervous' cough. Most if not all tics have their origin in a deliberate and significant movement, which later becomes unconscious, like a conditioned reflex. Tics most often affect insecure children. They generally vanish in time, but if a tic becomes a nuisance it may have to be treated as a neurosis.

Tic douloureux (trigeminal neuralgia) is not really a tic (◊ *neuralgia*).

tick. A small creature like a wingless insect, related to the spiders; a few species attach themselves to human skin and transmit varieties of typhus and relapsing fever.

tincture. Alcoholic solution of a drug.

tinea. Fungal infection of the skin; ◊ *ringworm*.

tinnitus. Ringing, buzzing, or hissing sound in the ear; it can arise from almost any disorder of the ear or its nerve. Wax in the ear-hole, blockage of the Eustachian tube with a common cold, and irritation of the auditory nerve by an overdose of aspirin are among the commonest causes, and often no cause can be found. The patient's distress is not relieved by being told that the symptom is imaginary. Hearing is awareness that nervous impulses have reached a particular area of the cerebral cortex. The impulses are no less real for having originated within the ear and not from vibrations of the outside air which others can also hear. There is no sort of connection between tinnitus and auditory ◊ *hallucination.* ◊◊ *Ménière's syndrome.*

tissue. Living matter of any one particular type, both structural and functional; a tissue is composed of more or less uniform *cells* which may or may not be surrounded by a homogeneous ground-substance or *matrix*. The cells of blood are suspended in a fluid matrix, *plasma*; those of bone in a hard solid.

An *organ* is a distinct structural unit (e.g. muscle, gland, eye), made of different kinds of tissue: the *parenchyma* is the specialized working tissue of the organ, and the *stroma* is the less evolved supporting tissue which holds the parenchyma together.

The many tissues of the body appear to be derived from four primitive cell-types: epithelial, mechanical, amoeboid, and nerve cells (but they can be classified in other ways).

Epithelial tissues include true epithelium such as the outer layer of the skin (*epidermis*) and the lining membranes of hollow organs, and also the parenchyma of glands. The cells are closely packed, with little if any ground-substance.

The mechanical tissues include muscle with its highly specialized cells, and various tissues in which the ground-substance is more important than the cells which produce it, such as bone, cartilage, and connective tissue.

The characteristic of amoeboid cells is independent movement in a fluid medium, and the tissues with which they are associated are the body-fluids blood and lymph.

Nerve cells arise in the embryo from the

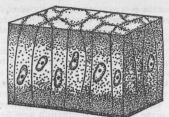

epithelial tissue

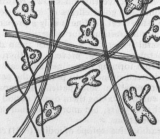

connective tissue

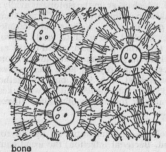

bone

same layer of tissue as the outer skin, but they behave so differently from any other cells that they must be separately classified.

Tissues were first described by ◊ *Bichat* in 1800.

◊◊ *histology.*

tissue fluid. Watery fluid percolating all the minute spaces among the cells of the body. Chemical supplies for the cells diffuse out of the capillary blood vessels into this fluid, from which they are absorbed by the cells. Waste products are transferred from the cells via the tissue fluid to the blood. The walls of the cells and of the capillaries act as filters, impermeable to anything as large as a protein molecule but allowing free passage to smaller molecules.

A solution in which the molecules are free to move tends to become uniform; in other words dissolved substances diffuse from zones of high concentration to zones of low concentration. Supplies, e.g. of oxygen, diffuse from the blood where they are concentrated to the cells where they are lacking. Waste products, e.g. carbon dioxide, diffuse in the opposite direction. If the blood ceases to flow the concentrations become balanced and diffusion stops: the cells can no longer be kept alive.

If all the molecules are not free to move the solution still tends to become uniform, but the movement is in only one direction and therefore exerts pressure. Protein cannot diffuse out of the capillaries in any quantity, but water from the tissue fluid can diffuse in to dilute it creating an osmotic pressure ($\diamond$ *osmosis*) of about 25 mm. of mercury.

Blood is pumped from the heart at a pressure of around 100 mm. of mercury, reduced in the arterioles to 32 mm. This exceeds the osmotic pressure; therefore at the entrance to a capillary water is forced out. As blood flows through the capillary the pressure falls to 12 mm. Since this is less than the osmotic pressure, water now returns to the capillaries. Thus the tissue fluid circulates, leaking from one end of the capillaries and returning to the other end.

Not all of the fluid returns to the capillaries. Some enters the thin-walled $\diamond$ *lymphatic* vessels and is ultimately returned to the blood in the veins at the root of the neck. This part of the fluid, the $\diamond$ *lymph*, carries away the small amounts of protein that leak from the capillaries, and any solid particles (e.g. bacteria) that find their way into the tissue spaces.

The tissues become swollen by an excess of tissue fluid if the hydrostatic pressure in the capillaries rises, or if the osmotic pressure falls ($\diamond$ *oedema*).

tobacco. The catalogue of diseases said to be caused or made worse by tobacco is so long and varied as to be unconvincing at first sight. Most people would be willing to blame tobacco for one or two diseases but will not accept a crime-sheet that includes indigestion, blindness, bronchitis, heart failure, gangrene of the feet, and several kinds of cancer; and because the campaign against smoking sounds like hell-fire propaganda or an advertisement for a quack remedy it is apt to be rejected. Yet each item on the list is backed by very sound evidence.

Tobacco smoke has at least three highly poisonous ingredients, each with complex effects on the body: tar, carbon monoxide, and nicotine.

Tobacco tar is an irritant. It causes chronic inflammation of mucous membranes, and is the most important of the various factors that lead to chronic bronchitis. In this condition the lining of the air-passages not only produces more mucus than it should but loses the ability to clear the passages of mucus and dust particles. The heavy smoker can inhale smoke in comfort only because the protective cough reflex is suppressed. The devitalized mucous membranes are an easy prey to bacteria. In time, breathing becomes so inefficient that the patient becomes a respiratory cripple. The condition of the lungs puts an increasing strain on the heart and may cause it to fail.

The degenerative change in mucous membranes is in some unknown way a precursor of cancer. The chance of developing lung cancer is in strict ratio to the amount of smoking. Nobody smokes enough or lives long enough to be quite certain of developing a tobacco cancer, but one can paint enough of the tar on a mouse's ear to be certain of producing cancer. Smoking does not make lung cancer inevitable, nor is it the sole cause of lung cancer. What it does is to convert a rare disease into a very common one.

Some tobacco cancers arise in the mouth or throat instead of the lungs.

Carbon monoxide displaces oxygen from the blood. In heavy smokers it may reduce the efficiency of the blood by about 10 per cent, so that in effect the patient is slightly anaemic. This would not ordinarily be enough to cause symptoms, but must aggravate shortness of breath from bronchitis. Carbon monoxide may be partly responsible for the defective eyesight (*tobacco amblyopia*) of some heavy smokers.

Nicotine interferes with the ganglia (relay stations) of the autonomic nervous system. Since this system is distributed throughout the body and is responsible for the reflex control of most organs, nicotine has very wide-spread effects. Small doses stimulate these nerves indiscriminately. The possible effects include the faintness and nausea of the novice, from stimulation of parasympathetic nerves; but as the habit develops these effects are largely superseded by stimulation of sympathetic nerves, causing over-activity of the heart, suppression of appetite, and constriction of small blood vessels near the body surface.

A rare form of arteriosclerosis, *Buerger's disease*, seems to be a direct result of smoking added to some unknown predisposing factor. This disease can cause gangrene of the feet, treatable only by amputation, when a susceptible person continues to smoke.

It is not certain whether tobacco contributes to the usual form of arteriosclerosis with *atheroma*, but people with atheroma (i.e. most of the population) greatly increase the risk of its more dangerous complications, such as coronary thrombosis, by smoking. The reason is not known, but nicotine is the likely cause.

The effect of nicotine on mood is hard to define. Most habit-forming drugs produce drowsiness or some kind of elation, or both – alcohol, for instance, elates by dulling the higher levels of consciousness with their uncertainties and inhibitions. But nicotine in the doses that can be got from smoking neither stupefies nor cheers. It has none of the soothing effects that are sometimes attributed to it. At the most it causes a fleeting confusion and a vague, equally fleeting sense of excitement. Even these trivial effects can only be produced after some hours' abstinence, e.g. with the first cigarette of the day, for nicotine is subject to *tachyphylaxis*: doses repeated at short intervals have less effect than the first dose.

A habitual heavy smoker gets little positive pleasure from the habit. The only obvious effect is the morning cough that he may call clearing his throat but is in fact a sign of bronchitis and serious trouble to come. The pleasure is negative; it is a very brief respite from the sense of physical deprivation that the smoker feels when he has not smoked for a while. This is the 'soothing' effect of tobacco. In other words some (though not all) regular smokers depend on tobacco for their sense of wellbeing. To insist, as some purists do, that these people are not addicted is quibbling. Addicted or only 'habituated', the majority of heavy smokers can give up smoking only with the greatest difficulty. It may take

them several months to feel at ease without tobacco, and even years later a single lapse may be enough to restore the old habit. The one certain remedy is not to start in the first place. As to giving up an established habit, any chest clinic or psychiatric department will offer advice and moral support, but everything depends on the smoker's determination to give it up completely – cutting down is almost bound to fail.

Cigarette smoke is more noxious than cigar or pipe smoke. This is partly because pipe and cigar smokers tend to inhale less and partly because of chemical differences in the smoke, but as regards heart attacks the difference is so great that some ingredients of cigarettes other than tobacco may play a part.

Snuff and chewing tobacco cause some chronic irritation of the nose or mouth, but most of their ill effects are confined to the actions of nicotine.

◊ *addiction.*

tocopherol = ◊ *vitamin E.*

tolazoline. A drug used to block certain actions (alpha effects) of sympathetic nerves; its main action is to prevent constriction of small arteries. It is used for chilblains and other similar defects of the circulation.

tolbutamide. A synthetic drug used instead of insulin in some of the milder types of diabetes. It seems to potentiate the patient's own insulin; if he has none, tolbutamide does not help him.

tolerance. Gradually increasing resistance to the effects of a drug given over long periods, typically seen with drugs of addiction such as morphine.

tomography. A technique of X-ray examination: the X-ray tube is moved during the exposure in such a way that only structures in a selected plane of the body cast clear shadows.

tongue. The tongue consists almost entirely of muscles, attached to the base of the skull below the ears, to the lower jaw, and to the hyoid bone above the larynx. These muscles are controlled with remarkable precision to adapt the shape and position of the tongue to the needs of eating or speech.

From their attachments it will be clear that the tongue is much larger than it appears to be – an important matter for an unconscious patient, whose tongue can easily obstruct his airway. But because of the attachment to the inside of the jaw the airway can be kept clear by drawing the chin forwards.

Quite apart from the special sense of ◊ *taste* the ordinary senses of touch and temperature are more acute on the surface of the tongue even than on the finger-tips.

Minute projections (*papillae*) from the surface give the tongue a velvety texture. Like all the other covering membranes of the body, that of the tongue is constantly shed and replaced. The debris, together with dried mucus and food particles, is more liable to accumulate on the tongue than on the perfectly smooth membranes of the rest of the mouth. Normally it is cleared by the saliva, but if the flow of saliva is deficient the tongue becomes coated or 'furred'. Fever, thirst, or merely loss of appetite reduce salivation, and a furred tongue is therefore a poor guide to the state of a person's health.

The tongue is seldom infected by microbes: competition from harmless bacteria in the mouth, the antiseptic action of saliva, and a very rich blood supply all contribute to this immunity. On the other hand the tongue is very sensitive to deficiency of iron or of various vitamins, of which a smooth, sore tongue may be an early symptom. The two commonest types of anaemia are due to lack of iron and lack of vitamin B_{12} so that a sore tongue often accompanies a naemia.

The tongue is susceptible to syphilis, but now that this disease is regularly treated with penicillin syphilis of the tongue is no longer common.

About 1 per cent of all cancers are found in the tongue. Syphilis used to be an important cause. Irritation from a rotten tooth has often been blamed, but there are many more rotten teeth than cancers of the tongue and the association need not be causal. Generally speaking the further forward the cancer the better the outlook. A cancer near the tip of the tongue is recognized early and is easily accessible for surgery or radiation. If treatment is sought at the first sign of trouble – pain, swelling, ulceration – the chance of cure is good.

tonsil. A mass of lymphoid tissue, in health about the shape and size of an almond (and called *almond* in many languages), at either side of the back of the mouth: the soft palate rises as an arch of which the supporting columns are split to embrace the tonsils. ◊ *pharynx*.

tonsillar. Of the tonsil.

tonsillectomy. Surgical removal of the tonsils.

tonsillitis. Inflammation of the tonsils, usually from infection by streptococci. ◊ *pharynx* (1).

tooth ◊ *teeth*.

tophus. A chalk-like deposit in the tissues, consistingly mainly of uric acid or its salts, characteristic of *gout*.

topical (of medication). Applied directly to the affected part, e.g. ointments, eye drops, injections into painful joints; as opposed to *systemic* medication, where the drug is given by mouth, by injection, by inhalation etc. so that it will enter the circulation to be distributed throughout the body.

torticollis. Wry-neck. ◊ *sternomastoid*.

torulosis (cryptococcosis). A rare but dangerous infection with a kind of yeast; similar to *blastomycosis*. Cases are occasionally reported from most parts of the world. The antibiotic amphotericin-B has much improved the outlook.

tourniquet. A constricting band placed tightly enough round a limb to stop the entry of blood in case of severe bleeding. Its use has been discouraged because a tourniquet left in place for more than half an hour is likely to destroy the limb. If possible it is better to control bleeding either by compressing the edges of the wound or by direct pressure over the artery. If a tourniquet is applied in desperation it must be as broad as possible – a scarf, not a piece of string. It must be no tighter than is needed to stop the bleeding – but if it is not tight enough it may increase bleeding from veins without checking the flow in the arteries; and it must *unconditionally* be completely released at intervals of not more than half an hour, preferably less, and only reapplied when the limb is seen to be flushed with blood. Since cut vessels usually seal themselves fairly quickly, it will often be found that the tourniquet is no longer needed, but in that case the wound has to be constantly watched for renewed bleeding.

toxaemia. Literally: blood-poisoning; illness due to *toxins* in the blood-stream, usually toxins formed by bacteria in some localized seat of infection. The fever and general illness with an abscess are due to this type of toxaemia. Some bacteria, e.g. those of diphtheria and typhoid, cause severe toxaemia while themselves confined to a relatively small area of tissue, and the symptoms of tetanus are due entirely to toxins, the bacteria themselves doing no apparent harm to the tissue where they establish themselves.

toxaemia of pregnancy. A mysterious and, it seems, exclusively human ailment affecting many women during pregnancy and disappearing as soon as the pregnancy is over. The term toxaemia implies more than is known, because although the symptoms suggest some such cause, no toxic substance has been identified. If there is indeed a toxin it is most likely to come from the placenta.

The symptoms are very like those of Bright's disease – accumulation of water in the tissues, first noticed as undue swelling of the ankles; loss of protein in the urine; and high blood pressure. Because of water retention the patient gains more weight than she would be expected to. At this stage the patient is carefully watched for any increase in the symptoms, or new symptoms, and kept quiet; most cases settle down and the pregnancy runs its normal course. Salt rather than water has to be restricted because the retention of water is an effect of failure to eliminate salt from the kidneys. The danger is that if the trouble progresses the patient may develop *eclampsia* at the end of pregnancy; this is a kind of epilepsy that can be fatal to the baby and sometimes to the mother too. If there is any threat of eclampsia, hospital treatment becomes mandatory: the pregnancy may have to be terminated at short notice, and intensive treatment may be needed to prevent fits.

toxic goitre (Basedow's disease; Graves'

disease) ◊ *thyroid* (2); *Basedow's disease*.

toxicology. Study of poisons, an extension of pharmacology.

toxin. A poisonous protein, such as many bacteria form. Bacterial toxins are roughly divided into *endotoxins*, incorporated in the bacteria and damaging tissues in the immediate vicinity of the infection, and *exotoxins*, which are released by the bacteria and pass into the blood-stream or elsewhere and produce harmful effects remote from the site of infection. Toxins act as *antigens*, i.e. antibodies are formed to neutralize them as a natural defence against disease (◊ *immunity*).

toxoid. A toxin extracted from bacteria and chemically modified so that it loses its poisonous effect but keeps its ability to evoke immunity. Diphtheria toxoid is injected to confer immunity to diphtheria.

toxoplasmosis. Infection with the protozoon *Toxoplasma gondi*; it seems to be common and in most cases almost harmless, but unsuspected toxoplasmosis is occasionally transmitted from a mother to an unborn child and seriously damages the nervous system.

trachea (windpipe). A straight vertical tube extending from the larynx to the level of the angle of the sternum, immediately above the heart, where the trachea divides into the two main *bronchi*, one to each lung. It is an elastic tube, held open by hoops of cartilage. A gap at the back of each hoop is bridged by muscle; only the uppermost cartilage, the *cricoid*, is a complete ring. The lining membrane of the trachea secretes mucus, which keeps it moist and traps inhaled dust. The mucus is constantly moved upwards by the undulation of the *cilia*, fine processes which give the lining a velvety pile.

The trachea lies immediately in front of the oesophagus. Behind the sternum, the innominate artery and vein cross in front of it. In the neck, the trachea lies under the skin except at the upper end where the thyroid gland intervenes.

Inflammation of the mucous membrane, *tracheitis*, often accompanies bronchitis, causing soreness in the mid-line.

The trachea itself is seldom blocked, but the larynx may be obstructed by injury, inflammation (e.g. diphtheria), or paralysis, or, in an unconscious patient, simply by the dead weight of the tongue against the back of the throat. Since the tongue is attached to the jaw, it can be drawn out of harm's way by pulling the jaw forwards – often a life-saving measure. During anaesthetics and with other types of unconsciousness an adequate airway can be ensured with a rubber tube passed between the vocal cords into the trachea.

Tracheostomy is an operation to by-pass the larynx. The trachea is opened and a metal tube is inserted. This operation is used when the larynx is blocked or liable to become blocked, as in diphtheria, and also when a patient is unable to cough because of severe coma or paralysis and the trachea must be cleared of mucus by mechanical suction.

tracheal. Of the trachea.

tracheitis. Inflammation of the ◊ *trachea.*

tracheostomy. Surgical operation, opening the ◊ *trachea* to relieve an obstruction and maintain a clear airway.

tracheotomy. 'Cutting the trachea': ◊ *tracheostomy,* 'making an opening (mouth) in the trachea', describes the operation better.

trachoma. Severe and prolonged inflammation of the membrane lining the eyelids and covering the front of the eye (conjunctivitis), due to a microbe resembling a virus but probably a degenerate bacterium (◊ *Bedsonia*). The microbe is closely related to that of the 'swimming-bath conjunctivitis' or pink-eye of temperate climates, but real trachoma is a disease of hot dry regions. It leads to scarring of the eyelids; the lashes may turn inwards and constantly irritate the eyes, or the patient may be unable to close his eyes properly, or a *pannus* – an opaque membrane of inflammatory tissue – may encroach on the cornea and obstruct vision. Although the infection tends to burn itself out, the victim is often partly or totally blind by the time it does so. The number of people blinded by trachoma runs into millions.

Unlike the true virus diseases, trachoma responds well to treatment with sulphonamides or antibiotics. Deformity of the eyelids in advanced cases may need surgical

correction. Blindness is of the type that can be treated by corneal grafting. The problem is not how to cure the disease but how to provide treatment for several hundred million patients in underdeveloped countries.

tranquillizer. A kind of drug, used to calm the emotions. Emotional agitation is a common symptom of ailments ranging from minor anxiety states to severe episodes of mania or schizophrenia. Until 1953 the only drugs that helped were *sedatives* such as bromides and barbiturates. A sedative was merely a small dose of a hypnotic drug generally used in larger doses to procure sleep. If the dose was large enough to relieve agitation it was also large enough to make the patient drowsy and inefficient. Agitated schizophrenics had to be almost anaesthetized before they were effectively calmed.

In 1953, *rauwolfia* was introduced to Western practice from traditional Indian medicine, and became the first of a new class of drugs, the tranquillizers or ataractic drugs. These induce a calmer mood without making the patient sleepy. Rauwolfia also lowers the blood pressure, and is now used more for this effect than as a tranquillizer.

Some of the antihistamine drugs used to control allergy were found to calm the patient's mood. This effect was investigated, with a view to finding a compound of which it would be the main effect, and in 1954 a *phenothiazine* compound, *chlorpromazine,* was introduced. With this or one of the many other phenothiazine drugs very severe mental disturbances can be controlled, and patients such as advanced schizophrenics, hitherto kept for years in mental hospitals, can lead ordinary lives.

Haloperidol is unrelated to the phenothiazine tranquillizers, but it has similar effects and is used in the same way. A further class of drugs, the minor tranquillizers, are used for controlling tension in less serious conditions such as anxiety states. Some of them probably relax physical, muscular tension as well as emotional tension. The first of them, *meprobamate,* introduced in 1955, is derived from mephenesin, a drug intended to be a muscle relaxant. Two more recent introductions, *chlordiazepoxide* and *diazepam,* are very widely used.

None of the tranquillizers appears to

cause addiction, and they have an added advantage over the older sedatives that accidental or deliberate overdoses are much less dangerous – an important consideration with mentally disturbed patients.

Tranquillizers have many special uses, including preparation for surgery, the control of vomiting (e.g. *travel sickness*), and overcoming some of the difficulty of breaking a drug habit.

transfusion. The transfer of blood from a healthy person to a sick one is an ancient and fairly obvious idea. It is in this sense that the word 'transfusion' is used here. A similar use of salt or sugar solutions is an 'infusion'.

Nobody would have known where to put the blood until Harvey's discovery of the circulation (1616) showed that it must be injected into a vein. The architect Wren suggested the injection of drugs into veins, and two other early Fellows of the Royal Society, John Wilkins and Richard Lower, carried out blood transfusion between dogs. A French physician, Jean-Baptiste Denys, successfully gave lamb's blood to a human patient in 1667, but soon after a second patient died, and no further attempt was made for 150 years.

Then James Blundell of Guy's Hospital, London, showed that blood could not be safely transfused from one species to another. He gave several of his patients human blood, the first in 1818, and transfusion became an accepted if unusual form of treatment.

Two problems remained. Firstly, the blood was apt to clot while it was being given. This can be prevented by adding a small amount of sodium citrate, which diverts calcium, an essential factor in clotting. Secondly, many of the patients had severe reactions, sometimes fatal. This was not overcome until Landsteiner discovered blood groups in 1900 (◊ *blood* (5)).

Some of the chemical components of the shell of a red blood cell differ slightly in different people. A particular factor and its two or three variants form a *system*. People whose red cells have the same variant belong to the same *blood group* as regards that system (though they may belong to different groups as regards other systems).

The most important blood-group system was the first to be discovered. There are three variants: A, B, and O. Everyone inherits a gene for one variant from each parent. O behaves as a blank, simply as absence of A or B. A man who inherits A from each parent, and one who inherits A from one and O from the other both belong to group A. Thus the 6 possible pairs (AA, AO, BB, BO, AB, OO) resolve themselves into 4 groups (A, B, AB, O).

A positive factor, A or B, that the blood does *not* contain is treated as a foreign substance which has to be neutralized. This is done by an *antibody*, a protein in the blood whose sole function is to react with that particular foreign substance. In the ordinary way, antibodies are formed only when a foreign substance has found its way into the body. They are a defence against infection by bacteria (◊ *immunity*). These blood group antibodies are unusual in that they are present at birth. All group A people have antibodies against B, group B against A, and group O against both. Group AB people have, of course, neither antibody – otherwise they would destroy their own blood cells.

If a patient is given blood against which he has antibodies he will destroy the transfused blood. Not only is the transfusion useless, but the destroyed red cells set up a severe reaction, occasionally leading to kidney failure and death. If the patient can be tided over, e.g. with an artificial kidney, the kidneys usually recover.

The dangerous reactions are between *patient's antibodies* and *transfused cells*. Transfused antibodies seldom do much damage to the patient's cells because they are rapidly diluted in the patient's body. Hence group AB people, having neither antibody, are universal recipients, and group O people, having cells against which neither antibody can act, are universal donors. But transfusions from other groups are not entirely safe, and in practice a donor of the same group is always sought.

In Britain the distribution of groups is O 46 per cent, A 42 per cent, B 9 per cent, AB 3 per cent. The figures are very different in some parts of the world.

Another system of blood groups (◊ *rhesus factor*) is important because incompatibility of rhesus groups between husband and wife may endanger their new-born children. This danger is much increased if a rhesus-negative mother has ever had a rhesus-positive transfusion.

Blood groups are determined by mixing the cells with serum known to contain antibodies against A and against B. If the cells stick together in clumps in both samples they must be group AB, because both antibodies react with them. If they clump only with the anti-A serum, they are group A. If both samples are unaffected, they are group O.

Blood can be stored for about 3 weeks at 4° C., the temperature of a kitchen refrigerator. It cannot be actually frozen without damaging the red cells.

One person in a hundred carries a virus in his blood which does him no harm but causes jaundice in susceptible people, and there is a small danger of transmitting this virus by blood transfusion. In the tropics there is the same risk with malaria. Syphilis was a worry in the early days of transfusion. It is much less common today; all blood banks test blood for syphilis before storing it; in any case this infection does not survive refrigeration.

In cases such as severe anaemia with heart failure, blood transfusion may overload the circulation. The risk is overcome by separating the blood cells and giving them without the plasma, the fluid portion of blood. On the other hand with severe ◊ shock, e.g. after extensive burns, plasma leaks out of the patient's blood vessels, leaving the cells with too little fluid. In this case, plasma without cells is transfused. Plasma can be stored for months as a dried powder.

transplantation. The transfer of a tissue or organ from one subject to another, as opposed to simple grafting of tissue from one part to another of the same person.

With the exception of the nervous system, where function depends on strict continuity between the centre and the periphery, almost any part of the body could be successfully grafted. The surgeon has only to ensure an adequate circulation of blood in the new site, and the technical problems of doing so can be overcome.

An organ can be grafted from one to another of identical twins with no more trouble than simple grafting. But a transplant from anyone other than an identical twin meets a hostile reaction from the recipient's tissues. This is due to the trivial chemical differences between different people. Any protein introduced to the

tissues that differs, however slightly, from its counterpart in the recipient's body is liable to be destroyed by *antibodies*. This is the ordinary mechanism for dealing with unwelcome invaders such as bacteria (◊ *immunity*). After a technically successful transplantation of, say, a kidney the recipient's blood flows freely through the vessels of the new organ; it is alive and begins to form urine. It may be threatened at once by the sort of destructive reaction that any foreign body in the tissues might provoke, but it is likely to survive this initial attack. The real danger comes some days or weeks later, when antibodies have been formed specifically to react with any of its proteins that are strange to the recipient. If the differences are extensive, the transplanted organ is likely to be rejected – it ceases to function and dies.

The easiest tissue to transplant is blood (◊ *transfusion*). There is the same possibility that transfused blood will be rejected, but the important points of difference between bloods have been identified, and a donor can be chosen whose blood is sufficiently like that of the patient to be accepted: the donor and recipient belong to the same group.

The chemical make-up of other tissues is more complex. Factors leading to rejection have not all been identified, and there are so many that an ideal donor may be hard to find. But it is already possible to choose donors from whom an organ stands at least a fair chance of surviving in the patient's tissues. Steps can then be taken to minimize the patient's reaction. These include giving corticosteroids and drugs that interfere with the formation of new antibodies. A class of white blood cells, the *lymphocytes*, are especially concerned with immunity and the rejection of foreign substances. When a transplanted organ seems likely to be rejected it may be saved by suppressing the lymphocytes, either by X-ray treatment or by drugs, or by removing the thymus gland and spleen where many of the lymphocytes are formed.

The price of suppressing the patient's reaction to the new organ is that his resistance to infection is also suppressed, and elaborate precautions are needed to prevent infection while the treatment lasts. A great deal of research is being directed to means of selective suppression that will leave the natural defence against bacteria and viruses intact.

Even when the problems of transplanting organs are solved, the problem of finding donors will remain. Kidneys have been successfully taken from living donors – one healthy kidney is enough – but the propriety of doing so is questionable. A blood donor replaces what he has given, but one cannot grow new organs. At present the usual source is a person who has just died suddenly. In time, it may become possible to store organs in a central bank, as blood is already stored. Another hope is that it may become possible to transplant organs from animals, and there has already been some success with livers taken from animals. There are already elaborate devices for use in hospitals that can take over the work of heart, lungs and kidneys, and modifications of these may after all prove to be more suitable than living transplants. It would be unrealistic at present to expect a machine to take on all the functions of the liver.

The cornea at the front of the eye is a special case. It has no circulation; lymphocytes and antibodies do not invade it, and a cornea from anyone who has given permission for his eyes to be used after his death can be grafted without any problems of immunity and rejection. These tissues can be preserved in banks and used to restore sight lost from damage to the front of the eye.

Some burns are so extensive that it is impossible to find enough intact skin on the patient to prepare ordinary skin-grafts. In such cases, skin can be transplanted from someone else although it will later be rejected: in the meantime it has provided a scaffolding where the patient's own new skin can grow. This compromise has to be accepted because any measures to prevent rejection would also suppress the process of healing, and also make serious infection of the raw areas a certainty.

transposition. Transposition of the great vessels is an uncommon fault in the development of the heart: the aorta arises from the right side of the heart instead of the left, and the pulmonary artery from the left instead of the right, and the circulation of blood is ineffective. The condition can now be corrected by an extremely elaborate operation.

Transposition of all the organs from left to right is interesting but unimportant (◇ dextrocardia).

trapezius. Large triangular muscle of the back; the two trapezii together are kite-shaped. The muscle rotates the shoulder-blade when the arm is raised (◇ shoulder). At rest the trapezius muscles are important in maintaining the ◇ posture of the shoulders.

trauma. A wound; damage to the tissues by any physical agency (burns, fractures etc.); emotional upset as a cause of mental illness.

travel sickness. The motion of ships, cars, aircraft, swings etc. disturbs the balance organ of the inner ear and sets up a chain of reflex action that may radiate to the vomiting centre in the *medulla oblongata*, the lowest part of the brain. The same reflex can be set off by artificial stimulation of the balance organ, e.g. by squirting cold water into the ear. The reflex appears to be a pure accident; one can hardly suppose that it was useful to some remote ancestor.

Travel sickness may become a conditioned reflex: a person who has learnt to expect it may be sick before the ship moves. But it cannot, as is sometimes suggested, be wholly psychological because it affects babies and animals. On the other hand the psychological or emotional element is not to be lightly dismissed. An attack can often be averted by occupying the patient's mind – in small boats a spell at the tiller can work wonders, or in larger boats a walk on deck, provided that the patient keeps warm – but if the attack has already begun the patient can seldom think of anything else.

In a ship or aircraft the see-saw motion is least at the point of balance, amidships. The view through a porthole is distressing, because the conflict of sensation between a deck that should be horizontal and a swinging horizon contributes greatly to the sickness. The ears are disturbed least with the head tilted back as in a dentist's chair. Aircraft seats can nearly always be adjusted to the right position, and car-sick passengers are more comfortable with head-rests.

Small but frequent snacks are better than no food. Alcohol is a traditional stand-by. It does nothing to help the physical factor of motion sickness but may allay the emotional factor. People who do not normally drink are better without it.

Of the many drugs that relieve travel sickness, *hyoscine* is the oldest and still among the most effective. Some of the antihistamine drugs and tranquillizers (the groups overlap) are also effective and cause less drowsiness than hyoscine; they include cyclizine, dimenhydrinate, and derivatives of phenothiazine. All these drugs are better at preventing than curing motion sickness: they work best when the first dose is taken an hour or so before the journey begins.

People who use car ferries may need to be reminded that any of the drugs can make them temporarily unfit to drive.

tremor. Trembling or shaking of a part of the body; a symptom of many disorders, trivial and serious. Occasionally the kind of tremor is a clue to the diagnosis, e.g. the rather slow shaking of parkinsonism (shaking palsy) or the fine quivering of the hands with an over-active thyroid gland; but often a tremor is no more than a hint that the case warrants further investigation.

trench fever. An epidemic disease among infantry in the First World War, probably a kind of typhus.

trench foot (immersion foot). A result of prolonged exposure to cold, especially to cold water. Water conducts heat away from the skin and aggravates the effects of a cold environment so that temperatures well above freezing become harmful. The natural response to cold is for blood vessels in the skin to contract, reducing the flow of blood and thus the loss of heat. If the reaction has to be sustained the skin suffers; it becomes waterlogged and numb and is then an easy prey to slight injury or infection.

trench mouth = ◊ *Vincent's disease.*

trepan; trephine. A trepan is a very ancient instrument for cutting a round hole in the skull; it is simply a cylindrical or crown saw. A trephine is a trepan with a central pin to guide the saw.

Prehistoric skulls have been found with signs of successful trepanning – when the margins of the hole are sealed with compact bone the patient must have survived the operation – and some primitive modern people still do the same operation to let evil spirits out of the head.

The ancient Greek surgeons used the operation as it is still used, to relieve pressure on the brain from bleeding after severe head injuries. Hippocrates gave detailed instructions in a treatise on wounds of the head, explaining how to avoid any risk of damaging the brain.

To avoid leaving a large hole in the skull, which would not heal, surgeons expose the brain by using a very small trephine at several points and joining the holes with a wire saw, so that a small trap-door can be raised.

Treponema. A kind of spirochaete or spiral bacterium. Species include *T. pallidum*, the cause of syphilis.

triceps. The muscle of the back of the arm: its three 'heads' (◊ *biceps*) arise (1) from the scapula just below the shoulder joint, and (2) and (3) from the back of the humerus. The whole mass is attached below to the olecranon process of the ulna, which juts out behind the elbow. Triceps extends (straightens) the elbow. ◊ *shoulder.*

trichiniasis (trichinosis). Illness due to a very small worm, *Trichinella*; this is a common parasite of pigs passed to man in undercooked pork. A week or two after infection, when the parasites breed, there is a feverish reaction, often with sore eyes and a variety of other symptoms that may represent a kind of allergy. The tiny larvae find their way into the circulation. Most of them, together with the parent worms, die and cause no further trouble, but some become embedded in muscles and may persist for months or even years, causing rather vague aches and pains. Trichiniasis is only rarely a serious disease. There is still no way of hastening recovery.

trichlorethylene. A volatile liquid, much used as a solvent and cleansing agent; medicinally, it is an effective anaesthetic especially suited to minor operations.

Trichomonas. An animal microbe (◊ *flagellate*) that commonly infects the mucous membrane of the vagina and causes irritation and discharge; since it can also infect the male urethra the patient's husband may also need treatment to prevent reinfection. Various antiseptic local applications may cure the condition , but the best drug seems to be *metronidazole*, which is taken by mouth.

trichophyton. Kind of fungus with an affinity for hair, causing some forms of ◊ *ringworm.*

trichotillomania. A bizarre neurosis: the patient pulls out tufts of her own hair.

Trichuris. An intestinal parasite, the whipworm. ◊ *worms.*

trigeminal. The *trigeminal nerve* (5th cranial nerve) emerges from the root of the brain and crosses the floor of the skull to a point close to the inner ear, where it bulges to form the *trigeminal ganglion,* a relay station for its sensory fibres. The 3 branches of the nerve spring separately from the ganglion. They are (1) the *ophthalmic nerve,* carrying sensation from the upper part of the face, (2) the *maxillary* nerve, carrying sensation from the middle of the face, and (3) the *mandibular* nerve, carrying sensation from the lower part of the face and also controlling the jaw muscles.
Trigeminal neuralgia (tic douloureux): ◊ *neuralgia.*

trinitrin. Glyceryl trinitrate, nitroglycerin; a standard remedy for angina pectoris.

trismus. Spasm of the jaw muscles, e.g. as a result of inflammation from an abscess around a tooth or a throat infection. Trismus can also arise from irritation of the nerve cells controlling the muscles – this is the symptom that gives *lockjaw* (tetanus) its name.

trochanter. One of two large knobs (greater and lesser trochanter) near the upper end of the femur, to which are attached various muscles acting on the hip.

tropical diseases. A few diseases can flourish only in a tropical climate, usually because they are carried by creatures confined to the tropics. For instance, the tsetse fly that carries sleeping sickness does not tolerate temperatures much below 25° C. (77° F.), and the snails that carry bilharzia have to live in fairly warm water. But most of the important tropical diseases are tropical mainly because the countries of the temperate zones have had the resources needed to eradicate them, while most tropical countries have not. In the past, malaria, leprosy, smallpox, plague and cholera have all been pestilences in Western Europe.
Preventive medicine cannot claim all the credit for confining these diseases to hotter and poorer countries. Nobody has the least idea why plague suddenly retreated in the 17th century, or why cholera waited until the 19th century before invading Europe. Epidemics are unpredictable. But there is not much doubt that vaccination controlled smallpox, and hygienic water supply and sewage disposal prevented intestinal infections from spreading.
Practically all tropical diseases are infectious, and most are curable, and can be eradicated by treating every case. For example, mosquitoes able to transmit malaria can be found in most of Europe, but they are harmless while there is no untreated malaria for them to transmit. Simultaneous treatment of the millions of people with malaria in the tropics would be impossible, and in practice malaria has to be tackled mainly by controlling mosquitoes. Large areas have been freed from malaria in recent years.
With the drugs now available for arresting leprosy it should be possible to reduce the number of active, infectious cases to a level where the disease can no longer flourish. But while leprosy recedes, a closely related disease – tuberculosis – advances, and tuberculosis is now well on the way to joining smallpox and the other diseases that have been more or less relegated to hot countries. Similarly yaws has been much reduced by effective drugs, while syphilis, which may well be a variant of the same disease, has increased.
Visitors to the main towns of tropical countries now run little risk of catching 'tropical' diseases, thanks to clean water, proper sewage disposal, control of insects and rodents, routine vaccination, and treatment of the sick. But in the poorer suburbs and in the vast rural areas these services are at best rudimentary. The greatest obstacle is lack of money: not only are most tropical countries poor, but the greater distances between settlements tend to make health services more costly than in industrial countries.
Most people in the tropics are underfed. Malnutrition is the greatest of all tropical diseases, and because of it people are less able to resist infection than they should be, and epidemics thrive.
Shortage of water is a common problem, making it difficult for people to keep themselves – let alone their environment – clean. At the other end of the scale, torrential rain

may wash away filth only to deposit it in the regular source of water. As often as not, villagers depend on a single stream for all their needs; they may even share it with their herds.

Polluted water can be made safe to drink simply by boiling it, but people will not always be persuaded to do so. The same obstacle, ignorance, stands in the way of all progress in preventive medicine. People readily accept curative medicine because it makes immediate sense – hospital beds do not stand vacant in the tropics – but the doctrines of hygiene make little impact, and may well conflict with cherished traditions. Health education is as necessary as clean water or insect control.

tropical ulcer. Chronic open sore, usually on the leg, common in the tropics. The ulcer begins with a minor injury and is infected with bacteria similar to those of ◊ *Vincent's disease*. Small, recent tropical ulcers heal if the infection is controlled with antiseptic dressings, but large ones often need skin-grafting.

truss. An appliance consisting of a pad and some means – a spring or an arrangement of straps – of holding it in place at a weak point in the abdominal muscles where internal organs are liable to protrude, i.e. to control a *hernia*. A truss is useful when there is some reason for not operating but as a rule hernias are best treated surgically.

trypanosome; trypanosomiasis. A trypanosome is a kind of *protozoon* or animal microbe, of which several species cause disease in men and animals. All types of trypanosomal infection (trypanosomiasis) are transmitted by insects confined to the tropics. Trypanosomes are related to the protozoa that cause leishmaniasis (kala-azar; oriental sore).

Sleeping sickness – African trypanosomiasis – is of two kinds. West African sleeping sickness is due to *Trypanosoma gambiense*, and is transmitted by the bite of a tsetse fly, *Glossina palpalis*. This fly breeds in damp forest near river-banks, and bites man for choice. Where the disease is endemic it may affect most of the population. After about a fortnight the site of the infection is marked by a firm lump, violet on a white skin but hardly visible on a dark skin; the patient is ill and feverish for some days;

lymph nodes swell, first in the area of the bite, later in all areas (armpits, neck, groins). A rash appears on a white skin but is seldom seen on African patients. In a week or two the patient seems to recover, and for many months or even years he suffers no more than an occasional bout of fever. Some patients probably overcome the infection, but in some the trypanosomes ultimately invade the nervous system. The drowsiness that gives the disease its name then follows. Often the patient sleeps little, but day and night he is dull and apathetic. He may starve for want of the energy to eat, or die of any passing infection. This disease is confined to the belt of rain forest along the West African coast and through the Congo basin to the Great Lakes.

East African sleeping sickness occurs in low-lying areas (below about 2000 ft) between Lake Victoria and Rhodesia. It is due to *T. rhodesiense*, and transmitted by several species of tsetse fly, notably *G. morsitans*. These flies breed in open country or sparse bush, generally away from human habitation; they bite antelopes and other wild animals for choice, and man only by chance. Infection is therefore sporadic. Even in the worst affected areas it is unusual for as many as 5 per cent of the population to be infected. The disease runs a much more rapid course than the West African type. Many patients die within a few months of infection. There is no 'sleeping' stage; in fact many patients are agitated.

Sleeping sickness is curable in the early stages before the nervous system is involved, but in the later stages the chance of cure diminishes rapidly, especially with the East African type. The drugs used include pentamidine, suramin, and various compounds of arsenic – these last offer the best hope in the late stages, but the doses required are themselves dangerous. Pentamidine has been used to protect people exposed to infection. The essential problem of treatment is that most of the patients are so used to fevers of one kind or another that they do not seek help until too late. The best chance of early diagnosis is to examine everyone in an infected area. Better still is to eradicate the tsetse flies.

Chagas' disease – South American trypanosomiasis – is due to *T. cruzi*, and is transmitted in the excreta of various bugs. After the initial fever, Chagas' disease often runs a fairly harmless course, but the trypanosomes may invade muscle and other tissues and cause them to be replaced by thin scars. If this happens to the heart, the disease is fatal. There are still no effective drugs.

Animal trypanosomiasis affects horses in South America and cattle and many other animals in Africa. One type, *nagana*, due to *T. congolense*, makes cattle farming impossible in much of tropical Africa. The relation of animal to human trypanosomiasis is not clear. Wild animals are often said to harbour *T. rhodesiense*, but opinions differ. These antelopes do not appear to develop any disease from their trypanosomes, but there is no reason why they should not act as a reservoir for the parasite. On the other hand nagana, which is deadly to cattle, does not seem to affect man. Attempts to control East African sleeping sickness by wholesale slaughter of wild animals have not succeeded.

tryparsamide. A compound of arsenic used against African trypanosomiasis.

trypsin. An enzyme from the pancreas for digesting protein.

tsetse fly. Blood-sucking insect of tropical Africa, like a small horse-fly, easily recognized by its fast, straight flight and abrupt landing, and the position of its wings at rest one over the other. Two species, *Glossina palpalis* in West Africa and *G. morsitans* in East Africa, transmit most cases of sleeping sickness, but at least a dozen other species are occasionally responsible.

TSH. Thyroid-stimulating hormone. ◊ *thyroid gland* (1).

tsutsugamushi fever. A kind of ◊ *typhus* transmitted by mites in parts of Asia.

tubal pregnancy. Pregnancy occurring in a Fallopian tube instead of the body of the uterus (◊ *ectopic*).

tubercle. 1. Small focus of inflammation and tissue destruction, the characteristic lesion of tuberculosis. **2.** Small natural promontory on a bone.
  Tubercle bacillus: the bacterium that causes tuberculosis.

tuberculin. A protein derived from tubercle bacilli, used in various diagnostic tests. A small amount is injected into the skin; a patch of inflammation indicates that the subject reacts to tuberculin and therefore has some immunity to tuberculosis, either from previous or current infection or because he has been artificially immunized.

tuberculosis. A common and dangerous infectious disease. A cautious estimate by WHO puts the number of new cases of tuberculosis in the world at 2–3 million and the deaths from tuberculosis at 1–2 million every year.

1. CAUSES

The immediate cause of tuberculosis is infection by the tubercle bacillus, *Mycobacterium tuberculosis*. There are five known variants of this bacterium: human, bovine, avian, murine, and piscine. The first two are common parasites of man.

Human bacilli are spread by coughing. Still air may remain contaminated for several hours. The bacilli are killed by sunlight, but in damp dark surroundings they may live in dust for weeks. The bacilli are inhaled, and the infection begins in the lungs.

Bovine bacilli infect cattle, and are passed to man in milk (or, rarely, through handling infected animals). The infection spreads from the intestine or, less often, the throat. It may be carried to any part of the body, most often to lymph nodes or bones.

Avian bacilli are adapted to the high body temperatures of birds and seldom trouble man, and piscine bacilli are adapted to the low temperatures of fish and are harmless to man. Murine bacilli (vole bacilli) do not cause human disease but confer immunity to the harmful variants; they can be used as a vaccine in the same way as the cowpox virus was used to protect against smallpox in the original method of vaccination.

There is no tuberculosis without tubercle bacilli, but most people who are infected never develop the disease. A generation ago, most people in industrial countries and nearly everyone in the cities had been infected in childhood or adolescence. The number has declined recently, but even in the fortunate countries where active tuberculosis is becoming a rare disease millions of people show clear evidence of having had a mild, possibly symptom-free attack. The predisposing causes that make the difference between a trivial unnoticed incident and protracted, often fatal illness are as important as the bacillus itself.

1. Although in theory a single bacillus could multiply and spread infection throughout the body, in practice many bacilli are more likely to take hold than a few, and repeated exposure is more dangerous than a single exposure. The main danger of *over-crowding*, *bad ventilation* and *lack of sunlight* lies in the number of infecting bacilli.

2. The *hereditary factor* has been over-estimated. Tuberculosis runs in families mainly because families live together and infect each other. Like all infections, tuberculosis is especially violent in populations to which it is new, as in some tropical countries; but many natives of the tropics are an easy prey because their resistance is lowered by malaria and malnutrition rather than because of their race.

3. Resistance changes with *age*. It is low at birth, but a baby is seldom infected unless its mother has active disease. After a few months resistance develops, but it falls off at puberty, especially among girls. 'Phthisis [pulmonary tuberculosis] most commonly occurs between the ages of 18 and 35 years' (Hippocrates, *Aphorisms*, 5th century B.C.). Old people are also susceptible, probably because their resistance is lowered by other illnesses.

4. *General health* at the time of infection is perhaps the most important factor of all. Tubercle bacilli thrive in the presence of malnutrition, or infection by other bacteria. Whooping cough is a notorious precursor of tuberculosis. In most people who have overcome an initial infection without apparent illness a few tubercle bacilli probably remain alive and may suddenly become active under the influence of illness, injury, or severe emotional strain – i.e. of *stress* in the widest sense.

2. EFFECTS

(i) *Pulmonary tuberculosis* (phthisis: consumption) is the commonest form of the disease. The *primary focus* is a small patch of inflammation in a lung, usually near the top. This forms a small abscess, with a central zone where tissue is destroyed surrounded by inflammation and healing. The lymph nodes at the root of the lung are also inflamed. In most cases the trouble goes no further. The focus dwindles to a small scar. The scar is revealed by X-rays, and a *tuberculin* skin test proves that the person

has developed a defensive (allergic) reaction to tubercle bacilli.

In a few cases, the primary focus spreads and causes a fever lasting some weeks, from which the patient generally recovers even without special treatment. The dangers with this type of tuberculosis are (1) rapid and fatal spread through both lungs (the 'galloping consumption' of 19th-century writers), (2) dissemination of bacilli throughout the body in the blood-stream (miliary tuberculosis), and (3) tuberculous meningitis.

The usual adult disease may not begin in earnest until months or years after the primary infection. It may be either a revival of the primary focus or a fresh infection. The defensive reaction – immunity or allergy to tubercle bacilli – acquired from the primary infection confines the disease to the lungs and prevents any rapid progression, but like an ill-disciplined army of liberation it does as much damage to the infected lung as the tubercle bacilli themselves. Pockets of infection enlarge and form cavities – chronic abscesses – in the lungs. Healing more or less keeps pace with the damage that is being done, but the balance is delicate. Any of the predisposing causes described above can tilt it in favour of the bacillus, or by dealing with the causes the disease can be arrested.

The symptoms may include fever, sweating at night, cough, blood-spitting, and loss of weight. None of these is peculiar to tuberculosis, and any may be absent from a particular case. Continued ill health is probably the most constant symptom, but some cases of active disease are discovered by chance during a routine X-ray examination. X-rays give the best evidence of the extent of the disease. The presence of active pulmonary tuberculosis is proved by finding tubercle bacilli in the sputum.

(ii) *Miliary tuberculosis* is spread of infection from the primary focus by transport of bacilli in the blood-stream. In some cases the patient is quickly overwhelmed. In others, the bacilli establish small colonies, and signs of tuberculosis appear simultaneously in various parts of the body with the formation of very numerous small abscesses (*milia* = millet-seeds). Or the disease may settle in one or two organs – bone, joint, kidney, nervous system, lymph nodes. In some cases, miliary tuberculosis settles with few if any symptoms.

(iii) The *lymph nodes* are to some extent

involved in all forms of tuberculosis. If the bacilli are swallowed and not inhaled (usually from milk infected with bovine tubercle bacilli) the disease may be confined to lymph nodes in the neck after infecting the throat, or to abdominal lymph nodes after infecting the intestine. Tuberculous glands in the neck used to be a common disease of childhood. The *scrofula* (king's evil) of earlier centuries was a spread of this infection to the overlying skin.

(iv) *Tuberculous meningitis* arises only as a complication of other forms of the disease. It was invariably fatal until the discovery of streptomycin in 1944.

(v) *Tuberculosis of bones and joints* is usually a very slow process, but since even in favourable cases the structures are gradually replaced by unstable fibrous tissue it always led to disability before the discovery of effective drugs: the least movement kept the infection alight and the best treatment was to immobilize affected joints. Tuberculosis of a vertebra (Pott's disease) leads to collapse of the bone, angulation of the spinal column, and injury to the spinal cord unless it is treated.

(vi) *Tuberculosis of the skin*, of which the commonest form is *lupus vulgaris*, a destructive inflammation of the skin of the nose and cheeks, is a reminder that the tubercle bacillus is closely related to the leprosy bacillus.

(vii) *Abdominal tuberculosis*, affecting intestine and lymph nodes (tabes mesenterica), and sometimes leading to a low-grade inflammation of the whole peritoneal lining of the abdomen, can arise either from drinking infected milk or from the patient's own infected sputum, some of which anyone with pulmonary tuberculosis must swallow. The disease is often surprisingly free of symptoms: the patient is vaguely unwell with some sort of digestive disorder, and loses weight, but the diagnosis is sometimes made almost by intuition, or by chance, when the infection is discovered during an abdominal operation. Any of the abdominal organs can be infected on occasion, particularly the kidneys, bladder, and reproductive organs.

3. TREATMENT

Until 1944 there was no means of attacking the tubercule bacillus, and treatment was directed at the contributory or predisposing causes. Since nobody knows how these causes act it is not possible to say why the older methods worked, or which were the effective ingredients, but with careful, sometimes prolonged nursing many patients recovered or at least improved who would certainly have died without treatment. The balance could be tilted against the disease and in favour of the patient. But many patients seemed to recover only to relapse later, and in some the disease could be slowed but not stopped. If the bacilli were already firmly established, as with tuberculous meningitis or any rapidly spreading infection, the case was hopeless from the start.

Rest is probably the most important of the older remedies. Sanatorium treatment relies greatly on physical rest, but the emotional rest of a calm, ordered environment could be as valuable, for in essence rest is absence of *stress*. In addition to resting the patient as a whole, a diseased lung can be rested by letting air into the pleural space around it, so that it deflates and only the good lung is expanded by each breath, or by surgical interference with the phrenic nerve on the diseased side so that that half of the diaphragm is temporarily or permanently out of action. These operations are akin to splinting a septic finger. They have the special merit of allowing the walls of an abscess cavity in the lung to cave in, stick together, and heal.

Anyone with tuberculosis needs a good mixed diet with enough protein and vitamins. The continous process of healing has to keep ahead of damage to tissue, and makes its own demands on the diet; and the raised body temperature means that food is consumed at more than the normal rate.

Fresh air is a traditional cornerstone of the treatment. Its greatest value may be to lessen the risk of infection to others. *Climate* has little if any direct influence, but a *change* of climate can make it much easier for the patient to relax.

Tuberculosis of lymph nodes in the neck, a single kidney, or a joint, often due to bovine (milk-borne) tubercle bacilli, was formerly known as 'surgical tuberculosis' because it could be cured, if the disease was inactive elsewhere, by removing the affected glands or kidney or by immobilizing the joint.

Excepting cases where the patient's natural resistance is clearly getting the upper hand, all types of tuberculosis are now treated with drugs acting directly against tubercle bacilli. The first to be used was streptomycin (1944). It was followed by para-aminosalicylic acid in 1946 and isoniazid in 1952. These three are still the standard remedies. Two or all three are given together because the bacilli quickly develop resistance to one alone. Other drugs are available for resistant cases, including pyrazinamide, ethionamide, cycloserine, and viomycin.

The effect of drug treatment has been remarkable. Even the severest types of infection can usually be arrested. In countries with effective medical services the remaining deaths from tuberculosis are mostly among older patients. For instance, in England and Wales in 1946, when streptomycin was still confined to a few experimental units and the other drugs were unknown, 900 girls aged 15–19 died of tuberculosis. In 1961, 9 died.

4. PREVENTION

Since many (in some places most) people are likely to be infected at some time, but only a minority will develop the illness, anything that increases people's resistance to the point where they can be infected without symptoms is in effect prevention. In English cities *infection* was still almost universal in 1910, but the *death rate* had been halved in 50 years. In the next 35 years it was halved again despite the setbacks of two World Wars. No single factor can explain the decrease (as vaccination explains the decrease of smallpox, or clean drinking water that of typhoid). Better diet, better housing, better working conditions, and better care of the sick must all have contributed. Recent campaigns against tuberculosis all over the world have shown that as long as people suffer from malnutrition nothing has much effect on the disease.

Infection of the lungs can be prevented only to a limited extent. But the greatest danger is from a sudden heavy infection, and this can be reduced by treating the source – the people with severe disease. In the past, hospital treatment automatically took these people out of the community and helped to reduce the danger. At present drug treatment renders nearly all patients non-infectious after a short time. An important element in any campaign is that as far as possible it should cover the whole community, which not only ensures that people who themselves need treatment will get it but protects those who are not yet infected.

For many years before the discovery of the new drugs, the number of new cases notified in Britain did not vary much. Probably a real decrease was cancelled by increased accuracy of diagnosis. The number of deaths had been falling steadily but slowly, and seemed to be levelling out at some 20,000 deaths annually. During the few years since the drugs have been in general use, this figure has fallen to 2000, and most of the deaths are of older people. At the same time, with fewer active cases to spread infection, the number of new cases has been halved.

Bovine tuberculosis can be eradicated by eliminating tuberculous cows from dairy herds, or by pasteurizing all milk. Pasteurization has practically eradicated bovine tuberculosis in much of Western Europe and the United States, and non-pulmonary tuberculosis has become fairly uncommon, occurring only as a complication of pulmonary disease.

Vaccination with a modified bacillus that evokes immunity without causing disease (BCG; bacille Calmette-Guérin) is now a part of all major campaigns. An alternative to BCG is the vole bacillus, which causes tuberculosis in rodents but not in man. Vaccination does not entirely prevent tuberculosis, but it greatly reduces the risk of a dangerous attack. A simple skin test (◊ *tuberculin*) shows which people have no immunity and need to be vaccinated.

tubocurarine. Active principle of ◊ *curare*.

tularaemia. An infectious disease related to *plague* but affecting rabbits insteads of rats. Human cases have occurred in the USA, Japan, and Russia, mostly from handling wild rabbits.

tulle gras. Netting impregnated with petroleum jelly and sterilized; a useful non-adhesive dressing for burns and wounds.

tumour. Any swelling, but especially a *neoplasm* (new growth), which is a collection of cells that have, as it were, seceded from the general community of cells that make up the various tissues and organs of the body, no longer serve any purpose useful to the rest of the body, and grow at the expense of their healthy neighbours.

A *benign* tumour is simply a growing mass of useless but essentially harmless tissue. It keeps within its own bounds, and becomes a nuisance only if it is unsightly or if it obstructs or otherwise interferes with neighbouring tissue. It is cured by removal. A common example is the ◊ *fibroid*.

A malignant tumour is the same thing as a ◊ *cancer*.

twins. *Fraternal* (dizygotic, binovular) twins develop when two ova are fertilized at the same time. As a rule a woman's ovaries release only a single ovum each month, but if two or more happen to be released together they can be fertilized together. A tendency to shed more than one ovum can be inherited, so that fraternal twins occur more often in some families than others. If pituitary hormones or the synthetic drug clomiphene are used to stimulate the ovaries in case of infertility several ova may be released.

Identical (monozygotic, monovular) twins develop from the two halves of a single ovum, formed as the first step in the growth of an embryo.

About one pregnancy in 90 produces twins; and according to Hellin's law one in 90^2 produces triplets and one in 90^3 quadruplets.

tympanic. Of the (ear-)drum.

tympanites. Flatulent distension of the abdomen.

typhoid. Prostrated and mentally numbed by fever. The *typhoid state* differs from *delirium* in the absence of excitement.

Typhoid fever is an infectious disease due to *Salmonella typhi* (typhoid bacillus), a bacterium of the same genus as those of paratyphoid fever and various types of food poisoning. Unlike the salmonellae of food poisoning, *S. typhi* seems to be exclusively a parasite of man, and the infection is always acquired from someone else. The usual source is drinking water or food that has been contaminated from someone either suffering from typhoid or harbouring the bacteria without symptoms (i.e. a carrier). In countries with poor sanitation, flies may carry the bacteria from excrement to food or water.

After infection the bacteria invade the wall of the small intestine and multiply in collections of lymphoid tissue (Peyer's patches) there, at this stage causing no symptoms. After 1–2 weeks they invade the blood-stream and cause fever, often with severe but ill-defined illness. Many patients develop a rash of pink spots about a week later when the fever is at its height. Without the help of a laboratory, typhoid can be indistinguishable from other severe fevers. Since the bacteria circulate in the blood they may settle anywhere and cause symptoms of inflammation in any organ. They have a particular affinity for the spleen and bones. Other species of salmonella regularly cause diarrhoea and vomiting, but neither is typical of typhoid; constipation is seen twice as often as diarrhoea. But the greatest danger is from the intestine, where the infection may erode a blood vessel and cause profuse bleeding, or perforate the wall and cause leakage into the abdominal cavity and peritonitis. Without treatment, at least 10 per cent of patients die. The others recover gradually. They may not completely overcome the infection, and second attacks are not uncommon; or they may remain symptomless carriers of the bacteria. Some people become carriers without going through any obvious illness.

The diagnosis is confirmed by finding the bacteria in the blood in the early stages or in the stools or urine later – these are the source of infection to other people. From about the second week of the attack, *antibodies* against typhoid can be demonstrated in the blood.

Nearly all cases respond well to treatment with chloramphenicol or some other antibiotic.

Typhoid can be prevented in the community by proper sewage disposal, controlled water supply, and clean food-handling. The system breaks down when an unsuspected carrier handles food or drinking water.

The individual can be protected by vaccination, usually with a combined vaccine (TAB) against typhoid and paratyphoid.

typhus. A group of infectious diseases caused by very small bacteria of the genus *Rickettsia*. Typhus was first distinguished from typhoid fever by an American physician, W. W. Gerhard, in 1837. There is still confusion with the names: in German, typhoid is *Typhus*, and typhus is *Flecken-*

typhus or *Fleckenfieber* (spotted fever). And in English spotted fever can mean either typhus or epidemic meningitis.

Louse-borne typhus affects only man. It is transmitted by body-lice, and outbreaks can occur whenever people are dirty and crowded together. It is rare in times of peace and plenty, but devastating epidemics can occur during wars or famines or after natural disasters, anywhere in the world.

The related diseases include *Rocky Mountain spotted fever* and several kinds of *tick fever*, transmitted from rodents to man by tick-bites; *murine typhus*, transmitted from rats by fleas; and *tsutsugamushi fever* (scrub typhus), transmitted from rodents by mites. These cause sporadic cases in infected regions (generally hot countries), but not major epidemics.

All forms of typhus cause a prostrating fever within a fortnight of infection, lasting one or two weeks. Skin rashes are common: red spots followed in some types of disease by pin-point bleeding into the skin. Many patients develop a kind of pneumonia. Some of these diseases are not very dangerous, but with untreated louse-borne typhus and Rocky Mountain spotted fever as many as 20 per cent of the patients die.

Fortunately all these infections respond well to good nursing and treatment with antibiotics.

tyramine. A substance found in cheese and some other foods. It imitates the effects of adrenaline in the body, perhaps by increasing the natural secretion of adrenaline in the nervous system. This may explain why cheese disturbs sleep in some people.

A class of drugs (monoamine oxidase inhibitors) given for ◊ *depression* increases the available adrenaline. The effect of tyramine added to that of these drugs sometimes causes a dangerous excess of adrenaline activity, with a sharp rise of blood pressure. Cheese is therefore forbidden to patients taking the drugs.

U

ulcer. A persistent breach in a body surface (skin or mucous membrane) that fails to heal because of defective circulation (e.g. ulcer of the leg with varicose veins), continued injury (e.g. an ulcer on the tongue beside a jagged tooth) or irritation (e.g. duodenal ulcer from an excess of acid), tumour formation (e.g. rodent ulcer), or infection – which can be the primary cause or can be added as a complication of any other. The primary cause of some ulcers, e.g. those of the intestine with ulcerative colitis, is unknown.

For gastric and duodenal ulcers ◊ *peptic ulcer*.

ulcerative colitis ◊ *colitis*.

ulna. The inner of the two bones of the forearm. Its upper end is the point of the elbow, and it can be felt under the skin throughout its length to the little-finger side of the wrist. Since the ulna and radius work in all ways as a unit they are discussed together under ◊ *radius*.

ulnar. Of the ◊ *ulna*.
Ulnar artery. In front of the elbow the brachial artery divides into two branches, *radial* and *ulnar*, which run parallel courses to the hand, roughly following the lines of the two bones of the forearm (radius and ulna). Of the two, the ulnar is more concerned with the blood supply of the forearm and the radial with the hand.
Ulnar nerve. One of the two nerves of the front of the forearm and hand; the other being the *median* nerve. The ulnar nerve enters the forearm by passing behind the elbow, where it is exposed to injury. Even a slight jar to the bone ('funny bone') at this point is very painful.

ultrasonic waves (ultrasound). Vibrations of the same kind as sound waves, but too rapid to be heard (above 20,000 cycles per second). Ultrasound has a limited use in diagnosis, for examining internal structures by the principle of radar (◊ *echo-encephalography*). In the treatment of disease, an ultrasonic beam can be focused at a given depth below the surface of the skin, where the energy of the vibrations is dissipated as heat; the method is used for relieving pain in joints and muscles. A more intense beam can be used to destroy very small segments of tissue. For instance, in disease of the inner ear with disturbance of balance (vertigo) ultrasonic waves have been successfully used to put the balance organ out of action without disturbing the adjacent organ of hearing.

ultraviolet radiation. Waves of the same kind as light, but with a higher frequency than the visible spectrum (but a lower frequency than X-rays).

Ultraviolet radiation in sunlight converts inactive steroids in the skin to vitamin D, but unless there is a deficiency of this vitamin (rickets) it does nothing to promote health. Artificial ultraviolet radiation is used for treating skin diseases (*acne; psoriasis*). It increases the rate at which the outer layer of the skin is shed and replaced.

An excess of ultraviolet is harmful; it can provoke severe inflammation and, in time, even tumours of the skin. Protective lotions can be had to filter off the radiation.

Bacteria are quickly destroyed by ultraviolet radiation.

umbilical cord. A bundle of two arteries and a vein and some vestigial structures, surrounded by a clear gelatinous material and a thin membrane, connecting an unborn infant with its placenta. The cord is normally sealed with a ligature and cut soon after birth, and the remaining stump withers and falls off.

umbilicus (navel). The scar in the centre of the abdomen where the umbilical cord entered.

A weakness in the muscles at this point may allow a bulge (umbilical hernia) to appear. ◊ *hernia*.

Infection of the umbilicus at birth is unusual with proper midwifery, but is common with primitive methods. In parts of West Africa many babies die of tetanus contracted in this way.

unconscious. The unconscious (subconscious) mind is a fundamental concept in Freud's psychology and, in one form or another, in most other schools. The mind is said to work at different levels. The conscious mind, i.e. the mind in the ordinary sense, examines events in the light of reason and experience. The unconscious mind is a great store of events that are forgotten as far as the conscious mind is concerned, and perhaps of events or impressions that have never reached consciousness. But it is not a passive store; it is continuously active, and its activity modifies the conscious mind, and it affects the functions of the body in similar ways to conscious thoughts and emotions. At times it may be in direct conflict with the conscious, reasoning mind. Such conflict is thought to be a major source of disturbed behaviour and physical health.

◊ *anxiety*; *psychoanalysis*; *psychosomatic disease*.

unconsciousness ◊ *coma*.

undine. A vessel like a small retort, for rinsing the front of the eye.

undulant fever. An infectious disease due to the bacterium *Brucella abortus*; this is primarily a parasite of cattle, in which it causes *contagious abortion*. Human disease is contracted either from handling infected cattle or from milk. Where milk is pasteurized, the disease is rare.

Two other species of *Brucella* are occasionally transmitted from animals to man: *Br. melitensis* from goats (Malta fever) and *Br. suis* from pigs.

Often the disease is so mild as to pass unnoticed unless a bacteriological examination for some other purpose shows that the patient has been infected with *Brucella*. In an average case an intermittent fever lasts 2 or 3 weeks and then clears completely. The disease gets its name from a tendency for episodes of fever to recur, sometimes over several months. There are no characteristic signs, and the diagnosis is impossible without the help of a bacteriological laboratory.

Although it can be a great nuisance, undulant fever is seldom dangerous. Most cases respond to treatment with antibiotics.

The commonest complication is chronic inflammation of a bone. Human infection does not cause habitual abortion.

unsaturated fat. A fat of which the component fatty acids are chemically unsaturated, i.e. able to take on additional hydrogen atoms. A certain amount of unsaturated fat seems to be necessary to health, especially to prevent disease of the arteries (◊ *atheroma*). Meat and milk products are deficient, while vegetable and fish oils contain plenty. It further seems that the proportion of unsaturated to saturated fat is more important than the quantity. A large amount of fat, such as most affluent diets contain, is tolerated provided that it includes enough unsaturated fat. The evidence is not conclusive, but it is fairly strong.

uraemia. Excess of urea in the blood, from defective function of the kidneys. Urea is not itself poisonous, but an excess of it implies an excess of other waste products that are poisonous. ◊ *kidneys* (3).

urea. Carbamide; $CO(NH_2)_2$, an end-product of the chemical breakdown of protein in the body, excreted in the urine at a rate of 20–30 grammes daily.

ureter. Tube leading from kidney to bladder. ◊ *kidneys* (1).

urethra. Tube carrying urine away from the bladder. The female urethra is short, passing below the pubis to open in front of the vagina. The male urethra passes downwards through the prostate gland before turning forwards to run the length of the penis. Because of the long urethra the male bladder is better protected against infection (*cystitis*) than the female.

urethritis. Inflammation of the urethra, commonly caused by *gonorrhoea*. But many other kinds of infection, not necessarily venereal, can also cause urethritis. They usually respond quickly to treatment with antibiotics. ◊ *Reiter's disease*.

uric acid. An end-product of the digestion of nucleic acids, excreted in the urine at a rate of about 0·6 grammes daily. People with ◊ *gout* either have an abnormality of body chemistry that causes them to form more uric acid than can be easily disposed of by the kidneys, or one that prevents them from getting rid of uric acid at the normal rate.

urine. A watery fluid formed by the kidneys as described under ◊ *kidneys* (2).

Normal urine is a solution in water of

numerous waste products of body chemistry, and of necessary substances (including water itself) of which there is at the time an excess. The principal waste products are from the digestion of protein and other nitrogen compounds. They are urea, uric acid, and creatinine. (The only waste product of fat and carbohydrate is carbon dioxide, which is excreted by the lungs.) In addition there is a variable amount of sodium chloride and other salts. If the body is short of salt, e.g. after profuse sweating, there may be none at all in the urine, but if there is an excess the amount in the urine can be increased to 2 per cent. By selective excretion of acid or alkaline salts the slight alkalinity of the blood is kept constant. The urine is usually, but not always, slightly acid. The yellow colour of urine is due to a substance *urochrome* of which neither the source nor the composition is known.

Abnormalities of the urine are often valuable clues in diagnosis. Even a very simple examination can give much information.

The *colour* can be affected by bile pigments, which do not normally appear in the urine but may do so with some disorders of the liver ($\diamond$ *jaundice*); or by blood with disorders of the kidneys or bladder. A few coloured substances in foods or medicines find their way into the urine.

Normal urine has only a faint *smell*. The unpleasant ammoniacal smell of stale urine is due to the action of air and bacteria. If there is infection in the bladder (cystitis), the urine may have an offensive smell.

The *concentration*, estimated by measuring the specific gravity, does not usually signify much in a single specimen, but inability to vary the concentration at different times is a sign of defective kidneys.

Normal urine contains no *protein*. The presence of albumin, of which a crude test is to curdle it by boiling, does not indicate any particular diagnosis, but does show that there is something to be investigated further.

Most simple tests for *sugar* (glucose) depend on the change of colour when a blue copper salt is reduced by glucose to red-brown copper. The chance finding of a small amount of glucose in the urine does not prove that anything is wrong, but the likeliest reason for it is diabetes, and many cases needing treatment are first recognized in this way.

urticaria (nettle-rash (*urtica* = stinging-nettle); **hives).** One of the commonest manifestations of $\diamond$ *allergy*.

Nettles release *histamine* and other poisons that cause the capillary blood vessels to leak fluid (but not blood cells) into the tissues, and also evoke sensations such as itching or burning. An allergic reaction against a substance to which the patient is sensitive (usually a food) causes similar poisons to be formed in certain tissues, and as a result itchy blotches appear on the skin. Typically they are fleeting, and disappear from one part of the skin only to reappear in another.

Urticaria usually responds to antihistamine drugs. In severe cases, adrenaline or corticosteroids may be needed. If the irritant can be identified and avoided, so much the better; but this is not always easy.

uterus (womb). A hollow muscle about the size of a duck's egg, lying in the pelvis immediately behind the bladder. The narrow lower end is the *cervix* (neck), which opens into the vagina. The upper part or *body* of the uterus opens at each side into a *Fallopian tube*, like an outspread arm above the ovary.

The uterus is slung from various ligaments, none of them efficient. Its real support is the muscular floor of the pelvis.

The lining of the uterus (*endometrium*) is shed each month during the thirty-odd years of fertility, and replaced by a new endometrium, which rapidly grows thick enough to provide a bed for the fertilized ovum if pregnancy occurs ($\diamond$ *menstruation; pregnancy*). During pregnancy, menstruation stops and the endometrium remains intact.

The muscle fibres that form the bulk of the uterus have a remarkable ability to adapt themselves. During pregnancy their weight increases from about 30 grammes (1 oz.) to 1 kg. (2 lb.), and their automatic contractions during labour exert a force of some 10 kg. (which a strong woman may double by voluntary contraction of her abdominal muscles). After pregnancy the uterus reverts to little more than its original size in a few weeks.

The embryonic uterus grows in two halves, each with its own Fallopian tube and ovary. In some mammals the later fusion of the two halves is incomplete, so that the cavity of the uterus is Y-shaped (bicornuate); and occasionally a human uterus develops in this way. This particular anomaly does not matter, but some others may interfere with conception or pregnancy and need surgical correction. The most difficult cases are those where the uterus is simply underdeveloped. Hormone treatment may encourage it to grow to a normal size, but the patient's chances of bearing children are not good.

Two common disorders peculiar to the uterus are ◊ *prolapse*, from weakening of its muscular support after childbearing, and ◊ *fibroids*, a sort of benign tumour.

The uterus is one of the commonest sites of cancer in women. This type of cancer is among the few that can usually be prevented. Most uterine cancer starts in the cervix, and for a long time (probably 10 years) before anything dangerous happens, characteristic changes can be detected in the lining of the cervix if a few cells are scraped off and examined microscopically. The operation takes only seconds and is pain-

less. If these changes – *carcinoma-in-situ* – are found, the affected part of the cervix can be removed and no cancer develops. The woman can still bear children.

Since the uterus has no function but childbearing, its removal for certain disorders does not affect general health.

uveitis. Inflammation of the *uveal tract*, a layer of tissues in the eye comprising the *iris* and its supporting structures and the *choroid* membrane behind the retina. ◊ *eye* (3).

uvula. The small projection of the soft palate in the mid-line. An irritating cough at night is sometimes attributed to a long uvula that tickles the back of the throat, and is treated by removing the uvula. This sort of cough is more likely to be due to a trickle of infected mucus from the back of the nose.

V

vaccination. The original meaning was infection with vaccinia (cow-pox) to confer immunity to smallpox, introduced in 1796 by Jenner (◊ *immunity*). About a century later Pasteur suggested that as a tribute to Jenner the term should be applied to the principle of using modified germs to confer immunity to more dangerous ones. Vaccination is now synonymous with ◊ *immunization*.

vaccine. A virus or bacterium so modified (e.g. by culture in an unnatural environment or treatment with formaldehyde) as to be no longer dangerous, yet able to confer immunity in the same way as infection with the actual disease.

vaccinia. 1. Cow-pox: a contagious disease of cattle that can cause a mild infection in man. The virus is so like that of smallpox that an attack of one confers immunity to the other.
2. An attenuated form of smallpox, produced by infecting calves with the virus, which then undergoes some modification that makes it comparatively harmless; now used in preference to natural cow-pox for vaccination. A few people have an attack of vaccinia after vaccination. It is usually like mild chickenpox – but it is dangerous to people with eczema.

vagina. Passage from the uterus to the vulva, behind and below the bladder: it is a tube surrounded by muscles, normally flattened to form a transverse cleft at right angles to the vertical cleft of the vulva. It is adaptable, allowing free passage to the baby during childbirth (the obstacles are at the entrance and exit of the vagina).
The lining membrane is controlled by *oestrogens* (sex hormones). In women after the menopause the lining may become thin and fragile, and in girls before puberty it is vulnerable to bacterial infection. In either case medication with oestrogens strengthens it.
Bleeding from the vagina other than normal menstruation always requires investigation. During pregnancy it may be the first indication of a threatened or inevitable miscarriage. At the end of pregnancy, it is likely to be a sign of ◊ *placenta praevia*. Bleeding after confinement may be due to a fragment of placenta that has remained in the uterus, or to an injury of the cervix. All these conditions need treatment to prevent further and possibly serious bleeding. Bleeding between menstrual periods, or after the menopause when the periods have stopped, has many possible causes, some trivial and some, such as cancer, very serious. This is a symptom that calls for expert advice as soon as possible.

vaginismus. Spasm of the muscles around the vagina, making coitus difficult or impossible (◊ *dyspareunia*).

vaginitis. Inflammation of the vagina. During the years of fertility the sex hormones seem to protect the vagina from most of the common bacteria, and the likely causes are *Trichomonas*, and *Candida*. Girls and older women are more liable to bacterial infection.

vagus nerve. Tenth cranial nerve; the most important component of the ◊ *parasympathetic* nervous system.
The nerve arises from the brain-stem, passes through the base of the skull, and accompanies the internal jugular vein down the neck. In the thorax the vagus nerves run down the sides of the oesophagus. In the abdomen their branches are distributed to the main digestive organs. On its way the vagus gives branches to the heart and lungs.
The *sensory* fibres convey (unconscious) sensations of *stretch* from the lungs, of *pressure* from the heart and aorta: these initiate appropriate reflexes to modify breathing and circulation. The *motor* fibres constrict the bronchi and slow the heart, and stimulate the digestive organs (◊ *respiration*; *heart*; *digestion*).
In addition the vagus conveys ordinary nerve fibres, unconnected with the parasympathetic system, controlling speech and swallowing.
Numerous drugs modify the activity of the vagus (◊ *parasympathetic*). *Vagotomy* is the operation of cutting the nerves for the relief of ◊ *peptic ulcer*.

valgus; varus. In Latin, *valgus* is bow-legged and *varus* is knock-kneed; but in current usage the meanings have changed places. The words are now used to describe several kinds of congenital deformity of the limbs. *Valgus* has the general meaning of outward angulation and *varus* of inward angulation: thus *coxa valga*, splayed hip; *genu valgum*, knock-knee, with the lower leg splayed outwards; *talipes valgus*, club-foot with the sole turned out in an exaggeration of flat-foot; and corresponding *varus* deformities in the opposite direction.

Valsalva, Antonio Maria (1666–1723). Professor of anatomy at Bologna; the teacher of Morgagni and a pupil of Malpighi. He was among the first to recognize the importance of studying the appearance of diseased organs after death, and many of his observations are recorded in Morgagni's great text-book on the sites and causes of disease.

Valsalva's experiment: inflation of the Eustachian tubes by holding the nose and trying to blow down it.

Valsalva manoeuvre: if the pressure in the chest is raised by blowing hard against resistance or by a static muscular effort such as straining at stool, blood is prevented from returning to the heart; the output of the heart is thus reduced and the subject may faint.

valve. Several body-tubes are provided with valves which restrict flow to one direction. The important ones are the valves of the heart and of the veins.

A valve consists of two or three *cusps* or flaps attached to the vessel wall like pockets. The flow of blood in the right direction presses the cusps flat against the wall. Reflux opens the pockets, brings their edges together, and blocks the vessel. The valves between the atria and ventricles of the ◊ *heart* (right: *tricuspid*; left: *mitral*) are prevented from turning inside out like an umbrella in a storm by strong threads attached to muscles which contract with the ventricles.

Disorders of the heart valves are described under ◊ *heart* (5). Failure of the valves in the veins causes ◊ *varicose veins*.

valvular disease ◊ *heart* (5).

varicella = ◊ *chickenpox*.

varicocoele. Varicose swelling of the veins from a testis, usually the left side, perhaps because the left spermatic vein joins the renal vein at an awkward angle so that the circulation of blood is less efficient than on the right. Most varicocoeles are of no significance. A few ache, especially if the patient's attention has been drawn to them; removal of the redundant veins is then a simple and harmless operation.

varicose veins. Abnormal swelling of veins, usually in the legs. Blood is returned from the legs in two groups of veins. The *deep* veins accompany the arteries. They are surrounded by muscles, which support them and squeeze the blood along them. The ◊ *saphenous veins* lie directly under the skin, and at intervals communicate with the deep veins. A system of one-way ◊ *valves* ensures that the flow is *upwards* in the principal veins and *inwards* in the communicating branches. If these valves are defective, the blood stagnates, the pressure in the saphenous veins rises, and the veins become swollen and tortuous. Aching and fatigue are the commonest early symptoms. Because of back-pressure on the ◊ *capillary* blood vessels fluid collects in the feet and causes them to swell. The skin above the ankles may become thin and discoloured and even break down to form a varicose ulcer.

The weakness of the valves which leads to varicose veins is sometimes hereditary, but the most important direct cause is prolonged standing – not walking, but standing still. Policemen and housewives are especially vulnerable. Obesity is a contributory cause; pregnancy has the same effect with the addition of pressure on the veins in the pelvis. Obstruction of the deep veins (e.g. with ◊ *phlebitis*) causes overloading of the saphenous veins.

Supporting bandages or elastic stockings relieve the swelling and discomfort, but to cure varicose veins surgery is needed. Either the vein is sealed off with ligatures or, more drastically, it is actually removed. Small varicosities can be treated with injections of irritant fluids which cause their walls to stick together. A first operation may be disappointing because other veins, previously unsuspected, may swell when the principal vein has been closed.

variola = ◊ *smallpox*. *Variola minor* = alatrim, a mild variant of smallpox.

variolation. Deliberate infection from a mild case of smallpox to confer immunity, superseded by ◊ *vaccination.* ◊◊ *immunity* (1).

Varolio, Constanzo ◊ *pons.*

varus ◊ *valgus.*

vascular. Of vessels, especially blood vessels.

vas deferens. The duct of the testis; it carries spermatozoa by a tortuous route up the neck of the scrotum, obliquely across the groin, through a gap in the abdominal muscles, behind the bladder and through the prostate gland to the urethra. In the groin the vas deferens lies directly under the skin, where it is easily accessible to the surgeon, and male sterilization by sealing it with a ligature is a very simple operation.

vasectomy. The operation of closing the vas deferens. ◊◊ *sterilization.*

vasoconstriction; vasodilatation. Reflex narrowing or widening of blood vessels; the principal means of regulating blood pressure. Selective constriction or dilatation of vessels in the skin adjusts the body temperature.

vasomotor nerves. ◊ *Sympathetic* nerve fibres regulating the calibre of blood vessels. They are controlled by nerve cells in the *vasomotor* centre in the brain-stem.

vasopressin. The *anti-diuretic hormone* (ADH) of the ◊ *pituitary.*

vector. Animal – often an insect – transmitting infection from person to person or from infected animals to human beings. Mosquitoes are vectors of malaria and yellow fever, lice of typhus, and tsetse flies of sleeping sickness.

vegetarian diet. Man has evolved as an omnivorous animal; his 'natural' diet contains both animal and vegetable foods. A good mixture provides all the necessities that cannot be synthesized in the human body (vitamins; essential amino-acids). All these things can be found in vegetable foods, but to avoid deficiency of one or other the diet must be as varied as possible.

vein (Lat. *vena*). Vessel by which blood returns from the periphery to the heart.

The high pressure of the blood in the arteries is expended by the time the blood has passed through the capillaries to reach the veins, and the average pressure in the veins is very close to atmospheric pressure, i.e. effectively nil. The veins accordingly have much thinner walls than arteries, but their diameter is much greater to accommodate the more leisurely flow. Veins are both wider and more numerous than arteries, but their structure is similar. Their thin walls contain a few muscle fibres, activated by sympathetic fibres, which enable them to contract in response to diminished return of blood and so ensure that the flow is maintained.

The column of blood in a vein is broken into short segments by valves which prevent any back-flow. Each consists of two opposed flaps like a pair of sluice gates. The continuous, imperceptible activity of muscles all over the body gently squeezes the veins and keeps the blood moving from valve to valve. If part of the body has been perfectly still for a time the blood tends to stagnate, but movement such as stretching or shifting the weight from heels to toes restores the flow.

An artery is usually accompanied by two veins, its *venae comitantes.* Strangely, the very largest of the arteries are accompanied by single veins (jugular, subclavian, iliac, venae cavae). In the limbs, the principal veins are supplemented by large subcutaneous veins.

1. DISORDERS

An injured vein bleeds much more slowly than an artery of the same size, but it is less muscular and cannot retract so well. On the other hand, the lightest pressure is enough to stop the bleeding while the blood clots. The *average* pressure in the veins is atmospheric, but gravity creates a positive pressure in veins below the heart and a negative pressure – suction – in veins above the heart. If the injured part is raised to the level of the heart there is no pressure in the veins, which stop bleeding. Above the heart the air pressure outside the vein is greater than the blood pressure within: the veins on the back of the hand collapse when the arm is raised. If a vein in this position is cut it usually closes, but with a hole in a large vein (jugular) air may be sucked in. This is more dangerous than bleeding for a large air-lock can stop the circulation in some vital organ. Serious cases are rare. Small quantities of air must often get into veins without harm; the fatal injection of air with a hypodermic syringe of popular fiction is mythical.

The commonest disorder of veins is failure of the valves in the veins of the leg; the resulting back-pressure stretches the vessels and causes ◊ *varicose veins*. Varicose veins in the rectum are ◊ *haemorrhoids*.

Inflammation of a vein (◊ *phlebitis*) is important because it is associated with obstruction by clotted blood (◊ *thrombosis*). Obstruction of a small vein does not matter. There are plenty of others. But if a very large vein is blocked by clot the part which it should drain becomes congested. The clot may break away and be carried through the heart to create a blockage (◊ *embolism*) in an artery of the lung. In the normal way, however, the clot is slowly absorbed, and either the vein resumes its function or a neighbouring vein takes over.

◊ *circulation; portal vein.*

vena cava. One of two great veins opening into the right atrium of the heart: the *superior vena cava* above, and the *inferior vena cava* below. Between them they receive the whole of the circulating venous blood (except the blood from the heart muscle, which drains directly into the atrium).

The superior vena cava is formed from the two ◊ *innominate* veins, by which it receives blood from the ◊ *jugular* and ◊ *subclavian* veins. It also receives the ◊ *azygos* vein; thus it drains the head, upper limbs, and thorax.

The inferior vena cava is formed from the two common ◊ *iliac* veins. It lies in front of the lumbar vertebrae, to the right of the aorta. Its largest tributaries are the ◊ *renal* and ◊ *hepatic* veins, from the kidneys and liver.

venene = ◊ *venom.*

venereal disease. Infectious disease usually transmitted by sexual contact. Any infection can be and presumably is transmitted sexually on occasion. The peculiarity of venereal diseases is that they are seldom transmitted in any other way. The common ones are *gonorrhoea* and *syphilis*, both world-wide, and *chancroid* and *lymphogranuloma venerum*, seen mostly in the tropics but increasing in temperate climates. All are discussed under their own headings.

All known venereal diseases are curable with antibiotics or sulphonamides, but when treatment is delayed, established damage may not be reparable. The early signs, especially among women, may be so slight as to pass unnoticed, unless the patient undergoes medical examination. Treatment of one partner without attention to the other is largely a waste of time, and one of the unsolved problems is how to trace and treat the patient's contacts.

Both World Wars greatly increased the incidence of venereal diseases. After the second, the incidence declined under the influence of effective drugs; but since the late 1950s venereal diseases have become commoner in most countries. One of the worst features of the newest epidemic is that the average age of the patients has steadily fallen, especially among girls.

venesection. Cutting a vein to draw off blood. ◊ *blood-letting.*

venom (venene). Poison injected by an animal by stinging or biting. Venomous animals include various insects (bees etc.), spiders, scorpions, reptiles, and fish.

Venoms are proteins. They can be neutralized by *antibodies* (antivenenes) in the same way as bacterial poisons (toxins), and effective preparations are available against most of the common and dangerous ones.

◊ *insect*; *snakebite.*

ventricle. A cavity, especially (1) in the ◊ *brain* or (2) in the ◊ *heart*.

1. The nervous system is developed from a simple tube. This structure persists in the spinal cord with its narrow *central canal*, but as the more highly developed parts of the brain grow the canal expands into a series of bubbles connected by narrower passages. In each cerebral hemisphere is a lateral *ventricle*, opening into the *third ventricle* at the centre of the brain. The cavity of the midbrain is a slender tube (*aqueduct of Silvius*), which broadens in the hind brain into the *fourth ventricle*, between the cerebellum and the brain-stem. The fourth ventricle narrows to the central canal of the spinal cord. The system is filled with cerebrospinal fluid, and communicates with the space around the brain and cord (◊ *meninges*) by holes in the roof of the 4th ventricle.

2. The two major compartments of the

heart are the right ventricle, pumping blood through the lungs, and the left ventricle, pumping blood through the rest of the circulation.

venule. Minute vein, receiving blood from capillary vessels (cf. ◊ *arteriole*, delivering blood to capillaries).

veratrum. Kinds of plant, including the ancient remedy ◊ *hellebore*, yielding alkaloids used to lower the blood pressure.

vermifuge. Any drug used to expel intestinal ◊ *worms*.

vernix caseosa. A greasy substance covering the skin of a new-born baby.

verruca = ◊ *wart*.

vertebra. Segment of the backbone (vertebral column). The human backbone has 33 vertebrae, of which the upper 24 are separate bones, the next 5 are fused to form the *sacrum*, and the lowest 4 form the *coccyx*, which represents the tail.

There are 7 *cervical* vertebrae in the neck, of which the uppermost, the *atlas*, makes a joint with the base of the skull. Then come 12 *thoracic* vertebrae, each carrying a pair of ribs, and 5 *lumbar* vertebrae. The backbone is described as a unit under ◊ *skeleton* (4).

The weight-bearing *body* of a vertebra is roughly cylindrical. An arch of bone, the *neural arch*, projects from the back of the body to enclose the *spinal canal*, which protects the spinal cord. Three projections from the neural arch provide anchorage for the muscles of the back: the *spinous process* in the mid-line and the *transverse processes* at the sides. The neural arch forms interlocking joints with the vertebrae above and below.

1. INTERVERTEBRAL DISCS

The flexible pads between the bodies of the vertebrae, or intervertebral discs, make up a quarter of the length of the backbone. Each disc consists of a jelly-like core, the *nucleus pulposus*, enclosed by dense fibrous tissue, which is firmly attached to the bodies of the vertebrae. This arrangement allows a certain amount of movement without loss of strength, and the discs are effective shock-absorbers.

The tough shell of a disc is weakest behind. Severe strain may cause a bulge here. The nucleus pulposus is squeezed into the bulge and causes symptoms from pressure on nerve fibres. If the bulge is to one side of the mid-line the pressure is on the nerve roots; if it is in the mid-line the spinal cord itself is affected.

This disorder is known as *slipped disc*, prolapsed disc, or hernia of the nucleus pulposus.

The usual cause of a slipped disc is strain while the backbone is flexed, e.g. bending forwards with the legs straight to lift a heavy object. This is a common type of industrial injury. Housewives suffer a similar type of back-strain from constantly working with their backs bent, e.g. working at a sink that is too low, leaning across a bed to tuck in the far side, or bathing the baby. The discs injured by this kind of strain are those between the lumbar vertebrae. The symptoms include backache and ◊ *sciatica* from compression of nerves running from the lumbar region to the leg. Weight-lifters avoid strain by keeping their backs straight, squatting, and lifting by straightening their legs.

The thoracic vertebrae are so well splinted by the ribs that their discs are unlikely to be strained. But the cervical discs are commonly damaged, perhaps by a combination of faulty posture (letting the neck sag and jutting the chin) and the processes of ageing. This is one of the many causes of pain, tingling, and numbness in the hand or higher up the arm, and also of some of the aches round the shoulder-blades that pass for 'fibrositis'.

A slipped disc is a mechanical defect, and its treatment is also mechanical. Postural training and manipulation may be enough. In acute cases the patient may have to lie flat for some weeks, or the affected part of the spine may have to be splinted, e.g. with a surgical collar. When simpler treatment fails, the protrusion of the disc can be removed surgically.

2. MOVEMENTS

The two uppermost vertebrae are very mobile. The joint between the atlas and the base of the skull is adapted to nodding the head. The next joint down, between the atlas and the second cervical vertebra (axis), is for shaking the head (rotation).

The movement of the other joints are comparatively slight, but added together they give the backbone a good range of movement. If a few of the joints become fixed as a result of disease, injury or surgery, the effect on the backbone as a whole may not be serious. Flexion (bending forwards) and extension (straightening or bending backwards) take place mainly in the cervical and lumbar regions, and rotation in the thoracic region, where the ribs prevent flexion.

3. INJURIES

Since the joints between the vertebrae interlock, and the fibrous part of the discs is very tough, it is easier to break these joints than to put them out of joint. But a kind of dislocation does occur between the 5th lumbar vertebra and the sacrum or between two lumbar vertebrae (◊ *spondylolisthesis*).

A direct blow or a sudden wrench can crack a spinous process or a transverse process. But the serious fractures are those of the vertebral bodies. If the body of a vertebra is broken it is liable to collapse. The backbone then bends forwards at a sharp angle, over which the spinal cord is stretched. This can cause paralysis below the level of the fracture. The damage to the spinal cord may occur not at the time of the original injury but as a result of attempts to move the victim.

When there is even a suspicion of injury to the back it is safest to leave all movement of the victim to trained first-aiders. If he has to be moved before expert help arrives it is best to carry him in the position in which he was found, or else face down so that any accidental movement of the backbone will tend to straighten it rather than increase the angulation.

These fractures heal well when they are immobilized, but a torn spinal cord cannot be repaired.

4. OTHER DISORDERS

The most important congenital disorder of the vertebrae is ◊ *spina bifida*, a defect of the neural arches.

Deformities are very common. They can be caused by faulty posture (when cause and effect are hard to distinguish); to defective muscles, e.g. after poliomyelitis; to deformity elsewhere, e.g. lateral curvature to compensate for deformity of one hip; or there may be no apparent cause.

With advancing years some degree of *osteoarthritis*, a degenerative condition,

seems almost inevitable. Many old people have *osteoporosis*, which is a loss of bone substance.

Pott's disease, tuberculosis of the vertebrae, was once a common cause of hunchback. The damage to the vertebral bodies caused angulation and injury to the spinal cord in the same way as a fracture.

Ankylosing spondylitis is a kind of inflammation affecting the backbone (and sometimes the sacroiliac and other joints). The typical symptoms are pain and extreme stiffness of the backbone. This disease is often regarded as a variant of ◊ *rheumatoid arthritis*.

vertigo. Giddiness with a definite sensation of movement; the subject feels that he or his surroundings are rotating. The ill-defined dizziness that many people feel if they suddenly stand up, or if they are tired or feverish, is not vertigo.

True vertigo arises from disturbances of the organ of balance (◊ *ear* (3, ii)) or its nerve (◊ *ear* (4)).

Vesalius (van Wesel), Andreas (1514–64). The most celebrated of all anatomists. Born in Brussels, he studied in Louvain and Paris, and became professor of anatomy at Padua at the age of 23.

Vesalius found anatomy more or less where Galen had left it in A.D. 200, and in 5 years of careful dissection and experiment he established anatomy as a modern science. He wrote several minor works, and one towering masterpiece, *De humani corporis fabrica*, published at Basle in 1543. This work, generally known as the *Fabrica*, is said to be the first modern treatise in any science – the first account of things actually seen, after centuries of arid speculation. Since no rational medicine is possible until the structure of the body is understood, the *Fabrica* was a turning-point for all branches of medicine. Vesalius knew that this would be so. He ascribed the decadence of medicine to the fact that the physicians of the Middle Ages had delegated to menials all surgical work and with it all knowledge of anatomy. He set himself two tasks: first, to revert to Galen by making anatomy the foundation of all medicine, and second to correct Galen's anatomical errors, of which he mentions over 200. He succeeded almost beyond belief.

The *Fabrica* is systematic, not regional anatomy, i.e. it deals with the organs according to type and not situation. Its 7 books describe (I) bones, (II) muscles, (III) blood vessels, (IV) nerves, (V) abdominal organs, (VI) heart and lungs, (VII) brain. Modern reference books are arranged in much the same way, as opposed to practical manuals or guides to dissection which describe the arrangement of organs in the various regions of the body. And Vesalius insisted that his book was for reference. Like any professor of anatomy today, he told his students that they would learn anatomy only by doing their own dissections and seeing for themselves, not from books or lectures.

The superb illustrations, drawn from Vesalius's dissections, are matched only by Leonardo's anatomical drawings, which remained hidden for 200 years.

Vesalius was the most practical of scientists. In his work, perhaps for the first time, natural science was divorced from philosophy. He decided what he was to investigate and described what he found, presenting unadorned facts for others to interpret. He produced no theories to obscure the truth, and perhaps that is why for once the truth was readily accepted by other scientists. Having completed his life's work at the age of 29, Vesalius resigned his post and became court physician to Charles V, later to Philip II of Spain. He founded a dynasty of brilliant anatomists at Padua, culminating in Fabricius and his pupil Harvey.

vesical. Of the bladder.

vesicle. Blister.

Vibrio. Genus of curved (comma-shaped) bacteria, including the cause of *cholera*.

villus. Minute finger-like protrusion from the lining of the intestine. The millions of closely packed villi give the lining a velvety surface.

Electron microscopy has shown that the villi are themselves coated with *microvilli*.

vinblastine; vincristine. Drugs isolated from *Vinca rosea*, the periwinkle, used to inhibit the growth of abnormal cells in Hodgkin's disease and some related forms of cancer.

Vincent's disease (Vincent's angina; trench mouth). (H. Vincent (1862–1950), French physician.) A bacterial infection of the gums, occasionally spreading to the throat. The bacteria are *Fusiformis* and a species of *Borrelia* resembling the spirochaete of relapsing fever. Both can often be found in healthy mouths, and it is not certain whether they cause the ulceration and inflammation or merely thrive in the presence of some undiscovered infection. Vincent's disease is associated with poor general health and physical exhaustion (hence 'trench mouth' in the First World War). The condition may clear up with simple cleansing and attention to general health, but it responds more quickly to treatment with metronidazole or with penicillin.

vincristine ♢ *vinblastine.*

viomycin. An antibiotic used in cases of tuberculosis in which the infecting bacilli have developed a resistance to streptomycin or the patient himself reacts unfavourably to the standard drugs.

Virchow, Rudolf (1821–1902). Prussian pathologist, anthropologist and statesman, a pupil of Müller in Berlin. For some years after taking his degree (1843) Virchow worked as a pathologist in Berlin. In 1847 he and his colleague Reinhardt founded what is still a leading medical journal, now known as *Virchow's Archiv*. A year later he investigated an epidemic of typhus, and his report strongly criticized the living conditions of the people affected. The government of 1848 was having more than enough trouble with revolutionaries, and Virchow was promptly dismissed. He became professor of pathology at Würzburg. In 1855 he returned to Berlin as professor, and held the chair for the rest of his life.

In politics he kept his liberal views. He was a co-founder and for many years the leader of the Progressive Party. He sat in the Prussian Parliament from 1862 until his election to the Reichstag in 1880. For what it was worth he opposed many of Bismarck's policies. To considerably more purpose he put the public health service of Berlin on a sound basis.

Virchow published numerous works on anthropology, and he assisted the archaeologist Schliemann in the exploration of Troy.

His detractors criticized him for opposing new ideas other than his own, such as Darwin's theory of evolution and some of the new discoveries about bacteria and infection. In fact he did nothing of the sort. He merely insisted that new theories should be proved before being allowed to displace the old ones, and he asked no less of his own theories.

Virchow's great fame rests on a simple principle: *omnis cellula e cellula*, every cell comes from a cell. From this germ a new science of pathology, a new understanding of all medical science and indeed all biology were to grow.

Until about 1850 pathology had been content to record the appearances of disease: this heart was enlarged, that liver was scarred, those kidneys were pale. It was an extension of the work of Morgagni in the previous century.

Another pupil of Müller, Theodor Schwann, made the important discovery that animals, like plants, were composed of living cells, which he thought arose spontaneously in a formless ground substance or *blastema*. Schwann's theory was published in 1839. The great Viennese pathologist Rokitansky concluded that disease caused the blastema to produce abnormal cells and tissues.

During his short exile at Würzburg, Virchow recognized that every cell in the body, healthy or diseased, was derived from an earlier cell and, at many removes, from one cell, the fertilized ovum – itself derived from cells of parents and ancestors. All diseases were manifestations of changes, active processes, that had taken place in cells derived from cells. This was like discovering for the first time that the population of a country is composed of individual people who are the children and parents of other people, who eat, sleep, grow, work, help each other, commit crimes against each other, and finally die yet still live in their offspring. It is only in such terms as these that history makes sense, and it was only in Virchow's terms that pathology at last began to make sense.

Virchow's greatest work was published as early as 1858 with the title *Cellular-Pathologie*. For the rest of his life he developed his theme. Every known disease had to be studied afresh. Instead of the old question 'what has already happened to this organ?' pathology had to ask 'what is at present going on in these cells?'. It was no longer a static science, but a dynamic one.

virus. The smallest microbe and the smallest known living creature – if indeed it is living. Viruses can be examined with an electron microscope, but most types are too small to be seen with an ordinary microscope. In size, they range between 0·0005 mm., about half the size of a small bacterium, and 0·00001 mm., the size of a very large molecule.

All viruses are totally parasitic. An isolated virus is an inert speck of matter. It cannot feed, grow, or multiply; it shows no more sign of life than a doornail. A few very small viruses have actually been crystallized. But when a virus becomes attached to a living cell of an appropriate organism (like other parasites, it can live on only one or two species of animal or plant) it diverts the cells' functions to its own needs and can multiply.

The essential difference between a virus and an undoubtedly living creature such as a bacterium or a plant or an animal is that a virus is not equipped with all the chemical components needed for life. It cannot provide its own energy, but must borrow from a better endowed organism. What every virus does contain is nucleic acid. The smallest viruses are parcels of nucleic acid and nothing else; it is because they are pure substances that they can be crystallized. Nucleic acids are the substances that control the synthesis of living matter: they are the very essence of life. All nucleic acids are made up of the same few substances strung together to make relatively huge molecules. The sequence of sub-molecules in the chain determines the kind of living matter that will be formed in the cell. Differences between species, between individual members of a species, and between the various types of cell in an individual represent differences in the structure of their nucleic acids.

Given a supply of chemical energy and raw material, a nucleic acid can form an exact replica of itself.

When a cell is infected with a virus, its resources are squandered in helping the invader to reproduce itself and prepare fresh virus particles to invade neighbouring cells. This futile activity is harmful to cells. A few viruses can produce toxins or poisons, in the manner of bacteria, but on the whole it seems that the harmful effects of virus infection are due to the mere presence of the virus.

It is impossible to say whether a virus is a living creature or not. Self-reproduction is characteristic of life. Viruses could be said to reproduce themselves, in which case they are alive. Or they could be considered as inanimate objects of which living cells make copies, in which case they are not alive.

1. TYPES OF VIRUS

No rational classification of viruses is yet possible. They are usually named after the diseases they cause or the sites where they are found. Animals, plants, and even bacteria are subject to virus infections, so the number of different viruses must be very great.

Human virus diseases include the common cold, influenza, measles, mumps, chickenpox, smallpox, poliomyelitis, herpes, intestinal upsets, and many others.

Obviously no virus can be grown like a bacterium on an artificial medium; a preparation of living tissue is needed. Certain viruses, e.g. smallpox, can be identified by their mode of growth in fertile eggs. More often they have to be identified by showing whether they react with ◊ antibodies isolated from men or animals who have developed immunity to them.

Some important virus diseases can be caused by several distinct types of virus, and infection confers immunity only to the one type. Furthermore viruses may change their character in the course of time by mutation: they are subject to evolution, and the diseases they cause can change their character.

A few groups have names unrelated to diseases. Among the enteroviruses (viruses found in the intestine) are Coxsackie viruses, named after the town in which they were first discovered, and ECHO (enteric cytopathic human orphan) viruses, called orphans with inappropriate pathos because for some time no disease could be found for them. This has been put right – various fevers have now been ascribed to them.

Myxoviruses, which include those of influenza, have an affinity for mucus. Arbor viruses are arthropod-borne, i.e. transmitted by insects and the like. They include those of yellow fever and dengue (mosquitoes), sandfly fever, and tick fever.

The largest viruses, not much smaller than bacteria, include those of trachoma (a common cause of blindness in hot dry countries), and ornithosis (a kind of pneumonia transmitted to man by certain birds). These are chemically more complete than other viruses, and some microbiologists classify them as ◊ Bedsonia, an intermediate form between viruses and bacteria.

The gradation from tiny viruses such as poliomyelitis virus to large viruses (smallpox), rickettsiae, bacteria, and fungi might suggest that evolution has followed a similar path, but this is unlikely to be so. Certainly viruses as we know them cannot be the earliest form of life, because they cannot live without higher forms.

2. VIRUS DISEASES

Some of the common virus diseases have already been mentioned. They are considered further under their own headings. In addition, many ill-defined fevers are caused by viruses. What used to pass for pneumonia in infants, unexplained diarrhoea at any age, and vague, short illnesses are often virus infections. True influenza is a serious epidemic disease due to a known group of viruses. The word 'flu' is applied to common colds and other minor virus diseases. Purists object, but since the particular virus is not likely to be identified in such cases 'flu' is as good a word as any, as long as it is not confused with true influenza.

Most viruses have an affinity for a particular type of cell, in which they produce a characteristic type of damage, with recognizable symptoms. One case of measles is very like another. Like bacteria and other foreign matter in the body, viruses provoke ◊ immunity by causing antibodies to be formed; these chemical substances inactivate present infection and prevent future infection. Some symptoms of virus disease are due to the body's defensive reaction and not directly to the virus. Viruses may stray from their usual haunts with serious results. Poliomyelitis is a common and mild infection of the intestine, but in 1 per cent of cases it involves the nervous system.

The drugs used against bacteria affect only the very large viruses mentioned above as being probably small bacteria.

A few drugs, none of them generally applicable, have some effect on virus infections. These include the thiosemicarbazones, a prophylactic against smallpox, and idoxuridine (IDU), which interferes with nucleic acid formation and may be effective with certain virus infections of the eyes. Drugs such as IDU could only be used against surface infection, because in the blood-stream they would interfere with the body's own nucleic acid. Sometimes virus infections are treated with ◊ *gamma-globulins* from the serum of someone who is immune to the disease. Several common virus diseases can be prevented by vaccination.

3. VIRUSES AND CANCER

Cancer is abnormal behaviour of cells, especially as regards multiplication. While reproducing themselves excessively, cancer cells tend to lose the functions of their healthy neighbours. But some viruses cause cells not only to produce more viruses, but to multiply themselves, all at the expense of their normal functions. The common wart is an abnormal proliferation of cells in the skin, caused by a virus. A wart is by no means a cancer, for it has no tendency to spread beyond the skin or set up colonies in remote parts of the body.

A few types of cancer in animals are certainly caused by viruses, e.g. the Rous sarcoma of fowls, but these are rarities. One form of human cancer, Burkitt's sarcoma, first reported in Uganda, may be due to a virus transmitted by mosquitoes.

Against any general virus theory is the lack of evidence that cancer is infectious: people simply do not catch cancer from each other. But this does not rule out the theory. If cancer were an occasional effect of a virus that most people carried it would be impossible to trace infection. Nearly all of us have chickenpox at some time. Only the unlucky few later develop shingles from the same virus, and if the virus had not been positively identified with that of chickenpox nobody would suspect shingles of being an infectious disease.

For viruses to cause cancer they would have to induce permanent changes in the nucleic acids of the infected cells, for one of the features of cancer is that the change in cell behaviour is irreversible. Studies of bacteria infected with bacterial viruses (bacteriophages or *phages*) show that this can happen. Changes induced by phages are transmitted to succeeding generations of bacteria. So it is quite conceivable that viruses might induce cancerous changes in human cells that would be transmitted to the successors of these cells. But proof is still lacking, and even if viruses are found to cause some cancer it is unlikely that they cause all.

◊◊ *cancer*; and the historical note under ◊ *microbe*.

viscus (pl. *viscera*). Any of the specialized internal organs – heart, lung, stomach, liver, kidney etc., but not muscles, bones, nerves or other parts of the general framework of the body.

vision. The structure, function, and common diseases of the eyes are considered under ◊ *eye*. The following notes are concerned only with refraction, on which sharpness of vision (visual acuity) depends.

Light entering the eye is refracted, and so brought to a focus, by the *cornea* – the window at the front of the eye, which cannot be adjusted – and the *lens* behind the pupil, which is flexible and can be adjusted.

When this optical system is correctly adjusted (*emmetropia*) a healthy eye can resolve two points subtending an angle of about one minute. The limiting factor is the distance apart of the sensitive nerve-endings (rods and cones) of the retina at the back of the eye, exactly as the resolution of a camera, however good its lens, is limited by the grain of the film.

The standard lettering used for testing visual acuity is made up from units subtending an angle of one minute at a known distance. The line of type for 'normal' vision is what an emmetropic eye can easily read at the prescribed distance of the chart, often 6 metres. On a 6-metre chart the line above should be legible at 9 metres, and the next at 12 metres. If this is the smallest type that the patient can read his vision is 6/12, or 0·5 in metric notation. With a 20-ft chart it would be 20/40. People with very sharp vision can do rather better than the arbitrary standard, and most charts include smaller type representing 6/5 and 6/4 (1·5 metric).

A common cause of poor visual acuity is a slight asymmetry of the cornea (◊ *astigmatism*), which is corrected with lenses that are asymmetrical in the opposite sense. More serious deformity of the cornea can be corrected with contact lenses.

The common defects of focusing arise from discrepancies between the focal length of the lens system and the actual length of the eye, causing short or long sight.

Short sight (*myopia*) is due to too strong a lens (or too long an eye). Distant objects are focused at a point in front of the retina. Near objects, which need a stronger lens, can be focused on the retina and seen sharply.

Long sight (*hypermetropia*) is caused in the opposite way. With the eye at rest, even distant objects are focused behind the retina. The muscles of the lens can shorten its focal length, i.e. strengthen it, and if the discrepancy is not too great distant objects can be focused sharply; but the lens is not so adaptable that near objects can be focused on the retina. (◊ *squint*.)

Presbyopia is a normal process of ageing. From childhood the lens gradually becomes less flexible, so that the muscles can adapt it less and less. In old age it is virtually a fixed-focus lens set at infinity.

A child with normal refraction can focus objects held a few inches in front of his eyes. This distance, the near point, gradually increases. In middle age he may be holding his book at arm's length to focus the print, which is then too far away to be read. Distant objects can still be focused because the lens does not have to be adapted for them. Short-sighted people, on the other hand, may still be able to read comfortably in old age.

All these defects are corrected by suitable glasses: short sight by concave (negative) lenses to weaken the refraction of the eye, and long sight by convex lenses to strengthen it. Presbyopes need separate glasses for distant and near vision.

These are the usual causes of poor eyesight. But it must be emphasized that many other disorders, needing treatment very different from glasses, can interfere with vision. All defects of vision therefore require expert examination before glasses are even considered.

visual acuity. Sharpness of ◊ *vision*.

vital centre. Collection of nerve cells by which some activity immediately essential to life is regulated, e.g. the respiratory, cardiac, and vasomotor centres which govern breathing, heart rate, and blood pressure. These centres are in the *medulla oblongata*, the lowest part of the brain immediately above its junction with the spinal cord. Serious injury to the vital centres is immediately lethal, whereas life may continue after loss of higher parts of the brain.

vitamin. Essential accessory to the main ingredients of the diet. A proper diet contains the raw materials of which the body is made and continually remade, together with fuel to provide energy. The main ingredients are protein, fat, and carbohydrate. Smaller quantities of inorganic matter are also needed: sodium, potassium, calcium, iron, and traces of several other metals; phosphates, chlorides, iodides, and fluorides. In addition, certain compounds are needed which the body cannot make from their raw materials (i.e. it lacks the enzymes needed for their synthesis); these are the vitamins. Only small amounts are needed. Most of them serve as minor reagents in major chemical reactions (◊ *enzyme* (4)). The system might be compared with the workshop of a versatile carpenter. He can fashion all the parts of a piece of furniture and makes his own glues and varnishes. But he cannot make screws; these he must buy ready-made. If he cannot buy screws he turns out rickety furniture held together only with glue and nails. So it is with vitamins. One may survive without them, but not in good health and not for the full span.

Some of the diseases due to lack of particular vitamins have been known for a long time, such as beri-beri in Asia, rickets in England, and scurvy among sailors. The 16th-century explorer Jacques Cartier cured his crew of scurvy with leaves, a remedy he learnt from the Canadian natives. In 1753 James Lind of Edinburgh showed that scurvy could be prevented or cured by fruit juice: '. . . as greens or fresh vegetables, with ripe fruits, are the best remedies for it, so they prove the most effectual preservatives against it.' No other 'deficiency disease' was recognized as such until the end of the 19th century, when Takaki in Japan and Eijkman in Batavia showed the connexion between beri-beri and diet. Children with rickets were given cod-liver oil in the 19th century, but nobody knew why until after the First World War.

That deficiency diseases were due to lack of 'accessory factors' was first suggested by (Sir) Frederick Gowland Hopkins of Cambridge in 1906. Later Funk named the factors 'vitamines' (because he thought they were chemically amines; when they were found not to be the 'e' was dropped).

As each new vitamin was discovered it was given a letter. It is not a very good notation, because several of the original vitamins were later found to be groups of different compounds. Now that all the known vitamins have been analysed they are often given their chemical names. But for ordinary discussion it does not matter that 'vitamin A' is actually two compounds, or that the B complex is a dozen or more.

The exact number of known vitamins cannot be given, because experiments with the diet of laboratory animals do not necessarily apply to man. For instance, rats deprived of vitamin E are sterile, but there is no evidence that humans need this vitamin. Humans do, on the other hand, need vitamin C, which rats can make for themselves from sugar or starch; in other words vitamin C is not a vitamin to a rat. (Returning to the carpenter's shop: his neighbour may have a lathe for making screws but no means of making his own glue.)

A good mixed diet contains enough of all the vitamins. Too much vitamin A or D can be harmful, and an excess of the others is at best useless. Nobody expects his car to run better with an extra quart of oil when the sump is already full, yet synthetic vitamins added to a good diet are widely expected to do wonders. Extra vitamins are really needed to correct malnutrition (which may be the result of poor diet or of faulty digestion), and to supply an extra demand such as pregnancy or regeneration of tissues after an operation or serious illness. Even then adjustment of the diet may suffice. There are also special circumstances in which a particular vitamin may be needed; some of these are mentioned in the following sections.

vitamin A (retinol). A complex alcohol found in fish oils, butter, and meat. Plant pigments include *carotenes* from which vitamin A is formed after digestion; hence carrots and other vegetables are a rich source. Since vegetable oils contain little or none, vitamin A is added to margarine.

Vitamin A forms part of the pigment *visual purple* in the eye and is essential for seeing in poor light. Night blindness is the earliest symptom of deficiency. With severe deficiency the skin and mucous membranes become dry and hard. The conjunctiva – the transparent membrane in front of the eye – may become opaque.

Deficiency can be due to very poor diet but is more likely to arise with diseases such as coeliac disease which interfere with the digestion of fat; vitamin A is absorbed from the intestine together with fat.

The Ebers papyrus (16th century B.C.) recommends liver – a good source of vitamin A – for night blindness.

vitamin B. Not a single vitamin, but a complex made up of at least a dozen totally different substances. They are grouped together because originally two extracts from food were found necessary for health, one fat-soluble (now known to have contained vitamins A and D) and one water-soluble, called vitamin B. More refined analysis revealed several components which were named B_1, B_2 etc. The struggle was abandoned when even these were found to contain more than one substance, and new discoveries are now given simplified chemical names.

Each vitamin is needed by a particular ◊ *enzyme* to take part in a particular chemical process; if the vitamin is missing the process is defective. Since various tissues use similar processes for different purposes, deficiency of a vitamin may cause diverse symptoms. The effects of lacking single B vitamins have been studied with experimental diets, but in any natural diet these vitamins are found in the same foods. If there is a shortage of one there is likely to be a shortage of several. But they are so widely distributed that no mixed diet is seriously deficient. The richest sources include yeast, liver, and the germ of cereals (which is lost in refined milling). In addition, the bacteria in a healthy large intestine can synthesize most of the B vitamins.

The complex includes *thiamine* (B_1, aneurin), *riboflavin* (B_2), *nicotinamide*, and *pyridoxine* (B_6), all of them involved in the use of oxygen by various tissues, and *cobalamine* (B_{12}) and *folic acid*, used in the synthesis of nucleic acids and therefore essential for the formation of new body-cells – e.g. those of the blood, which need frequent replacement.

Two diseases are ascribed to lack of B vitamins in the diet: ◊ *beri-beri* (mainly B_1) and ◊ *pellagra* (nicotinamide and other factors). Chronic alcoholics are nearly always short of these vitamins, partly because they eat poorly, and partly because they cannot properly digest what they do eat. Vitamin B deficiency may follow intensive treatment with antibiotics, which destroy not only harmful bacteria but also bacteria usefully engaged in synthesizing vitamins. Probably no diet lacks vitamin B_{12}, but pernicious anaemia ($\diamond$ *anaemia* (B.2)) is a result of inability to assimilate this vitamin from the food. Pyridoxine has a special place in the treatment of morning sickness.

vitamin C. Ascorbic acid, of which a deficiency is the cause of $\diamond$ *scurvy*. Long before other deficiency diseases were recognized it was known that scurvy was due to faulty diet and could be cured by eating fresh fruit. But Vitamin C itself was not identified until 1932 (by Szent-Györgyi, who was awarded a Nobel Prize in 1937). Ascorbic acid is needed in forming the fibres of connective tissue. Since these form part of all organs except the nervous system the effects of deficiency are wide-spread, but the most obvious and often the only serious trouble is weakness of the smallest blood vessels, which are liable to give way and bleed.

Most animals have the necessary enzymes for making ascorbic acid from glucose. For them it is not a vitamin, since by definition a vitamin cannot be synthesized in the body and must be supplied ready-made. Calves cannot, then, have scurvy, and cow's milk contains much less ascorbic acid than human milk. Bottle-fed babies can therefore be short of the vitamin. The healing of tissue damaged by disease or of wounds is in the first place a matter of laying down connective tissue. It creates a special demand for ascorbic acid.

All fruits and vegetables contain ascorbic acid, but it can be destroyed by elaborate preparation or cooking. Rose-hips, currants, and paprika are especially rich sources.

vitamin D. A factor necessary to the formation of healthy bone. Rickets, a disorder of bone formation, was treated with cod-liver oil as early as 1782, but the practice was not wide-spread – surprisingly, for no better medicine could have been found. As late as 1918 when Mellanby clearly proved that some factor in cod-liver oil (not then separated from vitamin A) cured rickets many people were unconvinced. It had been shown in Glasgow that lack of sunlight was the cause of rickets: how, then, could fish oil be of any use? In 1919 Dame Harriet Chick studied the severe outbreak of rickets in Vienna, and found that either cod-liver oil or sunlight would cure it. The explanation is that cod-liver oil and other foods contain a true vitamin – i.e. one which the body needs but cannot make for itself – and that sunlight transforms an inert substance in the skin (ergosterol) into *calciferol*, which is one form of the vitamin, known as vitamin D_2. *Cholecalciferol* in fish liver is D_3. Vitamin D_1 was an early mistake which proved not to be a vitamin.

Vitamin D promotes the absorption of calcium from the intestine and its excretion in the urine, but its most important effect is on the movement of calcium in bone. The hard substance of bone is composed of insoluble calcium salts. As bone grows these salts are removed from the inside and deposited on the outside. Lack of vitamin D impairs the process.

All the effects of this vitamin – absorption, excretion, bone growth – can be described as *mobilizing* calcium, which amounts to making it soluble. Calcium dissolved in the body-fluids is in two forms. Most salts of calcium, and of any other metal, dissociate when dissolved in water into electrically charged particles (*ions*). Calcium ions have important effects on muscle contraction; if their concentration in the body-fluids varies, the performance of muscle is seriously impaired. The $\diamond$ *parathyroid* hormone maintains a constant level of calcium ions. But *calcium citrate* is a soluble salt which does not dissociate and so has no electrical properties. In this form, calcium is merely a passenger in the blood. The amount can be varied to suit the needs of the moment.

Vitamin D is known to prevent citrates from being destroyed in the tissues. Its other effects could well be due to maintaining an adequate supply of citrates.

A gross excess of vitamin D causes too much calcium to be mobilized; this unwanted calcium may form bony deposits in the kidneys and elsewhere.

In summer, butter and eggs are good sources, and vitamin D is usually added to margarine. Fish oils contain very large quantities. But sunlight is the most reliable source.

$\diamond$ *rickets*; *osteomalacia*.

vitamin E (tocopherol). A vitamin discovered in 1936. Male rats deprived of tocopherol become sterile, and female rats cannot bear live young, though they conceive normally. In many animals tocopherol plays some part in the development of muscle and the processing of fats.

On the basis of these experimental findings vitamin E has been tried for various human ailments: infertility, repeated miscarriage, and disorders of muscle and nerve. The results have been disappointing, and there is little evidence that man is ever short of this vitamin.

vitamin K. A vitamin required for the formation of the enzyme thrombin, without which blood cannot clot. Two equally effective forms of the vitamin occur naturally, one in green vegetables and the other formed by intestinal bacteria. Various synthetic drugs can be used instead.

Since the vitamin is provided by food and also by bacteria a shortage is extremely unlikely; but it can be absorbed only in the presence of bile. If the flow of bile is obstructed (◊ *jaundice*) vitamin K is poorly absorbed. The clotting of blood is delayed and the patient is liable to bleed heavily if, for instance, he has a surgical operation. Obstructive jaundice often needs surgical treatment, which was dangerous before vitamin K was discovered.

Drugs such as dicoumarol oppose the action of vitamin K. They have been used to prevent unwanted clotting (◊ *thrombosis*).

New-born babies are sometimes short of vitamin K. To prevent them from bleeding they are given the vitamin until bacteria in the intestine (there are none at birth) take over.

vitiligo. Patchy loss of pigment from the skin. The white patches are unsightly, especially on a naturally dark skin, and they are very liable to sunburn, but otherwise the condition is harmless. The cause is unknown, and no treatment except the use of cosmetics has any effect.

vitreous humour. The clear jelly filling the larger part of the eye, behind the lens. (The part in front of the lens is filled with the watery *aqueous humour*.)

vivisection. Surgical operation on a living animal for experimental purposes. This highly emotive word is applied by opponents of animal experiment to any procedure, even dietary experiments.

In all civilized countries, these experiments are subject to laws about who may do them, compulsory anaesthetics and so on. The argument that they are scientifically unsound is not really valid, because nobody is more aware than the biologists who do them of their limitations – what is true of one species may not be true of another. But without animal experiments there would be little scientific background to medicine.

vocal cord ◊ *larynx.*

volvulus. Twisting of a loop of intestine so that its contents are obstructed and, if it is tightly twisted, the blood is prevented from flowing through its vessels. It is most likely to occur if the *mesentery* – the fold of tissue in which the intestine hangs – is unusually long. Volvulus has to be treated by immediate operation to untwist the loop and, in some cases, stabilize it to prevent a recurrence. If the circulation has been obstructed for any length of time the loop may be irreparably damaged; it has then to be removed.

vomiting. A reflex action with reversal of the normal movements of the muscles in the wall of the stomach; at the same time the voluntary muscles of the abdomen are brought under reflex control to hasten emptying of the stomach.

The reflex is clearly protective when it is set off by an irritant in the stomach, or by overloading. Vomiting can also be set off by over-activity of the intestine further down; hence anything that causes diarrhoea may incidentally cause vomiting. This can be regarded as a sort of radiation of impulses in branches of the *vagus* nerve, which controls both intestine and stomach. The nausea, salivation, pallor, and sweating that often precede vomiting are not governed by the vagus nerve. The whole system of reflexes is controlled by a centre in the brain, which evidently has a complex set of relays. It can be activated by conscious centres of the brain in some emotional states – disgust in adults, or mere excitement in many children.

Repeated or sustained vomiting is always a serious symptom. On the one hand, the causes include emergencies such as obstruction of the intestine and poisoning. On the other hand the vomiting itself can quickly lead to a dangerous loss of water and salt.

Vomiting can often be controlled by the anti-emetic drug *metoclopramide*. ◊ *travel sickness; hyperemesis.*

von Recklinghausen's disease. (F. von Recklinghausen (1833–1910), German pathologist.) = ⇨ *neurofibromatosis*.

vulva. Female external genitalia, bounded at the sides by the *labia majora*. These thick folds of skin and fat enclose two smaller folds, the *labia minora*, which in turn enclose the clitoris and the openings of the urethra and vagina.

W

wart. Small, rough tumour of the outer layer of the skin. Warts are of great theoretical interest because they are the only human tumours that are certainly caused by virus infection, and this might throw some light on the origin of cancer: ◊ *cancer* (1); *virus* (3).

The most important difference between warts and other tumours is their habit of disappearing spontaneously. But when a wart does disappear, the virus sometimes lies dormant and resumes its activity later. This unpredictable behaviour makes it difficult to assess the value of treatment. Warts are often 'charmed' away by people who claim special gifts for the work, but one can never be sure that the wart was not about to vanish of its own accord.

Warts can be cut out or destroyed by freezing or corrosive fluids. Skill and experience are needed, for unless the treatment is applied correctly it may cause the virus to spread and set up new warts.

As a general rule, warts are best left alone to vanish in their own time. But those on the sole of the foot (plantar wart, verruca plantaris) are painful and have to be treated.

Wasserman reaction (WR). A blood test for the diagnosis of syphilis. When the bacterial cause of syphilis was discovered in 1905, several kinds of infection could be diagnosed by showing a characteristic reaction between the patient's blood and a preparation of the appropriate species of bacteria. The reaction showed that the patient had acquired immunity to the bacteria as a result of infection. In 1906 the German bacteriologist August von Wasserman (1866–1925) introduced such a test for syphilis, using tissue from a patient who had died of congenital syphilis as the reagent. The test gave reliable results, but for the wrong reason. The effect of the reagent depended not on syphilis in the tissue but on the tissue itself, for by pure chance healthy liver and heart muscle contain a substance that reacts with the blood of a person who has syphilis.

The Wassermann reaction does not distinguish syphilis from yaws or other diseases due to species of *Treponema*, but nor does any other known test apart from observing the course of the disease. A few other infectious diseases also give a weakly positive WR.

The Kahn test is a modification of the WR, and gives similar results.

water. Water accounts for about 60 per cent of a man's body weight and 50 per cent of a woman's. The difference is due to the average woman's larger proportion of fat, which contains no water.

Of an average man's 40-odd litres (9 gallons) of water, the *plasma* of the blood contains rather more than 3 litres, and the *tissue fluid*, permeating the whole body and bathing each of its millions of cells, about 12 litres. Together, these 15 litres make up the *extracellular fluid*. The rest of the water, the *intracellular fluid*, is incorporated in the cells.

Although the balance between blood, tissue fluid and cells remains almost constant there is a rapid and continuous exchange of water between them (◊ *tissue fluid*).

The body inevitably loses about 1·5 litres of water daily. The kidneys *must* form at least 600 c.c. of urine to get rid of poisonous waste products. Evaporation from the skin (insensible perspiration) takes 500 c.c., and evaporation from the lungs 300 c.c. Only a small amount is lost in normal faeces, say 100 c.c.

Eating replaces some of the lost water. All food contains water. An average diet may provide 600 c.c. of free water, and in addition the end-products of combustion are carbon dioxide, excreted by the lungs, and water, say 300 c.c. The remaining 600 c.c. – a pint – is replaced by drinking. This pint is the very least that must be drunk daily in cool surroundings.

Sweating can greatly increase the loss. In extreme conditions the sweat glands can pour out as much as 10 litres in a day.

The balance is regulated almost automatically. Any reasonable excess passes into the urine, and a deficit arouses the sensation of thirst.

Shortage of water begins to cause obvious changes when the water in the body is reduced by about 10 per cent (4 litres). The plasma suffers least, because a deficit lowers the blood pressure and, by concentrating the plasma, increases its osmotic pressure. Both effects tend to keep water in the plasma at the expense of the tissues by the mechanism described under ◊ *tissue fluid*. The skin looks dry and pinched, and loses its elasticity. When the deficit reaches 25 per cent (10 litres) the blood is so viscous and the blood pressure so low that the circulation stops. Even under ideal conditions water is lost at a rate of 1·5 litres daily, so a man can live only a few days without drinking.

The commonest danger arises from diarrhoea and vomiting, to which sweating is often added. Severe vomiting makes drinking impossible, and the nausea that accompanies many illnesses makes it difficult. The extreme case is ◊ *cholera*, which can be fatal in a matter of hours. In all these conditions the associated loss of salt makes matters very much worse.

Children are particularly susceptible to loss of water; sick children may not feel thirsty although they are short of water, and they need encouragement to drink. Any child losing fluid needs the closest attention.

There are many situations in which drinking does not suffice, and fluid has to be injected. It is usually given into a vein. As well as ensuring that the right amount of water is replaced, injected fluids can also be made up to restore lost salts and other necessities.

It is possible to take in too much water, but water intoxication is a rare accident. On the other hand an excess of tissue fluid is a fairly common symptom (◊ *oedema*).

Weil's disease (leptospirosis). (Adolf Weil (1848–1916), German physician.) An infectious disease of animals occasionally transmitted to man, caused by various species of *Leptospira*, a spirochaete (spiral bacterium).

The usual form is due to *L. icterohaemorrhagica*, a common parasite of rats. The rats seem to carry the spirochaetes without being sick, as some humans carry diphtheria. The infection is mainly in the rats' kidneys, and is acquired by contact with anything (usually water) contaminated with rat's urine. Weil's disease is an occupational risk of sewermen, rat-catchers and miners, and cases occur from bathing in rat-infested canals and rivers.

Other species of leptospira infect dogs and farm animals and are sometimes passed to man.

Weil's disease is an acute fever, usually lasting a week or 10 days. In severe cases the liver, kidneys, and heart muscle may be heavily infected, and the combination of jaundice, nephritis, and heart failure can be fatal. Some patients have a tendency to bleed into the skin and elsewhere.

The variants of the disease caught from dogs and farm animals cause meningitis rather than jaundice. They are seldom if ever fatal.

Unlike other spirochaetal diseases (syphilis, yaws, relapsing fever, Vincent's disease), leptospirosis responds poorly to penicillin and other antibiotics. It is best dealt with by prevention: rubber boots and gloves for workers unavoidably exposed to rats; rodent control; surface drainage; and not bathing in dubious waters.

wen. ◊ *Sebaceous* cyst.

white matter. Parts of the brain and spinal cord composed mainly of nerve fibres. ◊ *grey matter*.

whitlow. Septic finger-tip, especially *paronychia*, a small abscess at the side of the ◊ *nail*, with a tendency to creep under the nail. If this happens part or all of the nail may have to be removed to release the pus.

whooping cough (pertussis). An acute infectious disease of childhood. The main symptom is coughing, in violent and uncontrollable outbursts, often followed by vomiting. The ◊ *incubation* period varies, but is commonly about a week. An attack confers immunity, and most children are exposed to infection at some time. The disease is thus rare in adults.

In the ordinary way, anyone about to cough first takes a deep breath. The cough of pertussis comes on so suddenly that the child may be caught at the end of expiration with no time to breathe in. The cough reflex closes the glottis, and the child cannot take a breath until the outburst is over; he thus appears to be suffocating. He then learns the trick of drawing in air against the resistance of the glottis, which produces the 'whooping' sound. With a mild attack, there is no need to whoop, and the disease may pass for a bad cold. Small babies

483

WITHERING

sometimes fail to learn the knack of whooping and get no air while the outburst lasts.

Pertussis is seldom dangerous in older children, but may be serious in babies, both in itself and in its complications such as pneumonia and mechanical damage to the lungs. A child with whooping cough is unusually susceptible to tuberculosis.

A small bacillus, *Haemophilus pertussis*, is supposedly the germ of pertussis, but its relation to the disease is less clear-cut than, say, that of the haemolytic streptococcus to scarlet fever. It is a difficult organism to grow in the laboratory, and its effects are not easy to prove. Other organisms are probably involved as well.

Immunization against *H. pertussis* does not entirely prevent attacks, but since it makes them less likely and less serious it is well worth doing.

The infection responds to antibiotics, which probably have more effect on other germs complicating the disease than on *H. pertussis* itself. Even with the best treatment, pertussis can be a protracted and debilitating illness.

Wilms' tumour. (Max Wilms (1867–1918), German surgeon.) Nephroblastoma. ◊ *kidneys* (4).

Wilson's disease (hepatolenticular degeneration). (A. Kinnear Wilson (1878–1937), British neurologist.) A rare hereditary disease with cirrhosis of the liver and disordered control of movement of the same kind as parkinsonism (shaking palsy).

Certain tissues need a trace of *copper*. All diets contain the minute amount required; copper deficiency is unknown in man, though it has been described in sheep. The fundamental disorder in Wilson's disease is faulty distribution of copper in the body: abnormally large amounts are deposited in the liver and parts of the brain and cause local poisoning.

Drugs such as BAL take up an excess of copper and are used to prevent further damage to brain cells.

wintergreen ◊ *methyl salicylate.*

Withering, William (1741–99). English physician. He practised in Birmingham. His *Account of the Foxglove* (1785) is among the most celebrated of all medical texts.

In 1775, Withering was asked for his opinion of a family receipt for the cure of the dropsy, long kept a secret by an old woman in Shropshire. It was said to act by producing violent vomiting and purging. It contained 20 or more herbs, but Withering quickly identified the root of the foxglove (*digitalis*) as the active herb.

At that time there was no science of pharmacology. Drugs were used because they had always been used or because someone of importance had recommended them. No drug had ever been properly studied a bare handful of the hundreds of remedies used would have withstood even cursory investigation.

Having shown that the drug had powerful effects, Withering set about finding a way of preparing it that would allow accurate dosage. The leaves were more reliable than the root, and because their properties changed during the year they had always to be collected when the plant flowered.

Withering soon recognized that purging and vomiting were not the useful actions of the drug but symptoms of overdosage. He recorded every known symptom of digitalis poisoning: 'sickness, vomiting, purging, giddiness, confused vision, objects appearing green and yellow; increased secretion of urine, with frequent motions to part with it; and sometimes inability to retain it; slow pulse, even as slow as 35 in a minute, cold sweats, convulsions, syncope, death'. He gave detailed instructions to avoid these dangers – 'the effects of our inexperience'. He recognized the important peculiarity of digitalis that its action is slow and sustained, so that repeated doses have a cumulative action.

Far ahead of the times is Withering's insistence on a large number of observations before drawing conclusions. This was made possible by his setting aside an hour or more each day for giving free advice to the poor – two or three thousand of them annually. He also drew many of his colleagues into the investigation.

Withering was unusual in trusting his chosen drug and giving it alone. Any ordinary prescription of the time contained a score or more of ingredients, and there was no way of knowing which, if any, of them had helped the patient. Withering added no more than flavouring to his digitalis, or occasionally a small dose of opium 'to restrain its action on the bowels'.

Not content with setting a standard for all future studies of drugs, Withering pointed out that chemistry (then in early infancy) might in the future come to the prescriber's aid, and that the actions of drugs on 'insects and quadrupeds' might be studied with profit.

worms (helminths). A diverse and ill-defined collection of primitive animals. Many species are parasites, and some cause human ailments. The mere presence of a parasite need not denote illness. Some parasitic worms live at peace with their hosts and cause no disturbance. Nearly all worm infestations clear up in time, though it may be a long time.

The worms to be considered here are those that live in the intestine. Some worms that live in other parts of the body are discussed under ◊ *bilharzia; filaria; Guinea worm; hydatid disease; trichiniasis.*

The common intestinal worms of childhood are passed from person to person: faeces contain the eggs; a child's fingers become contaminated; he swallows the eggs and the cycle is repeated. The worms of this type include the roundworm *Ascaris*, the threadworm *Enterobius* (both worldwide), and the whipworm *Trichuris* (mainly tropical). The eggs of the threadworm are laid on the skin around the anus, where they cause itching. The child scratches and reinfects himself when he sucks his fingers. Otherwise these worms cause little trouble, except that rare cases of blockage by a tangle of worms in the intestine are described. Of the many available drugs, piperazine is the most used.

Hookworms (*Ankylostoma duodenale*; *Necator americanus*) can occur in most parts of the world, but because of the mode of infection they are common only in warm countries. The larvae live in soil contaminated by faeces, and enter the body through the skin of the feet. Therefore the infection thrives only where sanitation and personal hygiene are defective, and people walk bare-footed. Under these conditions, whole populations suffer from hookworm disease. The worms attach themselves to the lining of the duodenum and cause very slight but persistent loss of blood. The resulting anaemia is not severe, but it is enough to keep the patient's general condition below what it should be. Hookworm disease used to be treated with chenopodium or tetrachlorethylene, both very unpleasant drugs. The newer bephenium hydroxynaphthoate is more reliable and easier to take.

Of the tapeworms – long segmented ribbons – *Taenia saginata* is a parasite of cattle, *Taenia solium* of pigs, and the very long *bothryocephalus* (*diphyllobothrium latum*) of fish, mainly in the Baltic. With adequate meat inspection these parasites do not often reach the consumer, and with thorough cooking even infected food is rendered harmless. Most tapeworm infections cause few symptoms, but all kinds of intestinal disturbance are ascribed to the first two on occasion, and the third is said to cause a sort of pernicious anaemia. Tapeworms are expelled with quinacrine or dichlorophen.

wound. The traditional classes of wound are *contusion* (bruise), *abrasion* (graze), *laceration* (tear), and *incision* (cut). Perhaps *puncture* should be added. A *penetrating* wound is one that enters a body cavity (skull, chest, abdomen). No such classification is of much use. What matters is which particular structures have been damaged (e.g. whether nerves or vital organs are damaged) and the effect of the local injury on the body as a whole.

With most wounds the most urgent problem is bleeding, discussed under its own heading. Broken bones and damaged nerves can wait; bleeding cannot.

With multiple injuries and unconscious patients, even the control of bleeding is less urgent than ensuring that the patient can breathe. In these circumstances his tongue may fall back and completely block his throat. But the tongue is attached to the jaw, and drawing the chin forwards and upwards clears the airway. This simple manoeuvre is more important than artificial respiration.

Apart from the control of bleeding by firm yet gentle pressure around the wound or on the appropriate artery the only essential first aid is to avoid infection. Antiseptics are only of limited value; a clean dressing does all that can usefully be done. Further treatment of all but minor wounds needs an operating theatre where the damage can be assessed, the wound thoroughly cleaned, and injured tissues repaired.

wrist. The joint formed by the ◊ *radius* and 3 of the small bones of the ◊ *hand*. The lower end of the radius is hollowed out to receive the *scaphoid* at the base of the thumb, the *triquetral* at the base of the little finger, and the *lunate* between them. These three bones are firmly bound together by ligaments and move as one in their socket. The ulna, which at the elbow is more important than the radius, does not take part in the wrist joint. Its joints with the radius are described under ◊ *radius*.

The capsule is reinforced by ligaments at the sides and in front of the joint. More than 20 tendons on their way from the forearm to the hand surround the wrist Most of them are bridged over by strong fibrous bands attached to the bones. These bands prevent the tendons from straightening like bow-strings as the wrist bends. Under them the tendons move in lubricated sheaths like the synovial membranes of joints.

Sprain (torn ligament) is not very common in the wrist, but other injuries are easily mistaken for sprains. The small bones – especially the scaphoid – are liable to fractures which are little more than cracks and are difficult to see in an X-ray film. Such fractures cause no deformity, but roughen the joint surface and so cause pain and stiffness. Part of the bone may be cut off from its artery and die. This is less likely to happen if the fracture is immobilized, because arteries then have a chance to grow across from the sound fragment, but even with the best treatment fractures of the scaphoid are sometimes troublesome. The lunate bone may be dislocated forwards, and this injury is sometimes complicated by pressure on the median nerve. Manipulation is usually easy, but if the artery to the bone is damaged there may be some lasting disability. Removing the bone relieves the pain but weakens the wrist. The ligaments around the wrist are apt to be stronger than the bones to which they are attached, and a sudden strain may tear off a chip of bone. These small fractures generally heal quickly if they are immobilized.

The commonest injury at the wrist is fracture of the lower end of the radius, ◊ *Colles' fracture*.

There is only just enough room for the ◊ *tendons* as they pass under their fibrous bands. Any inflammation of their sheaths (*tenosynovitis*) is immediately painful. The band across the base of the palm encloses the median nerve with a leash of tendons, and pressure here involves the nerve (◊ *carpal tunnel syndrome*).

wry-neck. Torticollis. ◊ *sternomastoid*.

X

xanthoma. Small soft yellow deposit of cholesterol and other fatty substances in the skin, especially common in diabetics and people with a tendency to *atheroma* (arteriosclerosis) and its complications. With a rare hereditary disorder these deposits occur all over the body; but the common type is confined mainly to the eyelids. The exact significance of these deposits (except that they indicate an excess of cholesterol in the blood) is not known, but in view of the association with arterial disease many physicians advise reducing the cholesterol in the diet (restricted animal fat and eggs). ◊ *atheroma*.

Xenopus test. Hogben test for ◊ *pregnancy*.

xeroderma. Abnormal dryness of the skin; ◊ *icthyosis*.

xerophthalmia. Dryness and, in extreme cases, opacity of the front of the eye, from deficiency of *vitamin A*.

X-rays. Electromagnetic radiation of shorter wave-length than ultraviolet rays. (◊ *Roentgen*.)

1. DIAGNOSIS BY X-RAYS

X-rays differ from light only in their much shorter wave-length. As some kinds of matter are translucent and others are opaque, so some kinds of matter allow X-rays to pass while others obstruct them to a greater or lesser extent. Dense, heavy substances are the most impermeable to X-rays (*radiopaque*). For instance, lead glass is radiopaque because it contains a heavy metal.

Radiopacity is a matter of degree, and different textures can be distinguished by the density of their shadows on a photographic plate or a fluorescent screen.

Bones are so much denser than other tissues that they can be examined in great detail. On the other hand the lungs, consisting mainly of air, cast very little shadow, and therefore abnormalities such as patches of inflammation are easily distinguished. With accurately judged exposure the shadows of many other tissues and organs can also be distinguished, though in much less detail.

Many organs can be examined with X-rays after suitable preparation. Barium sulphate casts a heavy shadow, and is so insoluble that it can be swallowed with no risk that any will be absorbed from the intestine. When a suspension of barium sulphate has been swallowed a series of X-ray pictures will show its progress along the oesophagus, stomach, and intestine. With a fluorescent screen the movements of these organs can also be studied.

Compounds of iodine are also radiopaque and can be used to study many organs. Those that are excreted into the urine cast shadows of the kidneys. Others, excreted into the bile, are used for examining the gall bladder. These methods not only provide clear silhouettes of the urinary passages or bile passages; they also indicate the efficiency of these systems by the rate at which the radiopaque substance is excreted.

Instead of a radiopaque substance, air can be injected into a space such as the ventricles of the brain to provide contrast in an X-ray picture. By one or other method, most organs can be studied.

2. X-RAY THERAPY

X-rays are used in the treatment of cancer. Some superficial cancers can be cured in this way. With deeper cancers, X-rays can be focused to a determined depth below the surface. They are used alone or as an adjunct to surgery, with the objects of picking off cancer cells at the periphery of the field of operation, reducing the risk of mechanical spread of cancer cells by the operation, and reducing the amount of tissue that needs to be removed. The X-rays used for this purpose are generated at a much higher voltage than those used for diagnosis.

In the past small doses of X-rays were much used for treating skin diseases, in the same way as ultraviolet rays, and also to remove hair for the treatment of ringworm, but this is no longer common practice. The use of X-rays to suppress over-activity of an organ such as the thyroid gland is practical-

ly obsolete, but there is still a place for
X-ray treatment of a few diseases in which
a tissue tends to proliferate, e.g. to suppress
the overgrowth of ligaments in ◊ *ankylosing
spondylitis* or of red blood cells in ◊ *polycythaemia*. When an organ has been transplanted, the natural process by which it
tends to be rejected can be suppressed by
treating areas of bone marrow with X-rays,
but this technique is being superseded by
less harmful methods.

◊ *radiation.*

Y

yaws (framboesia). An infectious disease of humid tropical regions, due to *Treponema pertenue*, a spiral bacterium indistinguishable from that of syphilis.

The early stages resemble syphilis, except that there is no history of venereal infection, and the primary lesion may be anywhere on the body. In the late stages the infection is practically confined to the skin, where it forms unsightly excrescences and ulcers, and the bones.

Yaws always responds quickly to treatment with penicillin, and in many areas where it was once common it has now become a rare disease – only to be replaced by syphilis.

The infection is transmitted either by direct contagion or on the feet of flies.

The relation of syphilis to other diseases caused by species of *Treponema* is not known. Only syphilis is regularly transmitted venereally. *Bejel*, a disease confined to small areas of North Africa and the eastern shores of the Mediterranean, cannot be distinguished from syphilis, yet it runs through families and communities without sexual contact. *Pinta*, a South American skin disease without serious complications, is a similar kind of infection. It is strongly argued by opponents of the theory that Columbus imported syphilis from the New World (◊ *syphilis*) that the four conditions, with their different natural histories, are variants of a single disease, and that the other three have evolved from yaws, which originates in the African rainforest. From the rain-forest to the northern desert there is said to be a gradual transition from yaws to bejel; and apart from the mode of transmission there is no difference between bejel and syphilis.

Against the theory that bejel and syphilis are modifications of yaws, and in favour of the Columbus theory, is the absence of any reference to syphilis before Columbus's voyage and the sudden epidemic immediately after his return.

yellow atrophy. Rapidly fatal damage to the liver by, e.g., poisoning or overwhelming infection.

yellow fever. A dangerous infection of tropical Africa and America, due to a virus transmitted by *Aëdes* mosquitoes. It is primarily a disease of monkeys and other forest creatures, but has caused epidemics in towns.

The liver bears the brunt of the infection, and may fail at the end of a short, violent fever with profound jaundice. The kidneys and heart are also affected. Mild cases are common among people who live in the forests where yellow fever is endemic; but during urban epidemics the death rate has been very high.

Mosquito control and vaccination have made yellow fever a rare disease, but public health departments throughout the tropics remain vigilant. An infected traveller, or an infected mosquito carried by aircraft, could start a disastrous epidemic. In 1940, thousands of people died in the Sudan during such an epidemic, and yellow fever had previously been unknown there. There has never been a case in Asia, but Aëdes mosquitoes abound. New arrivals must prove that they have been vaccinated. Yellow fever vaccine affords complete protection from getting the disease or carrying it.

Z

zinc. A small trace of zinc is among the essential ingredients of the body. No disease has been ascribed to either deficiency or excess of zinc.

Zinc oxide is a bland, mildly antiseptic substance much used in ointments and lotions to protect inflamed skin. *Calamine* is a preparation of zinc oxide or zinc carbonate.

Zinc sulphate is sometimes given internally to promote the healing of wounds and leg ulcers.

Zollinger-Ellison syndrome. Peptic (duodenal) ulcer caused by over-activity of the digestive part of the pancreas, which stimulates the glands of the stomach to secrete an excess of acid.

zoonosis (zoönosis). Any infectious disease of animals that may affect man. Most parasites have a preferred host but occasionally infect another species. A few appear to have no difficulty in changing their allegiance. The many zoonoses mentioned in this book include *anthrax, cat-scratch fever*, kinds of bacterial *food poisoning, ornithosis, plague, rabies*, kinds of *relapsing fever, tuberculosis* and *typhus, undulant fever, Weil's disease*, and many kinds of *worm* infestation.

zoster. Herpes zoster: shingles. ◊ *herpes.*

zygoma. Cheek-bone; a bridge of bone from the *maxilla*, below the eye, to the *temporal* in front of the ear.

zygote. Cell produced by fusion of male and female germ cells; fertilized ovum.

zymosis (archaic). Contagious or epidemic disease (literally = fermentation; the secondary meaning recognizes the similarity of infection and fermentation, finally explained by Pasteur's research into both phenomena).

FOR THE BEST IN PAPERBACKS, LOOK FOR THE

In every corner of the world, on every subject under the sun, Penguins represent quality and variety – the very best in publishing today.

For complete information about books available from Penguin and how to order them, write to us at the appropriate address below. Please note that for copyright reasons the selection of books varies from country to country.

In the United Kingdom: For a complete list of books available from Penguin in the U.K., please write to *Dept EP, Penguin Books Ltd, Harmondsworth, Middlesex, UB7 0DA*

In the United States: For a complete list of books available from Penguin in the U.S., please write to *Dept BA, Viking Penguin, 299 Murray Hill Parkway, East Rutherford, New Jersey 07073*

In Canada: For a complete list of books available from Penguin in Canada, please write to *Penguin Books Canada Limited, 2801 John Street, Markham, Ontario L3R 1B4*

In Australia: For a complete list of books available from Penguin in Australia, please write to the *Marketing Department, Penguin Books Australia Ltd, P.O. Box 257, Ringwood, Victoria 3134*

In New Zealand: For a complete list of books available from Penguin in New Zealand, please write to the *Marketing Department, Penguin Books (N.Z.) Ltd, Private Bag, Takapuna, Auckland 9*

In India: For a complete list of books available from Penguin in India, please write to *Penguin Overseas Ltd, 706 Eros Apartments, 56 Nehru Place, New Delhi 110019*

FOR THE BEST IN PAPERBACKS, LOOK FOR THE

PENGUIN HEALTH

Audrey Eyton's F-Plus Audrey Eyton

'Your short-cut to the most sensational diet of the century' – *Daily Express*

Caring Well for an Older Person Mulr Gray and Heather McKenzie

Wide-ranging and practical, with a list of useful addresses and contacts, this book will prove invaluable for anyone professionally concerned with the elderly or with an elderly relative to care for.

Baby and Child Penelope Leach

A beautifully illustrated and comprehensive handbook on the first five years of life. 'It stands head and shoulders above anything else available at the moment' – Mary Kenny in the *Spectator*

Woman's Experience of Sex Sheila Kitzinger

Fully illustrated with photographs and line drawings, this book explores the riches of women's sexuality at every stage of life. 'A book which any mother could confidently pass on to her daughter – and her partner too' – *Sunday Times*

Food Additives Erik Millstone

Eat, drink and be worried? Erik Millstone's hard-hitting book contains powerful evidence about the massive risks being taken with the health of consumers. It takes the lid off the food we eat and takes the lid off the food industry.

Pregnancy and Diet Rachel Holme

It *is* possible to eat well and healthily when pregnant while avoiding excessive calories; this book, with suggested foods, a sample diet-plan of menus and advice on nutrition, shows how.

A Complete Guide to Therapy   Joel Kovel

The options open to anyone seeking psychiatric help are both numerous and confusing. Dr Kovel cuts through the many myths and misunderstandings surrounding today's therapy and explores the pros and cons of various types of therapies.

Pregnancy   Dr Jonathan Scher and Carol Dix

Containing the most up-to-date information on pregnancy – the effects of stress, sexual intercourse, drugs, diet, late maternity and genetic disorders – this book is an invaluable and reassuring guide for prospective parents.

Yoga   Ernest Wood

'It has been asked whether in yoga there is something for everybody. The answer is "yes"' Ernest Wood.

Depression   Ross Mitchell

Depression is one of the most common contemporary problems. But what exactly do we mean by the term? In this invaluable book Ross Mitchell looks at depression as a mood, as an experience, as an attitude to life and as an illness.

Vogue Natural Health and Beauty   Bronwen Meredith

Health foods, yoga, spas, recipes, natural remedies and beauty preparations are all included in this superb, fully illustrated guide and companion to the bestselling *Vogue Body and Beauty Book.*

Care of the Dying   Richard Lamerton

It is never true that 'nothing more can be done' for the dying. This book shows us how to face death without pain, with humanity, with dignity and in peace.

PENGUIN HEALTH

The Penguin Encyclopaedia of Nutrition John Yudkin

This book cuts through all the myths about food and diets to present the real facts clearly and simply. 'Everyone should buy one' – *Nutrition News and Notes*

The Prime of Your Life Dr Miriam Stoppard

The first comprehensive, fully illustrated guide to healthy living for people aged fifty and beyond, by top medical writer and media personality, Dr Miriam Stoppard.

A Good Start Louise Graham

Factual and practical, full of tips on providing a healthy and balanced diet for young children, *A Good Start* is essential reading for all parents.

How to Get Off Drugs Ira Mothner and Alan Weitz

This book is a vital contribution towards combating drug addiction in Britain in the eighties. For drug abusers, their families and their friends.

The Royal Canadian Airforce XBX Plan for Physical Fitness for Men and The Royal Canadian Airforce XBX Plan for Physical Fitness for Women

Get fit and stay fit with minimum fuss and maximum efficiency, using these short, carefully devised exercises.

Pregnancy and Childbirth Sheila Kitzinger

A complete and up-to-date guide to physical and emotional preparation for pregnancy – a must for prospective parents.

Alternative Medicine Andrew Stanway

Dr Stanway provides an objective and practical guide to thirty-two alternative forms of therapy – from Acupuncture and the Alexander Technique to Macrobiotics and Yoga.

Naturebirth Danaë Brook

A pioneering work which includes suggestions on diet and health, exercises and many tips on the 'natural' way to prepare for giving birth in a joyful relaxed way.